THE HISTORY OF HOSPITALS IN IRAN
550–1950

Willem Floor

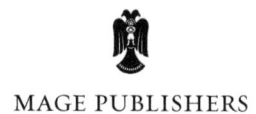

MAGE PUBLISHERS

Copyright © 2021 Willem Floor

All rights reserved. No part of this book may be reproduced or retransmitted in any manner whatsoever, except in the form of a review, without the written permission of the publisher.

Mage Publishers Inc
www.mage.com

Library of Congress Cataloging-in-Publication Data
Available at the Library of Congress

First hardcover edition
ISBN: 978-1-949445-24-4

Visit Mage online: www.mage.com
Email: as@mage.com

CONTENTS

Introduction xi

Hospitals In Sasanian Iran, 224–651 1

Hospitals In Abbasid Iran, 750–1258 7

Hospitals In Buyid Iran 934–1062 13

Hospitals In Seljuq Iran 1106–1194 19

Hospitals In Ilkhanid Iran 1256–1335 23

Hospitals In Timurid Iran 1370–1507 31

Hospitals In Aq-Qoyunlu Iran 1378–1501 33

Hospitals In Safavid Iran 1501–1736 37

Hospitals In Afsharid Iran 1736–1794 51

Hospitals In Qajar & Pahlavi Iran 1794–1950s 55

Appendix: List of American Medical Missionaries . . . 478

Bibliography 482

Index 511

TABLES

Table i: Foreign hospitals and private modern physicians in Iran in 1920. . . xviii
Table ii: Number of modern Iranian hospitals and their capacity in 1920. . . xix
Table 1: Hospitals founded in Iran between 550 and 1460 34
Table 2: Wages and other expenditures of the *dar al-shafa* of Mashhad
in 1747. 52
Table 3: Monthly budget of the Dowlat hospital (1919) 69
Table 4: Number of Outpatients, Inpatients, Operations and Receipts
American Hospital in Tehran(1882-1917) 85
Table 5: Number of patients treated and of activities undertaken
in Abadan APOC hospital (1926) 120
Table 6: Attendance and operation at Ahvaz Civil Hospital (1918-1920) . . . 127
Table 7: The number of new out-patients treated and of operations
performed in the Bandar Abbas British dispensary (1908-31). 134
Table 8: Out- and in-patients and operations in the
Bushehr British dispensary-hospital (1873-1928) 143
Table 9: Male, female and child patients visiting the
Bushehr British dispensary (1899-1901). 145
Table 10: Contributors to the cost of the construction of
the hospital in Bushehr (1918) 149
Table 11: British Bushehr Hospital Receipts (1925-28) 153
Table 12: British Bushehr Hospital Expenditures (1925-28) 154
Table 13: Number of patients and operations in the
British Bushehr Residency dispensary (1929-1940). 164
Table 14: Patients treated and operations performed
American hospital in Hamadan (1887-1915) 175
Table 15: Expenditures of the Samsamiyeh hospital in Hesar
according to the endowment document. 197
Table 16: Patients seen and operated at the CMS Kerman hospital (1912) . . 209
Table 17: List of Medical Staff of the CMS Hospital Kerman (1902-46) . . . 211

Table 18: Number of patients seen, operations performed in
Kerman CMS hopital and house calls made (1910-1925). 214–15

Table 19: Women's Welfare Center Activities - CMS Kerman 1924-1935 . . . 221

Table 20: Patients seen and operations performed at the
Indo-European Telegraph Department Dispensary at Kerman (1912) . . 221

Table 21: Number of visits to the British charitable dispensary
of Lengeh (1912-1925). 257

Table 22: Staff of the *Dar al-Shafa* of Mashhad and their wages (ca. 1870). . . 277

Table 23: Number of patients treated in the British hospital
at Mashad in 1904-05. 297

Table 24: British Mashhad Consulate Hospital Patients for 1919 299

Table 25: Number of patients treated and of activities
undertaken in the Fields APOC hospital (1926). 347

Table 26: Number of out-patients treated at the
Mohammarah British dispensary (1911-1925). 349

Table 27: The common diseases treated in the
Mohammarah British dispensary (1911-1913). 349

Table 28: Annual budgetted expenses of the `Ezz al-Molk
hospital in Shiraz (1912) 403

Table 29: Patients seen, house calls made, receipts collected,
hospital days, and operations performed in the
American hospital in Tabriz (1884-1931) 418

Table 30: Number of in- and out-patients, house calls and
operations at the American Urumiyeh Hospital (1876-1925) 453

Table 31: In- and Out-Patients Treated in the CMS
hospital in Yazd (1898-1905) 459

Table 32: Location and capacity of the Railway hospitals
and dispensaries in 1938 469

ILLUSTRATIONS

Favus patients in Nishapur xxx
Map of Shiraz indicating the probable location of the *dar al-shafa* 29
The American Hospital in Tehran, 1900 84
Group photo of American missionaries 86
The American Hospital in Tehran, main entrance, 1915 88
Cataract operation, American hospital, Tehran, 1918. 93
Ahmadiyeh Hospital in Tehran 110
Ahmadiyeh Hospital ward patients and nurses pose for the photo. 112
Najmiyeh Hospital in Tehran. 116
Ladies at the opening of the hospital. 116
Administrative building and nurses residence, APOC Abadan hospital . . . 122
APOC Hospital dispensary. The operating room. 124
APOC Hospital "Persian" ward. 126
APOC Masjed-e Soleyman complex 128
Jondishahpur Hospital, Reza Shah period. 129
Hospital in Arak 132
Hospital staff in Arak 133
Deserted operating rooms at the former
    British camp at Shusf (near Birjand) 140
New hospital in memory of Showkat al-Molk, Birjand, 1946 141
Medical staff of the government hospital of Bushehr, 1933 146
Patients waiting at the government hospital of Bushehr, 1933 147
The quarantine and hospital building in 1939.
    Now the Abu'l-Fazl private health clinic. 162

Mrs. and Dr. Joe Cook, 1915 178
New American hospital in Hamadan 183
Lily-Reid Memorial Hospital, Hamadan, 1909 185
American missionaries in Hamadan, 1921 189
The new CMS women's hospital, 1905 199
A women's ward at the CMS hospital in Jolfa, Isfahan 202
A ward at the hospital in Jolfa, Isfahan 203
Patient being x-rayed at the CMS hospital in Jolfa, Isfahan 204
Orphanage in Kermanshah established by Dr. Stead 233
Breaking ground for the hospital, Kermanshah, 1932 235
New and old hospital building, Kermanshah. 240
Report from Ministry of Interior mentions the presence of
 Colonel Theodore Roosevelt (son of the U.S. President)
 at the opening of the Westminster Hospital, Kermanshah. 245
The American missionary drugstore at Lahejan
 opened in 1911 256
American missionaries meeting at mission residence in Malayer, 1925. . . 266
Mission residence in Malayer 269
The Zoeckler family 271
Transporting manure 279
Watering the streets using goat-skin water bags before there was paving.. . . 280
The Ark Gate of Mashhad (demolished in 1930) 285
Entrance to the Shrine hospital; in 1922 functioned as a dispensary only.. . . 286
Parts of the main building of the Shah Reza Hospital, 1938.. 288
Main entrance Shah Reza Hospital. An eight-bed ward with Emma
 Degner and nurses. 289
Shah Reza Hospital in winter, 1935. 292
Shah Reza Hospital nurses with Ms Degner 293
Charitable British dispensary, Mashhad. British Consulate's free dispensary. . 298
The first American hospital in Mashhad (1915-18) 304
Waiting room at the American hospital with patients, Mashhad, 1916. . . 305
American hospital Mashhad 1918 with Rev. Esselstyn and Dr. Hoffman . . 306

Wedding party of Khanom Sharifeh and Mirza Abdol-Hoseyn Khan, ... 312
Dr. Lichtwardt with Afghan (Barbari) patients at the
    Mashhad American Hospital 313
Men's ward with Dr. Hoffman in American hospital, a rented building, 1921. . 314
Erecting a windmill to supply electricity to the American hospital,. . . . .
    Mashhad, 1926 315
Drs. Hoffman, Lichtwardt, and Kibbe, 1932 318
Nurse Taillie, Dr. Kibbe, Dr. McDowell; Drs. Frame and Blair 319
Mashhad dispensary with Barbari patients 320
Children in the American hospital, Mashhad, 1928. 321
Building the American hospital and houses of the physicians, Mashhad, 1924. 323
Construction of the American hospital and houses of the physicians,
    Mashhad, 1924. 324
Finished American hospital and houses of the physicians, Mashhad. 325
The front of the American hospital, Mashhad. 325
Dr. Hoffman's house in Mashhad. 326
Pharmacy window with Sayyed Abu'l-Qasem.
    Scrub-up room with Naser Khan and Loqman (Malek al-Fatehi). . . . 330
Surgical instrument cases bought from the British army. 331
Hospital kitchen with Russian stove and Mohammad and cook Ebrahim.. . . 332
Mashhad American hospital staff in 1925 *(top)* and 1929 *(above)* 333
Mashhad American hospital staff in 1930. 334
A corner of the pharmacy room, where the druggist and his
    assistants prepare the medicines for use in the hospital.
    Drugstore room of the American hospital, Mashhad. 336
Kerbela'i Hoseyn, hospital servant for 14 years with his 2 boys. 342
Ajari, lab technician. Employees of the American Hospital, Mashhad, 1934. . 342
Ali the carpenter makes wooden bed-steads, 1930s. 344
American hospital Mashhad laundry at work. 344
American dispensary at Qazvin, 1912. 355
Behbudestan, Shiraz 409
Dr. Vanneman 414

Dispensary day at the Urmiyeh hospital.
    Dr. Cochran with Kurdish chiefs at the hospital of Urmiyeh (ca. 1900). . 434
American Red Cross ambulance at Urmiyeh, February 1918 444
Map of Urmiyeh indicating the location of the American Mission before 1919. 448
Map of Urmiyeh with the location of Galla and the location
    of the new missionary compound with hospital and schools. 1930. . . . 449
Entrance of the Cochran Memorial hospital, Urmiyeh with
    Dr. Jos.Cochran Jr. on the left. 454
Wards in the Cochran hospital. 455
Dispensary in Yazd. 460
Surgery in Yazd. 461
The house in which the missionaries lived in Zabul. 466
Front entrance of the former Russian Consulate, used as hospital, 1921. . . . 467
Railway hospital 471
Railway hospital 472
Railway health post 473

INTRODUCTION

Although the common wisdom is that history doesn't repeat itself, in the case of the 'hospital' in Iran, history certainly rhymes. For, it is interesting to observe that both around 550 and 1850 Christian institutions and practice stood as models for the establishment of hospitals by Iranians. After 550 CE, the *xenodokheion*, a Christian Byzantine charitable institution that cared for sick travelers and the poor, became the model of what became the Sasanian 'hospital' or *bimarestan* and the Islamic *dar al-shafa*. Fortuitously, by 1850, Christian hospitals stood again as a model for the first establishment of a government hospital along Western lines in Iran. This first 'modern' hospital and its follow-up by the Iranian government and private persons was shored up and sustained by the building of modern Western hospitals in many cities of Iran that were established and operated by (mostly) British and American physicians. One might say that by 1950 their task of leading Iran to the way of modern hospital practice had been achieved; their task was done and thus, not surprisingly a decade or so later, the medical missionaries all had discontinued operations in Iran. However, that did not mean that the medical missionaries believed that their task was finished, for they did not write: 'mission accomplished.' On the contrary, in 1955 they felt that their presence was still much needed, because "The few existing hospitals in the provinces are greatly overcrowded and handicapped by very low standards of medical practice and nursing care."[1]

The appearance of the hospital or rather infirmary, a Byzantine invention, was a novelty, because people were treated at home in case of

---

1. Presbyterian Church 1955, p. 50.

illness. Also, only the wealthy could afford the services of a physician. Initially (6th-8th centuries CE) those institutions that provided medical care were not hospitals, but were hospices, where strangers, travelers and the poor stayed for a while, received some care, and, either got better or died. The accepted wisdom is that the continuation of the institution of the Sasanian hospitals "was one of the most remarkable achievements in the Islamic East."[2] Despite this achievement, we know very little about the earliest hospitals, much of which, certainly concerning the alleged first hospitals such the one in Jundishapur, is fanciful and they may not even have existed. Although by 800 we are certain that there were 'hospitals' or *bimarestan*s in Iran, but we still know nothing about them such as what kind of medicine was practiced and taught in them. Even information about the hospitals during their heyday during 900-1100 is sketchy and spotty at best. In fact, more information is available about most individual phycisians than about a single hospital in Iran.[3] Nevertheless, it would seem that these hospitals in the 10th and 11th century offered medical care to men and women, employing physicians from various religious backgrounds with different specialties, and who, using the library and patients in the hospital, taught their students. This type of hospital, at least in Iran, may have existed until the late 11th century. Thereafter, for a variety of reasons, the development of medical science by challenging accepted wisdom was discouraged. Slowly, but surely, *bimarestan*s or *dar al-shafa*s lost the characteristics that made them unique. In fact, what usually is mistaken for a hospital in Iran after 1100 often was an entirely different kind of institution, i.e. they were but hospices. In fact, one could argue that they had reverted to the early Byzantine model of the *xenodokheion*. In the period after the 11th century, there is little information on the number of *dar al-shafa*s and what kind of medicine, if any, was practiced there. This situation did not change after Iranian society and physicians came into contact with Europeans in general and European science, including medical, in particular. Because of the presence of Europeans in Safavid and Afsharid Iran

---

2. Sajjadi 1989, pp. 257-259.
3. For a good example, see Tajbakhsh 1379.

we know somewhat more about the *dar al-shafa*s during that period, which confirms that they were merely hospices. Also, their number declined as did their function. During the Qajar period we only know of three *dar al-shafa*s, of which only one functioned after a fashion, be it that its funds were 'eaten' by the staff of the Imam Reza Shrine.

The first, although short-lived, European medical dispensary was established in Tehran by Dr. Salvatori, the physician of the French diplomatic Gardane mission in 1807-09.[4] It was the American Presbyterian mission that established the first permanent dispensary in 1835 in Urmiyeh.[5] It was only as of 1850 that in Iran an attempt was made to introduce training in modern scientific medical science as well as the establishment of European-inspired hospitals, be it with limited impact. A new chapter began with the establishment of the Dar al-Fonun in 1852, a government established high school in Tehran that taught medicine as one of its subjects. Also, some state hospitals were built along European lines, but neither the funding nor the staffing was adequate. However, it was only towards the end of the nineteenth century that more effective hospitals were those established by American and British missionaries as well as those by the British government in a number of Persian Gulf ports. These Western hospitals not only had an impact on the training of Iranian physicians and nurses as well as on the introduction of modern methods of medical treatments, surgery techniques and medicines, but they also made it more acceptable for Iranian patients to seek treatment in a hospital, an institution that traditionally was viewed not as a place to heal, but as a place to die. Therefore, formal sustained modern medical assistance to the poor (95% of the population), was only available to a very limited extent, both geographically and numerically, through physicians who were attached to foreign Legations, foreign agencies (Indo-European Telegraph Department, Russian Red Cross, etc.), or who were missionaries (American and British). In addition, there were

---

4. Elgood 1951, p. 441.
5. Elgood 1951, pp. 533-535.

a few physicians attached to the royal court and some to provincial governors, who also had other, but paying private patients.⁶

European doctors in Tehran not attached to missionary organizations only treated patients that could pay, with the exception of the British and Russian Legation doctors, who treated the poor free of charge.⁷ However, it was the missionary hospitals that treated the largest number of patients, until the establishment of the Anglo-Persian Oil Company (APOC) hospitals. The American missionaries, for example, had a total of about 188 beds by 1920 and treated more than 30,000 patients per year. They only charged money for drugs, if the patient was rich; the poor received both treatment and drugs free-of-charge.⁸ It was not only Europeans who provided medical assistance. For example, the medical assistance provided to the poor in the various British Consulates by British or Indian physicians, assisted by Indian medical orderlies, while the missionaries were assisted by Iranian (mainly) Christian physicians and nurses, whom they had trained themselves.⁹ Although many patients were treated free of charge at the mission hospitals and dispensaries, these nevertheless felt that the physicians also gained something, viz., an enhanced spiritual position

---

6. E`temad al-Saltaneh 1306, p. 390. By the end of the nineteenth century and the beginning of the twentieth century there were, e.g., the following French physicians: Dr. Coppin (Mozaffar al-Din Mirza), Dr. Sorel (Zell al-Soltan - Isfahan), Dr. Broussière (Customs Service in the Persian Gulf), Dr. Bongrand (Na'eb al-Saltaneh - Tehran), Dr. Roth (Shams al-Saltaneh - Fars) and Dr. Ferte (`Azod al-Soltan, Gilan), see Hassendorfer 1954, p. 61.
7. Serena 1883, p. 142; Collins 1896, p. 276; Andreeva 2007, p. 193.
8. `Eyn al-Saltaneh 1376, vol. 1, pp. 377, 865; UNESCO 1343, vol. 2, p. 1451; Elgood 1951, pp. 511-512, 534; Presbyterian Church 1919, p. 270, 280; Presbyterian Church 1920, pp. 321, 332, 327; Presbyterian Church 1922, pp. 372, 378.
9. Wright 2001, p. 118. Mrs. Rice writes, "During the war, when Europeans had to leave Persia, the Armenian helpers, both nurses and teachers, courageously carried on the work as well as they could." Linton *et al.* 1921, p. 16, note. For similar laudatory observations about the contribution made by the local medical staff, see Wood 1922, pp. 60-61; Cash 1930, p. 31. For the training of nurses, see Floor 2020, pp. 91–168.

because of having done a good deed or *thavab*.¹⁰ Rich Persian patients paid, of course, for their medical service and medicines. "In fact, what might be called the private practice of the doctors largely pays for the upkeep of the hospitals, with their thousands of patients."¹¹ Moreover, the construction of many of the mission hospitals and schools had been made possible by the largess of Persian merchants and other wealthy individuals, both Moslem and non-Moslem.¹²

The Indo-European Telegraph Department (IETD), which was established in 1865, employed a number of physicians, who also operated some dispensaries for the poor. Of course, the main task of these physicians was to keep the IETD staff hale and hearty. Some telegraph station managers also provided help.¹³ The quarantine stations operated by the British Government in the Persian Gulf and by the Russian government at the northern border on behalf of the Government of Iran also provided medical assistance to the local population, in particular the poor.¹⁴ However, this only happened when there was no room in the Consulate dispensary.

---

10. Malcolm 1911, p. 55.
11. Rice 1916, p. 134. This was not always the case, for Dr. Burlie at Bandar `Abbas said about his well-to-do patients: "The Persian gentleman's or lady's idea seems to be that if you get well it is the hand of God and so *Shukr Allah*!- thanks be to God. If you don't improve it is the fault of the Doctor-then why pay?", Cursetjee 2001, p. 44
12. Linton 1923, p. 73; Rice 1916, pp. 133-134; Stuart n.d., p. 19.
13. Wright 2001, p. 126; Rubin 1999, pp. 295-299; Collins 1896, p. 109; see also pp. 162, 276.
14. Sadid al-Saltaneh 1342, p. 169.

Table i: Foreign hospitals and private modern physicians in Iran in 1920.

Nationality	Type of organization	Location	Type of service	Staff
American	Presbyterian Mission	Urmiyeh, Tabriz, Resht, Tehran, Mashhad, Hamadan; Kermanshah; Qazvin+	Hospital (plus apothecary): Mashhad (50 beds); Tehran (45 beds); Resht (5 beds); Hamadan (25 beds); Kermanshah (25 beds); Tabriz (100 beds); Urmiyeh (40 beds); + dispensary	11 physicians of whom two were female
British	British Government	Tehran+, Mashhad, Torbat-e Heydari, Naserabad+, Bushire, Kermanshah, Lengeh+, Mohammarah+, Ahvaz	Small hospitals; + = dispensary	At least 10 of whom two female
	Church Missionary Society	Isfahan, Kerman, Yazd, Shiraz	Isfahan 180 beds (120 for men and 60 for women) Kerman 80 beds (60 for men and 20 for women) Yazd 80 beds (60 for men and 20 for women); Shiraz 50 beds (new hospital under construction in 1924)	At least 6, of whom two female
	APOC	Abadan, Masjed-e Soleyman, Ahvaz, Mohammarah+	The most modern hospitals in the Middle East; + = dispensary; >200 beds	>20
Russian (until 1918)	Red Cross; Government	Tehran; Mashhad, Torbat-e Heydari; Tabriz; Urmiyeh	Small hospital	At least four
German (until 1915)	Government	Tehran, Tabriz, Barforush, Resht, Hamadan, Senneh, Kermanshah	Legation physician and one that directed the government hospital in Tehran. In the other towns are German apothecaries	Two
French	Soeurs de charité	Khosrova	Small 8-bed hospital at Khosrova	A Nestorian doctor trained in France

Source: Grothe 1911, pp. 131-132; Aubin 1908, p. 71; Gilmour 1924, p. 30.

Introduction

In 1920, the situation of Iranian run hospitals is represented in Table ii. The number of foreign hospitals was reduced after World War I. Due to the Russian Revolution all Russian hospitals were closed, while the French missionary service interrupted its operations. The German medical staff did not return, which loss was more than offset by the vastly increased number of Russian and Armenian physicians in the North.[15] After the Great War the British Church Missionary Society (CMS) continued its operations in four locations where it had each one hospital,[16] while the American Presbyterian Missionary Society operated seven hospitals by 1920. A new operator was the APOC, which opened a number of new hospitals and dispensaries as of 1914.

Table ii: Number of modern Iranian hospitals and their capacity in 1920.

Town	Beds	Remarks	Nature of ownership
Tehran	172 (civil) 200 (army)	dispensary + pharmacy	State (3), municipal (1), army (2)
Enzeli	10 male + 5 female	dispensary + pharmacy	Municipal
Tabriz	30	-	Municipal
Hamadan	12	Only out-patients	Municipal
Mashhad	(i) 70; (ii) 20	-	Two Foundations (i) + (ii)
Qazvin	25-30	+ dispensary	Amini endowment
Mohammarah	20	-	Sheikh Khaz`al
Malayer	10	-	Foundation
Sabzavar	?	-	Built with locally raised funds

Source: Gilmour 1924, pp. 29-30; q.v. Qazvin and Sabzavar.

The number of modern Iranian hospitals grew especially after 1905, with the largest concentration in Tehran, both in number and size. At first, doctors of foreign legations were looked on with suspicion. But the hostile attitude changed over time. First and foremost there

---

15. According to Schmidel n.d., pp. 137, 164 there were thousands of Russian physicians in Iran in the early 1920s who, because there were too many of them, eked out a subsistence living.
16. See also Rice 1923, pp. 261-262 as to the equipment of the CMS hospitals. The CMS also operated a dispensary in Shahr-e Kord from 1920-1923; see Amir Hoseyni 1357, p. 47.

were many Iranian doctors and many mullahs who opposed foreign medical aid. The first because they feared competition, the second because they saw medical aid (especially missionary medical aid) as an instrument aiming to establish foreign domination over Iran and replace Islam with Christianity, an attitude that is still found in writings of Iranian scholars or authors of to-day. Mullahs, therefore, "expressed surprise that Christians should look after patients who could not pay,"[17] for this was further proof of their suspicions about the ulterior motives of these European physicians. Not only were the competitors for people's body and soul wary of the gifts borne by European physicians, so were many of the poor and terribly sick patients. Despite the long presence of the American mission in Christian Urmiyeh in the town itself the Jewish and Moslem communities in 1892 were still "very conservative and wish no European help."[18] These sentiments were reinforced, in the case of Moslems, by their deep-seated conviction that non-Moslems were ritually unclean, and therefore, had to force themselves to be touched and swallow medicines prepared by a Christian physician.[19] The same kind of reaction was present in towns such as Yazd and Kerman.[20]

However, initial stand-offishness if not hostile attitude soon turned into acceptance and appreciation. There were still problems such as in 1908, when rumors were spread that operations were carried out in the hospital in Kerman that should not be done. A high-placed British individual even lent credence to these rumors and sent "a vindictive report" to London and, as a result, the CMS considered closing down the Kerman hospital. When the town's people learnt about the pending closure in the autumn of 1907 "a letter was written

---

17. Rice 1916, p. 89.
18. Speer 1911, pp. 166, 270, 328-329. It was difficult for women to come and seek help, for their men said: "she's only a woman," and many had "to steal away from their homes to go to the hospital during the absence of their husbands." Presbyterian Church 1921, p. 338.
19. Richter 1910, p. 321.
20. Malcolm 1905, pp. 55-59; A Friend of Iran 1940, pp. 20-21; Hume-Griffith 1909, pp. 157-61.

and signed by all the *mujtaheds* or leading mullahs, with 700 seals of merchants and townsfolk affixed." The CMS then decided to continue its Kerman operation.[21] Dr. Emmeline Stuart, who elaborated on the initial difficulties to overcome Moslem prejudice with regard to the Christian doctors, wrote around 1923, "No longer have we the same prejudices to contend with. No longer is the *istikhareh*, or omen, indispensable before patients submit to the treatment. It is now as a rule, only consulted by the more bigoted Moslems, or by those who do not really want to come into hospital, or who are afraid to undergo an operation."[22] When Dr. Dodson died of typhoid fever, while caring for his patients in Kerman in 1937, "The Governor of the town, all the officials, and fifteen thousand people lined the narrow streets and went to the bare graveyard in the desert outside the town to do honour to the man who had served them for thirty-four years."[23]

Other beliefs that interfered with effective treatment were ritualistic in nature. The dispensaries and hospitals were almost empty during Ramadan, because the taking of medicine, or the use of drops into the eye, was tantamount to breaking fast. European doctors, therefore, had to be aware to tell the few patients that showed up to take their medicine twice a night instead of twice a day. Also, after Ramadan the dispensaries were full of patients who had overeaten at night after having eaten nothing during the day.[24]

The goodwill that was created by this kind of medical assistance was so impressive that a commercial commission sent by the Government of India to Persia in 1904 remarked: "In my journey through Persia I have noticed the very great influence that a medical man possesses, and the good that he does; the appointment of a medical officer, with Hospital Assistants, at all head-quarters is desirable, and I would further suggest that the Consular Agents at Sirjan, Rafsinjan and Bampore be selected from the subordinate medical staff, and have

---

21. A Friend of Iran 1940, pp. 55-52.
22. Stuart n.d., p. 23.
23. A Friend of Iran 1940, p. 73.
24. Malcolm 1911, p. 49.

dispensaries at these stations."²⁵ Similar sentiments were expressed by British consuls in Lengeh and Ahvaz, who for that reason, wanted to separate the dispensary from the quarantine stations so that the British government and nobody else would get the patients' gratitude, while it was expected to stimulate British trade. It therefore comes as no surprise that those Iranians who were already suspicious of foreign assistance found vindication for their strongly held feelings in these and similar observations.

The Mission Hospitals and dispensaries as well as the British government charitable dispensaries and Civil Hospitals treated tens of thousands of patients every year a number that by 1925 had grown to more than 350,00, many of whom were repeat visitors, not new patients.²⁶ The missionary physicians trained native physicians and nurses and also provided education in hygiene.²⁷ For both at home, in their towns, and in their villages, people lived in an environment that was a breeding place for all kinds of endemic and contagious diseases, the main cause for the many diseases with which people were afflicted. Therefore, "the utter lack of cleanliness" was the main problem, coupled with the need to overcome "the ignorance and prejudices of the people," according to the medical staff in Mohammarah.²⁸ It was a refrain repeated by their colleagues in Bandar 'Abbas, where it was observed that the inhabitants practiced no sanitation whatsoever.

---

25. Gleadowe-Newcomen 1904, p. 19. In the mid-1830s the British envoy to Iran, Sir John Campbell had made the same argument, but his advice was not heeded. Elgood 1951, p. 472. The Russians also noted the benefit of good-will due to medical assistance. Andreeva 2007, p. 193. In 1904-05, Sykes reported that "During the Mohurram riots it was understood that the British Consulate-General was held inviolable by the people on account of the great boon conferred on the population of Khorasan by the work of this [British] hospital." Sykes 1905, p. 22.
26. In 1907 the American hospitals treated 30,000 patients. Grothe 1911, p. 131, while the CSM in Yazd alone did more than 30,000; otherwise see entries per town in what follows.
27. Wilson 1895, p. 310.
28. Administration Report 1912, p. 65; Wilson 1932, p. 98

Introduction   xxiii

"Advice given on the dangers of these conditions receive a deaf ear."[29] In Urmiyeh the missionary medical staff also tried to teach patients about the importance of hygiene and sanitation, and made an effort to improve the medical knowledge of Galenic physicians and also counselled them to arrive at better medical treatments.[30] People were more susceptible to notions of prevention, when it was too late (when there was already another cholera epidemic) and invariably only for as long as the epidemic lasted. There was little preventive follow-up either by the government or the population at large.[31] The APOC made the most concerted sanitation effort in that area, as good public health was vital for its operations and its ability to attract workers. It had special staff to inspect and enforce public health measures; in fact, it performed many functions (such as inspecting the sale of meat and vegetables) that should have been carried out by the government of Iran.[32] A similar concerted effort was made by the British government, on behalf of the government of Iran from 1849 until 1928, by enforcing quarantine rules in the Persian Gulf through five stations to check the spread of epidemics. The costs were borne by the Iranian government. However, the hospitals and its physicians were mainly treating symptoms rather than the underlying causes of the diseases that gave rise to them.[33]

In Iran in 1924, there existed some 35 hospitals with more than 1,400 beds, 40 or more dispensaries, ten quarantine stations,[34] and 945

---

29. Administration Report 1922, pp. 19-20; Administration Report 1921, p. 20); Administration Report 1923, p. 36.
30. Wilson 1896, p. 275.
31. See for the panic reaction to a cholera epidemic by the population and the temporary positive reaction to "what to do" pamphlets, for example, Wishard 1908, pp. 220-221.
32. Williamson 1927, pp. 133-138 and Gilmour 1924, p. 29, both give an overview of the types of measures taken. For the towns that had an Iranian public health physician see Gilmour 1924, pp. 24-25 (map). On the APOC health care system, see Floor 2018 a, pp. 107-29.
33. On this subject, see Floor 2018 a, pp. 61-68, 85-89.
34. This number also includes the quarantine stations on the Caspian Sea (Enzeli, Mashhad-e Sar) and on the border with the Ottoman Empire

officially authorized physicians (both foreign and Iranian, of whom 323 practiced in Tehran). Of course, there was insufficient capacity to address the health needs of the 10 million inhabitants of Iran let alone preventing or reducing the prevalence of endemic and contagious diseases. But it was a beginning. However, as in Europe, the incidence and prevalence of most common diseases in Iran was spectacularly and most significantly reduced not by hospitals, but by the spread of sanitation and personal hygiene through public (uncontaminated water supply; effective sewage and drainage system, etc.) and personal (clean clothes, bedding and homes, washing hands, etc.) policy, practice, and actions after 1950. Neither the traditional *dar al-shafa*s, nor the modern hospitals could really solve that problem. The former's staff had no notion of sanitation and hygiene, and even though the latter's staff did, they knew that it was a difficult and different battle than for which they had been created and equipped.[35]

But changes were made under the Pahlavi regime, which improved the public health situation through the training of physicians, the construction of hospitals and dispensaries, and, most importantly, the formulation and application of public health measures. Dr. Hoffman summarized this new wave that spread over Iran in the 1930s as follows:

> Much has changed, the Government of Persia has reorganized the Department of Hygiene and Health, established free hospitals in all large cities and in some of the smaller ones, organized free smallpox vaccination, free medical service to the poor in many centers, establishment of a school for midwives in Tehran, etc. The medical school in Tehran has improved and government labs now produce typhoid vaccine and sera to prevent cholera and other diseases. Registration of birth is required by law, burial not permitted without the doctor's death report; hospitals and dispensaries have to

---

(Kermanshah, Qasr-e Shirin) and Russia (Astara, Jolfa). Gilmour 1924, pp. 21-26. Torbat-e Heydari (q.v. above) should also be listed among the quarantine stations.

35. Gilmour 1924, p. 14.

Introduction

> report all contagious diseases and quarantine is imposed when epidemics threaten from neighboring countries. Barbers, bath-attendants and all handlers of food, such as butchers, bakers, and candy makers, all must have regular health examinations, and secure a certificate of cleanliness before they are allowed to carry on their work. Children with evident trachoma, favus, whooping cough or other contagious diseases are forbidden to attend school until their disease has been cured.[36]

And indeed, concrete steps were made. In 1930, the Department of Health of Khorasan, for example, employed doctors in a dozen centers in the province to vaccinate for smallpox, typhoid, and, when epidemics threatened, for cholera, using vaccine made at the Pasteur Institute in Tehran.[37] There seems to have been some measure of control to see to it that no fees were charged for this gratis service. For example, it was reported that "Dr. Mahmud Khan Falu, the traveling medical officer at Mohammareh left for the Bani Turuf on 5 September 1930 to carry out inoculations. On his return on 16 September he was arrested by the police and sent under escort to Tehran for having collected fees from the Bani Turuf."[38]

The Department of Health had other tasks as well. It had to inspect eating places, slaughter-houses, barbershops, brothels, and baths for sanitations and to see that doctors, midwives, druggists and dentists had permits to practice. The latter requirement became a problem for the missionary physicians, because these permits were harder to get after 1933, when the Licensing Law was passed. The law was not so

---

36. RG 91-20-2, Mashhad Medical Report 1931-32; "The Department of Health has now doctors in a dozen centers in the province giving smallpox vaccination, reports epidemics etc." RG 91-20-2, Mashhad Medical Report 1929-30. A dispensary service for the whole country was initiated. Government of Great Britain 1945, p. 410.
37. RG 91-20-2, Mashhad Medical Report 1929-30. How effective the new Health Department was, given that it was constrained by staff and financial problems, requires a separate study.
38. Political Diaries vol. 9, p. 266.

much aimed at the missionary physicians, but rather to make it difficult for mainly Russian physicians, who had diplomas from unknown universities and inferior training, of whom many came to Iran. After 1933, there was also an influx of Jewish physicians, who were fleeing the Nazi threat in Europe.[39] Furthermore, the Health Department asked the hospitals for reports on the work done and required certificates of births and deaths.[40] The new public health rules also meant that the missionaries had to stop their medical itinerating, because "the new health department demands that even a temporary hospital must provide beds and not lay patients on the floor. Moreover, we must have a registered pharmacist to dispense medicines."[41]

Dr. Hoffman (Mashhad) and the other American medical missionaries welcomed these changes and the demand for accountability. Dr. Blair (Tehran) argued that the American missionary doctors needed to nurture friendship with Iran and this meant that they had to identify themselves "with Iranian interests, sometimes to the apparent detriment of our own."[42] They realized that this sometimes resulted in friction and bruised feelings, but rather than seeing this as an obstacle they saw the new developing circumstances as a challenge. Dr. Hoffman argued that the new reality was that "Persia is changing rapidly; it has a health department which demands a higher standard of medical practice. People are becoming critical of hasty, superficial work. We must begin to keep better records, to train nurses, to see fewer patients and, in short, modernize."[43]

This was easier said than done (although it was done), because it required time, money and more medical staff, which were all

---

39. RG 231-1-2 Rolla Hoffman Correspondence 1910-1919, Hoffman to McClanahan, 03/07/1932; RG 321-1-6, Pioneering in Meshed, pp. 110-11.
40. RG 231-1-6, Pioneering in Meshed, p. 120.
41. RG 231-1-6, Pioneering in Meshed, p. 91.
42. RG 91-19-11-1, Report Tehran Medical Work 1934-1935. Dr. Frame in Rasht had the same attitude, see RG91-19-9, Resht Medical Report 1924-25.
43. RG 231-1-6, Pioneering in Meshed, p. 91.

interrelated and in short supply. The missionary physicians were quite aware that sometimes they worked hastily and superficially. However, given the literally overwhelming demand for their services, so much so that they were forced to turn away many needy patients, and given the often rather obvious and repetitive nature of the diseases that patients were afflicted with, this pattern of work was understandable. Above, I have referred to the impossibility to see all patients and, thus, the unavoidable necessity to deny service. Here I have Dr. Hoffman describe the most common range of diseases that were seen by him in Mashhad, which did not differ from that of the other hospitals. This range of diseases makes it understandable why physicians, who were under great pressure, felt justified and compelled to spend less time with patients to be able to treat more. Of course, every possible disease was seen in both the dispensary and the hospital, and more or less time was spent with patients, depending on the type of disease.[44] In fact, Dr. Hoffman suggested that "Our patients, in Mashhad, 50,000 per year could be good research subject given the many diseases."[45] However, epidemics of influenza, typhoid, typhus and contagious diseases occurred without being evident from the hospital's annual performance statements. This was because the Christian Hospital increasingly was a consultative practice that did not deal with a cross-section of diseases in the community. Also, its doctors did not treat people at home or make house calls, except in case of consultation.[46] Doctors noted that patients coming from faraway places mainly suffered from chronic complaints, but the hospital lacked data on the occurrence of acute diseases in the rural communities concerned. Also, only one diagnosis was reported for each patient. This explained the prevalence of trachoma, intestinal worms, favus, strabismus and all

---

44. "Intestinal parasites are even more common than our figures suggest and the same it true for malaria in its latent form. You assume that adults have malaria and children have worms, not doing so one is often tripped up." RG 91-20-2, Mashhad Medical Report 1935-1936.
45. RG 231-1-2, Hoffman to Friends 10/03/1930.
46. RG 91-20-2, Mashhad Medical Report 1935-1936.

kinds of minor afflictions.⁴⁷ Some diseases were more common than others. Of the dispensary patients 25% suffered from trachoma; some from afar came for an operation for entropion. Some 25% had skin diseases (scabies, impetigo, 'eczema', favus, scalp ringworm). Colds and respiratory troubles came in winter in huge numbers. TB was alarmingly prevalent (some 10% of the patients). Malaria, syphilis, typhoid and typhus fevers, diarrhea and dysentery were constantly seen. Although syphilis was very prevalent it was neither systematically nor adequately treated, because patients could not afford the high cost of the medicines. Very few patients continued regular treatment for three months and many returned with active recurrence. Also, there were the incurables among the patients: the blind, the paralyzed, the idiots, the deaf, the deformed, and the insane.⁴⁸ Of course, "Malaria is still one of our most common diseases, for nothing is being done as yet for the prevention of this destructive and unnecessary ailment."⁴⁹

There also were regional differences in the incidence of certain diseases. Dr. Frame reported that the less common diseases in Rasht included boils, diphtheria, and a host of others. In 1942, due to people's flight to Tehran after the Russian invasion, many got infected with the so-called Delhi boils, a disease not found in Gilan. Iranians considered it untreatable, calling it 'the little year' from its duration. They were very surprised that with newer methods it was possible to usually be cured without leaving the usual scar.⁵⁰ In the winter of 1934-45, there was a diphtheria scare in Rasht and environs, although the epidemic was not severe. Frame did Schick tests on girls of the Girls School to test if there might be a universal natural immunity from contacts in early

---

47. RG 91-20-2, Mashhad Medical Report 1935-1936.
48. RG 231-1-6, Hoffman, Pioneering in Meshed, pp. 61, 78; RG 91-20-2, Mashhad Medical Report 1935-1936 (here 10% is given for trachoma in 1935). See also, Khakestar 1395, pp. 164-72. On the public health situation in Iran at that time, see Floor 2004.
49. RG 91-20-2, Mashhad Medical Report 1931-1932. On the incidence of malaria and the anti-malaria program undertaken in Iran, see Floor 2018 a, pp. 42-46.
50. RG 91-19-7, Resht Medical Report 1921-1922; Idem, Report Medical Work 1919-1920.

childhood. Fifty teenagers were tested. Normally, incidence was low in this group, but he got 28% positive reactions. He didn't know why he got this result, but he was glad that the disease was rare in Gilan.[51] Another special study Frame carried out was about amoebic dysentery to establish whether it endemic in Rasht or not, the more so as liver abscess was uncommon there. The first results were inconclusive and he decided that more lab work was required.[52] Many among the poor had chronically infected ears that needed daily treatment over a long period. Skin infections prevailed as well, especially on little babies.[53] Frame commented that, "Many of the skin editions are due to dirt, but of what use is it to tell a man in the midst of winter, 'Go wash,' when the only suit he owns consist of a blanket or pair of trousers made out of burlap!"[54] There also was more rickets than in the rest of Iran as well as a general vitamin deficiency. Malaria also prevailed and "it is often necessary to keep the patients needing surgery a week or longer, to get rid of malaria, before operating."[55]

But the missionary hospitals modernized; they kept better records, they trained nurses, and they saw fewer patients. They also upgraded their equipment (X-ray, laboratory), developed new treatment programs (obstetrics, pre- and post natal care, favus, ring worm, information sharing) and aimed to be the leading edge of medical care facilities.[56] The government of Iran, meanwhile, also took steps to improve medical care, among other things, via hospitals. In particular, in the 1930s many new hospitals and dispensaries were built, either by the

51. RG 91-19-7, Report Resht Medical Work 1934-1935.
52. RG 91-19-7, Rest Medical Report 1930-1931.
53. RG 91-20-8, Resht Hospital Report 1944-1945.
54. RG 91-19-7, Resht Medical Report 1921-1922; RG 91-19-7, Report Resht Medical Work 1919-1920.
55. RG 231-1-6, Personal Report 1949 and Hospital Report. On the prevalence of malaria in Gilan, see Floor 2018 a, pp. 34-35.
56. In fact, it was the missionary hospitals that were the first to establish training programs for nurses in Iran, while they also helped establish the government's nurse's training program. For their pioneering programs in the field of ob-gyn, pre- and post natal care, TB, and other areas, see Floor 2020, pp. 169–270.

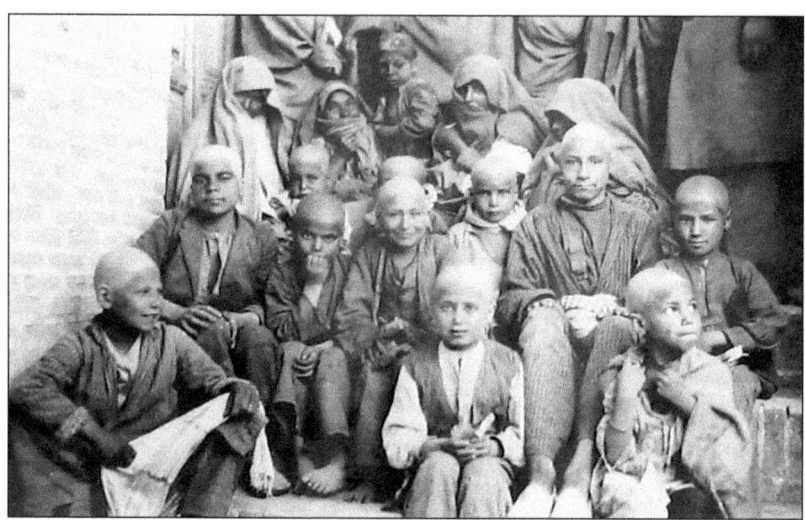

Favus patients in Nishapur

government or by private individuals. It was claimed that sixty-four hospitals were constructed during 1939-40.[57] This may well have been true, because the Department of Health operated all civil hospitals in Iran, except the military and missionary ones. In 1945, of 76 hospitals, 44 were government operated, eight were for the military, and eight were small quarantine hospitals. At that time there were five American missionary hospitals, four CMS hospital as well as a number of Anglo-Iranian Oil Company (AIOC) and private hospitals.[58] This was quite a change compared with the situation in 1924. It was not yet a transformation, but it was the beginning of a much more comprehensive public health policy as well as of national programs that were launched as of the 1950s. These programs (vaccination; anti-malaria campaign; better housing; safe piped water; education and public hygiene) would change the health of Iran's population, in which development of the growing number of hospitals, physicians and nurses played a supportive role. It still would take many years

---

57. Jarman 1997, vol. 1, p. 184.
58. US. Army Medical Service. Office of the Surgeon General, Department of the Army, *Preventive Medicine in World War II*, 1976, p. 225.

Introduction   xxxi

before modern scientific medicine would be the default setting for Iranians who fell ill, in particular in rural areas, where modern health care was still not available for most villagers and nomads before the 1970s. This was partly due to lack of access and partly due to lack of understanding. For example, in the early 1950s, even in the cities, blood transfusion was a misunderstood novelty to most people.

> A lad of twelve was brought to the Kermanshah hospital in a dying condition, accompanied by parents and relatives who were already beginning to wail in the traditional fashion. The father was found to have the right type of blood., but he collapsed and refused to risk his life in a lost cause. An older brother came forward, but the transfusion was interrupted by the mother's argument that the boy was dead and that there was no use doing anything further. Some relatives tried to pull out the needle, but a diminutive uncle stood guard and insisted that the doctors and nurses be given a chance. The boy continued to breathe, and a second transfusion the next day resulted in his sitting up and smiling. He went on to full recovery, and now patients are asking to see the doctor who takes blood from live people and with it brings the dead back to life![59]

Nevertheless, the hard work and sacrifice by the staff of these modern hospitals laid the groundwork for the necessary and comprehensive public health infrastructure and the health policies in Iran that were developed as of the 1930s and gained speed and size in application as of 1950. Therefore, it is important to learn the process of the introduction and development of Western hospitals and dispensaries in Iran and what conclusion one may draw from that experience. In what follows I give an overview of what is known about dispensaries (*darman-khaneh*), hospitals (*bimarestan* or *mariz-khaneh*) and hospices (*dar al-shafa*) in various Iranian cities between 550 and 1950. This inventory may divided into two periods. The first one, covering the period between 550 and 1850, is one where we have relatively little information about the functioning of 'hospitals', although more

---

59. Presbyterian Church 1955, pp. 50-51

information is available for the years after 1500 than before that date. The second period that covers the period between 1850 and 1950 is the one that constitutes the bulk of this study. This is due to the fact that much more information is available about hospitals during this period, because in particular reports and letters by American Presbyterian missionaries, give a detailed insight in hospital practice during this period. The study of this second period, unlike that of the first period, which is per force limited to a country-wide overview, discusses the hospital situation in Iran by city. It starts with the capital Tehran and thereafter alphabetically covers the hospital situation and experience in cities about which we have data. This part also serves, where data are available, to gauge the impact hospitals and dispensaries had and what the major problems were that they had to overcome to have some measure of success. Readers of my earlier foray into the history of hospitals in Iran will notice that part of that study is also to be found here, be it that the current study is much more comprehensive and adds much new information, a reason why it is also thrice the size of the 2013 study.

I wish to express my thanks to my friend Prof. Iraj Nabipour (University of Bushehr) for his encouragement to enlarge my earlier study on hospitals in Iran, which he was kind enough to translate into Persian. Further, to the staff of the Presbyterian Historical Society (Philadelphia) for facilitating my research by their very helpful attitude. Finally, I thank Finn Østrup (a former Kampsax engineer) for making the books by Boisen 1946 and Saxild 1971 available to me as well as to Mr. Mohsen Nia, who was so kind to bring the books by Khakestar and Sureshjani from Mashhad by way of the good offices of Dr. Mehdi Mojtahedi (Ferdowsi University).

HOSPITALS IN SASANIAN IRAN, 224-651

In the last four decades serious doubts have been raised about the early establishment of a hospital and medical school in Jundishapur.[1] The chain of events that resulted in the establishment of this hospital is in a nutshell as follows. After having defeated Emperor Valerian, Shahpur I (r. 241-274) settled Greek (Rumi) prisoners of war in Jundishapur. He also married Valerian's daughter; she settled in that city and brought two Greek physicians with her, who publicly taught Greek medicine in Jundishapur. Later Shapur I sent an Indian and Syriac-speaking physicians there. Moreover, Shahpur II (r. 306-80) endowed the town with a school, where medicine and other sciences were taught, and where scientific medicine was practiced. This school received an additional influx of scientific knowledge, when Khosrow Anushirvan I (r. 531-579) induced some of the Christian scholars, who, after having fled from Edessa (489), settled in Nisibis, to move to Jundishapur and engage in the translation of medical Greek texts. Therefore, it was no surprise that Harun al-Rashid, the alleged founder of the first Islamic hospital sent for Christian physicians from Jundishapur to supervise the establishment and manage the activities of his hospital. However, as shown by Dols, Conrad, Horden and others, the evidence for this story is partly fictitious, while the other adduced facts are fraught with historical problems. Also, there are no contemporary Pahlavi sources, while the above story is mostly based on 13th century Arab sources.

---

1. On the myth of the existence of a hospital in Jundishapur, see Abbott 1968, pp. 71-73; Dols 1987, pp. 369-70, Conrad 1995, p. 101; Prioreschi, Plinio 2001, pp. 362-65.

Before stating what we do know with some certainty, it is useful to define what may be understood by the term 'hospital'. Dols defined it "as a public charitable institution that takes care of the sick for some length of time." Such an institution, to care for pilgrims, travelers, widows, orphans, the aged and the sick, came into being in the fourth century CE in the Byzantium Empire. It was established jointly by the State and the Christian Church with a view to gain converts through charitable care. It was called *xenodokheion* (ζενοδοχεῖον), i.e. a hospice for strangers[2] and provided food and shelter. Many of these hospices also included a so-called *nosokomeion* (νοσοκομείων) or infirmary, where medical care was provided. It is thought that over time, because of their association, the two terms were used indiscriminately to refer to an infirmary. Prior to that time there were few facilities to care for the sick, but those were private institutions and only available for certain kinds of people such as soldiers and slaves. Also, it was contrary to cultural values and sensibilities to have an ill family member cared for outside the family. Whether you were wealthy and could afford the service of a physician or whether you were poor, the majority of people, who had to rely on folk medicine dispensed by family lore and/or traditional healers of various hues and kinds, all treated their sick relatives at home.

Thus, the public charitable institution that cared for the sick was a Byzantine Christian institution and its function was to care for pilgrims, travelers, and the poor, not for the public in general. Under the influence of this Byzantine practice the Synods of the Christian Syrian Church in Sasanian Iran repeatedly prescribed the adoption of a similar practice by establishing at many a church a place of shelter for strangers and the poor, known as *xenodokheion*.[3] Such a development was but a logical extension of the help given to the poor (in particular by monasteries) during famine and epidemics. Just as it was customary since Antiquity to endow or gift temples, later, Christian churches and church institutions such as a *xenodokheion* also received

---

2. From *xenon* or 'stranger, guest' and *dokhesthai* or 'to receive'. In modern Greek the term means 'hotel.'
3. Busse 1969, p. 530.

gifts from believers.[4] Whereas in Byzantium, the *xenodokheion* was a state-sponsored institution this was not the case in Sasanian Iran, where it was and remained a private establishment.

In Sasanian Iran the term *xenodokheion* was used in the meaning of infirmary, i.e. a place to care for the sick. According to the Chronicle of Zacharia the Rhetor, around 555 CE, after Khosrow Anushirvan I (r. 531-579) had been successfully treated by his Christian physicians, he, at the advice of these physicians, *departing from custom*, established a *xenodokheion* to which he attached 12 physicians and provided food and other needs. This remark, *departing from custom*, demonstrates that Sasanian kings had not been in the habit to establish 'hospitals', further making a stronger case that there is no evidence whatsoever of an earlier establishment of a hospital by the Sasanians such as that of Jundishapur. In fact, Khosrow Anushirvan only provided support for a Christian institution to which, and that is new, he attached medical staff, thus establishing that a *xenodokheion* was a hospital. What was not new was that Christian scholars working in Iran were engaged in translating Greek scientific, including medical, texts into Syriac and later also into Pahlavi. This translation activity that had begun as of around 500 CE became very important under Khosrow Anushirvan. This implies that these physicians were trained in Greek medical knowledge, and therefore, taught and practiced Galenic medicine or elements thereof.

The only contemporary document that shows light on the link between a teaching institution and medicine in Sasanian Iran are the statutes of the Syrian Christian school of Nisibis.[5] This theological seminary was headed by the *rabbaita* or major domus, who was assisted by a so-called *xenodeikh*, who received guests and, above all, was in charge of taking care of the seminary's sick staff and students. The Nisibis infirmary only served its own staff, students and guests. The reason was that the school did not want its students, when sick, to

---

4. Pigulevskaya 1963, p. 185.
5. Nisibis, a very ancient and famous city, the modern Nusaybin (Mardin province), Turkey, on the southern border, adjoining the Syrian city of Qamishli. Samuel Lieu, "Nisibis," iranica.online.org.

roam around neighboring towns and villages and become dependent on public charity, on which the school depended itself! The Nisibis statutes do not refer to the training of physicians (*malpana*) at the school, for this was not part of the regular curriculum. The main function of the school was to train students in Christian theology. Medical texts were studied at Nisibis, but those that preferred to focus on that kind of study, were not allowed to live together with the other students. Also, they were not allowed to study theology any longer. Moreover, Rule 20 of the school states: "The brothers who have left the scholarship and have departed for the (discipline) of medicine-if there is no good testimony about them, they are not allowed to hear in the school, except, however, the physicians, inhabitants of the town." In short, the school was a theology seminary, where medical books could be studied, and it had an infirmary for its staff, students, and travelers only, where Galenic medicine was practiced. This means that in the second half of the sixth century CE at the school at Nisibis Galenic medicine could be studied as part of the Greek sciences, and that it had a *bimarestan*, 'the place of the sick', the Pahlavi translation of the term *xenodokheion*, but it was not a medical school.[6]

There is no evidence that in Jundishapur a.k.a. Beth Lapat a situation existed like that in Nisibis; it is more likely that it had a theological seminary, nothing more. It is possible that later the seminary in Jundishapur like the one in Nisibis also had a *bimarestan*, where medical texts could be studied, but there is no evidence for it. There certainly was a hospital in Jundishapur in the first part of the ninth century, and therefore, perhaps already in the eighth century. Timothy, the Syrian Patriarch of Baghdad (780-823) wrote to his good friend Sergius, a physician as well as metropolitan of Elam and head of a school, that: "I have also sent you another youth for education, that is our Gabriel, for he too is very eager for the craft of medicine. So, hand him over to Zistq [?] and his establishment of education."[7] In his *Ferdows al-Hikmat*, `Ali b. Rabban al-Tabari (850) mentions that

---

6. Pigulevskaya 1963, pp. 249-50; Dols 1987, pp. 373-76.
7. Dols 1987, p. 377

in Jundishapur there was a *ra'is-e bimarestan* or 'head of a hospital.'[8] These two elements leave no doubt about the fact that in the first part of the ninth century there was a school and a 'hospital' in Jundishapur where medicine was taught.

The use of the term *bimarestan* by early Arab sources clearly indicates that Islamic medical institutions were modeled after the Syrian Christian *xenodokheion*, because in Syriac texts the Pahlavi term *bimarestan* is used as a synonym for the Syriac loan word *askenadaukin*. In 790 CE, a *xenodokheion* or *bimarestan* was established in Ctesiphon by the Syrian Christian church. In another letter from Timothy, the patriarch of Baghdad (780-823) to his physician friend Sergius writes that:

> We have built `ksndwkyn` [= *xenodokheion*], that is *bymrstan* [*bimarestan*] in the Royal Cities [al-Mada'in or Ctesiphon], and have spent more or less 20,000 [*zuke*]. It has been roofed over already and completed, and pray that our Lord may give in it healing to the sick and to those who are bodily or spiritually sick.[9]

Such a charitable act is not surprising as the majority of the population was still Christian and wealthy Christian patrons continued to make contributions to Christian charitable institutions such as the *xenodokheion*. The Syrian Christian origin of the institution is also acknowledged by Ibn Abu Usaybi`ah (1203-70), who states that Hippocrates:

> is said that he was the first one who conceived of and established a hospital. He used to work in a garden close to his house, a section of which was reserved for the sick; then he provided servants to take care of their treatment and called it *xenodocheion*, i.e. 'a place to host the sick'. This is also the

---

8. About 840, al-Jahez mentions the term *bimarestan*, when Bakhtishu described for him a fight in which he had been involved: "We met them in a space that was the size of a hospital courtyard." Dols 1987, p. 382.
9. Dols 1987, p. 379.

meaning of the Arabic term for hospital, *bīmāristān*, which comes from Persian: *bīmār* means sick and *stān* means place, and thus the meaning of *bīmāristān* is 'a place for the sick'.¹⁰

The Arabic *dar al-marza* was not used during the Abbasid period, in fact, according to Savage-Smith Savage Smith, "there was no Greek [how about *xenodokheion* or *nosokomeion*?] or Arabic word used for the institution at this time."¹¹

---

10. Ibn Abi Uṣaybiʻah 2020, 4.14.
11. Savage-Smith 2020. In a footnote she adds: "It was not until the modern period that the Arabic word *mustashfā*, 'place where healing is to be sought', became the normal word for 'hospital'.

HOSPITALS IN ABBASID IRAN, 750–1258

Caliph Walid I (r. 705-15) is often mistakenly hailed as the founder of the first Islamic hospital, but he only built a leprosarium in Damascus and provided food for its denizens. This act was but a continuation of Christian practice of charity for lepers in this former Byzantine bastion and it was not a medical facility, but rather a hospice to segregate and feed the afflicted. The first Islamic 'hospitals' were only built around 800 and thereafter. At that time, there were as yet few Moslem physicians, who were necessary to provide professional advice about the requirements of a hospital. By that time, Jundishapur had acquired a great reputation as a center of medical learning where allegedly the best physicians worked. This reputation, deserved or not, most likely was because the well-known Bukhtishu and the Musawaih families of physicians hailed from there, who dominated the medical profession in Baghdad and those physicians present at the caliphal court. Since they were very successful and were from Jundishapur, the school where they presumably had been trained was assumed to have been good. However, it is not known whether these famous physicians really received their training at the Jundishapur school. In fact, since they belonged to medical families, they most likely were home-schooled in the art of medicine. Given the above, it is not surprising that al-Jahez (ca. 840) blames the lack of success of a Moslem physician to the fact that he had a non-Christian name, wore a white cotton robe instead of a black silken one and did not speak the language of Jundishapur. This suggests that being a Christian physician from Jundishapur meant you were a member of the elite medical class as well as that the Syrian Christian school was famous. However, even if true, we still have no idea how the Jundishapur hospital and school functioned and what kind of medicine was practiced and taught there.

Because most medical training was still mainly a family affair, which meant that if you were not a Christian or a Jew, certainly in the Ummayad period, it was difficult to become a physician, unless you found a physician willing to accept you as his student. Initially, this meant that non-Moslem physicians had a strong market position. Furthermore, Syrian Christian physicians strengthened their professional position by translating Greek medical works into Syriac, although many Greek medical texts were also available in Pahlavi. Bukhtishu and Yuhanna b. Musawaih were important Syrian Christian physicians, who held posts in the hospitals of Baghdad and were involved with translating medical texts (either by themselves or as patron).[1] Likewise in the 10th century, physicians attached to the Azodi hospital (est. 982) in Baghdad continued translating Greek medical texts.[2]

As implied by al-Jahez, by 840 there were not yet many Moslem physicians, certainly not important ones. Because it is unlikely that Christian seminaries would allow a Moslem to study medicine there, the first Moslem physicians, therefore, must have been mostly converts to Islam. This may also explain why Galenic medicine was practiced in the first Islamic hospitals by Islamic medical practitioners. This suggests that there was no real alternative to Greek medical knowledge. Also, because there was as yet no Islamic medicine or *tibb al- nabi*, while Zoroastrian medicine was heavily imbued with Greek medicine, and Indian medicine, the only possible rival medical system, was only known to a few. There was an effort to make Indian medicine more accessible by the Barmaki brothers, who established the first Islamic hospital. It must have been founded before 803 CE, the date of the fall of Yahya b. Khalid. It was perhaps built to compete with the Christian *xenodokheion* built in 790 (see above). According to al-Nadim (d. 990):

---

1. Ullman 1970, pp. 108-15.
2. Ullman 1970, pp. 73-74.

Translators of India and the Nabateans ... He [Mankah or Kankah al-Hindi] translated from the Indian language into Arabic. Ibn Dahn, al-Hindi, who administered the Bimarestan (Hospital) of the the Barmak family.³

The same al-Nadim reports that Yahya b. Khalid "ordered Mankah [Kankah] the Indian to translate it [an Indian book of medicine] the Book of Sarsad, i.e. the Susruta-samhita] at the hospital and to render it in the form of a compilation."⁴ Indeed, Indian medicine was known to physicians and Ibn Usaybi`ah devotes his entire, be it a small one, chapter twelve to Indian physicians and also lists which books by Indian scholars al-Razi drew upon.⁵

The Barmaki hospital seems to have been the first Islamic hospital in Baghdad, moreover, one where Iranian-Indian medicine also was known. In this respect the Barmaki hospital possibly drew on the medical practice in Marv. This is suggested by the fact that the Barmaki brothers, who were descended from a family of hereditary Buddhist leaders in Balkh, had Indian medical texts translated. This hospital probably was continued after the fall of the Barmaki family by Harun al-Rashid, hence his claim to fame to have founded the first Islamic hospital.⁶

At that time, there were also two Christian schools in Baghdad that taught Greek philosophy and medicine. The pagan school of Harran and the Syrian Christian school of Nisibis were still influential in the medical field during the Abbasid period.⁷ There also was a number of Islamic hospitals, such as the one founded by the steward (*gholam*) of caliph al-Mu`tadid bi-Allah (r. 279–289/892 902), which was endowed by Shuja`, the mother of Mutawwakil `ala Allah.⁸ On 14 June

---

3. Ibn Nadim 1970. vol. 2, p. 589-90
4. Ibn Nadim 1970, vol. 2, p. 710. A major text of Ayurveda medicine and allegedly known to al-Razi.
5. Ibn Abi Usaybi`ah 2020, 12.2.
6. Najmabadi 1353, pp. 769-70.
7. Najmabadi 1353, pp. 682-83.
8. Ibn Abi Usaybi`ah 2020, 10.4.5.

918, the hospital of Shaghab, the mother of al-Muqtadir bi-Allah (r. 295-320/908-932), was opened at Suq Yahya at the Tigris, on which the Caliph spent monthly 600 dinars. In that same year he also opened a hospital at the Damascus gate, which was named after al-Muqtadir himself, on which he monthly spent 200 dinars.[9] In 302/924-25, Ali b. 'Isa, al-Muqtadir's vizier, founded a hospital at the Harbiyeh quarter.[10] In 313/935-36, mention is made of a hospital in al-Mufazzal lane, which was established by Ibn al-Furat (d. 371/981), several times vizier to al-Muqtadir.[11] Abu'l-Hasan Bajkam, the governor of al-Wasit also built and endowed a hospice or *dar al-ziyafat* in Baghdad around that time to nurse and treat the poor. However, Ibn Jawzi does not mention it, while al-Muqtadir's hospital apparently was not completed.[12] The fact that apparently all early Islamic hospitals only cared for the poor is also suggested by al-Tanukhi (d. 994), who related that part of the house of a wealthy Egyptian physician al-Qati` "had been turned into a sort of hospital to house the poor, whom he would treat, supplying that they needed in the way of drugs, food, attendance, and spending most of his earnings on it."[13] The fact also that famous physicians of whom it is reported that they were attached to a hospital also had a private practice confirms this as well as that those who could afford to cost of a physician did not come to the hospital for treatment.

In Iran proper, during the early Islamic period, not many hospitals were built; at least not many are mentioned in the surviving texts. There was a *bimarestan-e* Rayy, allegedly a big institution founded before 900, which, for a certain period, was headed by the famous physician al-Razi.[14] Another early establishment was the *bimarestan-e* Zarand, which, together with a mosque and a bazaar, was founded by

---

9. Ibn Abi Usaybi`ah 2020, 10.4.6.

10. Ibn Abi Usaybi`ah 2020, 10.16.

11. Ibn Abi Usaybi`ah 2020, 10.5.2.; Najmabadi 1353, pp. 771-2; Abu'l-Hasan Ali b. Isa b. Jarrah 772-4; Moqtaderi 774-

12. Ibn Abi Usaybi`ah 2020, 10.4.8; Busse 1969, p. 530 quoting Ibn Jawzi VII, p. 114..

13. Savage-Smith 2020.

14. Ibn Abi Usaybi`ah 2020, 11.5.7; Tajbakhsh 1379, pp. 65-66

'Amru b. Leyth al-Saffar (r. 879-901 CE).[15] However, it is uncertain whether it lasted after his death. Also, a hospital was established by the well-known physician 'Isa b. Maseh in ninth century CE in Marv.[16] These three are the earliest 'Islamic' hospitals in Iran. In all these cases, nothing is known about how these hospitals actually functioned and what kind of medicine was practiced, how many patients and diseases treated, and the success rate of each kind of treatment.[17]

As is clear from the above, the founding of a hospital was by patronage, royal or otherwise. It was an act of private piety and of charity to show that the philanthropic ruler or notable was pious and cared for the poor. An early example is that of Tahir b. al-Hoseyn, governor of Khorasan, in 821-22, who wrote to his son Abdallah on his appointment as governor of Diyar Rabia: "For sick Muslims you should set up hospitals [*duran*] to shelter them, people to attend them and doctors to treat their illnesses."[18] Thus, in the Abbasid era hospitals were not established by the state like in the Byzantine Empire, for Islamic hospitals were private charitable institutions that were maintained by private endowments (*owqaf*). The result was that Islamic hospitals were few in numbers and only existed in some major cities, although they were larger and better funded than the Christian *xenodokheion*. Also, initially, it seems that most of them were not attached to a religious institution like the *xenodokheion*, but were purely medical in nature.

---

15. Tajbakhsh 1379, pp. 89-91; Anonymous 1366, pp. 32-33.
16. Tajbakhsh 1379, pp. 75-76.
17. Savage-Smith 2020.
18. Dols 1987, p. 382.

HOSPITALS IN BUYID IRAN
934–1062

The Buyids were said to have established and endowed hospitals in Shiraz, Gorgan, and Baghdad.[1] The most famous Buyid hospital was the Azodi hospital in Baghdad, which was founded ca. 980 by Azod al-Dowleh, probably at the initiative of his Christian vizier Nasr b. Harun. It allegedly had twenty-four doctors. Ibn Abu Usaybi`ah, a 13th century source, mentions several classes of specialists that were employed in this hospital: oculists (*kahhalan*), surgeons (*jarrahiyyun*) and bonesetters (*mujabbirun*), a group of natural philosophers or physiologists (*taba'i`iyyin*), and a pharmacist and medicine store manager (*khazzan*), who prepared liquid an herbal medicines (*ashribah wa adviyah*). Also, lectures were given at the `Azodi hospital. The hospital director was called *sa`ur*, a Syriac loanword, indicating that the hospital was modeled after the Christian hospitals. Often the directors were also referred to as *motavalli*, such as in the case of al-Razi in Rey and Baghdad and al-Jorjani in Khvarezm, because these institutions were sustained by the revenues of endowments or *vaqf*s.[2] The Azodi hospital continued to be active after the fall of the

---

1. Hoffmann 2000, p. 235; Tajbakhsh 1379, pp. 99-100.
2. Ibn Abi Usaybi`ah 2020, 11.5.6; Busse 1969, pp. 531-32; Elgood 1951, p. 173; Tajbakhsh 1379, p. 91-93; Ibn Balkhi 1374, pp. 322, 406, p. 38; Mustawfi 1919, p. 114. "'Practice' in Syriac is sa`ūruthā [i.e. ܣܥܘܪܘܬܐ]; that is why someone who [tends] the sick in the hospital is called *sa`ur*, because he takes care of their treatment," see Ibn Abi Usaybi`ah 2020, 10.64.10 (Amin al-Dowleh ibn al-Tilmidh worked as *sa`ur* in the `Azodi hospital in Baghdad).

Buyids, although to what extent is unknown, until it was destroyed in 1252 by the Mongols. Ibn Battutta found it in ruins.[3]

There was allegedly also an 'Azodi hospital in Shiraz, the Buyid capital, which was founded and lavishly endowed by Azod al-Dowleh. Many physicians and other staff were reportedly attached to it and like the other hospitals the Buyids established it formed part of a large *madraseh* complex where medicine, astronomy, philosophy, and mathematics were also taught. However, the 13th century source for the information on this hospital is not contemporary and, according to Busse, not a reliable one for the Buyid period.[4] Be that as it may, there was a hospital with that name in Shiraz in the 12th century, which, according to Ibn Balkhi, was dilapidated (*khalal*), but in 1363 Zarkub reports that it was still functioning (*ma'mur*).[5]

During the Buyid period, in addition to those discussed above, a hospital is mentioned in Isfahan, which was founded by the famous physician Ibn Mandavayh al-Isfahani,[6] while Abdol-Karim b. Abi Othman Nishapuri (d. 1016) founded one in his hometown.[7] Ibn al-Balkhi mentions a fine hospital with a mosque at Firuzabad in Fars.[8]

It seems, although the information dates from the 13th century, that these Abbasid and Buyid hospitals, at which famous physicians worked or were in charge of, were rather large institutions, with separate sections for out-patients and in-patients, both separated for men and women. A patient, irrespective of religion, would either receive a prescription at the dispensary or would be accepted as an in-patient and then was referred to the hospital ward relevant to the diagnosed illness. The wards of the large hospitals were specialized in internal diseases, setting bones, surgery, and ophthalmology. The

---

3. Ibn Battuta 1962, vol. 2, p. 331.
4. Mustawfi 1919, p. 144; Busse 1956, p. 531.
5. Tajbakhsh 1379, pp. 91-92; Ibn Balkhi 1374, pp. 322, 406; Zarkub 1350, p. 51. For a list of physicians that may have worked in this hospital, see Tajbakhsh 1379, pp. 94-99.
6. Ibn Abi Usaybi'ah 2020, 11.16; Najmabadi 1353, p. 768.
7. Najmabadi 1353, p. 767.
8. Ibn Balkhi 1915, p. 46.

number of medical staff was in proportion to the number of beds. The staff consisted of physicians, male and female orderlies (*farrash; dayeh*) and helpers (*moshref*s and *qa'em*s), who seem to have been responsible both for treatment services and for collecting charitable funds. These funds were needed for the upkeep of staff and hospitals, as well as for bedding, clothes, food and heating fuel. There was also an administrative staff with a *motavalli* (the endowment manager) often the chief physician, a ward administrator (*vakil*), a supervisor (*nazer*), the medicine store manager (*khazanehdar*), and the doorkeeper (*darban*).[9]

The role of a hospital was such an important subject that al-Razi wrote a book about it with the title: *Sifat al-bimarestan*,[10] which unfortunately has been lost. In this book he described "the hospital and all the details of the patients who were treated there."[11] `Ali b. `Abbas Majusi Ahvazi (d. 994) wrote about the same subject that: "It is appropriate that a student of this art works at hospitals and at those places where hospitals are numerous and attends competent medical masters, and has regular interaction with patients and queries them about their situation."[12] The importance of a large hospital for developing medical science was fully realized even by well-read interested layman as `Unsur al-Ma'ali Kaykaus b. Iskandar b. Qabus b. Wushmgir b. al-Ziyar, the Ziyarid ruler of Tabaristan and Gurgan, who reigned from 1049 to 1087. He composed his *Qabusnameh* in 1082 for his son Gilan Shah (r. ca. 1087-90) and in chapter 31 dealing with medicine he writes:

---

9. Ibn Abi Usaybi`ah 2020, 10.4.2, 10.4.5, 11.5.6, 11.8; Sajjadi 1989, quoting Ibn al-Jawzi, *Montazam* VII, p. 112; Elgood 1951, p. 182.
10. Tajbakhsh 1379, p. 67.
11. Ibn Abi Usaybi`ah 2020, 11.5.5. Abu Sa`id Zahed al-Ulama also wrote a *Kitab f'il-Bimaristanat* (On Hospitals). Idem, 11.5.2; see also 8.5.4.
12. Tajbakhsh 1379, p. 83, quoting his *Kamil al-Sana`at al-Tibbiyah*, p. 9.

> The physician who undertakes therapeutics should make frequent experiments, though he should not experiment on men well known or of high repute. He must have seen service in hospitals, examined many patients and undertaken many treatments, so that rare diseases shall present him with no difficulty and diseases of the internal organs be no mystery to him. What he had read about in books he must actually see with his own eyes and never be at a loss for treatment.[13]

For indeed, through the systematic training of students and observation of patients in hospitals, the development of Islamic medicine by its leading scholars, although remaining faithful to Galen, showed that he had not known everything and therefore, Abbasid and later physicians sometimes prescribed entirely different and diverging treatments.[14]

Despite Kai Ka'us's open mind and advice that "the physician who undertakes therapeutics should make frequent experiments," physicians became more tradition-bound and did not experiment or try to open new avenues to better medical understanding. If they did, they ran the risk of being taken to task for their brazenness. Nezami Aruzi in his *Chahar Maqalat*, written about 1155, furiously attacks those who even dared to question Aristotle and Ibn Sina. "Whoever criticizes these two great men excludes himself from the array of men of wisdom, places himself among the ranks of idiots and shows himself to be among the group of fools."[15] This trend among the educated community also had consequences for the manner in which hospitals functioned, which had not yet shed all traits of their exemplary Abbasid medical model. However, over time 'hospitals' became hospices, where poor people and travelers came to die. Also, medical teaching

---

13. Kai Ka'us 1951, p. 171.
14. Swain 2020.
15. al-Nezami al-Aruzi al-Samarqandi, Ahmad b. `Omar b. `Ali 1927, *Ketab-e Chahar Maqalat*. ed. Mohammad b. Abdol-Vahhab Qazvini. Berlin: Iranschär, p. 80. Swain 2020 offers a nuanced appreciation of Galen's position as the *khatam al-atibba*, the seal of physicians, among Moslem physicians.

seems to have faded away as one of the hospital's functions as these institutions became at best dispensaries cum hospice. Whereas, the Islamic hospitals of the 9th-12th centuries AD, certainly in Baghdad, seem to have been mainly medical institutions serving patients, this changed during the Ilkhanid period.

Hospitals adhered to established tradition without going beyond it and did not play even a marginal role as to public health. After 1200, due to Orthodox opposition to the scientific methodology, i.e. challenging accepted wisdom, hospitals gradually became hospices that provided shelter, food and some care for pilgrims, travelers and the poor, but abandoned their medical and therapeutic functions. The fact that they were part of the mosque-madraseh-*dar al-shafa* endowment triangle, imitating the early Christian church-seminary-hospice trinity, ensured their acceptance. Henceforth, hospices rather than hospitals were built and/or operated, a reversal to the original Byzantine *xenodokheion*.

HOSPITALS IN SELJUQ IRAN
1106–1194

Nezam al-Molk, the vizier of the Seljuq rulers Alp Arsalan (r. 1063-72) and Malekshah (r. 1072-92) allegedly built hospitals in Nishapur, Balkh, Isfahan, and Baghdad (the Nezamiyeh),[1] but nothing is known about these institutions, which are merely mentioned in passing in chronicles. As Hoffmann points out, there are neither endowment nor other documents or archeological remains to attest to their existence, nor how they functioned.[2] It is as of this period, that quite often hospitals were located near *madraseh*s; in fact, most renowned *madrasa*s (e.g., the Nezamiyeh *madraseh*s of Nishapur, Isfahan, Balkh, and Baghdad) had hospitals attached to them.

Whether in all these places there actually were 'hospitals' is unclear. In fact, in the case of Nishapur, Sheikh Farid al-Din `Attar states that it was a dispensary or *daru-khaneh*, where daily 500 people came to have their pulse felt.[3] Also, allegedly, every day the endowment stipulated the distribution of one thousand dinars as alms, which indicates that it was not a hospital. The Nishapur 'hospital' was destroyed by the Mongols in 1220. Abu Sa`id Nishaburi, known as Khargush (d. 407/1016), one of the religious scholars and pious men of his time, endowed a hospital in Nishapur, perhaps the same one in the garden in which Khatib Samarqandi stayed during his visit to the city in 409/1018.[4] In 504/1110, Jorjani was *timardar* of the dispensary or *daru-khaneh*-ye Baha' al-Dowleh-ye Khvarezmi and allegedly 1,000 dinars per month

---

1. Najmabadi 1353767; Tajbakhsh 1379, p. 89.
2. Hoffmann 2000, p. 235.
3. Tajbakhsh 1379, p. 89.
4. Sajjadi 1989, p. 259.

were endowed to it. Based on Jorjani's own description it was not a hospital, but a dispensary as the term *adviyeh-khaneh* also suggests.[5] It is obvious that in case of *daru-khaneh*s and *adviyeh-khaneh*s we deal with dispensaries rather than with hospitals.

The Seljuq rulers of Kerman copied the policy of their predecessors by building complexes with a mosque, *khaneqah*, madraseh, bathhouse and *dar al-shafa* such as one endowed by Turanshah I 'Emad al-Dowleh (r. 1084-1096) in Bardsir, at that time the central place of Kerman. Mohammad b. Arsalanshah (r. 1142-1156) built similar complexes in Bardsir, Jiroft, and Bam. Bahram Shah (r. 1169-1174) built and endowed a *morestan* in Kerman, which fell into disuse, although its endowments continued to be managed by the physicians of Kerman. Nevertheless, in 595/1191, a *dar al-shafa* is still mentioned in Kerman.[6] Qotlogh Torkan Khatun, Qara Khetay, as of 1257 queen-regent of Kerman, for her minor son Mozaffar al-Din Hajjaj Soltan, built and endowed the traditional complex of mosque, madraseh, tomb, *khaneqah* and *dar al-shafa* in Kerman.[7]

Qazi Hamid al-Din Balkhi (d. 559/1163) mentioned that a *bimarestan* in Isfahan was so famous for the treatment by a famous physician of mental diseases (*tebb-e ruhi*) that people came from all parts of the Middle East to consult him and get his medicines.[8] In Shiraz, Atabeg Mozaffar al-Din built a *dar al-shafa-ye mozaffari*, probably around 1230.[9] Apart from treating in-patients with medicines, they were also given all kinds of fruit, while music was played to soothe the spirits.[10]

---

5. Elgood 1951, p. 192; Tajbakhsh 1379, p. 78. This hospital seems to be the same one visited in 733/1332 by Ibn Battutah, who mentions its Syrian physician, called Sayhuni. Ibn Battutah 1962, vol. 3, p. 542.
6. Tajbakhsh 1379, pp. 101-02; Ebrahim 1343, pp. 27, 52, 218.
7. Kermani 1362, p. 39.
8. Balkhi 1372, p. 112.
9. Zarkub 1350, p. 85. For a list of physicians who worked and taught in this hospital, see Tajbakhsh 1379, pp. 111-24.
10. Music therapy was not new and was subsumed into Islamic medicine. Horden, Peregrine 2016. *Music as Medicine: The History of Music Therapy Since Antiquity*. London: Routledge.

After the Mongol invasion this hospital fell to ruins. Amir Moqarreb al-Din Mas'ud and Amir Fakhr al-Din Abu Bakr, viziers of Atabeg Abu Bakr b. Sa'd built a complex with madraseh and *dar al-shafa* etc. in Shiraz, before 1265. Atabeg Abu Bakr b. Sa'd himself also built such a complex.[11]

---

11. Zarkub 1350, p. 84; Hedayat 1339, vol. 4, p. 612. It is not clear which one of these *dar al-shafa*s is to when Rashid al-Din writes that the *dar al-shafa-ye darvazeh-ye Salm-e Shiraz* was one of the buildings constructed by the Atabegs of Fars and had fallen into disuse for a long time. Rashid al-Din endowed this hospice again (the original endowments had been usurped). Hamadani 1358, pp. 232-33.

HOSPITALS IN ILKHANID IRAN
1256–1335

Under Mongol and Ilkhanid rule, *dar al-shafa*s tended all to be part of a complex of buildings with a religious function. Ghazan Khan (r. 1295-1304), the great-grandson of Hulagu Khan, attached a hospital to his mausoleum complex, and so did his brother and successor Oljaytu (r. 1304-1316) in Soltaniyeh, where Rashid al-Din founded a *dar al-marza* or house of the sick. However, in all of these institutions the *dar al-shafa* was not the main focus of the complex.[1]

This was also the case of the best documented Islamic Iranian *dar al-shafa* is the one established in Tabriz by Rashid al-Din, grand vizier to the Ilkhanid rulers, Ghazan Khan and Oljaytu. Rashid al-Din was a physician himself and member of a family with a long line of physicians. The Tabriz complex (Rab`-e Rashidi),[2] which included a mosque, a madraseh, a bathouse, a separate poor-house (*dar al-masakin*; *dig al-masakin*), where daily food was given to 100 poor people, as well as a *dar al-shafa*.[3] According to a letter allegedly written by Rashid al-Din, the *dar al-shafa-ye rashidi* was established near a *dar al-ziyafat*, a *dar al-mosaferin*, a *dar al-qoran* and a *dar al- hadith*, indicating the religious function of the complex, which allegedly was endowed, among other things, with the supply of 748,000 *man* of bread 320,000 *man* of meat (in addition to many thousands of chickens) per year, which food items had to be distributed among *arbab-e estehqaq va vazayef*. These last two terms suggest that the

---

1. Hamadani 1358, p. 213; Hoffmann 2000, pp. 112, 236.
2. For a short description of the Rashidi quarter, see Qazvini 1372, p. 55.
3. Hoffmann 2000, pp. 129-30, 212-13, 219-21, 231-34, 262-63.

food was destined for deserving members of the religious class rather than for the sick or the poor.[4]

The Rashidi endowment deed describes the formal functions of the *dar al-shafa* quite clearly. Of course, we don't know whether these prescriptive rules were adhered to in reality.[5] Although, the term *dar al-shafa* is often used in the endowment document, the institution is also referred to as *daru-khaneh* and *beyt al-adviyeh* and thus, the term was not used as meaning 'hospital' in strictu sensu, but rather as meaning 'dispensary.' The term *bimarestan* is not used in the endowment deed at all.[6]

A physician (*tabib*), an oculist (*kahhal*), who also performed the task of the surgeon (*jarrad*), a repetitor (*mu`id*), a pharmacist (*sharabdar*) or, a manager of the pharmacy (*khazin*) or, a *khadem* or *qayyim*, i.e. a medical orderly, plus support staff were attached to the Rashidi complex in Tabriz.[7] The physician and surgeon had an annual salary with a daily ration of bread, but the oculist had a monthly salary, be it that it was the same as that of the surgeon. The other staff also received annual wages, although these were paid monthly. The staff included a *sharabdar*, who prepared liquid medicines such as several opioids, including electuaries (*ma`ajin*), *taryaq-e faruq*, and *faluniya*, as well as various oils (*adhan*), eye medicines (*akhal*), unguents (*marahim*), suppositories (*shiyafat*) and instruments (*alat*) in the *sharab-khaneh* or *dar al-shorb*. In the kitchen (*matbakh*), which was located in the dispensary, the cook prepared a pea-lentil soup (*mozavvarat*) for the sick, which he brought to them. The orderlies had a day and a night service, presumably they alternated. Further there was a servant (*farrash*), a water carrier (*saqqa*), and a door keeper (*bavvab*).

---

4. Hamadani 1358, pp. 212-13. As to the reliability of this information, see Hoffmann 2000, pp. 236-37.
5. .The *dar al-shafa-ye rashidi* was established near the *dar al-ziyafat, dar al-mosaferin, dar al-qoran* and *dar al- hadith*. Hamadani 1358, pp. 212-13.
6. Hoffmann 2000, p. 129; Hamadani 2536, see Index.
7. Hoffmann 2000, p. 235, 237; Hamadani 2536, pp. 148, 159, 183, 224.

The physician had to treat patients in the morning and the evening. He explicitly was only allowed to treat and prescribe medicines to those persons who were residents (*sokkan*) of the Rab`-e Rashidi and of the Shahr-e Rashidi as well as to the neighbors (*hamsayegan*) of these two wards, as well as to travelers and the staff (*molazemin*) of the complex, who fell ill, but nobody else! In the pharmacy (*makhzan al-adviyeh*) herbal drugs were prepared and stored. Also, here, medicines were handed out. To that end, the physician had to be at the door of the *dar al-shafa* every Monday and Thursday. Patients presented themselves at the door, received a prescription from the physician, who gave it to the drugstore manager (*khazin*) and pharmacist (*sharabdar*), who worked inside the *beyt al-adviyeh*. On these two days only residents, travelers, staff and neighbors of the complex were entitled to treatment and receive medicines. There was a hierarchy in the handing out of medicines, because the residents and travelers had precedence over the sons of the founder, then followed his freed slaves and finally the staff. After this group the gardeners and farmers of the endowed lands around Tabriz and in the province were served, and finally the inhabitants and neighbors of the Shahrestan-e Rab`-e Rashidi had their turn. On other days of the week other people could present themselves, who did not receive the same (higher quality and/or expensive) kind of medicines as those who came on Monday and Thursday.[8]

Those travelers who had been assigned a room in the complex and had become bedridden were treated by the physician in their room. He had to instruct the *sharabdar* to bring medicines and the cook to bring food to the room of the bed-ridden patients. The endowment document states explicitly that important travelers with a suite had to be given a room and, if they fell ill, had to be treated in their room. However, if they were not belonging to this class of notables then they were allowed to lodge in the hospice or *dar al-ziyafat*. If they fell ill they would be treated there by the physician and they might receive a night robe.

---

8. Hoffmann 2000, pp. 129, 271-73; Hamadani 2536, pp.146-48.

The physician resided in the *dar al-tabib*, which was adjacent to the *beyt al-adviyeh*. Every day, he had to instruct his two students (*mota'allem*) together in medicine at the *rivaq-e beyt al-adviyeh* (store room), which was a.k.a. *rivaq dar al-shafa* or *rivaq al-adviyeh*, i.e. the place for healing or drugs, which also served as the residence of the medical staff. It was not part of the *dar al-shafa*, but was near to it, but it is unknown where.[9] The two students, who had to be pious and industrious, were allowed to study for a period of not more than five years. After this period they either received a diploma (*ejazeh*) attesting that they were authorized to practice medicine, or they had to leave, for two new students had to be engaged. The two students were lodged in one of the rooms (*hojreh*) at the back of the *beyt al-adviyeh*.[10]

In his purported letters, Rashid al-Din states that he had 50 physicians brought from India, China, Egypt, Syria and other lands who in total taught 500 students. He also employed eye doctors, surgeons and bone setters (*mojabberan*), who each had to teach five of the *vaqf*'s slaves.[11] These data are not borne out by the Tabriz endowment deed; in fact, it contradicts it, for Rashid al-Din's Tabriz dispensary cum hospice was small. Also, it only served the inhabitants and staff of the complex and important travelers, just like the *xenodokheion* of the Nisibis school. There were no in-patients, for important bedridden patients were treated in their own rooms, and all others in the hospice (*dar al-ziyafat*).[12] In short, the Rashidi *dar al-shafa* in Tabriz was not a hospital, but only a dispensary, which physically was separate from the hospice. Also, the Rashidi dispensary was of short duration as the entire Rashidi complex was given over to the Mongol soldiery when Rashid al-Din was sentenced to death in 1318. It was renovated during

---

9. Hoffmann 2000, pp. 237-38; Hamadani 2536, pp. 181-85 (when single, the *sharabdar* lived in a room in the *daru-khaneh*, the orderlies (*khoddam al-marza*) in the *rivaq al-morattabin*, the oculist/surgeon in the *sabat* or in the covered passage-way of the Rashidi complex. If they had a family they had to get a house in the Salehiyyeh quarter).

10. Hoffmann 2000, p. 238; Hamadani 2536, p. 174.

11. Hamadani 1358, p. 290.

12. Hoffmann 2000, pp. 237-38; Hamadani 2536, pp. 146-48.

the short vizierate of his son and thereafter lingered on. Abbas I (r. 1589-1629) allegedly ordered to repair the complex, but his successors abandoned this project so that it fell into ruins.

Rashid al-Din allegedly also founded a *beyt al-marza* in his home town of Hamadan. The *daru-khaneh va dar al-shafa* of Hamadan was explicitly established to care for the weak and poor and it was endowed with properties to ensure its function for eternity. Apparently, the donor's instructions were not respected for Rashid al-Din sent Malek al-Atteba to suppress the corruption that had arisen.[13] Rashid al-Din also allegedly founded and endowed a *bimarestan* in Basra, which like other such establishments was located near a *dar al-mosaferin* and a *dar al-hadith*. It is not clear why this establishment was called *bimarestan* and all his other hospices were referred to by other terms.[14] Rashid al-Din's charter further mentions a *beyt al-adviyeh* in Bastam.[15]

Tabriz, Hamadan and Basra were not the only cities where hospices were established. Yazd in particular attracted many patrons, who built the traditional religious-learning complex in that city, or perhaps, this seems to be the case, because more local histories of Yazd have survived than from other cities. The *dar al-shafa-ye Sahebi* in Yazd, named after its founder Khvajeh Shams-al-Din Mohammad Joveyni Saheb-e Divan (d. 1284), vizier of Abaqa (r. 1265-1282), was completed in 666/1267. Each year this patron paid all the expenses of the physicians and patients, and he also endowed the institution with the income from part of a village. It had good water supply, including a well. The *dar al-shafa* built by Khvajeh Saheb-e Divan was built at the entrance of the bazaar. It had houses, four *eyvan*s or porticos (*saffat*), an open-fronted summer room (*tanabi*), a wind-catcher (*badgir*), a *beyt al-adviyeh*, a *howzkhaneh*, a *mahbas-e majanin va marza*, a well, and a garden in the back with an ice-house. It was part

---

13. Hamadani 1358, p. 213 (20,000 head of chicken were allegedly endowed to *dar al-shafa-ye rab`-e rashidi*, the *dar al-marza-ye* Soltaniyeh and the *beyt al-adviyeh-ye* Hamadan for the sick); see, however, Hoffmann 2000, p. 237.
14. Hamadani 1358, pp. 22, 213.
15. Hoffmann 2000, p. 236; Hamadani 2536, p. 241.

of a mosque-madraseh complex.[16] The hospice fell into disuse, but it is not clear when. In 1310, Mohammad b. Mozaffar used the *dar al-shafa-ye sahebi* to display three captured emirs hanging from the building in a cage for the people's entertainment.[17] This may be an indication that the building was not used for its original purpose any longer, or this may have been an incidental event. However, in 1445, Khvajeh Ruhollah Mowlana Faraj established a workshop in the *dar al-shafa*, probably weaving silken fabrics or *diba* (ديبا), since he was the collector (*sahib-e tahvil*) of the government silk and headman (*moqtada*) of the *dabbaj* (دباج) weavers. Here a fabric was woven for dispatch to Mecca.[18]

Another *dar al-shafa* or *beyt al-adviyeh* in Yazd was attached to the madraseh-ye Rokniyeh. It had an observatory and a library. It was built by the famous scholar Sayyed Rokn al-Haqq va'l-Din Mohammad b. Nezam al-Hoseyni (d. 1332). There also was a *dar al-shafa* or *beyt al-adviyeh* at the madraseh-ye Kamaliyeh. It was built before 1336, the death of its builder Kamal al-Din Abu'l-Ma`ali, the vizier of Soltan Abu Sa`id (r. 1316-1335). It was part of a complex with a *khaneqah*, *beyt al-adviyeh*, bathhouse, caravanserai, and houses. The endower built a *qanat* towards it of which *beyt al-adviyeh* received two *dang*, i.e. one-third. It was finished in 720/1320.[19] In 747/1346, after Abu Sa`id died, Mohammad b. Mozaffar also built a *dar al-shafa* in Yazd.[20]

Under the Jalayarids (r. 1335-1411), a *dar al-shafa* (none are mentioned by name) was managed by a director, who was not a physician, and like the director of the `Azodi hospital in Baghdad was called *sa`uri-ye bimarestan*. This *sa`ur* (a Syriac loanword) was a religious official and his responsibilities were made known to the *motavalliyan* and *motassarefan* of the *dar al-shafa*. He had the authority to appoint and dismiss physicians, oculists and surgeons,

---

16. Ja`fari 1338/1959, pp. 89, 91, 150, 155; Kateb 2527, pp. 83, 131-33, 149.
17. Kateb 2527, p. 83.
18. Kateb 2527, pp. 83, 224.
19. Ja`fari 1338/1959, p. 87, 93, 150; Kateb 2527, pp. 125-26, 136.
20. Ja`fari 1338/1959, p. 33.

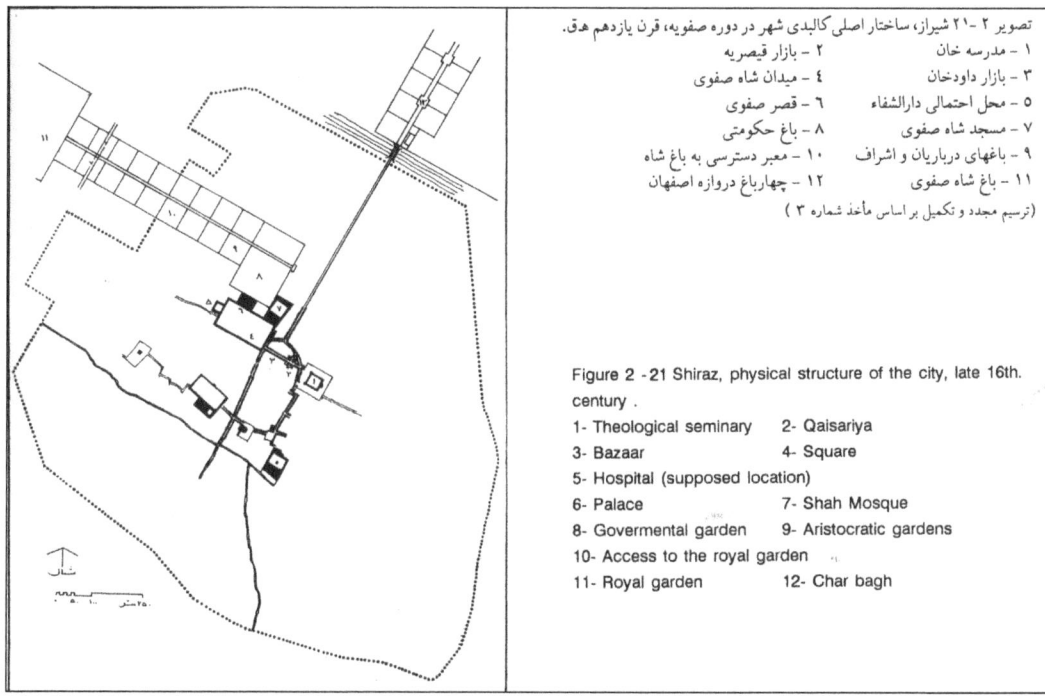

Figure 2 -21 Shiraz, physical structure of the city, late 16th. century .
1- Theological seminary 2- Qaisariya
3- Bazaar 4- Square
5- Hospital (supposed location)
6- Palace 7- Shah Mosque
8- Govermental garden 9- Aristocratic gardens
10- Access to the royal garden
11- Royal garden 12- Char bagh

Map of Shiraz indicating the probable location of the daral-shafa. From Tavassoli-Bonyadi 1371, *Urban Space Design*, Tehran, p. 68.

who also had to obey his directives.²¹ Shah Shoja` Mozaffari (r. 1358 to 1384) established a *dar al-shafa* in Shiraz. It still functioned in the Timurid period, but there is no report that it was still used as such during the Safavid period.²² In Tabriz reference is made to a certain Sheikh Nur al-Din *Bimarestani* about which no particulars are known, suggesting the existence of a *bimarestan* in that city.²³ The religious context of the *dar al-shafa* is also reflected in the poem that is found in the *Savfat al-Safa*.

---

21. Nakhjevani 1964, vol. 1/1, pp. 46, 52; vol. 2, pp. 235-37.
22. Fasa'i 1367, vol. 2, p. 943; Forsat 1312, p. 459; Mostafavi 1343, p. 385 (part of the madraseh still exists).
23. Ardabili 1373, p. 64.

*Dast-e `Isa dar in tasarrofgah-e dar al-shafa
ruh bakhshi kard az now in tan-e bimarra*

The hand of Jesus in this abode of healing
Gave new life to this sick body.[24]

---

24. Ardabili 1373, p. 338. In Islamic lore Jezus is depicted as 'the Healer.'

HOSPITALS IN TIMURID IRAN
1370–1507

In Timurid times, royalty and important officials continued to establish hospitals that likewise usually were part of a complex that included a mosque and madraseh. Timur himself allegedly had given orders that there should be at least one hospital in every city in his realm.[1] However, there is no trace of evidence that these actually were built let alone were functioning. In fact, it is more than likely that Timur never had such an intention and gave such orders. Of the Timurid hospitals, only those in Herat are known. In that city there were five hospices: *dar al-shafa-ye `Ali Shir*, named after the famous and learned vizier of Hoseyn Bayqara, which was part of his Ekhlasiyeh complex. Furthermore there was the *dar al-shafa-ye* `Abdollah `Amr; the *dar al-shafa-ye* Malikat Agha, as well as the *dar al-shafa-ye* Shahrokh and the *dar al-shafa-ye* Soltan Hoseyn, which latter two were outside city.[2] Allegedly, medical education still was offered at one of the hospices, for it is reported that the famous physician Mowlana Darvish Ali Tabib taught at the *dar al-shafa-ye Mahd-`Oliyah Malikat Agha*.[3]

---

1. Abu Taleb Hoseyni Torbati, *Tozukat-e Timuri*. ed. J. White, Oxford, 1783 (reprint Tehran 1342/1963), p. 371.
2. Terry Allen 1981, *A Catalogue of the Toponyms and Monuments of Timurid Herat*. Cambridge: MIT, p. 156; Khvandamir 1362, vol. 4, p. 342. The Malikat Agha hospice was headed by a Christian physician, Masih al-Din Habibollah. Khvami 1357, pp. 280-82.
3. Khvandamir 1378, p. 179. For a list of contemporary Herati physicians, see Tajbakhsh 1379, pp. 159-60.

HOSPITALS IN AQ-QOYUNLU IRAN
1378–1501

In Tabriz, there was a *morestan* (properly, [*bi*]*marestan*) that had been built by Uzun Hasan (r. 1453-1478), which was large, having many buildings, and "within it is even more beautifully ornamented than the mosque, having many large wards about ten yards long and four broad, each of them being fitted with a carpet to its measurement."[1] During the reign of Uzun Hasan and his son Sultan Ya`qub "more than a thousand people lived in the hospital."[2] In Shamakhi, Josapat Barbaro visited a small hospice, which apparently was attached to a religious building as there was a sepulcher with a dervish sitting there.[3] In Mardin, likewise was a hospice, which was visited by a dervish.[4] In particular the description of the 'hospital' in Tabriz as well as the fact that in the other two Barbaro did not mention the presence of sick people at all, suggests that these places were hospices rather than hospitals.

The number of known *dar al-shafa*s never had been large (see Table 1), despite the hype about their importance during the period before the fifteenth century. It is, of course, likely that there were many more of them than the few indicated by the existing sources, but even if we assume a ten-fold increase of the known ones their total number probably would still not exceed 100 at any given period. Most scholars agree that the number of *dar al-shafa*s greatly decreased after the Ilkhanid period, although the only evidence is *ex silencio*, because *dar al-shafa*s are hardly mentioned any more.

---

1. Barbaro 1873, part 2, p. 177.
2. Barbaro 1873, part 2, p. 178.
3. Barbaro 1873, part 1, p. 95.
4. Barbaro 1873, part 1, p. 48.

Table 1: Hospitals founded in Iran between 550 and 1460

Sasanians	224-651	
Ctesiphon ?	550 CE	Christian hospital
Nisibis	550 CE	Christian seminary/hospice
Jundishapur	Early 800s	Christian seminary/hospice

Abbasids	750-1258	
Ctesiphon	790	Christian seminary/hospital
Marestan-e Rayy	before 900	Moslem hospital
Bimarestan-e Zarand	about 890	Moslem hospital +
Bimarestan-e Marv	before 900	Moslem hospital
Bimarestan-e Barmaki	before 803	Baghdad
Bimarestan-e Badr Gholam Mo`tazed	before 900	Baghdad
Bimarestan-e Abu'l-Hasan Ali b. Isa b. Jarrah	before 900	Baghdad
Bimarestan-e Moqtaderi	918	Baghdad
Bimarestan-e Shaghab	918	Baghdad
Bimarestan-e Ali b. `Isa	924	Baghdad
Bimarestan-e Ibn al-Furat	930	Baghdad
Dar al-Ziyafat-e Bajkam	930s	Baghdad

Buyids	934-1062	
	934-1062	Shiraz, Isfahan, Nishapur, Firuzabad, and Baghdad (Azodi) +

Seljuqs	1016-1187	
Dar al-shafa/daru-khaneh		Nishapur, Balkh, Isfahan, and Baghdad +
Dar al-shafa	around 1090	Bardsir +
Dar al-shafa	around 1145	Bardsir, Jiroft, and Bam +
Dar al-shafa-ye mozaffari	around 1230	Shiraz +
Dar al-shafa	before 1265	Shiraz +
Dar al-shafa	before 1265	Shiraz +

Mongols/Ilkhans/Jalayers	1250-1432	
Dar al-shafa-ye Sahebi	before 1294	Yazd +
Dar al-shafa or bimarestan	around 1300	Tabriz, Basra, Hamadan, Bastam +
Dar al-Shafa	ca. 1310	Soltaniyeh
Dar al-shafa-ye Rokniyeh	before 1332	Yazd +
Dar al-shafa-ye Kamaliyeh	before 1336	Yazd +
Dar al-Shafa-ye Mozaffariyeh	1360s	Shiraz

Timurids	1370-1506	
Dar al-shafa-ye `Abdollah `Amr	before 1480	Herat +
Dar al-shafa-ye Malikat Agha	before 1480	Herat +
Dar al-shafa-ye Shahrokh	before 1480	Herat +
Dar al-shafa-ye Soltan Hoseyn	before 1480	Herat +
Dar al-shafa-ye `Ali Shir	around 1470	Herat +

Aq-Qoyunlu	1402-1501	
Marestan	around 1470	Tabriz, Shamakhi, Mardin

+ = part of a complex including mosque, madraseh, bathhouse, bazaar.

HOSPITALS IN SAFAVID IRAN
1501–1736

The situation under the Safavids did not differ that much from the preceding centuries in terms of the nature of medical services offered to the public. However, there is no evidence that the number of *dar al-shafa*s was less than in the preceding centuries. Allegedly one or two 'hospitals' existed in every city, according to Du Mans, which, if true, suggests that there may have been an increase in the number of *dar al-shafa*s. Unfortunately, we only have information about the existence of a few of these institutions, but that seems to confirm Du Mans' observation. According to Tavernier, there were no 'hospitals' in Iran as beautiful as the ones that existed in Europe.[1] Nevertheless, some of them were quite nice; at least that is what Chardin thought. He agreed with Tavernier that the one in Isfahan did not resemble anything like a European hospital. It was more like a two-storied convent around a garden, consisting of 80 rather nice, but small low rooms. This description is not unlike the one given by Du Mans.[2] The Isfahan 'hospital' was situated near the *Qeysariyeh*, behind the copper-smiths' bazaar that was also known as the *bazar-e dar al-shafa*, because its caravanserai had been built as an endowment to ensure the payment of the hospice's staff's wages. The hospice was part of the traditional complex consisting of a madraseh and mosque with facilities for pilgrims such as a hospice, which buildings, therefore, were referred to as *madraseh-ye dar al-shafa* and *masjed-e dar al-shafa*.[3]

---

1. Tavenier 1930, p. 277; see also St. Joseph 1985, p. 133.
2. Chardin 1811, vol. 7, pp. 389-390; Du Mans 1890, p. 219; Richard 1995, vol. 2, p. 171.
3. Chardin 1811, vol. 7, p. 391; Jaberi-Ansari 1373, pp. 147, 287, 341; Gaube

It is may be not superfluous to point out that usually the *dar al-shafa* mainly served pilgrims and other travelers (*ghoraba, zovvar, motaraddedin*) who came to the Shrine or mosque-madraseh complex, but not necessarily the inhabitants of the town in which it was located. In this respect its function is roughly the same as that of a hospital in the meaning as used in Europe during medieval times, viz., an almshouse for the poor and pilgrims.

Isfahan was not the only town with a *dar al-shafa*, for there was also a hospice or *morestan* (properly, *marestan*) in Tabriz that had been built by Uzun Hasan (r. 1453-1478). It was large, having many buildings, "and within it is even more beautifully ornamented than the mosque, having many large wards about ten yards long and four broad, each of them being fitted with a carpet to its measurement."[4] It still existed under the early Safavids. Some one hundred fifty years later, according to Chardin, there were three clean and well-maintained hospices in Tabriz.[5] In 1680, an additional *dar al-shafa* was built in Tabriz as part of the usual endowment complex consisting of a (founder's) tomb, a mosque, a madraseh and sundry buildings.[6] Elgood also mentions a 'hospital' in Ardabil, which was attached to the shrine of Sheykh Safi al-Din, as well as one in Qazvin, called the 'royal hospital', to which `Ali Afzal Qati` was attached as physician.[7]

There also were hospices or dispensaries elsewhere in Iran such as in Yazd where there was a so-called 'house of health' or *sehhatkhaneh*.[8] In 1515, in Astarabad, Khvajeh Mozaffar b. Khvajeh Ahmad Betekchi Astarabadi endowed the *dar al-shafa-ye Mozaffariyeh*,

---

- Wirth 1978, pp. 284-285; Nasrabadi 1361, p. 326; Monshi 1350, vol. 2, pp. 1070, 1110.
4. Barbaro - Contarini 1873, part 2, p. 177; Tajbakhsh 1379, pp. 162-164.
5. Chardin 1811, vol. 2, p. 324.
6. Werner 2000, p. 99 (*Zaheriyeh owqaf*), of which no trace is left.
7. Elgood 1970 p. 29; Tajbakhsh 1379, pp. 175-183.
8. Bafqi 1340, vol. 3, p. 398. Elgood 1970, p. 29 refers to this hospital as Dar al-`Ebadat or Place of Worship, which is wrong as his source, Monshi 1350, vol. 1, p. 168 only refers to the city of Yazd, which was known as Dar al-`Ebadat.

which he had established previously, with new endowments. A third of the endowment was to be used, among other things, to pay for a professor (*modarres*), students (*talabeh*), a repeater (*mo`id*), a servant (*khadem*), and an orderly (*sa`i*), and another third for the physician (*tabib*) and the sick. The deed further stipulated that the professor had to be knowledgeable about medicine, intimating that this was not always the case.[9] In Shiraz there was a *dar al-shafa*, which had been founded by Shah Shoja` Mozaffari in 1384 and functioned in the Timurid period, but there is no report that it was still used as such during the Safavid period.[10] According to an unpublished document, however, there still was a *dar al-shafa* attached to the mosque-madraseh complex in Safavid Shiraz located on the Meydan-e Shah (see map on p. 29 for its probable location at no. 1). This hospital perhaps still existed in the eighteenth century, for among the good works of Karim Khan Zand are mentioned the order to keep the streets and the bazaar lanes clean as well as to fund the *dar al-shafa*, which had to make its services available free of charge to the poor and orphans.[11] In 1695, the existence of a *dar al-shafa* is mentioned in Damghan.[12] There had been, or perhaps there still was, a *dar al-shafa* in Ashraf, because Rabino lists among the mosques of that town one that was called *masjed-e dar al-shafa*. Such a mosque or a hospice is not mentioned in similar descriptions of Ashraf.[13] There was even a hospice in Ben Esfahan (a.k.a. Esfahanak), a very large village near Isfahan.[14] There further existed a so-called charitable dispensary (*sharbat-khaneh-ye kheyriyeh*) which was managed by Hakim Yar `Ali Tehrani. He was known for his care of the poor and indigent, hence he was nicknamed

---

9. Setudeh 1366, vol. 8, pp. 184-186.
10. Fasa'i 1367, vol. 2, p. 943; Forsat-e Shirazi 1312, p. 459; Mostafavi 1343, p. 385 (part of the madraseh still exists).
11. Tavassoli-Naser 1371/1992, p. 68, quoting Naser Bonyadi, *Madarek-e montasher nashodeh-e tarh-e tarikh-e ejtema`i-ye Shiraz*, Tehran, 1358/1979; Asaf 1348, pp. 255-56.
12. Nasiri 1373/1994, p. 115.
13. Rabino 1928, p. 64; Setudeh 1366, vol. 5, pp. 615-16.
14. Jaberi-Ansari 1373, p. 323.

hakim-e kheyri or 'the philantropic doctor.'[15] All these instances suggest that the information provided by Du Mans about the prevalence of hospitals is correct, thus belying the generally held opinion that after the fourteenth century there was a decline in the number of hospices in Iran.

Most information about the formal functioning of a hospice concerns the *dar al-shafa* in Safavid Mashhad. Although it is not known when the hospice was established, the shrine itself already received endowments around the year 1034, according to Beyhaqi. Likewise, Ghazan Khan also bestowed properties on the shrine. Khvandamir reports that the the end of the ninth century the shrine had a beautifully embellished *dar al-hoffaz*, where each day the poor and orphans received food (*ta'am*), a function usually associated with a *dar al-shafa*.[16] It is possible that some medical care was provided, because in 1490, the existence of the shrine's *sharbat-khaneh* is mentioned in the *'Alamara-ye Amini* as part of the royal complex to care for the sick. This may indicate that a *dar al-shafa* existed at that time, because under the Safavids the hospice was directed by the *sharbatdar*.[17]

We are on firm ground as to the 16th century, for there was a *dar al-shafa* In Mashhad since the reign of Shah Tahmasp I (r. 1524-1576). At that time, assistance was given to the sick, because an endowment deed of 1524 states that part of the income of the endowed property had to be spent on the sick and strangers.[18] Shah Tahmasp I even appointed one of his court physicians `Emad al-Din Mahmud, an opium addict, as physician of the shrine, who spent some time there treating the sick.[19] The hospice was closed on Fridays and special

---

15. Monshi1350, vol. 1, p. 169; Savory 1978, vol. 1, p. 265. Tajbakhsh 1379, pp. 192-193 deduced from this physician's *nisba* that this dispensary was a hospital in Tehran, for which there is no evidence. He also notes that there was a dispensary in the royal train, when the shah was on the move. Idem, p. 194.
16. Khvandamir 1378, p. 179.
17. Sureshjani 1395, p. 75; for an organizational lay-out, see Idem, p. 76.
18. Mo'taman 1348, p. 401; Jashemi 1389, p. 5.
19. Monshi1350, vol. 1, p. 168; Savory 1978, vol. 1, p. 264. For other physicians employed at the Mashhad hospital, see Elgood 1970, p. 29.

holidays, such as *Nowruz*, when only in-patients were admitted.[20] The location of the *dar al-shafa* across from the Gowharshad mosque and near the madraseh suggests the continuation of the ancient pattern of the mosque-masdraseh-*dar al-shafa* complex. The oldest document concerning the *maraz-khaneh* or *mariz-khaneh* dates from 1013/1604 and deals with the cost of repairs (*bimar-khaneh*). The building measured about 183.5 *dhar`* or ells. In 1114/17, two rooms for the *nafkheh-khaneh* (house of phlebotomy) were added.[21]

Although the *dar al-shafa* fell under the responsibility of the *sharbatdar*, the *hakim-bashi* was in charge of *mariz-khaneh*. The physician and the *sharbatdar* worked as a team concerning patient care, i.e., they both had to sign the daily expenditure record.[22] However, the more we come toward the end of Safavid era the more the *dar al-shafa* had become independent and separate from the *sharbat-khaneh*.[23] Patients either received ambulatory help or were given a bed in the hospice and were there cared for by the *tabib* (physician) and the *bimardar* (*parestar-* orderly). The hospital had its own hammam, because the sick were banned from going to the public baths.[24] The hospice was divided into two parts, a male and a female section, although both shared the same space and were separated by a curtain. Therefore, the hospice employed both male (*bimardar* or *khadem-e bimaran*) and female orderlies (*khadameh-ye `owrat-e bimar*). The orderlies were paid in cash and kind, resp. 1/6 and ¼ of what a *tabib* was paid. The cash part varied between 7,500 dinars to 2 *tumans*/year; the female orderlies received less, of course.[25] In addition to the

---

20. Shahidi 1388, p. 65; Sureshjani 1395, p. 96.
21. Sureshjani 1395, pp. 73-74.
22. Sureshjani 1395, pp. 75, 79, 83; Shahidi 1388, p. 66; Jashemi 1389, p. 12.
23. Jashemi 1389, p. 8.
24. Sureshjani 1395, p. 81.
25. Sureshjani 1395, p. 122. Other employees employed included: *bimardar, bimardar-bashi*; *parastar, khadem*, and *khedmat-gozar*. In 1708, an *ayaghchi-bashi* (cup-bearer) is mentioned as part of the *khedmat-e bimardari*. Some of hospice positions tended to become hereditary. Jashemi 1389, pp. 12-13.

hakim or *tabib* (physician),[26] the *dar al-shafa* employed surgeons or *jarrah*, whose wages were paid in kind.[27] Other medical workers included: phlebotomists to which end there was a *nafkheh-khaneh* or a cupping house as well as a *dallak* to massage the head hair and/or body of the sick. The latter's wages were 330 dinars.[28] In addition, inside the Shrine was an ʿ*attar-khaneh* or *daru-khaneh* (pharmacy), while there also were many in the city. The ʿ*attar* had the technical responsibility of the *daru-khaneh*,[29] but the overall responsibility of he *daru-khaneh* was shared with the *sharbatdar* and he, with the *tabib* and the *daru-saz*, formed one team. Medicines were given per recipe that precisely detailed the ingredients and were prepared in the *daru-khaneh*.[30] The medicines prescribed, prepared and handed to patients included: *taraqiyat, javarshat, ayaraj; maʿajin, sefufat; hubbha, qorzha laʿuq* or *laʿuqat; shiyaf, falasafeh, taryaq-e faruq, qorz-e benefsheh, taryaq-e arbaʿeh, atrafil, foluniya, afiyun,* and *khashkhash*, which were all opoids In one week, 9,941 dinars were expended on medicines. In 1025/1616 the annual expenditure of the *sharbat-khaneh* was 69 *tuman*s and 3,656 dinars of which 45 *tuman*s and 2,785 dinars was for food and medicines or about 65% for the sick. In 1111/1699, about 70 *tuman*s were spent, of which about 52 *tuman*s were for food and medicines for the sick.[31]

The *dar al-shafa* also employed clerks or ʿ*azab*, who recorded the ambulatory (*bimaran-e motafarreqeh* or *bimaran-e sar-paʾi*) and

---

26. For a list of *hakim*s working in the shrine, see Sureshjani 1395, p. 116, who were paid in cash and kind. Sureshjani 1395, pp. 117-21; Jashemi 1389, p. 12.
27. Sureshjani 1395, pp. 125-32 (with a list of their names (126) and instruments (125) as well as of their wages); Jashemi 1389, p. 12 (*jarrahi-bashi*).
28. Sureshjani 1395, pp. 137-42. Also mentioned are: *ghossal* and *kahhal*. Jashemi 1389, p. 12.
29. Sureshjani 1395, pp. 89, 142.
30. Sureshjani 1395, pp. 102, 105; Shahidi 1388, p. 66; see also Chardin 1811, vol. 3, p. 136
31. Sureshjani 1395, pp. 97-100, 106-112; Shahidi 1388, p. 66. These medicines were all opoids, see Floor-Javadi 2019, pp. 479-98.

the in-patients (*balini*), and all their related expenses. They received a wage in cash (7,500 dinars) and kind (6 *kharvar*). All expenditures of the *dar al-shafa* were paid out of the income from endowments.[32] Therefore, the hospice also employed *nazeran* (supervisors) to supervise (i) the application of the rules of the endowments or *owqaf*, (ii) the performance of medical care, including of medicine preparation, (iii) the quality and correctness of food distribution, of expenditures as well as of the clothes and bedding of patients.[33]

Needy patients received meat as part of their food prepared in the shrines kitchen by cooks or *tabbakh*.[34] If patients could not chew, in particular in case of bed-ridden ones, they received a pottage called *shurba* or *mozavareh*, i.e. *ash-e parhiz*. Sometimes patients were served chicken with vegetables (*zereshk, sabzi, badam*) and fruit (*miveh-ye akhar-e ruz*). The cost was usually 90 dinars per day.[35] At night the rooms in the *dar al-shafa* were lit, while one family member or small child was allowed to remain with each sick person.[36] Bed-ridden patients were provided with new clothes. Men received: *pirahan, qaba, zir-jameh, kafsh, kolah* and sick women: *nim-taneh, rupak, pirahan, zir-jameh*, and *kafsh*.[37] Also, bedding for the patients was arranged, which were made of materials such as: *chit, karbas, pashm, nakh*, etc. which were prepared by the cotton carder or *hallaj*. In 1111/1699-1700, a barber (*dallak*) was paid 504 dinars for supplying five bed-coverings (*lehaf*) and matrresses (*toshak*).[38]

---

32. Sureshjani 1395, pp. 148-56. Other administrative staff incuded: *khazanehdar; zabet, `azab, kafil; moharrer, modir; moshref; maser.* Jashemi 1389, p. 12.
33. Sureshjani 1395, pp. 133-37; Jashemi 1389, p. 12.
34. Jashemi 1389, p. 12.
35. Shahidi 1388, p. 65; Sureshjani 1395, p. 82, 103. For the kinds of food given to patients, both with meat and meatless, see Sureshjani 1395, pp. 109-110.
36. Sureshjani 1395, pp. 142-43.
37. Sureshjani 1395, pp. 143-45. Patients' clothes were changed, which Chardin 1811, vol. 5, p. 82 says did not happen. These clothes were washed with soap. Sureshjani 1395, p. 147.
38. Sureshjani 1395, pp. 145-47.

Despite the detailed invoices and accounts one cannot be sure that these expenditures reflect the actual situation. If the situation in the Qajar period is an indication then it is quite likely that also in the Safavid period abuse and misue of Shrine funds was rampant. We know that the Shrine managers were greatly interested in promoting the Shrine's attractiveness, which partly may have been out of faith, but certainly partly also out of pecuniary considerations. Kaempfer remarked about this state of affairs the following:

> This city [Mashhad] owes its development and fame to his [Imam Reza's] sacred remains, to which Moslem pilgrims come to pray, but above all Persian Shiites. From among these, after Ali, the dear son-in-law of Mohammad, and his Ja`far they seem to attribute more saintliness to Reza than to the other Imams. In the first place they believe that blind people who have faith in prayer may have their sight restored at this place. In fact, quite often priests, to attract the faith of visitors, place somebody, who feigns blindness; when thanks to the fake prayers he recovers his sight they gather a crowd of admirers who accompany the sufferer with a procession, playing the cymbals and the drums across the places, as if in triumph and praise of his helper. Because during the procession each of the pilgrims wants to have a small token of the miracle they tear a piece of the clothes of the imposter, to wit that which covered his body, in which the initiate was found to be worthy. Once the spectacle is over, the actor receives new clothes and presents given by the chiefs of the [shrine's] treasury and is let go. This fable is enacted all the time, to the point that among the inhabitants of the city it rather gives rise to laughter than to faith and devotion.[39]

Royal supervisors

There seems to have been a court official, who is mentioned as functioning at the end of the Safavid period and who was known as the chief of the hospice (*timarchi-bashi*).[40] It is not clear what precise

---

39. Kaempfer 2018, p. 92.
40. Asaf 1348, p. 101. In medieval Khvarezm this official was known as

function this official had. There was not something like a hospice or dispensary in the royal palace grounds. May be the official was in charge of the hospices in Isfahan, of which one or two existed in Isfahan as well as in other large towns. It would not be the first time that a court physician was put in charge of the *dar al-shafa*. It happened to the one in Isfahan founded by `Abbas I, which was under the court physician for some time.[41] But it is more likely that he was in charge of the appointment of all physicians, who had to follow his instructions, just as the chief physician of the hospital (*sa`uri-ye bimarestan*) in Ilkhanid times had been in charge of all physicians.[42]

EUROPEAN HOSPICES

Apart from these Iranian hospices, there also was a European infirmary, the first of its kind in Iran, which was built by the Portuguese on the island of Hormoz in 1516. It was run by Augustinian friars and provided, among other things, charitable services to the poor. Its impact, of course, was limited. First, because at that time the type of medicine practiced by European doctors did not differ that much from that of Iranian ones. Second, Iranian physicians were more knowledgeable as to the diseases in the Persian Gulf and Iran than the Portuguese monks, who, certainly initially, therefore learnt more from Iranian physicians than the other way around. Third, the institute of a hospice per se was not unknown to Iranians. Also, the nature of the Portuguese infirmary was not that much different from that of a *dar al-shafa*, i.e., it was also a place to receive spiritual consolation and care and where one died, as indicated by the title of the manager of the Portuguese hospital (*provedor do esprital e defuntos*). Also, the capacity of the infirmary was very limited (certainly in the first few years of its existence) and often the sick had to stay on the ships due to lack of room in the infirmary. Its staff consisted of a physician,

---

timardar. Jorjani 2535, p. 644.
41. Du Mans 1890, p. 219; Richard 1995, vol. 2, p. 171; Monshi 1350, vol. 2, pp. 1070, 1110; Savory 1978, vol. 2, p. 1295; vol. 1, p. 536.
42. Nakhjevani 1964, vol. 2, pp. 235-236.

a surgeon, and a barber, while there also was a medical drug store (*botica*) in the fort.⁴³ All this suggests that the impact of this Portuguese institution on the medical situation in Iran, if any, was probably neutral.

The two hospitals in a hamlet near Bandar Abbas reported by Fryer, were no hospitals, although he used that term and Elgood took his remarks at their face-value. What Fryer actually referred to was the use of the natural sulfur springs at Ghinaw, near Bandar Abbas by infirm people. The use of hot springs for medical and other purposes was already known since Antiquity,⁴⁴ and they were widely used in Iran where they abounded.

> Nakoda Biram, the Dutch Broker, and Tockserey, our Banyan, have Built to these natural Baths, each an handsome Hospital: That of the first is an open one, Built Square, Capped with Four round Tubilated Cupilo's about an huge one in the middle, with Two Rows of Pillars to support it. The latter has made his more close, upheld by Nine Pillars on the sides, and Four in the middle, with a stately Portico at the Entrance, and a close Cell behind, commodious to Sweat in, besides a Stone Repository for Rain Water; they being both neat and durable Works.⁴⁵

From the above description it is quite clear that this was not a hospital, but an establishment to take the waters, of which there were many in Iran. Other travelers, who have written about this place, including Kaempfer, himself a physician, make no mention of a hospital at all, only of the beneficial qualities of the hot springs.⁴⁶ The Dutch who went there, not to get treated for illnesses, but to ease the pains of their aging bones, never referred to it as a hospital either. There was no physician attached to these hot springs, neither

---

43. Aubin 2000, pp. 401-403; Floor 2006, pp. 12, 27, 29, 54; Elgood 1951, p. 512.
44. On the merits of which Fryer 1909-15, vol. 2, pp. 330-335 expounds; see also the observation of Chardin regarding their use in Iran. Chardin 1811, vol. 5, p. 188.
45. Fryer 1909-15, vol. 2, pp. 329-330; Elgood 1951, p. 399.
46. Kaempfer 1968, p. 137; Hamilton 1930, vol. 1, pp. 60-61.

by the Dutch nor the English. But even if it had been a hospital it is clear that these baths were private establishments, inaccessible to those who had not been invited. Thus, their impact was very limited. The same remarks apply to the alleged hospital operated by the East India Company in Bandar Abbas in 1727 and in the 1770s in Basra, which, more than likely, was just a room where the sick could receive drugs and consolation, and die or recuperate, as the case might be, not unlike the alleged 'hospital' or rather sick room that the Carmelites operated in the 1660s in Basra.[47] Even if these establishments had really been hospitals then their impact on the medical situation in Iran was nil as their services were limited to a certain group of people only, i.e., Europeans and their Asian co-workers and there was no cross-fertilization with Iranian physicians.

How relevant were 'hospitals' in Safavid Iran?

In short, it is my contention that the number of hospices was too small to have had a significant impact on the public health situation in Safavid Iran. Even assuming that the number of *dar al-shafa*s was much larger than the number we know about, they could not have been very effective due to the limited number of doctors. Physicians, i.e., those who called themselves or were called *hakim*, practiced medicine that was Galenic in nature. Not only was their number limited, but often, they were attached to the families of the rich and mighty, thus leaving little time for others. Those that still had time and the inclination to serve patients in hospices would not have been able to serve many. I am leaving aside here the question whether these *dar al-shafa*s actually gave, or were able to provide, effective health care, or whether the population at large even wanted to go there to receive medical care. As we know, and is detailed hereunder, local people never went to the *dar al-shafa*, if there was one. The reality,

---

47. Elgood 1951, p. 341; Wright 2001, p. 122; Martin 1990, p. 427. Both the Dutch and English companies had an infirmary for sick personnel to which end the companies employed a physician. The most famous one was Engelbert Kaempfer, who worked in Bandar Abbas for the Dutch company from December 1685 to June 1688.

therefore, was that the majority of the population, whether rural or urban, relied on home remedies and folk medicine that was mostly pre-Islamic in nature and did not flock at all to the *dar al-shafa*s.[48]

The abovementioned analysis is borne out by the little we know about the actual functioning of Iranian *dar al-shafa*s in the Safavid period. For example, sick people did not come to the *dar al-shafa* in Isfahan to find healing, despite the fact that it had a staff that formally may have consisted of one doctor, a druggist, a mullah, a cook, a porter and a sweeper. There was no surgeon among them, "because surgery was not a specialty and moreover rather unknown in the east," according to Chardin. In the Isfahan hospice, the physician could be found at the hospital's door from 8 AM until noon, where he gave medical advice and prescriptions free-of-charge. Although the advice, drugs, and food were free, the few people who actually came there for treatment paid for the service and drugs. This was partly due to the fact that the hospital was badly endowed. It had 2,000 écus or 666 *tuman*s in rents to feed the sick, but these rents had been assigned on a source of income from which these were allegedly difficult to collect. Du Mans, Chardin and Ange de St. Joseph all agree that hardly anybody came to the *dar al-shafa* to find treatment. The only people they saw were some mad men who were chained to the wall or a poor moribund Indian. According to Chardin, as little as 1,800 écus or 600 *tuman*s[49] had been allocated for its medical staff, which may explain that not only was medical care limited in scope if not absent, but that the hospital's funds were stolen, or as Du Mans formulates it, the physicians and other staff "ate" all the allocated funds. This despite the fact that `Abbas I had assigned a rather reliable source of income for the 1,800 écus, viz., the income of the adjacent caravanserai of the copper-smiths, which the Shah had built at the same time as the

---

48. See for an analysis of the situation in Qajar Iran, Floor 2004.
49. Chardin qualifies this amount as being inadequate (*l'hôpital est fort pauvrement fondé*), but in fact it was an enormous amount, certainly if one takes into account the total amount of funds as well as the level of wages paid to the staff of the Shrine hospital at Mashhad (see Table 2) and that the average annual wages of an army officer were six *tuman*s at that time.

dar al-shafa. As a result, the hospice was not really charitable, while, moreover, the sick and mad men were badly treated and died there as a result. Poor people, travelers and strangers only came there to die, hence this and other *dar al-shafa*s were known in popular parlance as the 'house of death,' *dar al-marg* or *dar al-mowt*.[50] In Tabriz the situation was not much different. Chardin noted that hardly anybody stayed in its three *dar al-shafa*s. However, food was given twice per day to those who came there. Hence the three hospices were popularly known as *Ach-tacon* (*ash-maqam*) in Tabriz, i.e., the place where food (in this case soup or *ash*) was distributed.[51]

---

50. Du Mans 1890, p. 219; Richard 1995, vol. 2, p. 171 (*dar al-marg*); Chardin 1811, vol. 7, pp. 389-393; St. Joseph 1985, pp. 132-133 (*dar al-mowt*). A contemporary Persian text states that in Isfahan "the *dar al-shafa* is [built] in the form of a caravanserai; in it are sick people and madmen." Gaube - Wirth 1978, pp. 284-285.
51. Chardin 1811, vol. 2, p. 324.

HOSPITALS IN AFSHARID IRAN
1736–1794

The same system as in the Safavid period was in place with some changes during the remainder of the eighteenth century. The terms *dar al-shafa* and *sharbat-khaneh* are both used indiscrimnately in the Mashhad Shrine documents of that period, which probably indicates that, as before, both the *hakim* and the *sharbatdar* were in charge of the hospice, be it with separate responsibilities (respectively, for the medical and non-medical part). The *dar al-shafa* still had a male and a female part, served by respectively male and female orderlies or *bimardaran*.[1] The Shrine employed more doctors than in the Safavid period, because the endowments had increased. In the Safavid period their pay was 20 *tuman*s cash and 14 *kharvar* in 1111/1699-1700, but in the 1740s it was 20 *tuman*s cash and 110-120 *kharvar*. Also, the number of *nazeran* had increased as a result of the increase in endowments. As before, the staff of the *dar al-shafa* consisted of male and female *bimardaran, jarrah, dallak, `azab, tahvildar, anbardar, darban,* and *farrash*. The orderlies (*bimardaran*) in Safavid times earned 1-3 *tuman*s and 1-2 *kharvar* per year, but in the 1740s it was 4 *tuman*s plus 8 *kharvar*. Of course, female staff earned half of that. Instead of money some jewelry or *javaher* were given indicating the lack of money and bad economic times.[2] Among the *dar al-shafa*'s expenditures fabrics are listed that had to be bought to dress dead

---

1. Sureshjani 1395, pp. 168-69.
2. Sureshjani 1395, pp. 167-86 (for the list of physicians, see Idem p. 169).

patients such as *darabi* (a thick fabric), *refref* (a green fabric), *panbeh* (cotton [fabric]) and *karbas* (coton fabric).³

The endowment deed of the Shrine in Mashhad of 1747 suggests that its *dar al-shafa* was still functioning and assisting patients, although there is no way of knowing whether the money was really spent in accordance with the terms of the deed, as suggested by the reality in Isfahan. The deed states that in the past annually 94 *tumans* had been fixed for the expenses of the *dar al-shafa*, but now in view of the increased number of sick and poor it had been decided to add to that annual amount from the endowment funds as follows:

Table 2: Wages and other expenditures of the *dar al-shafa* of Mashhad in 1747.

Wages	Cash	In Kind
Physician	20 *tumans*	20 *kharvar* of wheat
Two overseers (*nazer*)	12.5 *tumans*	27 *kharvar* of wheat
Surgeon with the cost for ointments	8 *tumans*	2 *kharvar* of wheat
Orderly, porter, etc.	-	20 *kharvar* of wheat
Expenses for food, medicines, etc.	200 *tumans*	-
Total	240.5 *tumans*	69 *kharvar* of wheat

Source: Mo'taman 1348, p. 402.

There is no information available on the Mashhad hospice during the period after 1750 until the second decade of the nineteenth century, because of the unsettled times due to political unrest, upheaval and war.⁴

Given the fact that Iran before 1900, like all other countries on this planet, suffered from a lack of sanitation and thus, were a public health nightmare and remained so in the case of Iran well into the 1950s, the need for effective preventive health care is evident. However, there were neither enough real hospitals nor enough physicians to provide the necessary medical care. But even those hospitals that existed did

---

3. Sureshjani 1395, p. 165. For the textile terms, see Floor 1999.
4. Sureshjani 1395, p. 186.

not address the need for health care and as a result Iran remained a public health nightmare. The contribution of *dar al-shafa*s in Iran to the public health situation, therefore, was irrelevant and thus, we also need to re-assess our appreciation of the objective value of this institution in medieval Iranian society. This is further underlined by the limited impact that modern European dispensaries and hospitals had on the public health situation in Qajar Iran, despite much better clinical and diagnostic knowledge and much more effective treatment methods and medicines. This is mainly due to the fact that the real public health challenge in Iran, as in all countries all over the world, was and is the lack of sanitation and of personal hygiene. The answer to that problem of providing limited curative care, however effective that may have been in individual cases, could not and did not address the sanitation and hygiene problem. As a result, people remained sick or repeatedly fell sick, because of the continued existence of endemic and contagious diseases.

HOSPITALS IN QAJAR & PAHLAVI IRAN
1794–1950S

Until the Qajar period (1794-1925) there was no major change in the manner of treatment or of medical facilities. This began slowly to change through the employment of foreign physicians by the Shah and the royal princes after 1800. A major change took place through the establishment of dispensaries and later of hospitals by four major agencies, to wit: the government of Iran, the government of (British) India, American and British missionaries.[1] At the initiative of the prime minister, Amir Kabir, the government of Iran was the first to establish a hospital in Tehran that was opened in 1852. It was a hospital that was inspired by the European model, but it was not yet operated based on modern medical principles, because the medical staff was not trained in modern Western medicine. As a result, conditions in the hospital were not hygienic and treatment of patients left much to be desired. Thereafter, the government of Iran built two other military hospitals, also in Tehran (1854, 1874), while private Iranians, inspired by both their government's activities and by that of the three foreign agencies also established a few hospitals, in the beginning of the 20th century. The Iranian government's involvement in the building of hospitals was part of a home-grown modernization trend. It had started in the early 19th century, ran its course until the early 20th century, when it stalled for a while. However, its objectives were further developed and realized

---

1. There were other foreign agencies that also established dispensaries or hospitals, such as the government of Russia and other Christian organizations, but these were of much less importance and minor in comparison with the four agencies mentioned. Also, with one exception (in Arak), they did not last very long. Their activities are mentioned in the Introduction and/or under the heading of the cities discussed here.

under Reza Shah (r. 1925-1941). Although the first Iranian hospitals preceded the ones established by the Americans and British, the services they offered were limited. It did not include surgery, which was the comparative advantage of the foreign hospitals, in addition to other aspects of medical care the latter offered (better trained physicians, nurses, modern medical methods of treatment and instruments).[2]

The other state agency that founded dispensaries and hospitals was the government of (British) India. Because the British suspected that Russia wanted to extend its political and territorial influence southward, they feared for Russian encroachment, if not challenge, of their position in India. Given Iran's location between Russia and India, the British wanted Iran to act as a buffer between the two. To ensure that objective would be achieved, the British needed to increase their influence over Iran to avoid that the country would fall under the sway of Russia. The establishment of telegraph lines between India and Europe via the Persian Gulf and Iran in 1865 increased Iran's importance to British global strategic interests. Through the protection of its growing commercial interests with Iran, including the establishment of full maritime control over the Persian Gulf, the British exercised political influence over the government of Iran and its elite. Their diplomatic representative (first only in Tehran and Bushehr) were the executors of British imperial policy. Because of the health issues prevailing among the people in both the Persian Gulf and throughout Iran, the government of India attached a physician to its Residency in Bushehr. As of around 1873, this physician opened a dispensary where medical treatment was offered to the local population. When the government of India opened other consular stations in the Persian Gulf littoral (Bandar Abbas, Bandar-e Lengeh, Mohammerah, and Ahvaz) it likewise opened dispensaries there, some of which developed into small hospitals after 1907. Likewise, the government of India also opened dispensaries in Kermanshah, Mashhad, Zabol and Zahedan, where it had established consulates. Both British political and commercial circles considered the extension

---

2. On the introduction of Western medicine in Iran and the government of Iran's policy and investments to develop a domestic modern medical capacity and infrastructure, see Floor 2004 and Idem 2020.

of these medical services to the local population an important public relations instrument to enhance British influence.³ British companies such as the Indo-European Telegraph Department (IETD) and the APOC (Anglo-Persian Oil Company; after 1934 called Anglo-Iranian Oil Company or AIOC) also established dispensaries and hospitals at a number of locations where they were active.

The two missionary societies were primarily interested in saving souls and given that these souls were housed in bodies that were often stricken with disease, both the American and British missionaries soon realized that offering medical help was not only a Christian duty, but that it also might facilitate conversions. After all, waiting patients were a captive market, while healed patients would be grateful and perhaps more willing to listen to their message. The same missionary objective was targeted through the establishment of the missionary schools, which educated many of Iran's political, technical, medical and judicial and other professional leaders.

The American Board of Commissioners for Foreign Missions (ABCFM) began its missionary (evangelization, medical and educational) activities in Urmiyeh in 1835.⁴ As of 1872 it expanded its Mission to Tehran while additional missionary stations were opened at Tabriz in 1873, Hamadan in 1882, Qazvin in 1902, Rasht in 1903, Kermanshah in 1907, and Mashhad in 1911. Medical institutions were established in all these places. The first American missionary physician, Dr. Asahel Grant was active in Urmiyeh as of 1835, while Dr. Joseph Cochran was the first American missionary physician to build not only the first modern hospital, but also the fist medical school in Iran. Ms Mary Bradford was the first female physician in Iran (working in Tabriz), and she was soon followed by many others.

---

3. On the British methods and motives, see James Onley, *The Arabian Frontier of the British Raj: Merchants, Rulers, and the British in the Nineteenth-Century Gulf (Oxford Historical Monographs)* Oxford University Press, 2008, pp. 33-38.

4. For their considerations to start activities in Iran, see Thomas O'Flynn. *The Western Christian Presence in the Russias and Qajar Persia*, c.1760c.1870. Leiden: Brill, 2018, pp. 585f.

The CMS (Christian Missionary Society) had the same objectives as the ABCFM.[5] It began its missionary activities in Iran in 1869, when the Rev. Robert Bruce established a mission station in Jolfa, the Armenian suburb of Isfahan. Thereafter the CMS expanded its missionary activities to Kerman, Yazd (1893) and Shiraz (1900). Dr. Hoernle was the first British missionary physician to work in Isfahan in 1880, where he was soon joined by Mary Byrd, who opened a dispensary for women in Isfahan in 1891. In 1906, the first dedicated CMS women's hospital in Iran was realized by Dr. Emmeline Stuart, which was adopted as a model at other CMS hospitals in Iran.

---

5. On the CMS, its considerations and activities, see Stileman, Rev. Charles Harvey, *The Subjects of the Shah*. London: CMS, 1902, pp. 56-93.

TEHRAN

Tehran, the capital city of Iran since 1796, had a population of more than 220,000 (even 300,000 according to some) in 1920. Until 1852, when it had a population of about 100,000, Tehran had no real hospital. There was a *dar al-shafa*, which had been built by Fath ʿAli Shah (r. 1798-1834). As was usual for this type of institution it was attached to a religious school and mosque, where sometimes a few sick people stayed and were fed. It still existed under Mohammad Shah (r. 1834-1848), but fell into disuse. It was then turned into a madraseh, although the students did not receive stipends. It does not seem to have had any active medical function anymore under Naser al-Din Shah (r. 1848-1896).[1]

In 1850, at the instructions of Amir Kabir construction was begun of a state hospital (*mariz-khaneh-ye dowlati*), which was the first modern hospital built in Iran.[2] The new hospital, which was situated outside Tehran, was opened in January 1852. It also had a pharmacy and could house 400 patients. The first director was Mirza Mohammad Vali *hakim-bashi*, and Dr. Fortunato Casolani (1819-52), physician-in-chief of the army, a mere sinecure, was responsible for medical treatment. The doctors with three students were busy everyday till noon, and the patients were satisfied with the service offered and left the hospital in good health, according to the government newspaper.

---

1. ʿEyn al-Saltaneh 1376, vol. 1, p. 306; Sepehr 1377, vol. 3, p. 1183; Tajbakhsh 1379, p. 217. It was located opposite the Masjed-e Shah, part of it was situated in the Khiyaban-e Bozorjmehr. Shahri 1368, vol. 5, p. 700, n. 3. When the street was broadened the *dar al-shafa* was destroyed and a plaque was erected to commemorate its location, which was later occupied by a branch of the *Bank-e Bazargani*. Moʿtamedi 1381, pp. 104, 197, 629.
2. Ebrahimnejad 2000, p. 171, mentions an anonymous Persian manuscript (*Resaleh dar khosus-e taʾsis-e mariz-khaneh*), written in the early 1850s, that proposed, amongst other things, the establishment of a military hospital. It seems likely that this text was written at the suggestion of the Amir Kabir, in which case it must have been written in 1849, because construction work of his hospital had started already in 1850. For an English translation of this text see Ebrahimnejad 2004.

From January 1852 till January 1853, 2,238 patients were treated in the hospital, who suffered from difficult diseases.[3]

Dr. Polak, the Austrian physician and teacher, arrived on 26 November 1851 in Tehran and used the first weeks to establish the teaching program that would form the basis for the remainder of his activities at the Dar al-Fonun. He also wanted to do more than just teaching. Therefore, with some delight he wrote on 17 December 1852 that one week later he would "move to my well-equipped hospital." There he was assisted by his students, who thus acquired some hands-on practice.[4] Later Polak opened a small dispensary in the Dar al-Fonun, where after his daily teaching, he treated out-patients and performed minor operations. This broke the monotony of his teaching routine and, as a trained surgeon, allowed him to change theory to practice. Also, he later allowed them to perform small operations, first under his supervision and later alone. These type of operations even included amputations.[5]

It would seem that this military hospital was inadequate, for in 1854 Naser al-Din Shah ordered the establishment of another hospital in Tehran.[6] It was built outside Tehran at the instigation of Dr. Polak who had seen that sick soldiers were kept in dark cellar-like barracks, where they died like flies. Whether Polak referred to the first hospital

---

3. E'temad al-Saltaneh 1306, pp. 62, 73; Ruznameh 1373, vol. 1, p. 611 (no. 102, 8 Rabi` II 1269/19 January, 1853) states that 1,238 patients had been treated since Rabi` I of last year (i.e. Dec-Jan. 1851-52), but vol. 1, pp. 618-619 (no. 103, 10 Rabi` II, 1369/21 January, 1853) gives the higher number of 2,238 from Rabi` I of 1269 (December 1852); Elgood 1951, p. 512. After Dr. Casolani's death in January 1852, Polak succeeded him as physician-in-chief, see Ruznameh 1373, vol. 1, pp. 34, 64, 260, 303 (his death) and Adamiyat 1348, p. 327 who stated that he was the brother of Casolani the chief painter (*naqqash-bashi*), about whom I have found no further information. The Casolanis were a British family from Malta.
4. Polak 1853, vol. 3/14, p. 219. On the Dar al-Fonun, see Floor 2020 pp. 1–90
5. Polak 1854, vol. 3/25, p. 396.
6. E'temad al-Saltaneh 1300, vol. 3, pp. 218, 255; Polak 1859 b, p. 140; Hedayat 1338-39, vol. 10, p. 813.

that Amir Kabir had built in 1852, or whatever happened to that first hospital, is not known. Polak does not even explicitly refer to this first hospital, although he had worked in it. Polak's original design was a roomy and light building, that formed a square with a spacious courtyard, in the middle of which was the inevitable pond. Around the building he had planned that bushes and trees were to be planted, while a wall would surround the entire site. The rooms were three and a half feet high above the ground. The design was completely changed by the chief general during his absence, but Polak was able to get most of his way. Once the hospital had been built, the next battle began; how to get funds for its operation. The army doctors had an allocation for a large establishment, but spent most of it on themselves. They did not even buy the most necessary drugs, such as quinine. The doctors shared the hospital's operational budget with the army's officers and were not interested in changing this arrangement. Polak's students, whom he had entrusted with the management of food, clothing, instruments, and drugs, diverted the money for their own use. Instead of showing how a proper hospital might function, Polak received a demonstration of how Iran functioned. Nevertheless, it was not a wasted effort, because the students still were exposed to the concepts of hospital management, saw many patients, and learnt how much you could do for the soldiers with limited means. Hundreds of patients were treated at the hospital, and despite their initial mistrust of the hospital, the sick gradually begged for admission. Because Polak was appointed the shah's personal physician he only worked there part-time and the hospital was managed by an Iranian physician. When Polak came back later, he was shocked to see the conditions in which the patients were kept. It was like a scene from medical hell. "Patients with typhus and dysentery literally danced in their own feces and vomit." Also, all trees and bushes that he had financed with his own money had disappeared.[7] He became so disappointed about the work methods and conditions of the hospital that he discontinued

---

7. Polak 1859 b, p. 140; Idem., 1865, vol. 1, pp. 307-311; Idem 1862, p. 249. According to Elgood 1951, p. 512, the hospital was first put under the management of Drs. Polak and Schlimmer.

his work in the hospital. His students continued to work there for a period, but they at least had been exposed to, if not had learnt, the practice of a modern hospital. This included proper examination and the writing of a patient's history.[8]

Despite Polak's disappointment and disengagement he did not entirely abandon the hospital. Polak also insisted on appointing a number of physicians as sanitary inspectors of army barracks. It was their task to ensure that preventive measures were taken to maintain proper hygienic conditions in the barracks, and to acquaint new recruits with preventive medical rules. He was able to convince Naser al-Din Shah to order the military physicians to present themselves to the Dar al-Fonun in the mornings. During that time Polak taught them the basics of modern medicine and discussed with them the main diseases from which soldiers suffered such as malaria, dysentery, typhus and frostbite. To provide them with guidelines Polak had written instructions in Persian, which presented the most important information about the above diseases that the military physicians had to study. The pamphlet was also sent to physicians in the provinces.[9] By 1860, it did not deserve the name of a hospital anymore, according to Häntzsche, a German physician who had worked for many years in northern Iran.[10] Polak prior to his return to Europe in 1858 had wanted to establish a hospital for foreigners, but it met with Iranian opposition and the absence of finances.[11]

In 1874 or thereabouts a new military hospital was built after Naser al-Din Shah returned from his first tour to Europe. Hajj Mirza Hasan Khan Moshir al-Dowleh Sepahsalar-e A`zam, the grand vizier, took steps to build a hospital in Tehran like the ones he had seen in Europe to which end he assigned one section of the Madraseh-ye Naseri, later known as Madraseh-ye Sepahsalar, to be used as a hospital. It was not

---

8. Polak 1862, pp. 249-50.
9. Polak 1859 b, p. 140; Idem 1862, pp. 249-50.
10. Häntzsche 1869, p. 442.
11. Polak 1862, p. 249.

built in 1869 as Elgood and Wright have it.[12] According to Elgood, the old hospital was now dedicated for civilian use and was placed under the management of Dr. Albo, a German physician who taught at the Dar al-Fonun.[13] The new hospital, like the old one, was called the *mariz-khaneh-ye dowlati*. A director and assistant-director managed it. The staff consisted of three doctors, a manager (*mobasher*), a chemist (*davasaz*), two supervisors (*nazer*), one cook (*tabbakh*), one receiver, six nurses (*parestar*), one bathhouse attendant, one barber, and five washer-men.[14] The new military hospital may have been the same as the one described as the *dar al-shafa-ye jadid-e Naseri-ye tupkhaneh*, which had a staff of 15, consisting of two physicians, one surgeon, one chemist, one supervisor (*nazer*), four orderlies (*parestar*); two cooks/ washer-men, and four guards.[15] Whether the same or not, the new army hospital was a small building with only a few rooms with about 20 beds. It was ominously nicknamed 'the cemetery of the living,' reminiscent of the nickname of the *dar al-shafa*s in Safavid times (see above). There were no sick patients in it, for nobody came there, which explains its nickname. After the opening of the hospital it staff had left, because there was no money allocated for its operation, at least it was not made available to the hospital. The idea behind its creation was that the medical students at the Dar al-Fonun would receive part of their practical training at the hospital. However, after the death of the European professor, who only gave one course there, the project was abandoned. According to Mme. Serena, the Shah had charged his great-uncle `Ali Qoli Mirza E`tezad al-Saltaneh to manage the

---

12. Elgood 1951, p. 512. Wright 2001, p. 126 reports that the hospital was established with German help in 1869, but he does not provide any reference for that statement and this German assistance is nowhere mentioned in publications dealing with German-Persian relations.
13. Elgood 1951, p. 512.
14. E`temad al-Saltaneh 1306, p. 405.
15. E`temad al-Saltaneh 1306, pp. 349, 361. The chief army surgeon was Mohammad Nezam al-Hokama Tabib, Sepehr 1368, pp. 97-98.

hospital, which is contradicted by Nafisi. E`tezad al-Saltaneh used the funds for his own private use and let the hospital slowly deteriorate.[16]

The need for hospitals was something to which many among the Iranian elite were receptive. In February 1886, for example, Asaf al-Dowleh wrote that he intended to build a hospital in Tehran. The land had already been bought and land preparation had started. However, there is no further mention of this hospital in Asaf al-Dowleh's published documents. He further proposed to establish dispensaries in Sarakhs and Sistan and argued that such facilities should be established all over Iran.[17] Eqbal al-Saltaneh, another member of the elite, had built a hospital in Tehran, which `Eyn al-Saltaneh visited in May 1889. He commented that it was very clean and proper.[18] But it would seem that this hospital did not remain operational. The 1317/1899 census of Tehran recorded the existence of only two unnamed hospitals, both in the Dowlat quarter.[19] The census probably referred to the army hospital built in 1874 and the former army, but now civil hospital built in 1851. There also was a military dispensary in Tehran, "exactly opposite the entrance to the [Golestan] Palace," where soldiers went to be treated for minor injuries.[20] Afzal al-Molk reported that Mirza Mohammad Nazem al-Atebba, the chief army surgeon, was credited with having established effective army dispensaries (*dava-khanehha*) for which he had been awarded a diamond ring.[21]

---

16. Serena 1883, pp. 143-144; Nafisi 1325, p. 57; Curzon 1892, vol. 1, p. 606. For the introduction of modern European medical science in Iran in the nineteenth century see Floor 2004; Idem 2020.
17. Asaf al-Dowleh 1377, vol. 1, p. 220.
18. `Eyn al-Saltaneh 1376, vol. 1, p. 208.
19. Sa`dvandiyan-Ettehadiyeh 1368, pp. 353, 359, 451. For the location of the Dowlati hospital, west of the Meydan-e Tupkhaneh, see the map in Moghtader 1992, p. 47, figure 2.
20. Collins 1925, p. 221.
21. Afzal al-Molk 1361, p. 139. Prior to that time there had been surgeons attached to the army, who managed field dispensaries. Tajbakhsh 1379, pp. 214-216.

It is of interest to note that the Imperial hospital was still part of the traditional triad: mosque, madraseh, and hospital. The Shah put `Ali Akbar Khan, a recent graduate from the Dar al-Fonun, in charge of the construction of the *mariz-khaneh-ye dowlati*, who managed the hospital until 1880. `Ali Akbar Khan reported directly to the Shah or to the Prime-Minister. When he left (after his patron E`tezad al-Saltaneh had died), he was succeeded by Mokhber al-Dowleh, who was not a physician and who was director of the Dar al-Fonun at the same time. Therefore, after a short period Dr. Mohammad Khan Kofri was appointed as director of the hospital and remained in office until 1886. In that year he was succeeded by Dr. Abu'l-Hasan Khan Bahrami, who had just finished his studies in Paris. He occupied the post of hospital director until 1892. Because the directors also taught at the Dar al-Fonun students of that school reportedly received part of their education in the hospital.[22] As of 1892, the management of the hospital seems to have remained for more than a decade in German hands. Therefore, the hospital was sometimes referred to as the 'German hospital.' First, for a short period, a certain Dr. Loew (?) was in charge of the hospital and then a certain Dr. Kolnik (?). In 1896, Mozaffar al-Din Shah formalized this German relationship by a royal edict bestowing the directorship on Dr. Kolnik and ordering him to renovate the hospital. In 1897, Dr. Ilberg joined him as deputy, while later Dr. Becker became the director of the hospital. The Iranian government paid 12,000 *tuman*s for the hospital's upkeep. Germany only paid the salaries of its doctors. At the outbreak of the war Dr. Becker left. In November 1915 the German Legation left, including Dr. Ilberg, who was the remaining German doctor, who took many

---

22. Elgood 1951, pp. 511-512; Nafisi 1325, pp. 56-57; Idem, 1329-31, p. 19; E`temad al-Saltaneh 1306, p. 83; Idem 1298-1300, vol. 3, p. 31-32. The new hospital director later became Mirza Mohammad Doktor Mo`tamed al-Atebba, who also taught Western medicine at the *Dar al-fonun*. Rahnama 1332, p. 51. The hospital fell under the jurisdiction of the Minister of Science, Hospitals and Arts (*Vazir-e `Olum va Dar al-Shafa va'l-Fonun*), see Afzal al-Molk 1361, p. 5. The *shah* and his minister were not the only Iranians who were impressed with European hospitals, so was Shushtari 1363, p. 262, as is clear from his description of the sights of London.

instruments with him. After Dr. Ilberg's departure Dr. Zeyn al-`Abedin Khan Loqman al-Mamalek, Ahmad Shah's personal physician, was appointed as director.[23] In 1912, Mme de Warzée gives a rather rosy picture of the situation of the hospital under German management, which stands in stark contrast to Dr. Neligan's assessment (see below):

> It is now under the direction of a German doctor who belongs to the Prussian army, and he is aided by another German military doctor, a Persian doctor, a chemist, and a band of male nurses who are very well trained. The hospital has two good operating rooms, and has sufficient beds from from sixty to eighty patients. It has also rooms arranged so as to be able to take in Persians of a better class and Europeans. All the poor are given consultations, medicine and bandages free, and there is a free vaccination surgery attached to the hospital.[24]

According to Neligan, the Iranians were unsatisfied with the medical side of the German methods and, he opined, they had good

---

23. Elgood 1951, p. 546; Rahnama 1332, pp. 332-33. Vothuq al-Dowleh wrote to Neligan that the only arrangement with the German Legation was a *farman* to Dr. Muller in 1896 or 1897, appointing him as doctor to the hospital and that the Iranian government fixed the hospital's annual budget at 12,000 *tuman*s, when the late Loghman al-Mamalek was made director. FO 248/1291, Neligan to M (20/01/1919). The service of these and other German physicians is not mentioned by Olivier Bast, "Germany ix: Germans in Persia," iranicaonline.org. By 1914, if not earlier, the financial situation of the hospital was so bad that Dr. Ilberg paid 13,372 *tuman*s out of his own pocket to keep the hospital up and running. This money was not reimbursed when he left Tehran in 1915 or later, even though in 1918 Vothuq al-Dowleh promised to do so with 6% interest. Ebrahimnejad 2014, pp. 158, 216, n. 194.
24. De Warzée 1913, pp. 171-172. Wishard 1908, p. 234 reports on this subject that recently, the German government had opened a free general hospital in Tehran, which does not seem to be correct. He probably mistook German management of the Imperial hospital as this being a German hospital, which it was not. For example, Litten 1925, p. 404 only mentions the management of the Imperial hospital by Dr. Becker, and no other German involvement with the hospital.

reason to be. He further reported that the Iranians were also riled that the Germans always refused to show the hospital's accounts. Shortly after the German mission left in November 1915 the Russian Legation asked the Iranian government to appoint one of their physicians as director of the hospital. The German Legation protested, but the appointment was made and soon afterwards the hospital was taken over by the Russian Red Cross. Neligan didn't think that the Russian doctors had much to do with the hospital. Moreover, the appointed doctor died in 1916 and his successor in 1917. The Russian Legation's physician's post was not filled until January 1919, when an Armenian physician was appointed.[25] The Russian Red Cross used the hospital, its staff and its equipment rather roughly, so that by 1918 the hospital could only receive 30 patients. After General Baratov's army departure in early 1928, the hospital was returned into Iranian hands. As of then, two young Iranian physicians, former assistants of the German physicians, managed it. "They had been trained in Tehran and their attainments accordingly were limited." Officially, 30 beds were open for the poor, and 20 for paying patients, but in practice no patient 'escaped' without paying and it was practically useless to send destitute cases there, Dr. Neligan submitted. Thus, he concluded, in a city of some 250,000 inhabitants there had been for months practically no hospital in-patient accommodation for the very poor. The only alternative was the American hospital, which had been closed for two years and was always closed during summer. Moreover, the Imperial hospital had no up-to-date apparatus such as an X-ray machine and was short of ordinary instruments.[26]

Neligan had discussed a possible British role in the Imperial Hospital with the various British Ministers in Tehran since 1906, and noted that all of them had agreed that it was regrettable that the hospital was not in British hands. In fact, Marling, the British Minister, thought that the British should try to secure it.[27] Therefore, towards the end of

---

25. FO 248/1291, Neligan to Minister (i.e. ambassadors, 20/01/1919).
26. FO 248/1291, Neligan to Ambassador (20/01/1919).
27. FO 248/1291, Memo on a proposal to secure an English instead of a German administration for the Persian Government Hospital, Tehran,

1918, Neligan raised the issue again and submitted, given the fact that Britain wanted to increase its influence in Iran and block the Germans, that obtaining control of this hospital might be useful. His colleague Dr. Scott had the same opinion. Because the hospital would be run like a British one it would not only provide better service, but also clinical teaching could be given to Iranian students and doctors. To ensure the British Minister of the importance of his proposal, Neligan reminded him that if the British didn't do anything the Germans might well retake control over the hospital when they returned, given the existence of a pro-German party in Iran. To further bolster his argument, Neligan submitted that although the British dispensary did a good job for out-patients there was no in-patient facility attached to it. Therefore, British doctors had to send their serious cases to Iranian hospitals or the American one. The latter was adequate, but was poorly equipped and always closed in summer. Thus, British doctors had no facility for surgical cases in Tehran or for research, which a hospital made possible. Moreover, Iranians looked for education, but Great Britain was the only great power that had no teaching establishment in Tehran, the hospital thus offered an excellent opportunity to remedy this defect. The Imperial hospital could accommodate 100 patients, if funds were available. The buildings were old and not ideal, but it had a good operating theater and was centrally located.

As to government of Iran, the German *farman* was not an obstacle, Neligan argued. The Germans had abandoned the hospital in a not honorable way. To convince the Iranians how serious the British were as well as to address the hospital's immediate needs, Neligan argued that Britain needed to contribute 2-3,000 pounds/year for hospital upkeep, the balance to be paid by the Iranian government. Scott and Neligan were willing to take charge of the hospital. It was also the right moment to do something, because Neligan was very friendly with Prime Minister Vothuq al-Dowleh and with Loqman al-Mamalek, director of hospital, who was chamberlain in the royal court.

---

20 October 1918.

Table 3: Monthly budget of the Dowlat hospital (1919)

A. Traitement	Qrans/month	Qrans/year
2 Internists	1,000	12,000
1 Secretary-bookkeeper	300	3,600
6 Orderlies	600	7,200
1 Gardener	120	1,400
1 Laundryman	100	1,200
2 Cooks and kitchen help	120	1,400
1 Valet	100	1,200
2 Servants and water carrier	100	1,200
2 Cossacks	80	960
1 Steward	100	1,200
b. Various expenses		
Food, medicines for 30 patients (5 *qrans* each)	4,500	54,000
Wood and charcoal (2 *qrans*/day)	60	720
Telephone	40	480
Electricity light	120	1,440
Soap	60	720
Petroleum	300	3,600
Sugar and tea	300	3,600
Nurse	20	240
Burial cost, etc.	100	1,200
Repairs	150	1,800
Clothes for servants and office costs	220	2,640
Bonus for servants	30	360
Cost of water and dress for the 2 doctors		2,400
Total expenditures	9,020	110,640

Source: FO 248/1291, Neligan to Ambassador (20/01/1919).

The report showed that the Shah had made additional grants to the hospital and that one of 1,500 *tuman*s per year was for the German doctor's salary. Neligan asked Vothuq al-Dowleh whether the Iranian government would increase the hospital's budget, because 12,000 *tuman*s was quite insufficient for even 50 beds, given the then prevailing high prices. The best estimate Neligan had was for the Ahmadiyeh military hospital, to wit: two *tuman*s/bed/day or a total of 35,000 *tuman*s for 50 beds. Neligan further suggested that the British grant should have to be spent in Great Britain to buy new instruments. Also, the proposed grant was 2,500 pounds for the first year, but its continuation should be reviewed at the end of that year. Vothuq al-Dowleh agreed that 12,000 was not enough and said he would advice the cabinet to give 24,000 *tuman*s. Neligan further asked the Prime Minister whether his government would agree to a 25-year period of British management. Vothuq al-Dowleh's initial reaction was negative, because he feared that this would raise distrust. But after reflection he said that the cabinet might be displaced by an unfriendly one tomorrow and so he would propose that it would be accepted. In return, Vothuq al-Dowleh wanted written confirmation that the British government officially offered to assist in reorganizing the hospital, that two British doctors would be lend, that the Iranian government was not to be asked to pay a salary to the two British doctors and that it would make a grant of 2,500 pounds/year. In that case, he would propose to the cabinet that the Iranian contribution would be doubled to 24,000 *tuman*s. Vothuq al-Dowleh further agreed to send a copy of all hospital accounts. Neligan insisted that the late Loqman al-Mamalek would not be succeeded by his eldest son if the hospital was handed over to Great Britain. Vothuq al-Dowleh agreed and asked whether Hakim al-Dowleh, his other son, would be acceptable. He added that the shah was very fond of this family and would like to appoint a member of that family as director. Neligan told him it would be possible to work with Hakim al-Dowleh. He commented that "Logman al-Dowleh, the eldest son is regarded by Persians as mad and thought to smoke opium. He is senior physician to the Shah or was, for I think H.M. wants to get rid of him by appointing him dean of the faculty of medicine. At any rate he is impossible."[28]

---

28. FO 248/1291, Neligan to Ambassador (20/01/1919).

In an undated Memorandum from Neligan to the British Minister, but probably from February 1919, Neligan reported that Vothuq al-Dowleh told him a rescript (*dastkhatt*) had been issued appointing Hakim al-Dowleh, the son of the late Loqman al-Mamalek as director. He would get the 200 *tuman*s, the other 200 *tuman*s would go to a German or Russian doctor, in case any of them would be appointed chief-physician. Neligan reminded Vothuq al-Dowleh that the shah had given 150 *tuman*s to the second doctor, but this was not in the budget. He replied it would be in the reconstituted one, probably meaning the budget after the Germans had left. He said that the financing of the second doctor would be fixed in the new budget, and he was looking forward to the British Minister's proposal.

On 3 April 1919, Sir Percy Cox wrote to Vothuq al-Dowleh making a formal offer of British support for the *bimarestan-e shahenshahi*. Cox noted that the hospital had 30 beds for the poor and lacked many instruments and that its medical staff was partly trained. To improve matters British support intended to increase accomodation for the poor, reorganize and re-equip the hospital, and provide clinical teaching in medicine and surgery. If the offer would be accepted, two British doctors would be made available as well as a financial contribution, to begin with 2,500 pounds. The arrangement would be for 25 years, the Iranian budget had to be increased to 24,000 *tuman*s, if possible, and the buildings had to be maintained in a condition satisfactory to the medical staff. The senior doctor (A.R. Neligan) would receive an allowance of 200 *tuman*s, the junior (J. Scott) 150 *tuman*s/month. Given the need for a general refit of the hospital it was expected that the British contribution would have to be spend on instruments in Europe and an X-ray machine.[29]

On 11 May 1919, Vothuq al-Dowleh replied that the Iranian government agreed to the proposal and would increase its contribution to 24,000 *tuman*s/year and pay the two British doctors the allowance, who would be in charge of medical work and teach students of the Dar al-Fonun in their medical and surgical clinics. Moreover, "Three

---

29. FO 248/1291, Sir Percy Cox to Vothugh al-Dowleh, (03/04/1919).

days a week for two hours a day deserving patients who come to the hospital for consulation will be received gratis." Until the hospital needs required the hiring of a special full-time British physician the two doctors would continue their position with the Legation and the Indo-European Telegraph Department (IETD). As to the British financial contribution the Iranian government considered that this should be given in the form of medical and surgical instruments and medicine, which were needed every year. Thus, instead of cash, the British would supply the necessary instruments and medecins in the beginning for the hospital's reorganiation.[30] On 18 September 1919 the Britsh Legation informed Vothuq al-Dowleh that Dr. Neligan and Dr. Scott had entered hospital service immediately after having been received there on 2 June 1919. As to the allowance the doctors prefered to be treated equally, so that each would receive 175 *tuman*s/month, an arrangement endorsed by the Legation.[31] As a result, between 1919-23, the British government helped reorganize the government hospital at Tehran with 90 beds, and also supplied staff (Dr. A. R. Neligan, the physician of the British legation, and Dr. I. Scott, head of the medical staff of the IETD, as well as medical stores and equipment.[32]

On 5 August 1919, Dr. Neligan (at the instruction of the Iranian government) had written to the Overseas Nursing Assocation asking it to send a nurse (salary 80 pounds/year) and a matron (100 pounds) plus board, lodging, uniform allowance, and a 3-year contract. Because the matron was coming later than expected, Neligan had left a dossier with his substitute, which contained the written instructions (in Persian) from the Iranian government to hire a matron; the original of the contract between the matron and the Overseas Nursing Association on behalf of the Iranian government; the arrangement for board, which was made with the Iranian government by the Tehran branch of the Overseas Nursing Association for the two English nurses; the arrangement for lodging - a rented house; and a letter in which the

---

30. FO 248/1291, Vothugh al-Dowleh to Cox, (11/05/1919).
31. FO 248/1291, Cox to Vothugh al-Dowleh, (18/09/1919) (French and English versions).
32. Elgood 1951, p. 545.

Iranian government accepted to pay the outfit allowance.³³ Neligan also placed an order for medical equipment and supplies.³⁴

On their arrival Neligan and Scott found a dirty dilapidated hospital that required an Achilles or Rustam to clean up. Neligan reported about the hospital's condition as follows:

> The buildings were old, inconvenient, ill-ventilated, and badly lighted; sanitation and conservancy generally were very bad; repairs and cleaning were required everywhere; the material was absolutely insufficient; there was no separate section for women, no isolation wards, no rooms for special departments, no laundry, no proper baths, no laboratory, no murtuary; the nurses were untrained and were not of the class that could be trained. The hospital was badly thought of, was in debt, and had difficulty in obtaining payment of its budget. War conditions still prevailed, extravagant local prices, impossibiluty of finding at Teheran much that wa surgently needed, slow transport from abroad. Dr. Scott and I were in fact not a little dismayed at the prospect. We had, however, the goodwill of the Persian Government, of the staff, and of the Persians generally; the promise of a substantial increase in the budget and the certainty of a generous contribution from His Majesty's Government.³⁵

Unfortunately, Hakim al-Dowleh left one month later for Europe, and Scott and Neligan took their long overdue furlough. In their stead came Dr. A'lam al-Molk, Dr. Woollatt (IETD) and Lt. Col. A. Irvine Fortescue, a military doctor. It was then that problems arose. One Iranian assistant physician asked for a raise and without waiting for a reaction left the hospital without permission or warning. As a result, he was immediately dismissed, which upset the local Iranian medical fraternity. Attempts to provide students from the medical

---

33. FO 248/1291, Memo Neligan 30 November 1922: Comments on McLean's memo.
34. FO 248/1291, Invoices medical supplies (14/01/1920) and (30/03/1920).
35. Elgood 1951, p. 546.

school with clinical training in the hospital foundered, because no Tehrani physician was interested to participate, most likely due to anti-British sentiments. Finally, three Iranian physicians were hired, two of whom had been trained in Great Britain (Lesan al-Hokama, in charge of ophthalmology; Mohammad Khan Ala'i and Musa Khan). This enabled the staff to increase the number of beds to 88 and the number of out-patients to almost 4,000 in that year. [36]

In the absence of the two British doctors, on 4 February 1920, Lt. Col. Fortescue alerted the Minister about the hospital's worrisome financial situation. He urgently pressed for immediate payment of the British 2,000 pounds for 1920-21, because there were 35 cases of typhus and dysentery in the hospital, who all had been infected in Shahr-e Now. Moreover, the Hospital was in debt for more than 2,000 *tuman*s and would be unable continue to function if no funds were forthcoming. He stressed that just because of the absence of the cabinet or of the Minister of Public Works should not be allowed to endanger 30-40 lives. The money should be handed to Dr. Joseph Scott, who would distribute it appropriately, and on no account should the money be given to Hakim al-Dowleh. The 1919-20 contribution had also been handed to Dr. Scott and Dr. Neligan.[37]

Ms Oxley the matron arrived on 26 April 1920, but since then had received no salary. Although Hakim al-Dowleh was sympathetic he claimed to be unable to get pay from the Iranian government.[38] Because the matron complained about non-payment of her salary and other benefits, MacLean, a member of the Legation, looked into this matter, because neither Dr. Neligan nor Dr. Scott were in the country. On 7 August 1920, MacLean wrote a rather negative memorandum stating that the entire arrangement was unsatisfactory. Despite the contribution of 2,500 pounds/year to the hospital fund he did not find any stipulation that the British government or the British doctors had

---

36. Elgood 1951, pp. 546-47; Ebrahimnejad 2014, p. 158.
37. For 248/1291, Lt. Col. Fortescue to Ambassador, (04/02/1920).
38. FO 248/1291, Neligan to Overseas Nursing Association (05/08/1919); FO 248/1291, Memo Neligan (30/11/1922) Comments on McLean's memo.

any control or consultation in the management of the hospital and its funds or even the right to audit its accounts. This he considered to be unacceptable, because the British contribution was made

> for political objectives, clearly to benefit Persia and its people and to influence patients and students and public in favor of British methods and connections. But if the hospital was badly run, and it was, this objective was not achieved." Not only was the hospital badly run, but the arrangements provided "grounds for the accusation that Great Britain have secured lucrative billets for two British doctors paid for by Persia. [...] Our interests would be better served by the appointment of a resident doctor, who must receive slow and steady diplomatic support in effort to achieve effective management or at least a controlling influence on management and audit and publication of accounts.

MacLean added that he could not find any documentation regarding the contracts with the nurses.[39] Meanwhile, Lord Curzon informed the British Minister in Tehran that on 31 March 1921, the next 2,000 pounds would be allocated provided the Iranian government contributed the promised 24,000 *tuman*s.[40]

On his return from furlough, Neligan replied to MacLean's criticism by pointing out where he had erred. He pointed out that the British money was expended by the British doctors on behalf of the hospital. The hospital accounts were shown to them, when asked. Also, the hospital director consulted them about expenditures. It was true that the Hospital was frequently short of funds since he left on furlough in March 1922, because the arrangement by which its budget was paid in advance by the Customs had been changed. Since that time the Iranian government was desperately short of funds, but he believed that the old arrangement would be restored. In consequence, however, patients suffered. Nevertheless, students received better teaching than elsewhere in Tehran. Visitors of the hospital were impressed by the improvements made in the hospital.

---

39. FO 248/1291, Memo MacLean (07/08/1920).
40. FO 248/1291, Curzon to Cox (telegram 29/10/1920).

Neligan also reacted to the suggestion that the payment to him and Dr. Scott might be resented. He pointed out that the pay was the same as that accepted by the German doctors before the war. Moreover, "Persians seldom show their appreciation of getting something for nothing." The pay at ordinary rate was much less that it was when the arrangement was made; in any case the Iranian payment was in *qran*s and not in sterling. Also, to defend himself, Neligan pointed out that the hospital work was arduous when it was full.

> It is constantly unpleasant and dangerous owing to the nature of the cases (leprosy, typhus, anthrax, tetanus, tuberculosis) and the large amount of advanced surgical sepsis, venereal disease, advanced malignant growths etc. treated. There is no clause in the contract for loss of life or health by the medical officers in the event of infection. The work is important because of large number of surgical work and because until 1921 we were responsible for the clinical teaching of the Persian medical students. The French professors give 3 lectures/week with much higher pay and they are off duty three months/year, while our work is continuous. Personally I have spent 6 hours/day often. It reduced scope for private practice, leaving aside the question of transport. In the beginning we considered offering our services for nothing, and were advised by the Minister not to do so. Thus, we are not overpaid.

Neligan further submitted that indeed, a resident full-time British physician would be of great use to the hospital. However, he would cost more (salary, fares, house, furniture) than the present arrangement, and if he was changed frequently he would never acquire the depth of experience that Scott (25 years in Persia) and he (16 years) brought to the work. The arrangement was made hurriedly, because it was feared that the Germans might return and the Iranians were trying to get the post. Nevertheless, the arrangement pleased especially the local profession and there were no complaints at that time.

As to the matrons, unfortunately Scott and Neligan were on furlough when she arrived, but he had left all papers with his substitute and showed them to him. If he had shown them and the Legation had taken up the matter as soon as the matron was not paid all would have been well. Even McLean said that the contract was not disputed. In fact, the Iranian government doubled the matron's salary in January 1921. As to exchange matters. He had wanted to raise this point before leaving Iran, but the matron's arrival had been so much delayed that the Minister instructed him not to do so, as he would arrange it once she arrived. Neligan told the Director, who said that he had already passed the question to the government and that it would be settled in a satisfactory manner.[41]

According to the American missionaries, "the number of foreign doctors practicing has increased but we have no numbers. The number of hospitals doing surgery for the poor has increased. The Dowleh hospital under Drs. Scott and Neligan is doing good work. Its equipment has been extensively improved, so that can do any work. They employ a full-time pathologist and expect to have their own X-ray department."[42] As a result of the British involvement, the hospital soon became known as 'the English hospital.' Because the Iranian government did not provide any real financial support for the operation of the hospital, the unpaid and neglected Iranian staff blamed the British for their problems. The British doctors, however, were but advisers and had no decision-making authority. British involvement, therefore, became an embarrassment (especially as the political climate had become very anti-British), the reason why Great Britain withdrew its assistance in 1922. It asked the Anglo-Persian Oil Company (APOC) to take charge of the hospital. The Company accepted to do so, provided there would be a continued role of the British with the hospital, which the government of Iran refused. The APOC then dropped this condition and assumed charge of the hospital, but made it clear that it could halt its subsidy at any time without notice. It also accepted joint management of the hospital by APOC and Iranian physicians.[43]

---

41. FO 248/1291, Memo Neligan (30/11/1922) Comments on McLean's memo. img 8734-38
42. RG 91-19-11-1, Notes on medical work of Teheran station Jan. 1922.
43. Elgood 1951, pp. 546-554 (with details on the state of budget, patient care, the building and staff, and how it developed later). Litten 1925, pp.

Most patients treated at the Imperial hospital were those with acute malaria. During the summer many patients were treated in the garden under the trees. The staff consisted of a medical director, a surgeon, an assistant surgeon, a physician, an assistant physician, a surgeon aide and a physician aide, who dealt with patients who came for consultations. The nursing staff consisted of one trained nurse, two assistant nurses and 6 orderlies. The hospital had treated 499 hospitalized patients (450 men; 32 women; 17 children) during March 1923-March 1924. During the same period 6,450 outpatients were treated. Apart from in- and outgoing patients no database was kept.[44] A few years later the hospital was renamed *Bimarestan-e Sina* and as of 1940 *Bimarestan-e Ibn Sina* and served partly as surgical and partly as medical clinic of the medical faculty of the Tehran University as well as the main hospital for accidents to which end it had a well-equipped emergency room.[45]

6, 242; Wright 2001, p. 127.
44. Gilmour 1924, p. 26.
45. Karamati 1999, Iranicaonline.org.

American Missionary Hospital

The American medical mission in Tehran began in the fall of 1881 with the arrival of Dr. and Mrs. Torrence in Tehran. Before their arrival the health of the American mission personnel was in the hands of Dr. Baker of the IETD, who was paid £50/year for this service.[46] Presumably, Dr. Torrence first spent time learning Persian, which was standard procedure for arriving missionaries.[47] In 1882, helped by an Iranian assistant, Dr. Torrence ran a very active dispensary.[48] In 1883, his dispensary was open throughout the year, while he also made house calls, probably in connection with the outbreak of a measles epidemic in the summer, while in early winter there was a wave of diphtheria and scarlet fever.[49] In addition to his medical work, Dr. Torrence was given several tasks that in later years the Iran Mission would not give to young doctors. "He was selected Superintendent of the Girls' School, a position he held until 1884, when resigned stating that the school would be better served by a 'female' force. He also was charged with planning and building the boys' school and erecting the chapel."[50] In 1884, Torrence moved his dispensary from the Mission premises due to the danger of infection by contagious diseases. It was established in a suitable location in one of the streets in the so-called *Ferangi* or European quarter.[51]

In 1882 and again in 1883, Dr. Torrence reiterated that "we greatly need a hospital, where we may care for those needing surgical attention. Nothing has been done by me toward surgery, further than a few minor operations, reduction of dislocations, etc." Torrence wanted to start

---

46. RG 91-19-11-1, Historical Sketch. The American missionary station in Tehran existed since 1872.
47. Presbyterian Church 1882, pp. 56-57.
48. Presbyterian Church 1883, p. 66.
49. Presbyterian Church 1884, p. 70.
50. RG 91-19-11-1, Historical Sketch.
51. Presbyterian Church 1885, p. 77.

small, i.e. with a 6-7 bed hospital.[52] In 1885, Mrs. W.H. Ferry of Lake Forest, Ill. gave $5,000 for the construction of a hospital. The Board authorized the establishment of a hospital on condition that the Prime Minister would give the land. However, that never happened and the Board decided to buy land (24,000 sq. yards), near the Mission. The British objected to the proposed location of the hospital, it being too close to the British Legation, while the shah did not want it too close to the government hospital. Amin al-Dowleh then offered land for the site of the hospital near his home at a low price of one *qran* per sq. m. It concerned a piece of land of 20,000 sq. meters inside the city walls with valuable water rights. This low price was due to his friendship for the American Mission and esteem for Dr. Torrence. But even after the purchase and the granting of a royal *farman* or edict it took two years before the first hospital building was erected, because but there were as yet no funds for the construction. As of 18 May 1888 or 1889 actual construction started on the hospital (pavilion for 20 patients) and the doctor's residence. The Prime Minister's brother made a gift of 20,000 bricks.[53] Apart from his dispensary, Dr. Torrence, in the absence of a British doctor, also treated the British Legation staff against payment as well as the Shah and some of the royal palace staff due to absence Shah's physician.[54] In 1887, Dr. Torrence was decorated by the shah with order of the Lion and Sun second class. In 1888, the Shah asked him to accompany the new Iranian envoy to Washington and he was given five months' of absence. During his absence the dispensary was closed.[55]

In the fall of 1889, Dr. Mary Smith arrived. A female physician, the second of her kind in Iran, was a novelty for Tehran, in fact, a nine day's wonder. When the Shah visited the hospital he specially asked

---

52. Presbyterian Church 1883, p. 66; Presbyterian Church 1884, p. 70.
53. Presbyterian Church 1887, pp. 85-86; Presbyterian Church 1888, p. 88; Presbyterian Church 1890, pp. 180-81; RG 91-19-11-1, Historical Sketch.
54. Presbyterian Church 1886, p. 89; Presbyterian Church 1888, p. 88.
55. Presbyterian Church 1889, p. 90. Dr. Wishard also received the same decoration. RG 91-19-11-1, Historical Sketch.

to meet with the lady doctor. He said: "Feel my pulse, and tell me the state of my health."[56] Dr. Torrence first built the hospital wards, later dispensary rooms and a surgery were added, unconnected to the wards. This was awkward and so when a concert was given by the foreign community it gave the hospital a generous contribution. A long hall was constructed to connect the two units and a new surgery was erected on the north side of the hall. Until that time there was no women's ward.[57] Dr. Mary Smith acted as physician for the girls' school and boys' school and continued her language study. In 1890, she opened a women's clinic and held dispensary two mornings each week. Dr. Torrence reported treating 3,997 out-patients; Dr. Smith saw 117 patients outside of the school. Total receipts amounted to $685. In 1892, the new woman's dispensary was nearing completion.[58]

In 1890, Dr. Torrence reported an unusual amount of work due to the the influenza pandemic followed by an intermittent fever of a severe type. "The almost absence of sanitation and disregard of hygiene aggravated the disease." Torrence was helped by the British physicians Dr. Odling and Dr. Basil in all aspects of his work.[59] With two doctors and a building it looked as if there were no obstacles to go ahead, but complications arose that delayed work for several years. The main one was the 'hospital farman', when it was read and translated the Mission was dismayed to read that it contained stipulations to which it could not agree, e.g. that the entire hospital staff had to be Moslem, that a muezzin had to be appointed to look after the spiritual welfare of the patients, who had to be paid by the hospital, and finally, that no women patients were to be admitted. Dr.

---

56. RG 91-19-11-1, Historical Sketch.
57. RG 91-19-11-1, Historical Sketch.
58. Presbyterian Church 1890, p. 181; Presbyterian Church 1891, pp. 157-58; Presbyterian Church 1893, p. 161; RG 91-19-11-1, Historical Sketch.
59. Presbyterian Church 1890, p. 181; Presbyterian Church 1891, pp. 157-58. On the occurrence of influenza in Iran, see Floor 2018 a, pp. 93-106.

Torrence resigned and went into a business project in the city.[60] Dr. Torrence's resignation and the temporary transfer of Dr. Mary Smith to Hamadan seriously interfered with medical work in Tehran, the more so, because the hospital had just been completed. Dr. Odling (British Legation) filled in during Dr. Smith's absence.[61]

Given this situation, other missionary doctors also refused to take charge of the hospital. The building stood unused for some time. Amin al-Dowleh who wanted the hospital to function finally convinced the Mission that the *farman* was not binding and that he would see to the removal of the unacceptable stipulations. Then the Board was asked to send a doctor and a surgeon. Meanwhile, Dr. Mary Smith held dispensary two mornings each week. At that time, the new dispensary was nearing completion. While waiting for the new doctor, cholera struck Tehran in 1892. In this emergency the hospital wards were temporarily opened to care for cholera patients. Dr. Torrence accepted to be put in charge assisted by the British chemist Griffiths. A volunteer group of nurses, six boys (14-18 years old) from the US missionary Boys' school, cared for the patients. The hospital was the only institution in Tehran that helped the plague stricken. The total number of deaths in Tehran was estimated from 13,000 to 20,000. The American missionaries cared for 83 in-patients and 2,000 outside. Naser al-Din Shah expressed his appreciation for the work done during the cholera as did British Minister.[62]

In 1893, Dr. Mary Smith reported the move of the dispensary to the building erected for the purpose on the mission premises. It had three rooms, one drug room to prepare and dispense medicines, one waiting-room and one consultation room.[63] Dr. Smith also worked in the central dispensary and in the Jewish quarter.[64] On 10 May 1893, Dr. Wishard arrived and began studying Persian. On 20

---

60. RG 91-19-11-1, Historical Sketch.
61. Presbyterian Church 1892, p. 196.
62. Presbyterian Church 1893, p. 161; RG 91-19-11-1, Historical Sketch.
63. Presbyterian Church 1894, pp. 199-200; RG 91-19-11-1, Historical Sketch.
64. Presbyterian Church 1896, p. 184 (Receipts 545 Ts =$545.).

September the so-called Ferry hospital was formally opened, and it admitted more than 20 in-patients and Dr. Wishard did 20 operations, although he had little trained help. Wishard also spent several times with the Shah, when in the spring of 1894 he was called to the palace women's quarters. Dr. Tholozan, one of the royal physicians, visited the hospital and was highly pleased.[65] In 1895, the hospital added a separate building of six rooms, adapted to demand, the funds (1,215 *tuman*s) for which were raised in the field. Some 6,000 patients were treated, mostly Moslems. Almost every day the American medical staff had to refuse admittance due to lack of space. There were 120 in-patients (110 Moslems), of which 84 were surgical cases. Ms Dale was the matron. A commercial company offered to link the hospital by telephone with the central mission buildings accepting in payment the medical service of the hospital and dispensary for its workers, which added to the convenience.[66]

In 1898, Dr. Wishard held clinic three times per week in the central dispensary. He and three assistants saw 12,803 patients in that year. Moslem women seen at the dispensary numbered about 4,000, and 418 Jewish and Armenian women, or a total of 17,436 patients.[67] In 1899, Dr. Wishard's wife died and he temporarily returned to the US. Therefore, the hospital was not open, but work of the medical class and dispensaries was continued by Dr. Mary Smith and Dr. Funk, who together worked until Wishard's return in 1903.[68] At the beginning of winter, there were many applicants for admission to hospital, who did not understand why we could not take them. Not only was the hospital closed for men, but medical work was limited, due to the absence of a male doctor.[69] In June 1904, there was a cholera epidemic in Tehran, during which time there was no dispensary, only those who wanted

---

65. Presbyterian Church 1894, pp. 199-200; RG 91-19-11-1, Historical Sketch. For a bio of Dr. Tholozan, see Floor 2018 a, pp. 167-65.
66. Presbyterian Church 1896, p. 184.
67. Presbyterian Church 1899, pp. 187-88.
68. Presbyterian Church 1904, p. 238. In 1902, Dr. Funk had arrived in Tehran. Presbyterian Church 1903, p. 246.
69. Presbyterian Church 1901, p. 263; Presbyterian Church 1902, p. 221; Presbyterian Church 1903, p. 253.

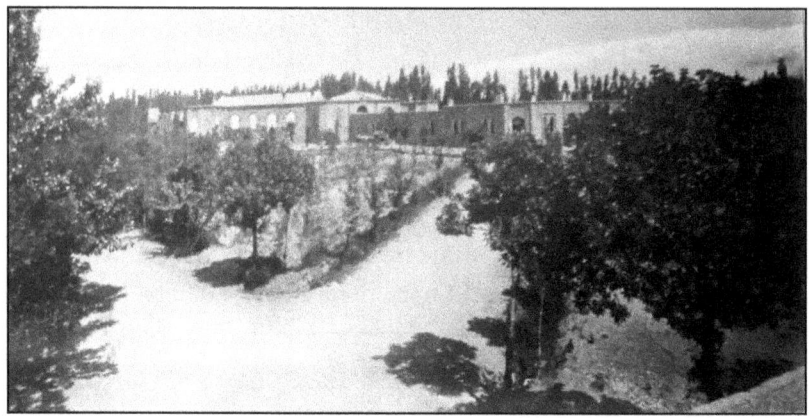

The American Hospital in Tehran, 1900

medicine came. This cholera epidemic was far more widespread than the one of 1894. To inform the public what cholera is and what to do, Dr. Wishard wrote a booklet: 'Asiatic Cholera- A Few Necessary Precautions with some hints concerning treatments in emergency.' It was printed both in English and Persian. Funds for the relief work were given by popular subscriptions. This time four relief centers were opened under the direction of the hospital, and during the three weeks of the height of the disease, these centers saved many lives. Dr. Wishard noted that the recovery rate in case of hospital treatment was 40% against 30% at home. After the epidemic was over the hospital needed to be disinfected. New floors were laid, walls were cleaned, replastered and repainted. The funds for the cleaning and repairs ($2,500) were donated by various banks, business corporations, the government and friends in Tehran.[70]

After the summer, as soon as the cholera epidemic was over, Wishard started again with regular hospital and dispensary work. Work on the new addition and waiting rooms, which had to be stopped because of the cholera, was resumed. "The new aseptic room, with hot and cold water, excellent light, and fully equipped, is a great comfort and help to the surgeon." Dr. Wishard was assisted by Dr. Scott as well as by Dr. Bedrosian and Dr. Ayob, two former graduates.[71]

---

70. Presbyterian Church 1905, pp. 274-75; Presbyterian Church 1906, pp. 289-90; RG 91-19-11-1, Historical Sketch. On the waves of cholera epidemics in Iran, see Floor 2018 a, pp. 16-28.

71. Presbyterian Church 1906, pp. 289-90.

Table 4: Number of Outpatients, Inpatients, Operations and Receipts American Hospital in Tehran(1882-1917)

Year	Outpatients	Inpatients	Operations	Receipts
1882	3,352	-	-	$412
1883	3,700	-	-	-
1884	2,500	-	-	-
1890	3,997	-	-	$685
1892	9,666	-	-	-
1893	2,000	20	20	-
1895	6,000	120	84	$545
1896	6,313	194	193	-
1897	16,936	208	201	-
1898	12,803	215	-	-
1899		239		
1903	5,000	78	58	-
1904	9,846	286	-	-
1906	17,200	201	504	20,897 *qrans*
1908		197	-	-
1909		250	74	$2,200
1910	-	285 (51 women)	-	-
1911	-	112 (51 women)	-	-
1913	6,900	(61 women)	-	-
1914	10,000	258	290	-
1915	19,000	399 (149 women)	115	-
1917	18,728	333	-	-

Source: Presbyterian Church 1883, p. 66; Idem 1884, p. 70; Idem 1885, p. 77; Idem 1891, p. 158; Idem 1893, p. 161; Idem 1894, pp. 199; Idem 1896, p. 184; Idem 1897, p. 157; Idem 1898, p. 178; Idem 1899, pp. 188; Idem 1900, p. 193; Idem 1904, p. 238; Idem 1905, pp. 274; Idem 1907, pp. 303; Idem 1909, p. 340; Idem 1910, p. 325; Idem 1911, pp. 325; Idem 1912, p. 351; Idem 1914, p. 326; Idem 1915, p. 314; Idem 1916, p. 293; Idem 1918, p. 280.

In Tehran only two rooms in the men's hospital were available for women. After Dr. Wishard had treated an Iranian noble woman, Amin al-Dowlehs' wife, she told him that she wanted to build a woman's hospital out of gratitude. She came to the hospital selected the site and

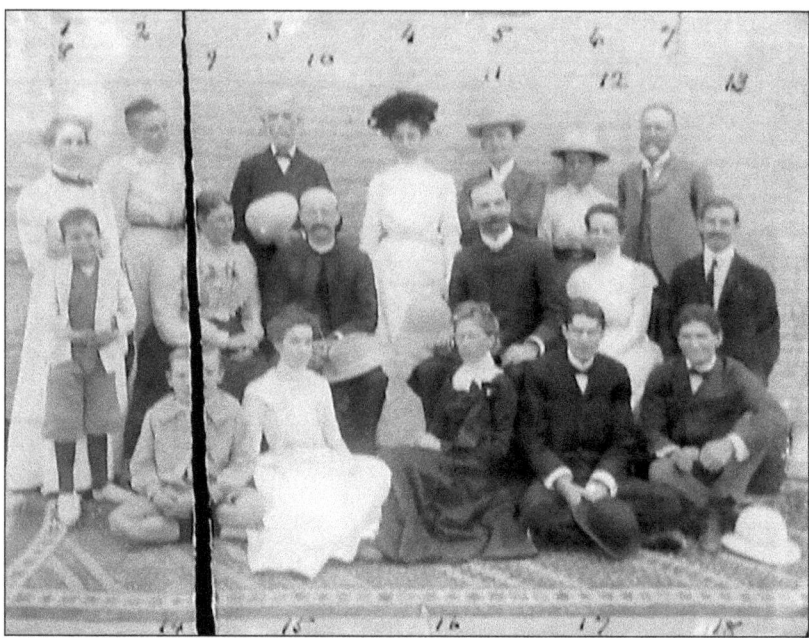

Group photo of American missionaries: 1. Mrs. Esselstyn. 2. Ms Bartlett. 3. Dr. Potter. 4. Mrs. Chas Douglas. 5. Rev. Chas Douglas. 6. Dr. Mary Smith. 7. Rev. Jas Hawkes. 8. Esselstyn boy. 9. Annie Montgomery. 10. Dr. L. Esselstyn. 11. Dr. Sm. Jordan. 12. Mrs. Hawkes. 13. Dr. Funk. 14. ? 15. Mrs. Jordan. 16. Dr. Mrs. Stead. 17. Mr. Stead. 18. Dr. Lawrence. Photo taken in 1910 or earlier.

gave the money of the estimated cost. In 3-months time the women's hospital was built and on 23 July 1906 the masons were whitewashing its walls. This donation was matched by Mrs. McCormick of Chicago and the Women's Court was erected and funds for the maintenance and furnishing of the hospital. Others gave money for the construction of rooms for the nurses, and one lady gave money for the maintenance and furnishing of the hospital.[72]

---

72. *Mercy and Truth* 1906, vol. 10, pp. 373, 375; RG 91-19-11-1, Historical Sketch; Wilson 1896, pp. 259-260; `Eyn al-Saltaneh 1376, vol. 1, pp. 377, 865; UNESCO 1343, vol. 2, pp. 1449-1451; Elgood 1951, pp. 511-512, 534; Wishard 1908, pp. 12, 99; Mo`tamed 1381, pp. 632-633; Richter 1910, p. 322.

In 1908, Wishard was on furlough and Dr. John Frame supervised the hospital during his absence assisted by Dr. Lindley (Shah's staff), Dr. Neligan and Dr. Scott (respectively British Legation, IETD).[73] Throughout 1908 attendance at the dispensary was rather small as low as 15 patients to 70-80 in the men's department, on average 35 patients. The Women's department under Dr. Smith did much better, who had a large dispensary all through winter.[74] Due to Dr. Wishard's resignation in the fall of 1910 work only started in mid-December; during the rest of year there was much work, including many house calls. There were two dispensaries, which were closed for two months in summer; otherwise the dispensaries were open for business: three mornings each week at the hospital and one afternoon at the Central Premises. As to the women's department, Dr. Smith reported that it was still closed for two months in summer. Otherwise dispensary work continued for three mornings each week at the hospital and one afternoon at the Central Premises. Attendance was often so large that it was impossible to give each patient the time and attention that should have been given. Also, many patients were more in need of good clothing and food than medicine. Some women were old patients, who came for a cataract operation on the second eye; their fear was gone and it was fun "to hear them giving advice and encouragement to the new-comers."[75]

Despite an increase in the number of foreign doctors and the opening of other hospitals there was no drop off in the number of patients in 1910. More than half of the 234 patients in men's ward were surgical cases. The burden of this workload was complicated by the fact that the surgeon had to train his assistant at the same time. Dr. Smith remained the summer and continued her dispensary and

---

73. Presbyterian Church 1909, p. 340; Idem, 1914, p. 326.
74. Presbyterian Church 1909, p. 340 (Dr. Frame, who substituted for Dr. Wishard, regretted very much that after having employed Mirza Ayub as pupil and assistant for 10 years that he joined the Bahais. He also was happy with the help given by Dr. Neligan and Dr. Scott).
75. Presbyterian Church 1910, p. 325.

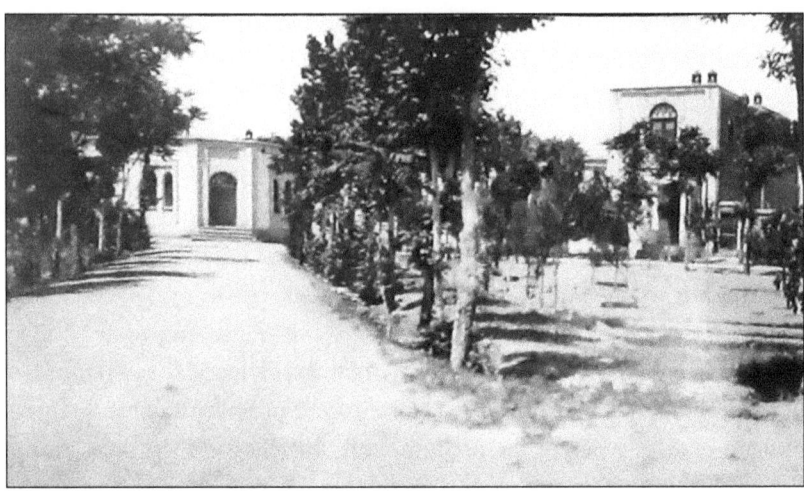

Above and opposite: The American Hospital in Tehran, main entrance, 1915

medical work.[76] Despite the loss of Dr. Wishard and the absence of a successor medical work was continued by Dr. Mary Smith and by the self-sacrificing, although temporary assistance of Dr. Joseph Scott of the IETD to keep the American hospital's doors open.[77] For the next 20 years the continuity of the hospital was much broken. During eight of these 20 years no male doctor was assigned and Dr. Smith worked alone. She provided the experience for five young, inexperienced male doctors, who served 12 of these remaining 20 years. With the arrival of Dr. McDowell in 1919 the hospital began unbroken service by a male doctor.[78]

A substantial part of admitted patients were surgical, many of which were cataract cases. Also, because the number of women applying for admission increased the need for a women's ward was sorely felt. One patient was troubled, because he had not 'sneezed' for a long time.[79] In 1911, in the hospital there were only surgical (mainly eye) and special cases. Mirza Musa and Mirza Qavam took care of

---

76. Presbyterian Church 1911, pp. 325-16.
77. Presbyterian Church 1912, p. 351.
78. RG 91-19-11-1, Historical Sketch.
79. Presbyterian Church 1905, pp. 273-75.

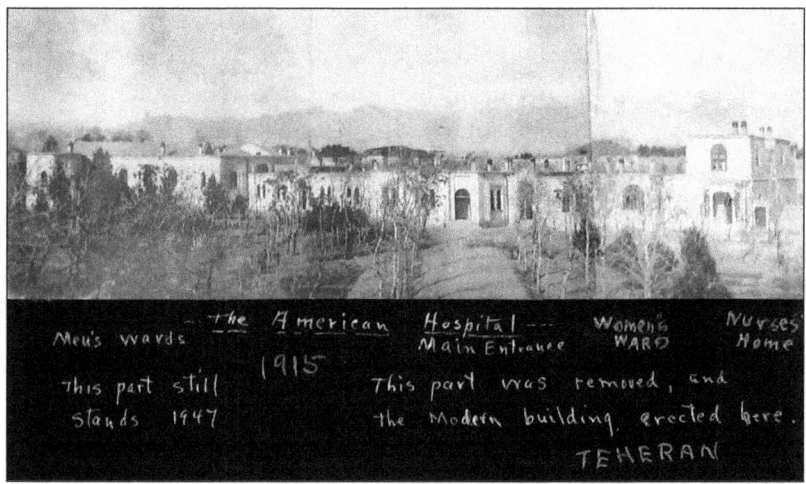

the dispensary and assisted in operations. Many patients came for eye operations.[80] In 1912, the male ward of the American Hospital for Men and Women was closed for business for almost one year, because there was no male physician. The male ward was closed again from 1917 until early 1919 for the same reason, when with the arrival of Dr. Post it was reopened. The female ward, however, had remained open all this time and was led by Dr. Mary Smith, who intermittently was assisted by an American trained nurse.[81] In 1913, soon after his arrival, Dr. Cook introduced the custom to give each patient a white card, with the following text on one side:

> The American Hospital, days and hours of dispensary, name of patient, date of coming, and number, with instructions to retain card and always bring it to the dispensary. On the other side is the following: Jesus said, the Spirit of the Lord is upon Me because He hath annointed Me to preach the Gospel to the poor; He hath sent Me to heal the broken hearted, to preach deliverance to the captives, and recovering of sight to the blind, to set at liberty them that are bruised.[82]

---

80. Presbyterian Church 1912, p. 351.
81. De Warzée 1913, p. 171; Presbyterian Church 1919, p. 259; Idem 1920, p. 310; Griscom 1921, p. 239.
82. Presbyterian Church 1914, p. 326.

In 1914, further improvements were made in the hospital. The operating room was enlarged, the building was painted and sanitary conditions were improved. In that year for the first time a hernia operation was done under spinal anesthesia. Thereafter, this patient sent three of his friends, who also had hernia.[83] During the summer of 1915 extensive repairs were made. The hospital was open from 5 October 1914 until 5 June 1915. The work done at the hospital was much appreciated as indicated by the fact that two Iranians offered to endow beds and one lady, who was already a donor, offered to build an additional room for obstetrical work.[84] In 1916, Dr. Cook and Ms Sutherland re-opened the Tehran hospital, but since the political situation had cleared up Dr. Cook went to Mashhad and Dr. Rolla Hoffman was left in charge of the Tehran hospital. Dr. Mary J. Smith had returned from furlough and had taken up her usual work two weeks later.[85] Dr. Cook returned from Mashhad to open the hospital in the fall of 1917 and the rush of patients was on immediately. However Dr. Cook had to leave in January 1918. The entire burden was on Dr. Smith, but the hospital was kept open, Dr. Scott of the IETD attending the surgical work.[86]

Dr. Cook was supposed to return that same year, but his arrival was delayed. Dr. Smith was helped by Dr. Petros, a Chaldean Catholic educated in the US, who took charge of the dispensary.[87] The women's dispensary had the same attendance as in 1917, during the time it was open. It was closed for three months, due to lack of funds and difficulties in getting supplies and food. Dr. Smith's dispensary in the central building was also only open during a small part of the year,

---

83. Presbyterian Church 1915, p. 314.
84. Presbyterian Church 1916, pp. 293-94.
85. Presbyterian Church 1917, p. 296; Dr. Cook left on 11 November 1915 ("I came on 4 October - since his departure I did 29 cataract operations, in total 60 operations, about 30 major ones, not counting trachoma, abscesses, etc."). RG 231-1-2, Hoffman to Friends, Tehran, 26/12/1915.
86. Presbyterian Church 1918, p. 280.
87. Presbyterian Church 1918, p. 280.

because it was difficult to get there. Carriages almost had disappeared and walking was impossible. Dr. Petros and Dr. Saeed Khan who lived nearby were willing to care for the needy ones, so the patients were not without care.[88] In 1918, two additional dispensaries were opened in the south of Tehran. The big question was whether they should be closed or not, given the doctors' inability to give them proper oversight. It was decided to keep them open to be used for Relief work for the sick and the poor for part of the year.[89] Dr. Mary Griscom, who worked there as of 1919, reported that

> At the dispensary I saw from fifteen to thirty patients, two or three times a week. Poor Armenians, beggars, members of Persian ministers' families and relatives of the Shah all rubbed elbows in the waiting-room. The majority of them had eye-diseases demanding operation. Persian ladies of high degree never expected to be seen ahead of the others. They took it as a matter of course that they were to be examined in their turn.[90]

Because Dr. Cook did not return, Dr. Scott again came to help and the hospital was opened on 15 October. Only the Women's hospital was kept open, given the difficulty in obtaining supplies and food for the hospital due to their low funds. Only private patients, who could take care of their own food, were admitted to the Men's department. In 1918, when famine and fever struck Tehran, the hospital helped many undernourished and typhus patients. Over time it became more

---

88. Presbyterian Church 1919, pp. 259-60.
89. Presbyterian Church 1919, p. 259; Idem 1920, p. 310; Griscom 1921, p. 239. Hence there were two dispensaries (male and female) at the same hospital. Presbyterian Church 1921, p. 326.
90. Griscom 1921, p. 239. By 1920 Dr. McDowell was also working in the hospital. Presbyterian Church 1921, p. 328. In 1918 there were four dispensaries in Tehran that treated 11,561 patients. Presbyterian Church 1919, p. 256 (with a picture of Dr. Mary Smith in an operating room). In 1921 it was noted that 80% of the patients of both the hospital and dispensary were from outside of Tehran, mostly from its nearby districts. Patients also included pilgrims coming from or going to Mashhad and Karbala. Presbyterian Church 1922, p. 364.

difficult to find bread; "we told women we would accept and them food, but no bread. Although they accepted it they found it difficult to do without. One room in the hospital was used for relief work, and on Fridays when supplies were handed out the street was so crowded that people could not get through. What they needed was food more than medicine."[91] The female ward of the hospital was closed for three months in 1918, while the main dispensary had been open irregularly due to the quasi-disappearance of droshkies from the streets, while walking was not possible. However, emergency cases on those days were taken care of by Drs. Petros and Saeed Khan, who lived nearby.[92]

Tehran hospital work was greatly hampered because Dr. Cook did not arrive due to sickness. Dr. Smith opened the Women's Hospital and had a busy year. The Men's Ward opened in March 1919 under Dr. Post, of the Relief Commission, but soon stopped due to his sickness and return to his work in Turkey. Dr. Griscom assisted in the dispensary.[93] In 1919, Dr. McDowell and Dr. Smith in Tehran took care of the in-patient service, which was small in numbers, and chiefly surgical in character. There were several deaths of pneumonia in hospital, because its policy did not deny admittance of the terminally ill.[94] "About 80% of patients are out-of-town, both in the dispensary and the wards, mainly from the nearby districts. Quite a few are pilgrims en route, who were are unwilling to stay long for proper treatment. Many surgical cases, especially those with incurable diseases, increase the mortality rate."[95]

It is of interest to observe that the discussion about the eventual closure of the hospital in Tehran, which took place in September 1942, already was foreshadowed in discussions that took place in 1921. In January 1921 of that year the Tehran medical staff drew attention to the fact that the situation in the capital city was different from that of

---

91. Presbyterian Church 1919, pp. 259-60; RG 91-19-11-1, Historical Sketch.
92. Presbyterian Church 1919, p. 260.
93. Presbyterian Church 1920, p. 310.
94. Presbyterian Church 1921, pp. 328-29.
95. Presbyterian Church 1922, p. 364.

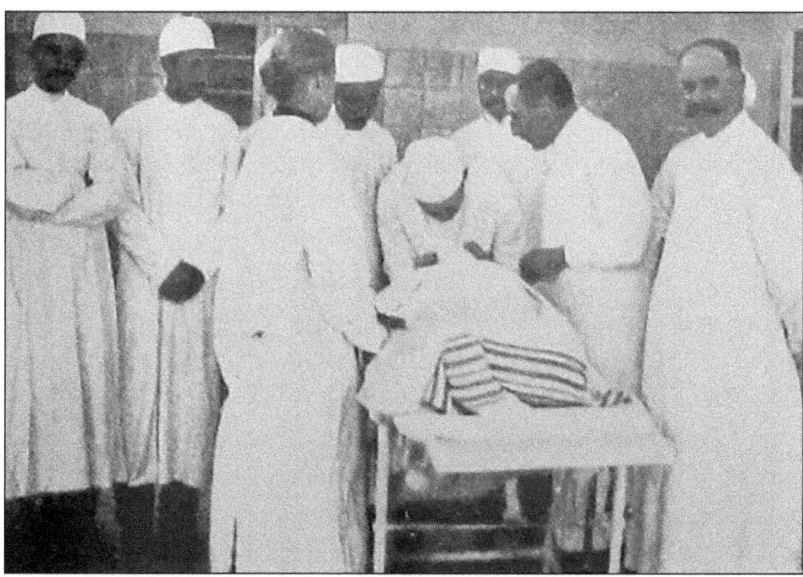

Cataract operation, American hospital, Tehran, 1918.
Dr. Mary Smith standing without a cap.

its environs. Whereas Tehran had changed over the last decades, its environs had hardly undergone any changes.

> The villages are untouched in their ignorance and isolation. They hardly know anything of modern medicine and science and are content with the native quack doctor. One advantage has been the establishment of vaccination center in the larger towns throughout Persia. They are under the Sanitary Council but are too few to reach the masses.
> Tehran is different through its contact with Europe, there is a growing no of Persians who have been to the West for business or education. Mode of living and dress has become farangified. Even amusements as shown by cinema and theater in Lalezar. Cars owned by Persian has grown significantly, Government is slowly making much needed reforms to control sanitation, the sale or narcotics and alcohol, and inspection of certain foods. Streets are repaired and some are lighted by electricity. Also, in medical field change. Persians went abroad for medical education and have returned to practice in Tehran. Very few educated people now consult the old traditional quacks. As a result the

average man in the street also knows about modern medicine, that microbes cause disease and that it may be cured. There are a great number of drug stores where you can buy almost any drug needed. Hypodermic administration is the most fashionable method of taking medicine. The patent medicine traffic, that sign of advanced civilization, has made its appearance.[96]

Given this analysis, the Tehran missionaries concluded that the Christian hospital needed to be better than any other hospital; else it would lose its comparative advantage, which would "adversely impact on evangelization." This meant that the hospital needed at least two male doctors and one lady doctor with a nurse. Furthermore, the hospital needed modern equipment, in particular diagnostic appliances. This would be a sine qua non, if it would be decided to attach a medical school to the hospital. If, however, it was decided that the hospital was no longer required in Tehran "then we should transfer all our energy to other parts of the country where there is actual need. This policy has merit and several years ago Dr. Cook proposed it."[97]

Although it was decided to continue with the hospital, be it without a medical school, the money needed to keep the hospital modern was not made available. In 1928, the hospital staff reported that the dispensary quarters were inadequate, resulting in slow treatments and congestion in the waiting rooms. "During spring and summer women overflowed into the men's waiting room - which was bad enough anywhere--doubly so in a Moslem land. Last year the missionaries raised the issue of a throat clinic and the growth of the nose, ear, throat practice so much so that the junior doctor McDowell had very little chance to see other patients during dispensary hours." The

---

96. RG 91-19-11-1, Notes on medical work of Teheran station Jan. 1922.
97. The missionaries also clearly stated that "there must be an evangelic worker in connection with the hospital." RG 91-19-11-1, Notes on medical work of Teheran station Jan. 1922. Dr. Cook started doing much itinerating in 1915, some 6 weeks/year, with temporary dispensaries. This work was abandoned in 1929. Better roads and transport made the city more accessible and work in the city absorbed all his time. RG91-19-11-1, Historical Sketch.

throat clinic was a mere cubbyhole of 7x10 feet with the outdoors as waiting room. "Toward noon it is almost as intolerable to keep patients waiting under the 'broad blue canopy' as it is in the cold and rain of winter."[98] Despite this tight financial situation, Dr. Edward Blair (1925-36) developed a nose and throat specialty, in addition to general medical work.[99]

Fortunately, in 1928, the wife of the new Amin al-Dowleh gave money for a TB ward, augmented by gifts from other Persian friends. It was a 2-storey building with wide verandahs. In 1930 the hospital roof covering everything but the last building was found to be riddled with white ants, making the building dangerous. Re-roofing was a major project and the old building was quite inadequate. So a new hospital was built in 1930. The men's wards built by Dr. Torrence were incorporated into the new building as was the long hall built with the concert money.[100]

In early 1931, Dr. and Mrs. Blair left on furlough for nine months, an extra burden for Dr. McDowell, who worked alone till Dr. Hoffman came in 19 March 1931 from Mashhad to replace him during most of this period. This timing was good since after *Nowruz* many patients came. Dr. Blair's temporary replacement Dr. Vassei contracted erysipelas and was unable to work for six weeks.[101] Dr. Blair returned on 3 July 1932, while Dr. McDowell and Ms Taillie left on furlough on 20 July 1932. Dr. Hoffman returned to Mashhad in March 1932 leaving matters in the hands of Drs. Vassei and Blair, and volunteer help from Dr. Davies and Dr. Aliasgharzadeh. Therefore, the hospital had to reduce work. During May-June 1933, Dr. Brinkman from Rasht replaced Dr. Blair due to his illnes. In the absence of Ms Taillie, Ms Haikows Minassian, a graduate from the Tabriz Christian hospital took over. She supervised the nurses, did the hospital records and also did nursing. The missionary doctors did not teach at the government

---

98. RG 91-19-11-1, Teheran Hospital Report 1927-1928.
99. Presbyterian Church 1930, p. 187.
100. RG 91-19-11-1, Historical Sketch.
101. RG91-19-11-1, Report Medical Work Teheran 1931-1932; Presbyterian Church 1936, p. 151.

medical school, but many of its students were an increasingly an important part of the hospital's personnel. At least one medical student was permanently on its staff the whole year. Three other students volunteered, and four to five picked up clinical instruction regularly, when they were free from classes.[102]

In early September 1933, Dr. McDowell returned, but there still was no American nurse. Apart from usual staff, the hospital benefited from the honorary services of Dr. Aliasgharzadeh, a Russian female physician, a specialist in children diseases. How long the hospital might be able to retain her was unsure, however. Hikowe Boghasian, continued as head nurse and two new additions were Hosmik Karapetian, a last year's graduate from Tabriz and Vartanush Minasian, who, after graduating from Tabriz, had worked some time in Mashhad and Kermanshah. She was doing only operation room (OR) and dispensary service. Astqiq Hosepian, the other OR nurse was crippled most of the year by an eye infection. A new development was that there was an alarming trend of criminal suits brought against well-known Iranian surgeons in the city for the death of patients. Therefore, some local hospitals "have a printed form for the patient and family to sign requesting treatment and releasing the surgeon and hospital from responsibility. Such a form cannot prevent suit from being brought, but Persian doctors think that most people think that when signed they don't have the right to sue."[103] In 1935 and thereafter, Dr. Aliasgharzadeh continued to offer her services. A new development was the eye clinic. Dr. Hamzavi, an eye specialist of Russian birth and training, donated several hours three afternoons to this work in the Christian hospital. She saw her patients in the room used as a children's clinic in the morning. Although her hours were not the most convenient she built up quite a clientele after four months' work. The men's staff was joined by a young man supported by the CMS, who was a student in the School of Pharmacy. He worked partly

---

102. RG91-19-11-1, Report of Teheran Hospital 1933.
103. RG91-19-11-1, Report Medical Work Teheran 1934. One medical student, Dr. Nejat graduated and went into private practice. RG91-19-11-1, Report Teheran Medical Work 1934-1935.

in the hospital's pharmacy, partly in the wards and dispensaries. Also, three medical students interned in the hospital work and were given serious training.[104]

In the summer of 1936, the Zoroastrian Dr. Faridun Varjavand, a former student and then teacher at the Alborz College, returned from his 5-year course at the Medical School at the American University in Beirut. He joined the staff of the American hospital as associate physician in the women's clinic, surgery and wards. He also opened an office in another part of the city and in his spare time he translated text material for the school of nursing. For several years Dr. Vassei had taken charge of the men's clinic, Dr. Blair, the ear, nose and throat cases, while he also acted as consultant in the men's and children's clinics. They both were assisted by a varying number of medical students. The medical school urged the hospital to take more students than its doctors felt they could do justice to. In 1936-37, there was an increase in stomach and thyroid surgery and a decrease in industrial and accident surgery, while Dr Vassei broke all records for the number of cataract surgery.[105]

In February-March 1936, there was a waiting list for men's private rooms. If the hospital had more rooms it could accommodate more paying patients, which would have been more than welcome given the reduced appropriation from the Board. It was possible to refit the basement where patients could be placed during the hot season and avoid the seasonal decrease of surgery and income, however that required funds that the hospital lacked.[106] It was not only the patients who needed more room, the same held for the nurses. Their living quarters left much to be desired; they were crowded and located into two different buildings. Also, there was no quiet place for the night nurse to sleep. Because of the growth of the nursing school adequate space for the nurses was urgently needed. Moreover, there was another bedeviling problem, viz., the waiting list for wards and private rooms,

---

104. RG91-19-11-1, Report Medical Work Teheran 1936. On the School of Pharmacy, see Floor 2020, pp. 63–69.
105. RG91-19-11-1, Report Medical Work Teheran 1937.
106. RG 91-19-11-1, Teheran Hospital Report 1928.

which only was becoming worse, because demand for hospital care was increasing. Furthermore, there was the problem of how to isolate cases with infectious diseases, and what to do with pneumonias, the need long-term nursing, of diphtheria, meningitis, etc.? The doctors raised these issues, because these types of cases were rarely referred to other hospitals, while there was no protection for the patient or the other children at home. "The men nurses and the resident medical students are tucked away in all kinds of odd corners. There is only a makeshift provision for a house for the American nurse." Despite the limited funds some improvements were made in the hospital such as the cementing of the floors, the whitening of the walls of the kitchen, the renovation of the staff dining room, the fixing of a bath for women in-patients, etc. As to instruments only a new sterilizer and a cautery were added. The furniture was repaired and the hospital received some new stuff from an Iranian friend. In September it received supplies from the US White Cross.[107] In 1937-38, the main hospital was improved by laying concrete floor in the man's wards, the large women's ward, the large waiting room for women and children, and the hallway of the women's hospital, as well as some smaller rooms. The other hallways and the ramp were asphalted enabled by the generosity of Farmanfarma, who donated $1,000. All beds in the women's hospital were raised to standard height to facilitate nursing. A rolling dressing table was designed and made which saved many steps. Many other changes were made as well. As there continued to be a shortage of private rooms the partition between the linen storeroom and ironing room was removed, thus getting another large room in which one or two patients could be accommodated. Other options to get more rooms were abandoned for cost reasons. The ratio private to ward beds was too small in view of the growing necessity to increase income. In fact, if the doctors continued to treat the same number of free patients, they would be forced to focus more on the well-to-do. Fortunately, Dr. Aliasgharzadeh and Dr. Faridun Varjavand continued their honorary services. Dr. and Mrs. Blair returned to the US in the summer of 1938, which meant that some of the surgery he did

---

107. RG 91-19-11-1, Report Medical Work Teheran 1936.

could not be done any longer; also he had been an excellent business administrator.[108] To replace Blair, Dr. Hoffman came from Mashhad. In 1940, Mrs. Hoffman started to repair the buildings. She renovated the nurses' quarter with improved sanitary facilities, screening and ventilation. She received a gift from an Iranian lady for a pump and some money for water piping from the Iran Presbyterian Mission, so that as of then the nurses had piped water. She also prepared a basement for use of the night nurse to sleep quietly, although the nurses' housing continued to be makeshift.[109]

Although the hospital would be closed in 1942, as early as 1938 its medical team foresaw that this was going to happen. In June 1938 they began their annual report as follows: "This report year in all probability marks the end of an era. We have reached the high tide mark as an institution so far as numbers of patients and receipts are concerned. Our road in the future leads downward- how long or how short it will be cannot now be foreseen." Why did the staff have such a pessimistic view of the hospital's future? They had good relations with the government and the local medical community. However, they observed that local demand for larger and better medical service was growing as was the cost of hospitalization. The early beginning of the hospital had been simple medical work, but since WW I, its doctors had progressed from that level to intricate and major operations of modern surgery, covering a large number of specialties. "We kept abreast of developments and hold a position of leadership, but we cannot hold that position without the needed financial backing to buy more modern equipment and introducing new methods." However, given constraints on staff and finances imposed by the Home Church, meant that one or more missionary hospitals had to be closed. Blair's departure had created a problem. Before his departure, the men's side had always been full. The ear, nose and throat clinic (his specialty) had always been busy, an indication that many health problems had to do with infected tonsils and sinuses. Without being able to perform this

---

108. RG 91-19-11-1, Report Teheran American Hospital 1937; Idem, Report Medical Work Teheran 1937-1938.

109. RG 91-19-11-1, Report American Hospital Teheran 1940-1941.

particular service the medical staff felt that it would be very difficult to continue, because the hospital's effectiveness would be reduced significantly. Nowhere else in the city a similar service was available to the public and within financial reach of even the middle class.[110]

This failure to address this question as well as that of the hospital's finances probably led to the resignations of Drs. Blair and McDowell, which caused a major crisis at the hospital. For given the high medical standards in Tehran mere survival was not an option. Either two American doctors were found or the hospital should be closed while its reputation was still creditable. In November 1940, Dr. McDowell went on furlough. Without other doctors work was impossible. Who, apart from Dr. Hoffman, were still there at that time? Dr. Faridun Varjavand lived in the mission compound. He attended many night maternity cases and did most of the emergency operations. However, he had an outside private practice and how long he was able to stay depended on the question whether the hospital could raise his salary. He had been McDowell's associate for four years and had considerable obstetrical experience in the government hospital for women in Tehran. Dr. Aliasgharzadeh also continued to work, but she did not do surgery, which Dr. Varjavand and Dr. Hoffman did. Apart from these two members of the hospital's regular staff, there were also outside doctors who worked in the hospital. Dr. Abdollah Vassei had worked there already for many years and had received there a good surgical training. For two years following Blair's resignation he had charge of the men's department, but as of 1940, he devoted all his time to his large private practice. He still referred his surgical patients to the American hospital, where he usually had 2-6 patients. There also were two female physicians, one Swiss and the other Czech, who assisted in the women's dispensary and OR as non-paid helpers. Furthermore, two doctors working in the government health department came when they had time to assist in surgery, while several other doctors also came.

Dr. Hoffman had daily rounds each morning and on Sunday morning when the staff and visiting doctors usually attended, the

---

110. RG 91-19-11-1, Report Medical Work Teheran 1937-1938.

regular hospital physicians systematically reviewed the entire inpatient population, checking each patient's status and discussing problems of diagnosis and treatment. Although there was a unified record system, which was in the hands of half a dozen persons, there was no index so that records lost track of patients and 'new' patients were really old ones. Hoffman, who had introduced an effective record system in Mashhad, made sure that there was a separate record room and somebody in charge of it as record clerk. As a result, as of 1940, there were records with a name index so that everybody's records could be found, even if the patient had lost his card. Thereafter the record room and clerk were a source of satisfaction. Names were indexed by both first and family names, because there was considerable uncertainty about both. Sometimes, patients gave as many as three family names: their father's, husband's and their own.

Hoffman also reopened a lab of sorts, run by a doctor of the military hospital. This was very convenient, although any profits went to the doctor not to the hospital. However, Hoffman stressed that if the Tehran hospital was to be continued it needed to have its own lab. Another problem child was the pharmacy, because the pharmacist was mentally unstable and a source of danger. Therefore, he was released. Temporarily an outside pharmacy, the *Namse*, filled the hospital doctors' prescriptions for free and bank (contract) cases. Furthermore, Dr. Islami, a medical student, who also was a graduate pharmacist, employed a helper and prepared intravenous solutions and other medicines for in-patients. According to Hoffman, Dr. Islami "is an unusual and valuable young man who works in the children's department; very cheerful, always willing to help, gives anesthesia, assists in emergency operations and does anything that is needed. He lives in the hospital and accumulates a very useful and varied experience for his future practice." There was no change in the lab situation thereafter. Because the outside army doctor was only available three mornings per week, Hoffman flagged the need for the hospital to have its own pharmacy. The more so, because the pharmacy had to do some dispensing of medicines as prices in outside pharmacies have sky-rocketed and esp. sulfonamide drugs are very scarce.[111]

In 1941 it seemed as is the crisis of the hospital's future had been averted. The year 1941-42 was a busy one. Dr. Hoffman was in charge of the women's and children ward and children outpatients were under Dr. Aliasgharzadeh. Dr. Varjavand again carried the men's department, handled the midnight to morning baby cases and the whole hospital during Hoffman's short vacation. Hoffman's hoped that the Board would appoint Dr. Faridun Varjavand as the first Iranian doctor full-time to replace an American doctor. A positive development was that under the new regime there was a more liberal attitude instead of over over-intense nationalism that was planning to close all foreign hospitals after the foreign schools. In 1942, the civilian camps of Polish refugees had serious sanitation problems with epidemics of typhus, typhoid and contagious diseases. Dr. Norem from the Christian hospital in Mashhad worked there with US Army medical men during the spring of 1942. Sanitation was established in the camps, while an Indian army hospital unit looked after the civilians, while the Pasteur Institute produced a typhus vaccine. The Iranian government gave a medal to the American doctor, who taught the Institute the technique of making typhus vaccine. The US Army claimed Dr. Norem and urged Dr. Hoffman to join as well. However, because he didn't want to leave his hospital without an American doctor he offered to make the hospital available for any US soldier who fell ill here, thus relieving the army from posting a doctor in Tehran. Some 20 soldiers and aircraft employees came to the hospital, mostly digestive upsets.[112]

In 1942, the hospital was closed, although at the beginning of the year it did not look that way, in fact fees were rising and the hospital's outlook was bright, if only it could find an American doctor. However, in August 1942 the Presbyterian Iran Mission had to decide which of its six hospitals had to be closed. Its medical force was depleted by furloughs from which doctors did not return due to WW II, by a death

---

111. RG 91-19-11-1, Report American Hospital Teheran 1940-1941; Idem, Teheran Medical Report, 1941-1942.
112. RG 91-19-11-1, Teheran Medical Report, 1941-1942.

and resignations (to the Army). Almost all remaining doctors were due to furlough. It was decided to sacrifice the Tehran hospital, because the remaining missionaries could get there better medical help than anywhere else in Iran. On 30 September 1942, the hospital closed after having served the community for half a century. The American staff was distributed to fill the thinning ranks in the other Christian hospitals. Ms Fulton went to Kermanshah and Dr. and Mrs. Hoffman to Mashhad. The employees were dismissed and given bonuses in proportion to their length of service. The nurses had no trouble finding employment, as they were in great demand. Some of the student-nurses went with Ms Fulton to Kermanshah, some to Mashhad to continue their studies. The compound plus two residences were turned over to the US government for the duration of the war. The US Army began repairs and alterations immediately, making the sorting, storing and disposal of equipment and supplies difficult. Very good was the sinking of a deep well from which water was pumped to a reservoir from which water was piped throughout the hospital. Also, the Army put in better flooring and wall-paint, showers and plumbing fixtures. The hospital had an overhaul that it never had before. The medicines and supplies were distributed over the other hospitals; much of the furniture was borrowed by the US government and some surgical instruments were loaned to Dr. Varjavand, who immediately opened a small private hospital, some others were 'loaned' to other mission hospitals; the rest was stored for future use.

The loss of the Tehran hospital was felt as a blow; not only missionaries came there to receive treatment that they could not get in the provinces, but the presence of two US doctors in Tehran was an advantage when having to approach the Iranian government and departments, the US embassy, the Red Cross, etc. The Red Cross gave the Christian hospitals many medicines and surgical goods, which it probably would not have done had not one US doctor be on the spot to confer with them.

The Iran Mission clearly wanted to reopen the Tehran hospital, but formulated as conditions that in that case there should be at least two, preferably three US doctors with emphasis on surgery and on accurate and careful diagnosis. One of them should be radiologist, another with experience in lab work, including serology, another in preventive medicine and health teaching. It also needed at least two US nurses to develop the school of nursing better than anything in the land. Also, better teaching materials and equipment as well as furniture and instruments for a 60-80 bed hospital were required. Furthermore, there should be an X-ray machine and technician as well as a lab technician with adequate lab equipment for serological work, blood chemistry and all other ordinary tests; the hospital also should develop a school for X-ray and lab technicians. Because at the end of the war much equipment would be available from the US Army, funds had to be set aside to buy it before it was sold elsewhere. Finally, each doctor should be assigned a car as a necessary part of his equipment.[113]

WOMEN'S PAVILION

Although in 1898 women came in large numbers to Dr. Smith's women's dispensary, she as yet feared to admit women in-patients, due to Moslem prejudice. However, at the same time, she noted that this prejudice was waning and that many women patients would come to the hospital if there was a place for them.[114] She also observed that a certain category of women did not even have the opportunity to visit the dispensary. Therefore, she opined that house calls were important, for "It is only by going to their homes that one can reach this class of [wealthy and influential] women, as they would never be allowed to come to the dispensary."[115] At first, during the first five years, hardly any women were admitted to the hospital. However, in 1906 it was reported that medical work had increased in quantity and quality, especially for women. Medical work for women was limited to eye cases and minor surgical ones. Women requiring major surgery were not admitted out of fear that a death might produce a severe prejudice against the missionaries' medical work. In 1906, an important courtier

---

113. RG 91-19-11-1, Teheran Medical Report 1942-1943.
114. Presbyterian Church 1899, pp. 187-88.
115. Presbyterian Church 1902, p. 221.

insisted that his wife be operated and that the Shah showed personal interest in this matter. Therefore, the hospital gave in and the operation was successful. Then other women also asked to be admitted. "I said for women we only have a small room; they said, but you treated a court official's wife, why not us?" When Dr. Smith was on furlough, there was only her young assistant Dr. McDowell. He was called to treat the mother of a nobleman. During the visit, he explained to her that there was a great need for a hospital for women in Tehran and it was difficult to treat women and children in one for men. She then told him to show her his plans and promised that if she would be in good health that she would give him the necessary funds (see above). For 20 years no other building was constructed, aside from a second residence at the Hospital compound. More well-to-do patients who were able to pay indirectly helped, as it allowed the doctors doing work for the poor without charge.[116]

The new addition, initially a 10-bed pavilion for women, was opened in October 1907. This addition had the advantage that more private male patients could be admitted, because the private rooms in the 25-bed men's hospital were not needed for women any longer. Higher class patients came to realize advantage of hospital over treatment at home, and "those who until recently thought it a disgrace to go to a hospital to stay, looking on it as a charitable institution for poor people without a home and friends, are now quite willing to honor us by coming."[117]

In 1928, a wealthy Persian family promised to finance building a new women's TB wing; they started hauling stones for the foundation, when the government pressed workmen to work on the shah's new summer palace and the widening of business streets. The result was an ugly pile of stones. The resignation of the female Armenian doctor, who had assisted for two years, made the workload heavier, and left the hospital interns with too little consultation or supervision in the men's clinic. Dr. McDowell was solely in charge of the women

---

116. RG 91-19-11-1, Historical Sketch; Presbyterian Church 1907, pp. 302-03.

117. Presbyterian Church 1908, pp. 342.

dispensary with two results. He built up large clientele of clinic and private patients and there were more women demanding surgery than the hospital had beds. If there had been more room in the women's wing for post-operative care the hospital could have done more urgent work. From begin April to midsummer 1928 there was not a day when there were not two or more patients waiting for a bed whenever somebody was discharged. It was felt that a female doctor to replace Dr. Smith, who retired in 1923, would increase the effectiveness of the women's department. Also, the male physicians would be able to spend more time supervising the men's department.[118]

The women's clinic continued to grow and, in fact, was the best known department of the hospital. For several years during spring and fall doctors had to turn away patients, because they could not properly care for them. The maternity service was popular among the well-to-do and prenatal care was experienced as accepted routine.[119] The amount of prenatal work was difficult to assess. "The majority of the poor who are delivered at the Nesvan, Zayeshgah, etc. are abnormal cases referred to by midwives. Probably ours is the largest prenatal clinic." The Christian hospital normally didn't accept cases that had not been seen in the clinic, thus avoiding infectious cases.[120] In 1940, the hospital employed two women doctors, one Swiss and the other Czech, who assisted in the women's dispensary and OR as non-paid helpers.[121] Obstetrical services continued to flourish until the closure of the American hospital.[122]

---

118. RG 91-19-11-1, Teheran Hospital Report 1928.
119. RG 91-19-11-1, Report Teheran American Hospital 1937 (Twice there were 11 newborns in the nursery this year. The number of confinements showed an increase of 30 over 137 last year).
120. RG 91-19-11-1, Report Medical Work-Teheran 1937-1938 (15 at a time is the largest no we had. 245 deliveries.).
121. RG 91-19-11-1, Report American Hospital Teheran 1940-1941. The female doctors probably had been unable to get a license to practice.
122. RG 91-19-11-1, Teheran Medical Report 1941-1942.

Other Tehran Hospitals

In 1904, at the suggestion of Hajj Sayyah a small hospital was established in Tehran to respond to the need for medical assistance created by the 1904 cholera epidemic. In collaboration with Mr. Naus, the Treasurer-General, and Mokhtar al-Saltaneh, the chief of sanitation (*mohtaseb*) of Tehran, a building was rented and Feylosuf al-Saltaneh Mirza `Abd al-Karim was hired as its medical director, at a salary of 250 *tuman*s per month. They also organized a system whereby sick people were transported to the hospital by droshky, all free of charge. Those that died were taken by the same service to the washers of the dead. The hackneys were paid one *tuman* per patient. Dr. Morel, a French physician, assisted in the operation, in particular in managing the women's hospital that had been set up. Some wealthy individuals such as Moshir al-Dowleh provided further financial assistance.[123] Ja`far Shahri, the historian of life in old Tehran, does not list this hospital, which, therefore, must have been a temporary solution (using a rented building) to an immediate and pressing problem, i.e., the 1904 cholera epidemic.[124] In fact, Shahri states that around 1920, there were only two Iranian hospitals in Tehran, the State or Imperial Hospital (then called *Ahmadi*, but later again *Dowlati* and ultimately *Sina*) and the *Najmiyeh* Hospital, in addition to the American and Russian hospital.[125] According to Mrs. de Warzée, in 1912 there was only one Iranian hospital, viz., the State or Imperial Hospital.[126] She

---

123. Sayyah 1347, pp. 536-540.
124. This supposition is confirmed by Wishard 1908, pp. 219-220 who mentions that during the 1904 epidemic his general hospital was converted into a cholera hospital; furthermore, "a house was taken as a refuge hospital on the west side of the city [Sayyah's hospital], and also a place was opened in Shiran [Shemiran?]. These three centres of work, together with a dispensary in the Jewish quarter of the town, were kept in operation day and night for nearly a month, when the epidemic ceased." On this epidemic see Burrell 1988, pp. 258-270.
125. Shahri 1368, vol. 1, p. 294.
126. De Warzée 1913, pp. 171-172. Wishard 1908, p. 234 reports on this subject that recently, the German government had opened a free general hospital in Tehran, which does not seem to be correct. He probably mistook German management of the Imperial hospital (see above) as this being a

mentions a second Iranian hospital, most likely the hospital built with funds from Vajihollah Mirza Sepahsalar (see below), but it did not function as such yet in 1912.

> A Persian sinner who had misdirected public funds repented of his sins at the eleventh hour and just before his death gave a large sum of money to build a hospital. He was told that by doing so he would gain Paradise. A great building was erected outside Teheran towards the mountains, but, unluckily, the money was not only insufficient to run the hospital, but also to complete the building, and until now it has stood unfinished and useless. It is to be turned into barracks for the new Persian gendarmerie.[127]

The Russian hospital, which was supported by the Russian Red Cross, practically only served Russians and was managed by the Russian Legation's doctor. According to Wishard, it was opened in 1907. There also was "an infirmary in the Russian (sic) Cossack Brigade buildings, where the brigade and their families are attended. There are over a thousand consultations monthly in this infirmary and the dispensary is free."[128] French nuns (*filles de charité*) also had a small hospital-dispensary in Tehran.[129] Finally, there was the dispensary of the British Legation, which had "consulting-rooms for men and women, and an operating room attached to the English Legation doctor's house; it is financed by the English Government and the consultations are free."[130]

By 1924, there were six Iranian civil and two army hospitals in Tehran. The largest and oldest was the Imperial or State Hospital

---

German hospital, which it was not. For example, Litten 1925, p. 404 only mentions the management of the Imperial hospital by Dr. Becker, and no other German involvement with the hospital.

127. De Warzée 1913, p. 172. There was indeed a military hospital at Yusofabad (see below).
128. De Warzée 1913, pp. 171-172; Grothe 1911, p. 131; Wishard 1908, p. 234.
129. Hassendorfer 1954, p. 61; Wishard 1908, p. 234.
130. De Warzée 1913, p. 172; Wishard 1908, p. 234.

(*mariz-khaneh-ye mobarak-e dowlati*), built in 1874 (see above) with a nominal capacity of 50 beds.[131]

In November 1903, Vajihollah Mirza Sepahsalar endowed 15,000 *tuman*s for the establishment of a hospital at Yusofabad, n.w. of Tehran on a piece land of 15,000 sq. *zar*. Furthermore, a total of 5,350 *tuman*s, representing the revenues of four *qanat*s and five mills, were assigned for the hospital's expenditures. He died in 1904 during the cholera epidemic, and although the endowment deed nominated a number of administrators, it is not known whether this hospital ever became operational (see below).[132]

The *Vaziri* Hospital had been made possible by Mirza 'Isa Tafarroshi Vazir (d. 1892), one of Naser al-Din Shah's ministers, who had bequeathed one-third of his wealth for the construction and operation of a small hospital as well as of a mosque, in which he was buried. The combination of a mosque, hospital and the founder's tomb was clearly modeled after that of the traditional *dar al-shafa*. The construction started in 1898 under the supervision of the cleric Hajj Sheykh Hadi Najmabadi, who had been made *motavalli* or administrator of the Vaziri endowment. The hospital with 10 beds and a medical and surgical section was completed in 1900. It had two physicians, Dr. Abu Turab for the medical department and Dr. Wolf (a German) who was in charge of the surgical section. After Najmabadi's death the hospital's work was hampered, because the foundations that Najmabadi had created questioned the hospital's finances. The hospital was then managed by Yusof Bozorgmehr ('Alem al-Saltaneh).[133] As a result, the hospital never functioned properly, a reason why the state took over its management in 1918. The hospital had 30 beds for both medical and surgical cases. The director of the hospital was the chief medical officer at the same time. He also taught at the Medical School, as did the hospital's surgeon. Three students in their last year functioned as their assistants. There were eight nurses, two of which were female.

---

131. Gilmour 1924, p. 26.
132. Rezai 2012, pp. 119-20.
133. Bamdad 1347, vol. 2, pp. 514-515 (with biography); Tajbakhsh 1379, pp. 240-242; Rezai 2012, pp. 118-19.

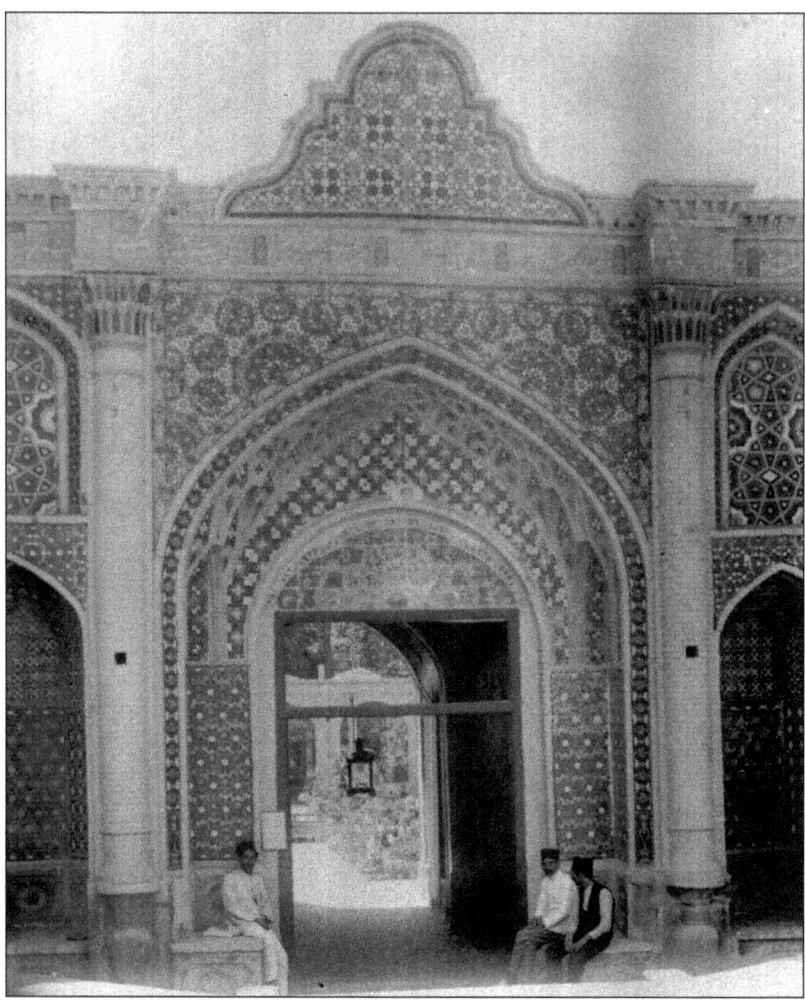

Above and opposite: Ahmadiyeh Hospital in Tehran

During 1923-1924 the hospital admitted 344 patients and treated 1,104 outpatients. In 1926, the hospital was transferred to the Ministry of Health.[134] In 1940, the Ministry transferred the 110 bed-hospital to

---

134. Gilmour 1924, pp. 26-27; Tajbakhsh 1379, pp. 240-42. Dr. Mehdi Malekzadeh was director for some time; in 1936 Dr. Jahanshah Saleh, a US-trained physician became director. Dr. Wilhelm and Dr. Roland, French physicians worked in the hospital until 1931. Dr. Mir then took over the surgical section and Dr. Mohammad Hesabi the medical section. Dr. Yahya

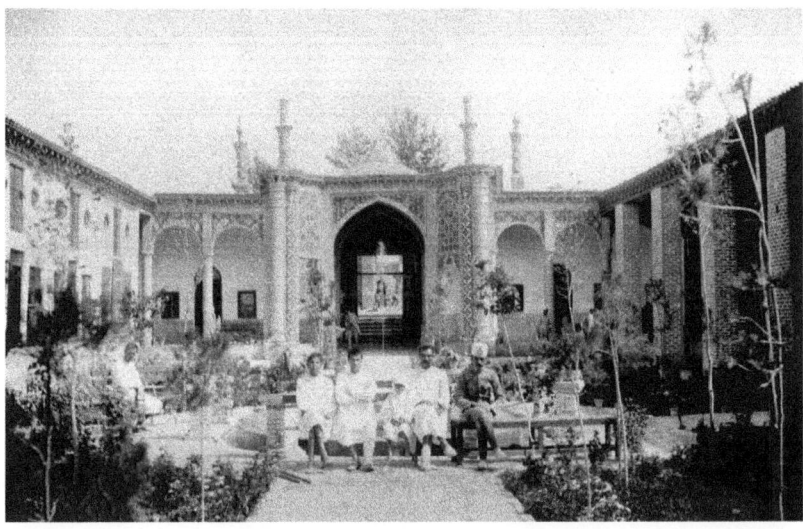

the medical faculty of the University of Tehran. The hospital became a leading medical institution and offered general medical services, obstetrics, had a dentistry polyclinic, X-ray facility, a laboratorium and pharmacy, specializing in otorhinolaryngology and ophthalmology.[135]

Third, the Women's Hospital (*Bimarestan-e Zanan*), a small one with 20 beds, had become really operational only in 1918. The proposal for the hospital had been submitted by Dr. Amir A`lam on 5 May 1915. The government adopted the idea already on 20 July 1915 and a government-owned building was assigned as the premises for the hospital. Two French midwives were supposed to have been hired to train Iranian midwives, but the outbreak of the Great War made that impossible. Instead the services of Mme Fraskina, who had been trained as a midwife in Europe and was working as such in Tehran, were engaged. When the hospital was officially opened much money was collected, but it was not enough to make the hospital functional. In 1916 there was no money to buy 50 beds and other equipment, but the Iranian government allocated 3,600 *tuman*s to pay for the staff. As a result the hospital functioned as a genealogical out-patients'

Mirza Lesan ol-Hokama established an ophthamology polyclinic in this hospital, which later was taken over by Dr. Bastan.

135. Karamati 1999, Iranicaonline.org.

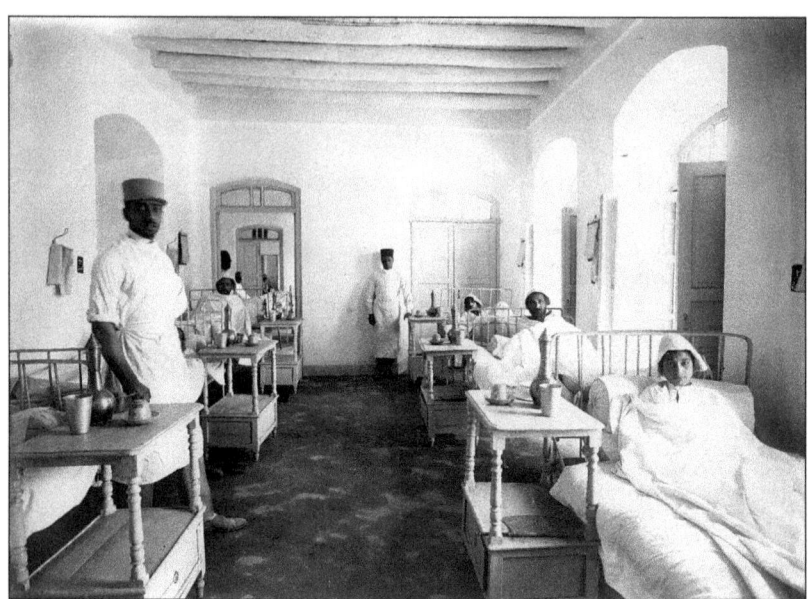

Ahmadiyeh Hospital ward patients and nurses pose for the photo.

dispensary, which, as of March 1916 until 1924, was managed by Dr. `Ali Reza Bahrami Mohadhdhab al-Saltaneh. In September 1918, the then Minister of Endowments (*Owqaf*) tried to raise funds to properly equip the building and turn it into a real hospital. He was only able to acquire funds to buy six beds, where from September 1918 until March 1919 about sixty women gave birth. During that period Mme. Fraskina trained 10 Iranian girls to become mid-wives. After the end of Great War funds became available to establish an internal medicine and surgical (obstetrics) department in the Women's Hospital, which was led by Dr. Sa`id Malek Loqman al-Mamalek. Mme Fraskina was replaced by a French female physician Dr. Dermes, who remained there until 1934. In that year Dr. Jahanshah Saleh became director of the hospital and was in charge of the obstetric department. Thereafter, the hospital served as training center for the Medical School for Women, while women continued to be admitted to give birth. During 1923-24, some 107 patients were admitted, 20 of whom suffered from malaria. Some 1,342 outpatients were treated, of whom 192 suffered from malaria. In 1921, the Medical School for Women had

13 students, who all belonged to the elite families; instruction was in French. They received a training of three years that was focused on women's diseases and obstetrics. On graduating the student received a diploma. They were not physicians, but more broadly trained than mid-wives.[136] In 1940, the hospital became part of the University of Tehran and in 1943 it moved to a new building, which was henceforth called *Jahanshah Saleh* Hospital (with 50 beds), while the old building was turned into the *Bimarestan-e Amir A'lam*, an otolaryngology clinic of the medical faculty.[137]

Fourth, was the *bimarestan-e baladiyeh* or Municipality's Hospital No. 1; it was renamed *Ruzbeh* Hospital in 1940 when it became affiliated with the Faculty of Medicine. In the mid-1950s it was turned into a psychiatric hospital with sixty beds, a clinic and a laboratory.[138]

Fifth, the so-called *Farabi* Hospital was situated in a garden, which the government of Iran acquired in 1921. Gilmour does not mention the Farabi hospital, but it was the same as what he called the *Municipality* Hospital. It had 72 beds (30 medical; 32 surgical; 10 isolation), one surgeon, four physicians, one ophthalmologist, one director of the laboratory, three medical interns, twelve male nurses, six nurses and two pharmacists. Its dispensary treated patients from all over Iran. In 1923 the hospital admitted 818 in-patients, while it treated some 50-80 out-patients daily. Like in the Imperial hospital many out-patients were treated in the open-air, some in tents, and others in the shade of the trees in the hospital garden. Although malaria was one of the major diseases none of the beds had a mosquito-net. The monthly budget for the hospital was 575 *tuman*s, of which 250 served to pay the staff.[139] From 1921 until 1940, with many interruptions it was the Municipality hospital, a.k.a. Hospital No. 2, and was then made available to the medical faculty of the University of Tehran, which renamed it the Farabi Hospital. The building was enlarged and

---

136. Gilmour 1924, p. 27.
137. Karamati 1999, Iranicaonline.org.
138. Karamati 1999, Iranicaonline.org.
139. Gilmour 1924, pp. 57-58.

became the ophthalmology clinic of the medical faculty, while it also housed part of the otolaryngology clinic.[140]

Sixth, the Sheikh Hadi hospital, which in 1921 had been revived and turned over to the French professors of the medical school to satisfy the French Minister's demand. This is probably the new government hospital mentioned by the American physicians, who reported that it was opened in Shahr-e Now giving free care to the poor. This meant that there were about 200 beds for the sick of the city, excluding the American hospital. The American physicians further reported in January 1922 that the municipality recently established a number of free dispensaries in different parts of the city and employed fairly well educated doctors. Patients were entitled to free examinations there. According to the local newspapers, they treated several 100 patients daily, but this number was expected to fall as the novelty wore off. As a result of these various development, the American physicians concluded that "we are no longer the only foremost center of modern medicine; ii, the practice of medicine in Tehran approximates that of Europe and the US."[141]

Under the Pahlavi regime more hospitals were built, both by the state and by private individuals. The *Najmiyeh Hospital* was founded by Dr. Mossadegh's mother Princess Malek Taj Firuz Najm al-Saltaneh as a charity hospital in 1928, and was located in the Khiyaban-e Hafez.[142] In 1933, the *Bimarestan-e Razi* was established in a large rented building. It had to serve the growing population of Tehran. In 1936, the hospital moved to a new large building that had been bought by Hajji Mohtasham al-Dowleh. From 1933 until 1939 the hospital director was Dr. Abbas Adham A'lam al-Molk. In 1940, the hospital became part of the medical faculty. It has 80 beds in the

---

140. Karamati 1999, Iranicaonline.org.
141. RG 91-19-11-1, Notes on medical work of Teheran station Jan. 1922.
142. Rosta'i 1382, vol. 1, pp. 532-539 (includes the text of the *vaqf-nameh*); Tajbakhsh 1379, pp. 242-243.

medical department, 80 in the surgical department, and 33 beds in the dermatology and VD department.[143]

The *Mo'tamed Hospital* in Khiyaban-e Sheikh Hadi, founded in 1930, was directed by its founder Dr. Hoseyn Khan Mo'tamed and a few leading physicians in Farvardin 1310/March 1931. It had 30 beds, private rooms and a men and women's ward, of which four were maternity/confinement beds and when the construction will be completed some 20 other beds will be added. Its polyclinic offers the following specialties: internal diseases, female diseases and obstetrics, VD, dental diseases and dentistry, pediatrics, and a chemical lab. Further, in 1932, the *Tutiya Hospital* under Dr. Mohammad Ali Khan Tutiya offered major and minor surgery such as hernia, appendicitis, bladder stone, gall bladder, fistula, hemorrhoids, goiter, tonsils, intestines and stomach (gastro-enterostomy), fractures, dislocated bones, etc. Dr. Tutiya further offered radioscopy, ultra-violet, as well as treatment for various forms of VD (with electricity), gynecology and obstetrics. The hospital also had a lab that could perform examinations of sputum, urine, stomach, feces, and do the Wasserman test, etc. Dr. Tutiya recommended people to read a book on VD to prevent being afflicted with it.[144]

In 1933, the *Hakim* Hospital was managed by Dr. Musa Khan (Hakim A'lam), a graduate from London University, who specialized in surgery, ophthalmology, VD and urology.[145] The Doctor *Rezanur Hospital* for radiology, electro-therapy, and hydro-therapy, occupied a three story building that was surrounded by a tree-lined garden, located in the Khiyaban-e Shah at the Rafael Cross roads and was officially opened in 1314/1935. It had public wards and private rooms and two beds with all modern accessories and German nurses. It offered a range of radiology and electro therapies. Dr. Musa Khan also offered treatment for TB with pneumo-thorax as well as rectosopic and systecopic examinations for intestinal diseases. The hospital had a full

---

143. Karamati 1999, Iranicaonline.org.
144. *Salnameh-ye Pars* 1311, Pt. 1, ads following p, 144.
145. *Salnameh-ye Pars* 1312, ad no 2, after p. 164.

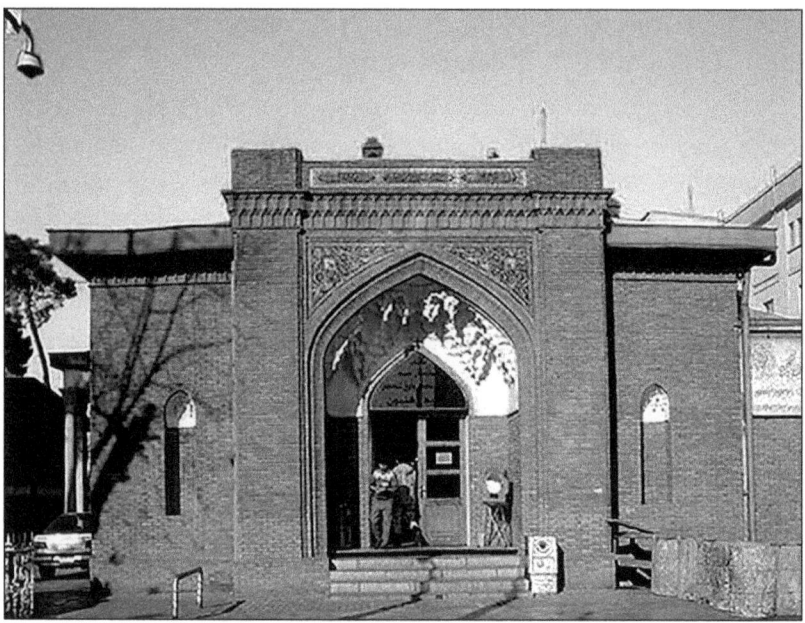

Above: Najmiyeh Hospital in Tehran.
Opposite: Ladies at the opening of the hospital.

lab for blood, urine, stomach acid, semen and feces exams. Dr. Musa Khan advertised his hospital as being the most modern of its kind in Tehran with equipment as recently used in France and manufactured by the German firm Sanitas. At great cost these machines had been transported to Iran. Dr. Musa Khan stressed the fact that there was no longer a need to go to Europe as the same treatment could be had there right in Tehran. Dr. Rezanur was a radiologist and internist who had studied in Germany and had been a deputy-physician in the Charité Hospital in Berlin, where he had become well-known.[146]

In 1934, two new hospitals were opened in south Tehran, which had a total of 150 beds. One of them was the *Firuzabadi Hospital*, which was officially opened in Shah `Abdol-`Azim on 25 Esfand 1313/16 March 1935. It was built by Mr. Firuzabadi, supported by the *Ettela`at* newspaper and obtained funds, which it channeled to the construction of this hospital. The state took responsibility of all cost

---

146. *Salnameh-ye Pars* 1315, pp. 190-94 [photos of hospital and machinery on 192 and 193

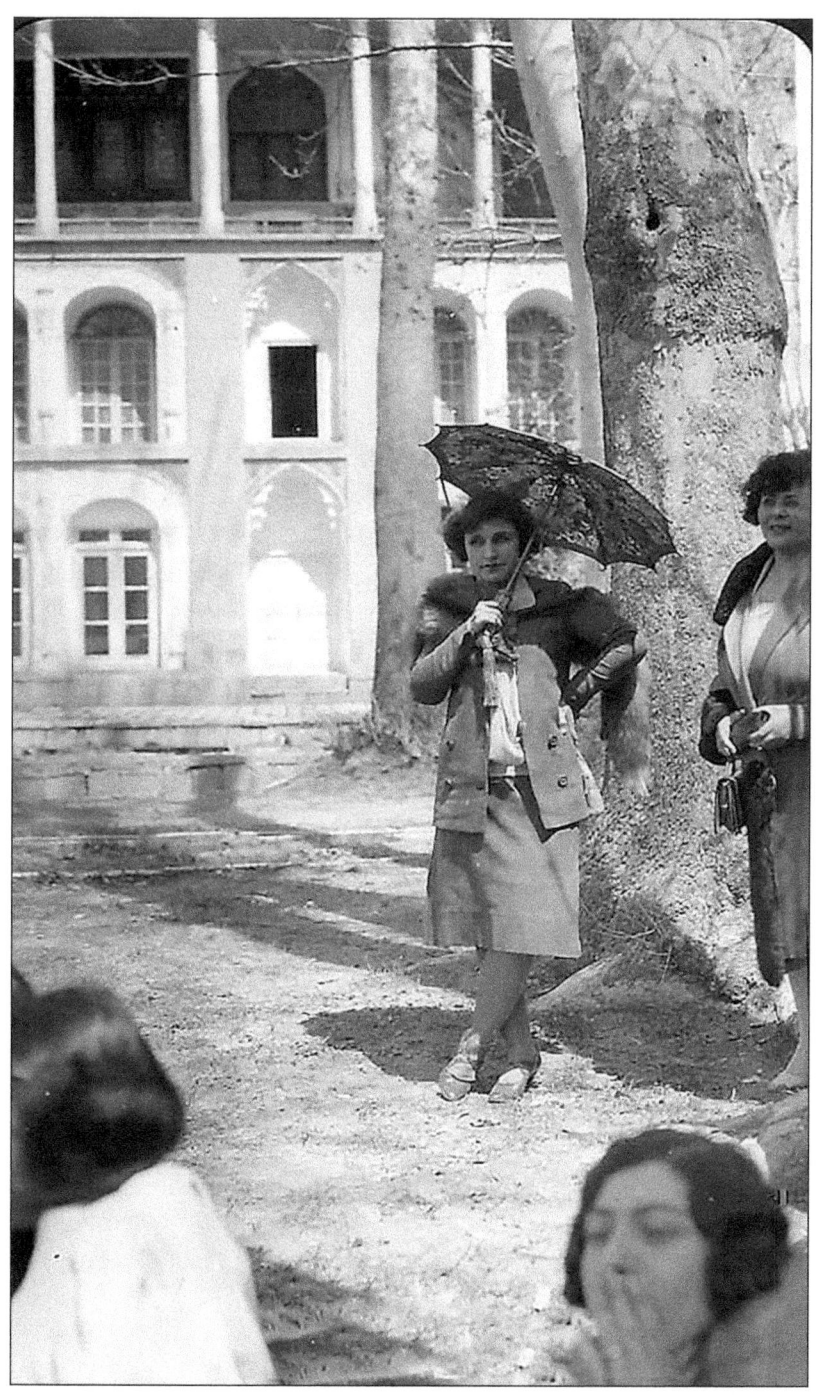

for staff, medicines and food.[147] The other may have been the *Baladiyeh Hospital* at Khiyaban-e Sirus under Dr. Aristu offered its services to the public, amongst which surgery and ophthalmology.[148] Many of the young Euro-trained Iranian doctors "can practice there and we hope that they will have the necessary equipment to carry on; at the moment they lack many of the essentials." Consequently, the presence of this hospital did not decrease the work of the other hospitals; in fact the American hospital experienced an increase of patients. This growth was seen as an indication of the growing appreciation for hospital treatment and care. Because the number of beds was still insufficient for Tehran's needs the government planned to build a 1,000-bed hospital outside and west to the city. The American doctors wondered whether the location was not too far from the city to attract patients, also, whether there would be sufficient staff for it.[149] This large hospital was completed in 1939 and called the Pahlavi Hospital. Originally designed for five hundred beds, it was further extended in the late 1940s-1960s and was one of the largest and best equipped hospitals in Tehran with over one thousand beds and various medical services.[150] In 1950, Ayatollah Hajj Sheikh `Abdol-Karim ordered that from the charitable offerings that he had received a hospital should be built. Initially it had only 12 beds. Religious leaders asked the Red Lion and Sun Society to support the extension of this hospital.[151]

---

147. Ettela`at 1329, p. 135. The hospital built by Hajji Sayyed Reza Firuzabadi was on a piece of land of 62,000 sq.m. and was situated on the old Shahr-e Rey road, above the `Abdollah Imamzadeh. He later built a mosque and an orphanage next to the hospital. Initially his salary as member of parliament was used to meet the operational cost of the hospital. Tajbakhsh 1379, pp. 243-244.

148. *Salnameh-ye Pars* 1315, part 1, p. 174 (photo of Aristu). Notes by Dr. `Allaj Aristu of the Municipal Hospital (*Baladiyeh*), *Salnameh-ye Pars* 1315, part 2, pp.111-46 a kind a medical guide.

149. RG 91-19-11-1, Report of Medical Work Teheran 1934; Idem, Report Tehran Medical Work 1934-1935.

150. Karamati 1999, Iranicaonline.org.

151. Ettela`at 1329, p. 57.

In addition, there were two army hospitals in Tehran, which exclusively treated army personnel. One, situated outside Tehran was housed in old barracks and had 150 beds although its capacity could be increased to 250 beds, and was led by three Russian civilians (administrator, surgeon and chief doctor) in 1924. These barracks had been transformed into a hospital by Dr. Amir Khan and opened its doors for business in 1914. The other army hospital, called the *Ahmadiyeh*, was in the center of Tehran and had a capacity of 50 beds, but was being extended to receive 100 in-patients. It had an important dispensary attached to it; the service was good and the patients were well looked after, but there was no regular disinfection of the clothing and bedding. Also, each regiment had a regimental physician as well as a dispensary, and thus the army had a better medical organization than civil society.[152] In 1950, the army hospital was opened by the shah on 4 Shahrivar (26 August 1950) and was named hospital no. 2, after hospital no. 1 at Yusofabad. This means that the *Ahmadiyeh* hospital had been closed down. It had a capacity of 200 beds and had a surgery, ophthalmology, internal diseases, contagious (*mosriyeh*) diseases, and a dentistry department. At the same time, a teaching facility for female nurses was opened, which lasted eight months. It also had a bathhouse and a kitchen.[153]

Finally, for completeness' sake, the existence of the mental asylum or *dar al-majanin* has to be mentioned. Until 1905 there was no facility in Tehran to receive and treat psychiatric patients. However, in that year, after complaints to the police about mad people going about naked in the streets, the Minister of Police, Sa`id al-Saltaneh sent them to the Imperial Hospital. In consultation with Dr. Luf [Loew?] and Dr. Abu Torab a psychiatric ward was constructed there at the minister's expense. This seems to have consisted of four to five small

---

152. Gilmour 1924, pp. 30-31; Rosta'i 1382, vol. 2, p. 125. For a picture and description of the first army hospital see Shahri 1368, vol. 1, p. 295. The Ahmadiyeh was situated in the Khiyaban-e Sepah and the other hospital (later known as Pahlavi) in Yusofabad, Rosta'i 1382, vol. 1, p. 179. The latter probably was the hospital built by Vajihollah Mirza Sepahsalar.

153. Ettela`at 1329, p. 116.

rooms closed with an iron door in an isolated part of the Imperial Hospital. Because psychiatric cases, who were a public nuisance, were the responsibility of the police it was at the initiative of general Westdahl, the Swedish chief of police of Tehran (1922-24) that a separate and larger mental institution was built in Akbarbad. The building had four rooms above ground and four below ground. In one of the rooms below ground there were four dark narrow cells to hold agitated patients. Treatment of the patients was harsh. There was one orderly per 50 patients. The orderlies, who were bullies, used violence to keep order, while the food that patients received was bad and insufficient. In short, the patients suffered not only from their illness, but also from poor treatment, hunger and bad food. According to Shahri, referring to a later period, apart from real mental cases, most of the inmates of the mental hospital were there for political, financial or other non-medical reasons.[154]

Abadan

Since 1914, the British APOC maintained its own medical service for its staff, although it also extended its gratis services (including dental treatment) to the local population who did not have any relationship with the Company. The Abadan hospital, one of the most modern in the Middle-East, was one of the three hospitals the APOC operated (see also Ahvaz and Masjed-e Soleyman), as well as 12 separate dispensaries: nine in the Fields, one at Mohammarah, one at Bawardah, and one at the refinery.

Table 5: Number of patients treated and of activities undertaken in Abadan APOC hospital (1926)

Activity	Number
Hospital in-patients	2,228
Out-patients (a) new cases	40,129
(b) attendances	137,169

---

154. *Ruznameh-e ye soltani va Iran* 1380, year 58, nr. 11, p. 2 (10 Jomadi II 1323/12 August 1905), p. 346; Shahri 1368, vol. 1, pp. 436-437; Rosta'i 1382, vol. 1, pp. 488, 522-524 (with more details about its lay-out and use of the various available spaces). For a photograph of the asylum see Afshar 1371, p. 349.

Activity	Number
Major operations	214
Minor operations	1,815
Pathological examinations	4,733
Dental cases	892
X-ray photographs	99

Source: Williamson 1927, p. 130.

The Abadan hospital had a capacity of about 100 beds (36 for administrative staff and 60 for workmen plus special private wards), an out-patient department and a dispensary, a dental surgery, an operation room, a pathology laboratory, a disinfection station and X-ray equipment. In 1926, the hospital at Abadan treated more than 180,000 patients, or some 500 per day. At that time, its population was about 30,000 and growing. The APOC employed a senior medical officer, two resident medical officers, a visiting medical officer, a consulting surgeon, a pathologist, and an ophthalmologist. These were assisted by 26 local nurses under a European matron and assisted by eight European nurses.[155] By 1940, the AIOC had a hospital had air condition with 140 beds, which could be extended to 160 beds. There was room for an additional 100 beds in the clerks' and other buildings. S.E. of Bawarda, there was an isolation hospital with 60 beds as well as as a segregation camp of two separate enclosures. This had cookhouses and latrines. The hospital had all the equipment and facilities mentioned above, but not as yet a portable X-ray machine. It was planned to enlarge the pathology lab. The hospital had a steam clothing disinfector, which took care of the hospital's laundry work.[156] Together with the hospital in Mohammareh it maintained dispensaries at Ahvaz, Kut Abdollah, Dorquain, Gach Qaragoli(Gach Saran), Ganaveh and Agha Jari.[157]

---

155. Williamson 1927, pp. 128-132; Gilmour 1924, p. 39.
156. IOR/L/MIL/17/15/24, 'Military Report on Oilfield Area', p. 49.
157. IOR/L/MIL/17/15/24, 'Military Report on Oilfield Area', pp. 49-50.

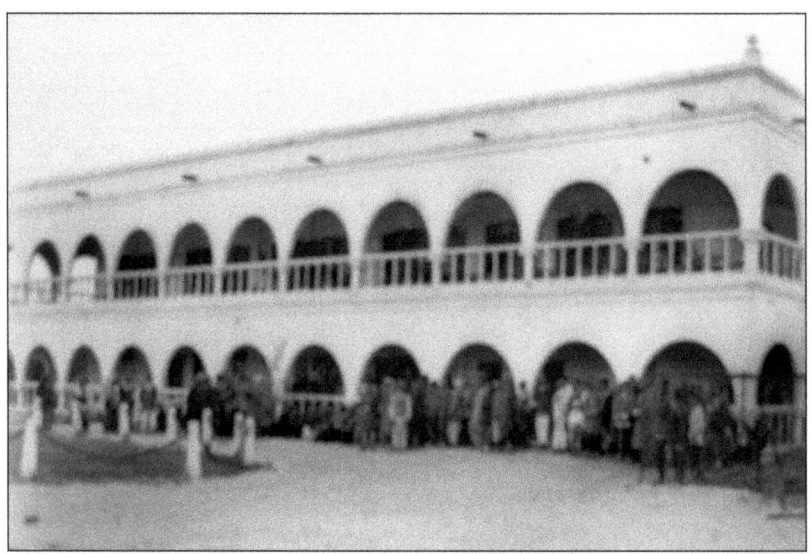

Above: Administrative building and nurses residence, APOC Abadan hospital, showing patients lined up early in the morning. *Opposite:* Staff of the APOC hospital.

Ahvaz

In 1914 or thereabouts, Ahvaz had an estimated population of 12,000 and no modern medical institutions.[158] In January 1906, a hospital assistant arrived at the British Consulate. However, as yet, no medical equipment had arrived. However, with the remainder of the drugs received in 1904, and with help from Mohammareh, it was possible to treat the gunshot wounds of 8 Persian soldiers.[159] In May 1906, medical supplies and instruments arrived with Capt. Crossle, IMS who was consular surgeon for the consulates in Ahvaz and Kermanshah. Because he could not stay long he was unable to immediately organize the dispensary arrangements. As of January 1907, suitable quarters were rented for "the joint occupancy of the Hospital Assistant, Dispensary, and Head Clerk." For the time being there only was one hospital assistant and one *farrash*. In June-July 1906, Capt. Crossle accompanied the vice-consul on tour and treated patients en route where

---

158. Administration Report 1919, p. 10.
159. Administration Report 1905-06, p. 36.

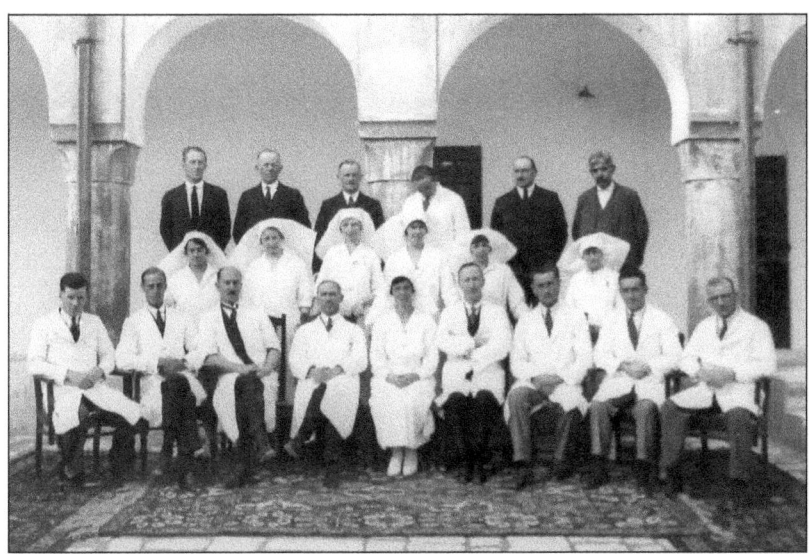

feasible. In February 1907, the superintendency of medical arrangement was transferred from Kermanshah to the Bushehr Residency surgeon. Daily attendance of the dispensary was 42 patients per day; no operations were performed.[160] The sick in Ahvaz also could receive gratis treatment at the dispensary. In 1907-08, the dispensary was open throughout the year. The daily average attendance rose from 44 during April-November to 84 patients per day during December-March. Those coming for treatment were not only local inhabitants, but also Bedouin Arabs and even people from Shushtar and Dezful.[161] In 1908, the dispensary was closed from 6 May to 17 December, because the hospital-assistant accompanied the vice-consul on tour. How much its services were appreciated became clear when the community of Naseri learnt that the dispensary would be temporarily closed. A number of community leaders then came to ask the vice-consul to leave Fazl Elahi, the hospital-assistant, "and painted in gloomy colours the fate which would otherwise befall them. Providence, however, does not appear to have combined with opportunity to rid the community of any of its leading lights." Average attendance during that year 93

---

160. Administration Report 1906-07, pp. 24-25.
161. Administration Report 1907-08, p. 29.

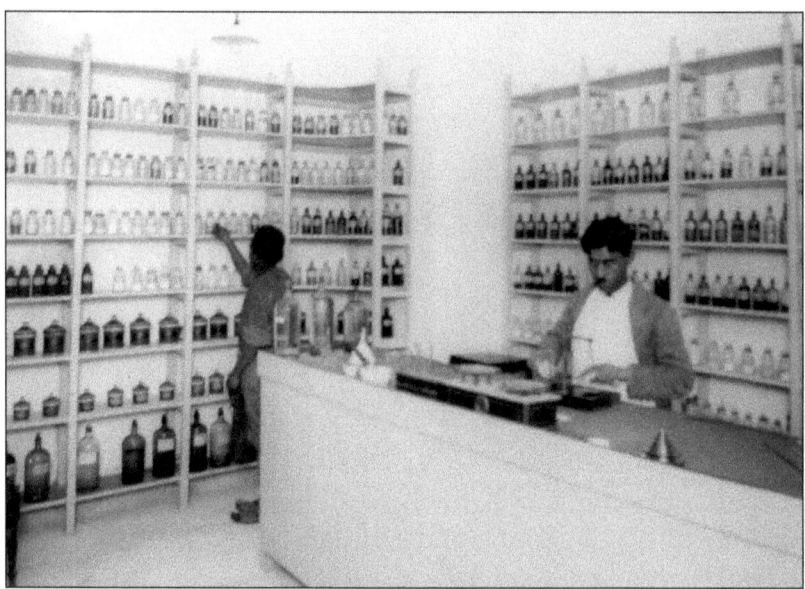

Above: APOC Hospital dispensary. *Opposite:* The operating room.

patients per day, a considerable increase compared with the preceding two years, an increase that the vice-consul ascribed to Fazl Elahi's "greater suitability" than his predecessor.[162]

In 1909, the dispensary again was closed for part of the year (24 May till 26 November) because the hospital assistant accompanied the consul on tour. During the time that the dispensary was open daily average attendance was 93 patients, while 67 operations were performed, i.e. 28 more than in 1908. During the tour the daily average patients treated was 12. The main diseases treated were eye diseases and malaria, both in the province and among the hill tribes. In the town itself epidemics of small-pox in the spring and malaria and dysentery" in the fall and winter months. Since the dispensary was opened the 1909 malaria epidemic was the first recorded.[163] In 1910, again the dispensary was closed from 27 March to 23 October due to the consul's tour. Daily average attendance was 105 patients per day, while 57 operations were performed. "On tour an average of

---

162. Administration Report 1908, p. 21.
163. Administration Report 1909, p. 52.

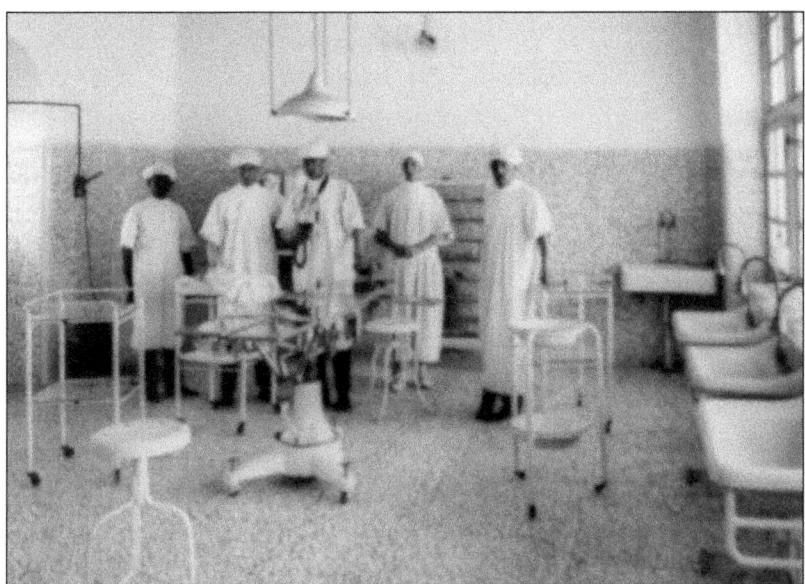

31 patients were treated per day. Eye diseases, malaria and worm are the most common diseases in the province and among the hill tribes; while in Ahvaz small-pox, measles, whooping cough, influenza and sporadic cholera in December 1910."[164]

In October 1915, sub-assistant surgeon Fazl Elahi was invalided to India. Dr. Moir of the APOC looked after the dispensary till the arrival of sub-assistant surgeon Atta Mohammad, who remained in charge of the dispensary throughout 1916. In 1915, the total number of new patients treated was 12,065 and 380 major and minor surgeries were performed.[165] Atta Mohammad remained in charge of the dispensary until 1 July 1917, when the dispensary was absorbed by the new Civil Hospital, which was managed by assistant surgeon K.S. Dick until the arrival of Captain T.H. Bishop, IMS as civil surgeon on 11 September.[166] Atta Mohammad continued to work at the Civil Hospital in 1918,

---

164. Administration Report 1910, p. 63.
165. Administration Report 1915, p. 35; Administration Report 1916, pp. 54, 59 (5,627 patients, 171 minor and 1 major operations).
166. Administration Report 1917, p. 37.

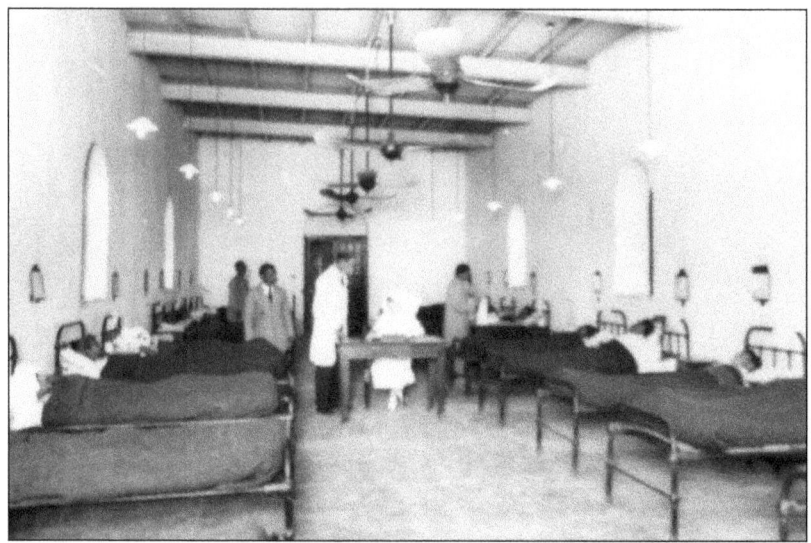

APOC Hospital "Persian" ward

1919, and 1920.[167] The Civil Hospital had grown from a charitable dispensary to a 30-bed hospital in 1919.

> Except for the pay of the Civil Surgeon, and a Sub-Assistant Surgeon, it is self-supporting and it is hoped to arrange for its activities to extend to Dizful and Shushtar in the future. The cost of drugs, however, a large item of expenditure, which has up till quite lately been bore by the Iraq revenues, will no doubt seriously hamper the work of the hospital if further local support is not forthcoming. Patients of all classes from Bakhtiari, Kuhgilu and Luristan attend, and its undoubted political value cannot be under-estimated.
> The Civil Surgeon is also responsible for the organisation of the Municipality and is thus able to

---

167. Administration Report 1918, p. 43; Administration Report 1919, p. 44; Administration Report 1920, p. 41, 44 (the civil surgeon continued to supervise the santation of the town, Capt. J.B. Lewis left for Great Britain on 30/03/1920 and was replaced by Major A.C. Oldham).

control the sanitation of the town, the cleanliness of which compares very favourably with any other in the East.[168]

In 1921 it was reported that "the Civil Hospital treated 2,236 outdoor and 221 indoor patients; 14 major and 175 minor operations." This was a good result as in that same year the civil surgeon died and there was no replacement for him. The consul, therefore, proposed to abolish the hospital and revive the old charitable dispensary.[169] As a result, the Civil Hospital was closed in March 1922, but probably due to lack of funds, the charitable dispensary closed as of November 1922. Efforts were then made to open a town dispensary funded by public donations.[170] This does not seem to have met with success as nothing more is heard about the matter. Perhaps the effort was abandoned, because in 1921 it was made public that the APOC would establish a new hospital at Ahvaz, staffed with one medical officer and two nurses, which hospital indeed was operational in 1922.[171] It was set up with similar equipment, staff and capacity as the APOC hospitals in Abadan and Masjed-e Soleyman (q.v.).[172]

Table 6: Attendance and operation at Ahvaz Civil Hospital (1918-1920)

	1916	1917	1918	1919	1920
Indoor patients	-	-	662	670	452
Outdoor patients	5,627	6,661	5,104	6,383	3,235
Major operations	1	8	29	55	60
Minor operations	171	296	189	358	420

Source: Administration Report 1916, p. 59; Ibid. 1917, p. 40; Ibid. 1918, p. 45-46; Ibid. 1919, p. 48; Ibid., 1920, pp. 44-45.

---

168. Administration Report 1919, pp. 44-45.
169. Administration Report 1921, p. 43.
170. Administration Report 1922, p. 43.
171. Administration Report 1921, p. 43; Williamson 1927, p. 124. However, in 1933 the British consul in Ahvaz refers to the move of a dispensary to another place. IOR/L/PS/12/3650, Consul Ahvaz to Amb. R.H. Hoare, Tehran, 27/03/1933.
172. Williamson 1927, p. 124.

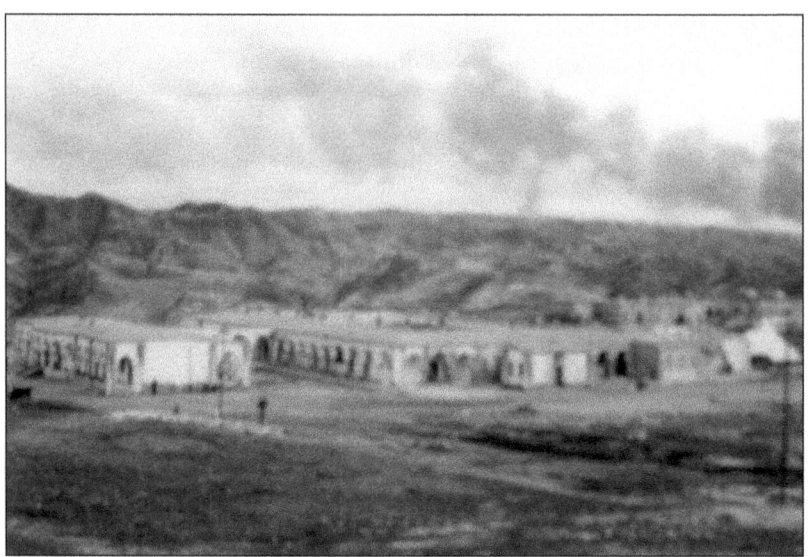

APOC Masjed-e Soleyman complex

In January 1931, a 10-bed hospital for the poor was opened by the Municipality of Ahvaz. In addition, there also was the APOC's Oil Fields hospital in the same town[173] as well as a military hospital[174] and a railway hospital.[175] The Anglo-Iranian Oil Company (AIOC) continued to operate a 'field hospital', which in 1942 was qualified as a dispensary, in Ahvaz with six beds that was associated with the hospital of Abadan. In other buildings there was room for 50 beds.[176] On 9 August 1933, news was received that Mirza Hoseyn Khan Moqavvar, deputy for Mohammerah had died in Tehran and had provided in his will for the construction of a charitable hospital at Ahvaz; cost estimated at 400,00Rls.[177] On 20 October 1933, a meeting was held of

---

173. IOR/L/PS/12/3400, Diary of HBM's Consul for Khuzestan, Ahwaz, no. 1, for the month of January 1931, p. 3.
174. IOR/L/PS/12/3400, Diary of HBM's Consul for Khuzestan, Ahwaz, no. 6, 1933 for the month of June 1933, p. 2.
175. IOR/L/PS/12/3400, HBM's Consulate for Khuzistan, Ahwaz, Diary no. 4 for the month of April 1933, p. 3.'
176. IOR/L/MIL/17/15/24, 'Military Report on Oilfield Area', p. 49.
177. IOR/L/PS/12/3400, Diary of HBM's Consul for Khuzestan, Ahwaz,

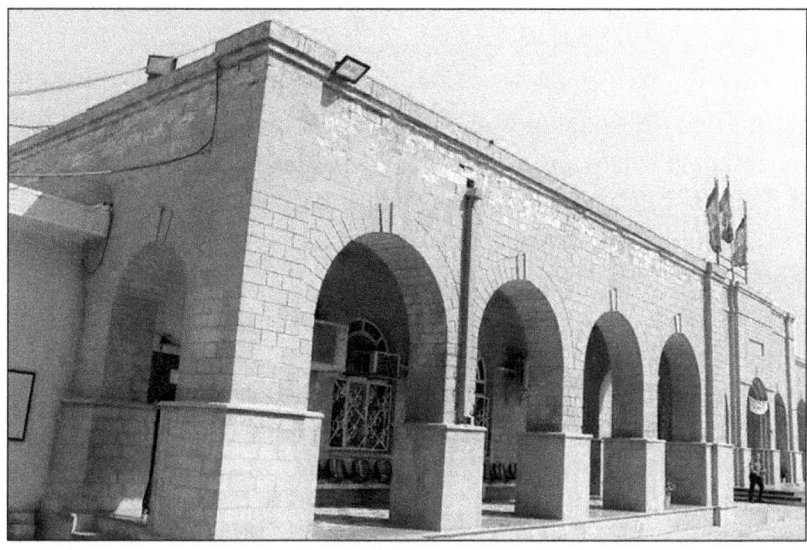

Jondishahpur Hospital, Reza Shah period.

department heads and notables to elect the members of the Red Lion and Sun Society. "The construction of a hospital from the estate of the late Aqa Moqavvar was discussed and also the expenditure of the sum of Tomans 13,500 which has been collected from the public. The majority of the Persian officials proposed that the existing Baladieh Hospital should be improved and enlarged from the funds standing to the credit of the Red Lion and Sun Society."[178]

In the 1930s, there also was a dispensary run by Dr. D'Souza, who also took care of the health needs of the British colony in Ahvaz, but as of 1935 he was not "allowed by the Iranian regulations to have his own dispensary or to dispense his own medicines."[179]

---

no. 6, 1933 for the month of June 1933, p. 3.

178. IOR/L/PS/12/3400, Diary of HBM's Consul for Khuzestan, Ahwaz, no. 9 of 1933 for the period of 21st October 1933 to 30th November 1933, p. 4.

179. IOR/L/PS/12/3400, Diary of HBM's Consul for Khuzestan, Ahwaz, no. 10 of 1933 for the month of December 1933, p. 2; IOR/L/PS/12/3592, copy letter no. 540 from vice-consul Mohammarah to Pol. Resident Persian Gulf, 07/06/1935 [Reduction of medical expenditure'].

Arak

In 1914 the British Church Missionary Society (CMS) allegedly established a hospital in Arak or Soltanabad, a town of some 20,000 inhabitants.[180] However, it does not seem to have been started or, if it did, not to have lasted very long for there is no mention at all to be found of this hospital or of activities by the CMS in the local histories of Arak.[181] Moreover, in various CMS tracts (Linton, Rice, etc.) no mention is made of any activity in Arak, while they list their medical facilities in Isfahan, Yazd, Kerman and Shiraz. However, in 1926, the Seventh Day Adventists, a Protestant denomination, opened a dispensary in Soltanabad led by the Iranian Dr. Arezu, who shortly thereafter, in 1929, established a 15-bed hospital. In the early 1930s, the dispensary treated 4,000 patients per year or 12,000 treatments. The in-patients had to pay a fixed amount per day per bed, which barely covered fifty percent of the variable operating cost of the hospital.[182] Apparently, by the end of the 1930s this hospital was "virtually inoperative."[183] In 1960, the same organization still operated a 10-bed hospital in Arak.[184] It is sad to see that this medical service of more than 45 years is not even mentioned in a book that claims to provide a complete overview of Arak.[185]

---

180. Elgood 1951, p. 535.
181. Tabrizi 1966-1967, pp. 362-460; Dehgan 1950.
182. The average daily pay of a worker in Iran was 60 *pfennig*, while the cost per bed was 100 *pfennig*, which was a great burden for patients, Rühling 1934, pp. 82-85. Already in 1913 there was a call to US physicians to fill a vacancy in Soltanabad. Muirhead 1913, p. 205; Anonymous 1913, p. 205. the missionary societies of the Students Volunteer Movements advertised with vacancies for physicians in Tehran, Soltanabad and Senneh, and one for the North Khorasan district. In Soltanabad, Dr. Arzo, a Seven-Day Adventist doctor, was working. RG 231-1-6, Hoffman, Pioneering in Meshed, p. 12. In 1929, he was assisted by a British engineer, Henry E. Hargreaves. *Yearbook Royal Society* 1932, p. xviii.
183. DeNovo, 1963, p. 315.
184. CARE 1961, p. 10.
185. Mohtat 1368.

ASHURADEH

There was a small hospital of 14 beds established by the Russian government on the island of Ashuradeh in 1848 to treat its naval as well as Russian consular staff in the Caspian littoral, although the date of its establishment may have been earlier.[186] In 1844 there were no buildings on the island. Holmes described it as follows at that time: "The only habitations are two large sail-cloth tents, occupied by the sick. [...] They were much exposed in these tents, and a building of wood was in the course of construction as an hospital."[187] Twenty years later Melgunof reported that there were some wooden buildings on the island, amongst which he mentioned "the hospital, a house for both physicians (one for the Russian, the other for the Persian)."[188] The hospital is not mentioned in a description of the island around 1900.[189]

BANDAR ABBAS

Given the fact that Bandar Abbas had 20,000 inhabitants by 1914, almost as many as Bushehr,[190] and no medical facilities or even an Iranian physician,[191] it was no surprise that the British consul submitted that, "A charitable dispensary was sadly required at Bunder Abbas owing to the large numbers of the very poor. One was opened under the charge of the Quarantine Medical officer in March 1906 and does an immense amount of good in reliving suffering, apart from the political

---

186. Elgood 1951, p. 512; Teymuri 1363, pp. 269-271, who also reports that Russia in addition obtained a concession for the establishment of a hospital in Astarabad. In 1848, the Russians had first asked for such a concession at Gaz, the port of Astarabad, while in 1850 they were again denied to build a hospital there despite a renewed request, although later (with more success) they asked for permission to build a hospital at Astarabad, see Kazembeyki 2003, pp. 55-57, 124. However, the Russians did not build a hospital in Astarabad, at least no published source mentions it.
187. Holmes 1845, p. 250.
188. Melgunof 1868, p. 75.
189. Adamec 1981, vol. 2, p. 32.
190. Administration Report 1919, p. 10.
191. Sadid al-Saltaneh 1342, p. 169.

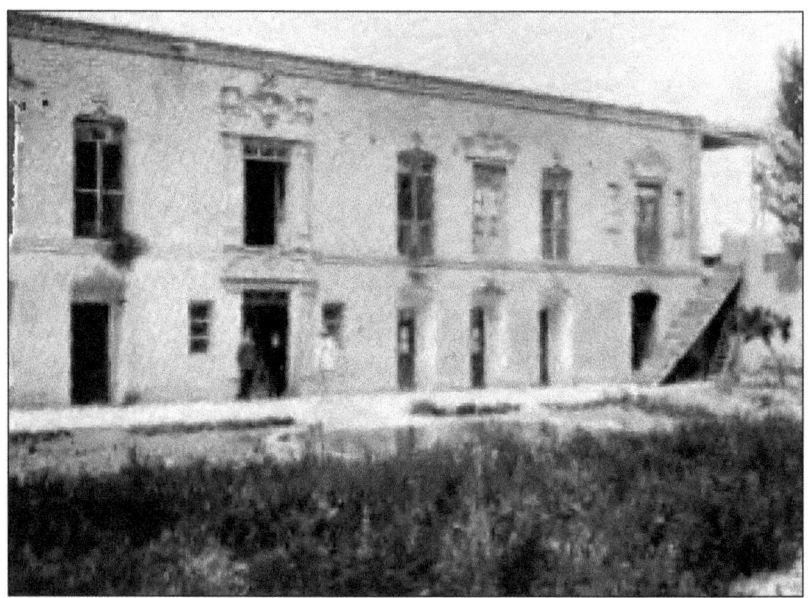

Hospital in Arak

influence which such institutions always bring in their train in Persia."[192] Although the dispensary was well received and was a great benefit to the population the consul opined, "At the same time, the advisability of placing the equipment for a charitable dispensary in the hands of a subordinate who is not precluded from taking fees and engaging in private practice, is thought to be open to question, while the fact that in this case, the individual is the Quarantine Medical Officer and as such a the servant of the Persian Sanitary Administration, has the effect of concealing the source of benevolence from those visiting the dispensary and thus there results no political influence."[193] The consul, therefore, argued that the dispensary should be moved from the Quarantine station to the new consulate that was to be ready in 1909. "The charitable dispensary is indeed a boon to the poor who swarm in Bunder Abbas and now that free treatment has become a regular feature, the shifting of the local from the Quarantine Medical Officer's house to the Consulate will bring yet more prominently before the

---

192. Administration Report 1905-06, p. 59.
193. Administration Report 1906-07, p. 50. However, Sadid al-Saltaneh 1342, p. 169 was quite aware that the British government, not the Quarantine Service, provided the medical services to the public.

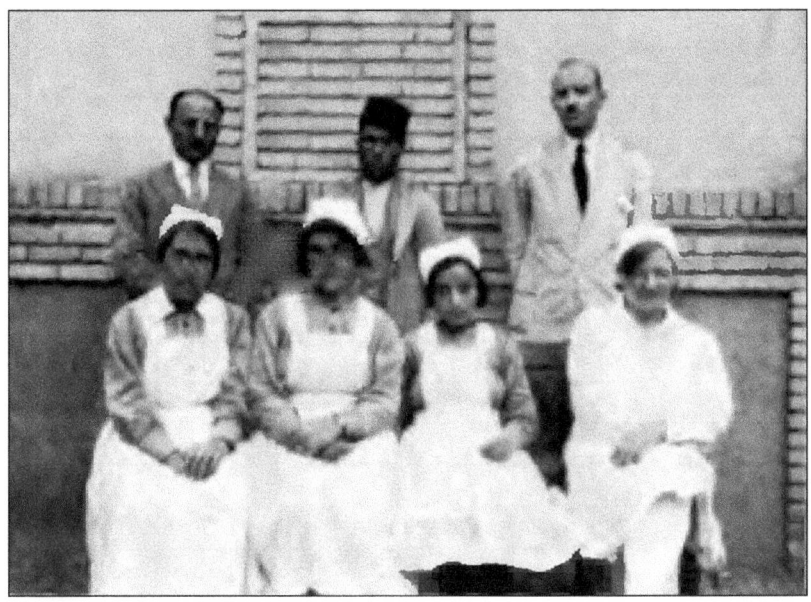

Hospital staff in Arak

public that their well-being is closely identified with the British flag."[194] Attendance remained steadily increasing thereafter, while the opening of the new charitable dispensary in 1920 provided a considerable additional boost to attendance.[195] In British administrative parlance it was a second class dispensary with an assistant surgeon Indian Subordinate Medical Department (ISMD), who was the quarantine officer of the port. From 1915 to 1921, at the British military camp at Naiband there was a 5th class dispensary with 30 beds under and IMS officer and two sub-assistant surgeons.[196]

---

194. Administration Report 1908, p. 63.
195. Administration Report 1920, p. 18.
196. IOR/L/MIL/17/15/6/1, 'Military Report on Persia. vol. iv, part i,' p. 79. The Indian Subordinate Medical Department (ISMD) was the uncovenanted branch of the medical service (as opposed to the covenanted Indian Medical Service). It was formed in 1812 to provide medical services to Indian natives. Initially, the senior positions were occupied by persons of British origin. Thereafter Anglo-Indians and later also native Indians were able to gain the more senior positions. The Indian Medical Service (IMS) was a military medical service in British-India. Many of its officers, who were both British and Indian, served in civilian hospitals.

Table 7: The number of new out-patients treated and of operations performed in the Bandar Abbas British dispensary (1908-31).

Year	New patients	Operations
1908	1,894	-
1910	2,855	-
1911	2,345	-
1912	2,879	-
1913	2,092	-
1916	3,122	-
1917	3,388	-
1918	3,889	-
1919	3,673	-
1920	4,279	92
1921	4,215	182
1922	4,526	195
1923	4,425	-
1924	4,419	-
1925	5,848	258
1926	7,450	280
1927	6,568	-
1928	7,620	-
1929	6,664	-
1930	7,432	-
1931	7,002	-

Source: Administration Report 1908, p. 63; Ibid., 1899-1900; Ibid., 1912, p. 47; Ibid., 1913, p. 48; Ibid., 1917, p. 13; Ibid., 1918, p. 16; Ibid., 1919, p. 19; Ibid., 1920, p. 18; Ibid., 1921, p. 19; Ibid., 1922, p. 19-20; Ibid., 1923, p. 35; Ibid., 1924, p. 27; Ibid., 1925, p. 36; Ibid. 1926, p. 21; Ibid., 1927, p. 18 (drop due to quarantine imposed due to cholera); Ibid., 1928, p. 29; Ibid., 1929, p. 24; Ibid, 1931, p. 28.

The major diseases treated at the dispensary were malaria, eye and skin diseases, which three accounted for 52.5% of total admissions in 1908.[197] Vaccinations were also given.[198] The British consul believed that the dispensary created if not political influence it most certainly would get good-will and he was right. For, although a British operated and funded institution, it filled an enormous need. It was the only medical institution in town and in the region and its services were free and therefore it also received local support from the most influential persons in Bandar Abbas. For example, in 1924, "The floor of the operation room was repaired and the expense met by Haji Sheikh Ahmed Galledary, a local merchant. A well was built in the compound of the dispensary which supplied a great need, the expense in this case being met by Haji Mukhtar Divani another local merchant. The latter is erecting at his own expense ten small cubicles for the purpose of accommodating poor persons coming in from distant villages for treatment at the dispensary. When completed the cubicles will be of great convenience to the poor."[199] Similarly, the next year, "The roof was replastered paid by Haji Mukhtar Divani, while Haji Sheikh Ahmed Galledary paid for the cost of extra drugs and dressings of Rs 520."[200]

D.L. Mackay IMD, who was the quarantine officer of the port, was also in charge of the British Consulate's dispensary and the town's charitable dispensary. When he went on leave in mid-July 1925 he was replaced by ass. surgeon A.L. Greenway, IMD. The number of operations increased from 246 (1923), 186 (1924) to 258 in 1925. These comprised incisions of abcesses, of tumors, extractions of cataracts, iridectomies, extraction of teeth, etc. A craniotomy was performed to remove a dead full term foetus. All operated cases recovered.[201] When D.L. Mackay returned to resume his functions

---

197. Administration Report 1908, p. 63; for further data see Administration Report 1921, p. 19; Administration Report 1922, p. 19; Administration Report 1923, p. 35, Idem 1925, p. 36.
198. Administration Report 1907-08, p. 74.
199. Administration Report 1924, p. 27.
200. Administration Report 1925, p. 36.
201. Administration Report 1925, p. 36. The Indian Medical Department (IMD)

in 1926, he found that the number of outdoor patients had increased considerably as compared with the previous years, which was partly due to the fact that caravan men coming from the interior also attended to dispensary for treatment.[202]

In the summer of 1927, cholera broke out in Minab, and through fleeing people almost reached Bandar Abbas. The central government sent three doctors by air from Tehran with anti-cholera vaccine. At the dispensary more than 10,000 persons came to be inoculated, as well as many others on the islands and nearby villages. As a result of these and other preventive measures only four deaths occurred and cholera did not reach the town. Contrariwise, in Minab and environs 4-5,000 people died. The gratis service by the dispensary was greatly appreciated by the half-starved people.[203] Dr. MacKay left after 7 years of service and was succeeded by Dr. J. E. Sweeney on 16 February 1928 as consular physician. On 1 August 1928 Dr. Sweeney was relieved by Dr. Mohammad Ali Khan Moayed Hikmat as quarantine officer of Bandar Abbas at orders from Tehran, which replaced all British quarantine physicians in the Persian Gulf ports.[204] Dr. Sweeney remained in charge of the British consular dispensary. The government of India continued to make its services available at no cost and also provided many medicines annually, but, because the funds for its maintenance were low the dispensary might have to close, the consul reported, unless the merchant community came forward with

---

dates back to 19th century. Initially starting as compounders and dressers in the three Presidency Medical Services they became Sub Surgeons and later on as Indian Medical Assistants in Indian Regiments. In 1868, they were redesignated as Hospital Assistants. In 1900, the Senior Hospital Assistants were granted the rank of Viceroy's Commissioned Officers and in 1910 the designation was finally changed to Sub Assistant Surgeons of IMD. They primarily worked with the Indian troops, see, e.g., Lt. Col. D.G. Crawford, *Roll of the Indian Medical Service 1615-1930*, 2 vols. London, 1930, vol. 1, p. xliv.

202. Administraton Report 1926, p. 20.
203. Administraton Report 1927, p. 18.
204. Administraton Report 1928, p. 29. For a discussion of this change of the quarantine guard, see Floor 2018 a, pp. 65-67.

subscriptions.[205] Dr. Sweeney remained in function until 10 August 1930, when he was relieved by sub-asstistant surgeon and Jemadar Abdur Rahim IMD. The dispensary continued to function well, but its poor finances made its closure seem inevitable. The leading merchants of Bandar Abbas, who so far had generously contributed could not be expected to continue to do so, given the adverse trade conditions plus the high taxes. Also, the dispensary was no longer a political asset for the British as was originally planned when it was established. "In my opinion the Persian Government is being encouraged to evade its obligations to the local community to whom no medical aid is afforded as a 'quid pro quo' for rates and taxes paid." The municipality did not contribute anything for its upkeep.[206] In 1931, Jemadar Rahim was in charge of the dispensary. Because funds had been running low for the past few years there was a need for further subscription to meet higher cost. Moreover, closing the dispensary would be necessary in the near future despite its benefit to the population, "especially as it is intended to withdraw the Medical Officer from the Consulate and to abolish that post."[207] Established at the urging of the British consul in 1919 by public subscription the dispensary/hospital remained under his control until 23 January 1932, when it was closed down, when the post of Consular medical officer was abolished, who used to be there daily at no cost. On 7 November 1932 the hospital was transferred to the governor. He was able to raise Rs. 24,000 by subscription to enable the re-opening of the dispensary. Dr. Kaikobad Hormisji Dumree, an ex IMD employee, and medical practitioner from Kerman, was negotiating with the governor to become its medical officer.[208]

The charitable dispensary, henceforth called *Sehhiyeh Baladiyeh* (Municipal Health Department), was reopened on 14 February 1933 with Dr. Dumree, as medical officer. However, those having given money did not like this name and insisted that it be called *mariz-khaneh-ye melli* (National Hospital). Because the dispensary was

---

205. Administration Report 1929, p. 24.
206. Administration Report 1930, p. 22.
207. Administration Report 1931, p. 27.
208. Administraton Report 1932, p. 20.

well-known from the past it was more visited than the quarantine office. Because of paucity of staff no operations were performed. It was intended to have six beds, but this was cancelled. Only serious cases were admitted as in-patients, who were then cared for by friends and relatives. Whether it would continue after March 1934 was unknown as Dr. Dumree, wo treated consular medical cases free of charge, did not like to work with so few staff.[209] At the beginning of the summer 1934 the dispensary was closed as Dr. Dumree resigned, because of low pay and too few staff. Henceforth, the British Consular staff had to go to the Quarantine physician, "who cares little for treatment and or recovery of patients but is ever ready to pocket their fees."[210] Dr. `Ali Khan Hamidi was recalled to Tehran at the end of December 1933; Dr. Ashraf continued.

The Quarantine Hospital was not the only medical institution in town, for in 1936 (and probably earlier) there was a military hospital in Bandar Abbas.[211] Although the charitable dispensary/hospital had been closed in 1934, some time thereafter a bigger hospital had been established. For in 1946, the British reported that in Bandar Abbas "there is a civil hospital with 50 beds, but it is not fit for Europeans, and has no qualified doctor."[212]

---

209. Administraton Report 1933, p. 21.
210. Administraton Report 1934, p. 23. names quarantine physicians, p. 31.
211. IOR/L/PS/12/3413, HBM's Consulate Kerman Diary no 11, 1936, p. 5 (*Sargord* Mahin was in charge of the Military Hospital of Bandar Abbas).
212. IOR/L/MIL/17/15/40, 'Persia Intelligence Report. May, 1946', p. 32.

BIRJAND

Probably around 1900, the British Consulate in Birjand had a small hospital and dispensary. In November 1909 it had an attendance of 2,937 out-patients.[213] The hospital still existed in 1935.[214]

There also was a municipal doctor in the town, who since 1928 received drugs and instruments from the government. In 1929, the local municipal authorities selected a site to erect a hospital,

> which will be fitted with an operation theatre and electrically lighted. It is doubtful however whether sufficient funds can be raised speedily. The Soviet Consulate also has been reinforced by a Medical Officer who dispenses drugs free of charge. At present, however, any major operations can only be performed in the British Consulate hospital.[215]

Indeed, as is clear from a later report the hospital that was finally erected was smaller and less electrified than intended or hoped for. In 1932, at Birjand "the new Electric Light Installation was formally opened on 1st July. A small hospital of 10 beds has been opened - cost of the upkeep is to be defrayed from Municipal funds." There was a real need for that hospital, because typhoid was increasing in the town, due to the piped water-supply that had been installed the previous year, which was infected. The British consul commented, "but such is the faith of Persians in everything modern that they decline

---

213. IOR/L/PS/10/328/1, Reductions in expenditure on Agencies and Consulates', p. 6. In 1912, it was operated by Mirza Mohammad Beg, Sub-assistant surgeon. IOR/L/PS/10/209, Consular Diary HBM's Consul for Sistan and Kain, no. 42, for the week ending 18th October 1913, p. 1. Idem, Diary no. 40 ending 4th October 1913, p. 1 (1,220 new cases in Birjand and 1,460 new cases Sistan dispensary. Old cases respectively, 443 and 1,097 and operations 1 and 51).
214. IOR/L/PS/12/3406, HBM's Consulate General Khorasan and Sistan. Diary for February 1935, p. 3 (the dispensary was run by Dr. Fazal al-Haq).
215. IOR/L/PS/12/3415, Annual Commercial Report for the Province of Sistan and the Kainat for the year 1928-29, p. 7.

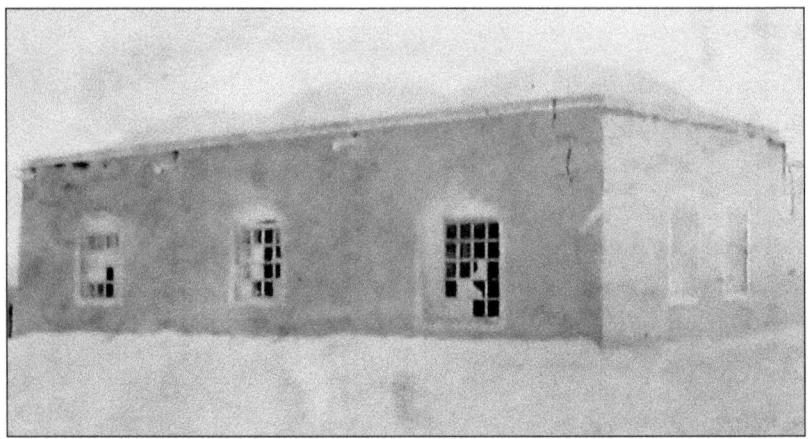

Deserted operating rooms at the former British camp at Shusf (near Birjand)

to believe that the water of an expensive pipe-system can possibly be unhealthy."[216] The hospital is not mentioned in a 1941 report that discussed the medical services that were available in Birjand. There was a Russian doctor, who had become a naturalized Persian citizen and who already had lived there for 25 years. It was unknown, however, what the quality of his services were. The Iranian government had appointed a doctor there to treat the workers who were constructing the Mashhad-Zahedan road, but the consul was advised, when he was ill, "that it would be definitely unwise to call him in." Another obstacle to medical treatment in the town was that "Medicines have long been virtually unobtainable in Persia, except perhaps at Tehran"[217] In 1946 Asadollah Alam, chief man of Birjand built a 30-bed hospital in his home town.[218]

In 1963, Birjand had 14,000 inhabitants and was reported to have 10 physicians, including army and gendarmerie doctors, who also had a private practice. One of them was trained by Dr. Adle (Tehran)

---

216. IOR/L/PS/12/3403, HBM's Consulate, Sistan and Kain, Diary for July 1932, p. 1.
217. IOR/L/PS/12/3561, Personal aspects of life as Vice-Consul, Zabul (December 1941), p. 6.
218. RG 231-1-6, Hoffman, Pioneering in Meshed, p. 147

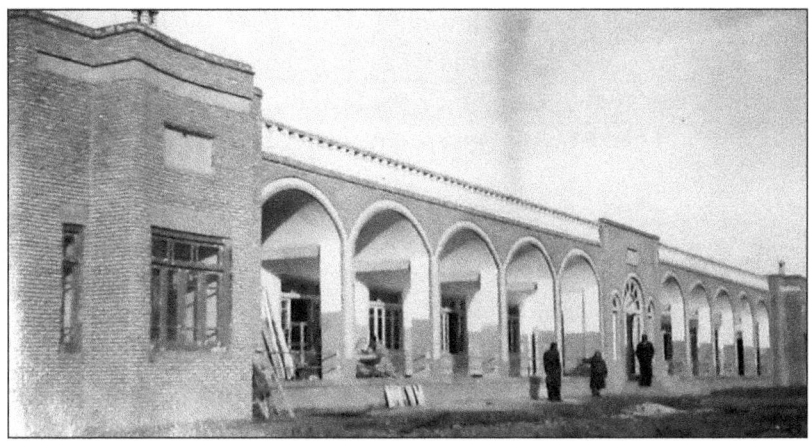
New hospital in memory of Showkat al-Molk, Birjand, 1946

but he had no operation facilities. Sometimes, he was allowed to use the facilities of the Red Lion and Sun hospital. The main hospital, the Alam Hospital, had two sections. The first was a single-storey building with about 50 beds, although it was in practice operating on an 18 bed capapcity. The second building was the maternity hospital, which had a midwife. At the time of the visit it was being repaired and thus, maternity cases were sent to the hospital. The hospitals's operating room had an excellent operating table, but instruments were limited, but more were ordered. The most common surgery was the Ceasarian section. Medicines were supplied to patients free of charge and seemed to be of good quality. The kitchen was clean and well-equipped. According to the staff, people were afraid to come to the hospital, reason for its below capacity occupation. The nursing matron (Mahareh Nuri) was a graduate of the Mashhad 3-year nursing school. The army hospital was neat and clean, well-equipped and was in the process of installing a dark room with X-ray. There also was an army dentist with a dentist chair. The hospital only served military personnel.

Neither hospital had an adequate laboratory, nor were these facilities available among the private practitioners. In the local dispensary, the physician had an X-ray that he used for chest and stomach fluorscopies, identifying foreign bodies, and diagnosis of fractured bones. In the city was a private, well-stocked drugstore, which was regularly visited by drug company salesmen and had the latest drugs (e.g. Grisovin). Local notables expressed the need for a medical dispensary (*darmangah*), which would make regular visits to neighboring villages.[219]

Bushehr

Prior to the opening of the British Residency dispensary, the population of Bushehr had no choice but to have recourse to the Galenic-trained physicians and in particular to folk-medicine. The latter was similar to the kind of superstitious methods that also prevailed in the rest of the country.[220]

British Residency Dispensary

For many decades, the British Residency's physician had issued medical advice and medicines free of charge to the people of Bushehr and environs as part of official British policy. As of 1873, the British had what they classified as a second-class dispensary at Bushehr.[221] It was a great success among the population, not only because it was the only modern medical facility in town, but its services were also gratis to the poor. "This boon is much prized by the natives, and if there was an arrangement for treatment of indoor patients, the results would be still more satisfactory than at present."[222] As a result, be it after initial reluctance about the Ferangis bearing gifts, the number

---

219. RG 280-1-14, Frances Zoeckler, Report on Medical Itineration, 1963.
220. On the practice of medicine in nineteenth century Persia, see Floor 2004.
221. This classification of dispensaries was administrative and financial in nature. The first two classes were funded and managed by the government of India. Whereas the first class dispensary was open to all comers, those of the second class only served a special section of the public, in this particular case the staff of the British Residency and the population of Bushehr. Government of India 1906, p. 36.
222. "It is the only place for free treatment in Bushire," Administration Report 1914, p. 12; Idem 1873-74, p. 7; Sadid al-Saltaneh 1371, p. 38.

of patients increased steadily (see Table 8). The statistics show that the largest daily attendance took place during the height of the hottest weather, i.e., June, July, and August.[223] Many of the patients were and continued to be women as well as children, whose numbers were also on the rise as indicated by the data available.[224] Bushehr, with 24,000 inhabitants around 1920,[225] had a much higher attendance at its dispensary that those in Bandar Abbas or Lengeh with a similar population size, probably due to the fact that people were longer accustomed to its service.[226]

Table 8: Out- and in-patients and operations in the Bushehr British dispensary-hospital (1873-1928)

Year	Total	Out-patients	In-patients	In-patients operations	Total operations
1873-74	19,056	19,056	-	-	-
1874-75	13,672	13,672	-	-	-
1879-80	7,022	7,022	-	-	-
1898-99	6,418	6,418	-	-	395
1899-1900	5,026	5,026	-	-	315
1900-01	8,050	8,050	-	-	525
1907-08	13,393	13,254	139	69	609
1908	8,821	8,734	87	-	476
1909	16,581	16,422	59	-	589
1910	13,094	13,045	49	-	389
1911	13,470	13,397	73	-	599
1912	13,747	13,716	31	-	589

---

223. Administration Report 1907-08, p. 19.
224. Administration Report 1914, p. 12; Idem, 1913, p. 34. "We found the doctor busy considering prescribing for and dosing a number of patients, among whom were a great many women and children." Cursetjee 2001, p. 114.
225. Administration Report 1919, p. 10.
226. Also, the service there had begun in 1907, see Floor 2010, p. 23 and Idem 2011, p. 43.

Year	Total	Out-patients	In-patients	In-patients operations	Total operations
1913	15,155	15,009	146	-	552
1914	13,295	13,190	105	-	636
1915	14,667	14,537	140	-	n.a.
1916	15,575	15,520	55	-	639
1918	14,759	14,696	63	63	583
1919	12,764	12,711	53	n.a.	n.a.
1920	12,374	12,302	72	69	709
1921	11,453	11,365	88	-	614
1922	13,571	13,461	110	-	945
1923	10,912	10,766	148	146	664
1924	18,852	18,747	105	94	1,169
1925	42,177	42,030	147	119	1,649
1926	59,198	59,056	142	135	2,263
1927	47,454	47,298	156	87	1,828
1928	40,308	40,160	148	n.a.	n.a.

Source: IOR/V/24/2639, Medical Report on Bushire ending 21 March 1875, p. 1 (in 1873-74 of the total 3,432 admissions were from fever, one year later that figure was 2,591); Government of India, *Report on the Administration of the Bombay Presidency for the year 1879-80*, pp. cclx-cclxi; Administration Report 1898-99, p. 15; Idem, 1899-1900, p. 11; Idem, 1900-1901, p. 11; Idem, 1907-08, p. 19; Idem, 1908, p. 12; Idem, 1909, p. 17; Idem, 1910, p. 20; Idem, 1912, p. 43; Idem, 1913, p. 34; Idem, 1914, p. 12; Idem, 1915, p. 10; Idem, 1916, p. 10; Idem, 1918, p. 8; Idem, 1919, p. 10; Idem, 1920, p. 7; Idem, 1921, p. 9; Idem, 1922, p. 9; Idem, 1923, p. 14; Idem, 1924, p. 8; Idem, 1925, p. 10; Idem, 1926, p. 6; Ibid, 1927, p. 7; Ibid, p.10.

In 1907, the dispensary was referred to as a hospital for the first time,[227] and usually thereafter as the hospital-dispensary and as of 1922 as the Bushehr Civil Hospital or Bushehr Residency Dispensary and

---

227. Administration Report 1907-08, p. 19; Sa`adat 1390, p. 23. It was situated on the eastern shore of the island of Abbasak. Lorimer 1915, vol. 2, p. 341.

Charitable Hospital.[228] The qualification of hospital was determined by the fact that as of 1907 in-patients were treated and what was qualified as major operations could be and were performed (e.g. lithotomy, removal of urethral calculus -i.e., removal of stones). Minor operations were mainly the extraction of the teeth, evacuation of abscess and removal of wax.[229] The most modern methods and treatments were introduced as soon as these became available. For example, with some pride, the Political Agent reported the "Successful treatment of leprosy cases by means of the new Nastine treatment inaugurated by Professor Deycke Pasha."[230]

Table 9: Male, female and child patients visiting the Bushehr British dispensary (1899-1901).

Year	Total	Daily attendance	Men	Women	Children
1898-99	6,418	58.5	2,849	1,959	1,610
1899-1900	5,026	27.7	2,266	1,652	1,108
1900-01	9,050	43.7	3,465	3,470	2,115

Source: Administration Report 1898-99, p. 15; Idem, 1899-1900, p. 11; Idem, 1900-1901, p. 9.

The Bushehr dispensary had so much success that in 1908 it was reported that "The hospital has been open the whole twelve months under report. Owing to the gradually increasing attendance the rooms hitherto occupied by the dispensary in the Residency building having become too small for requirements, and the congregation of patients in the Residency court-yard a source of considerable inconvenience, the government of India were pleased to sanction the renting of a capacious house next door to the town Residency and the hospital and dispensary were moved in."[231] The move made in 1912 to other premises was in hindsight not a good one, for although the building

---

228. Administration Report 1922, p. 9; Idem, 1925, p. 10; Nura'i 1385, p. 163 (*mariz-khaneh* in June 1914).
229. Administration Report 1898-99, pp. 15-20.
230. Administration Report 1908, p. 12.
231. Administration Report 1907-08, p. 19.

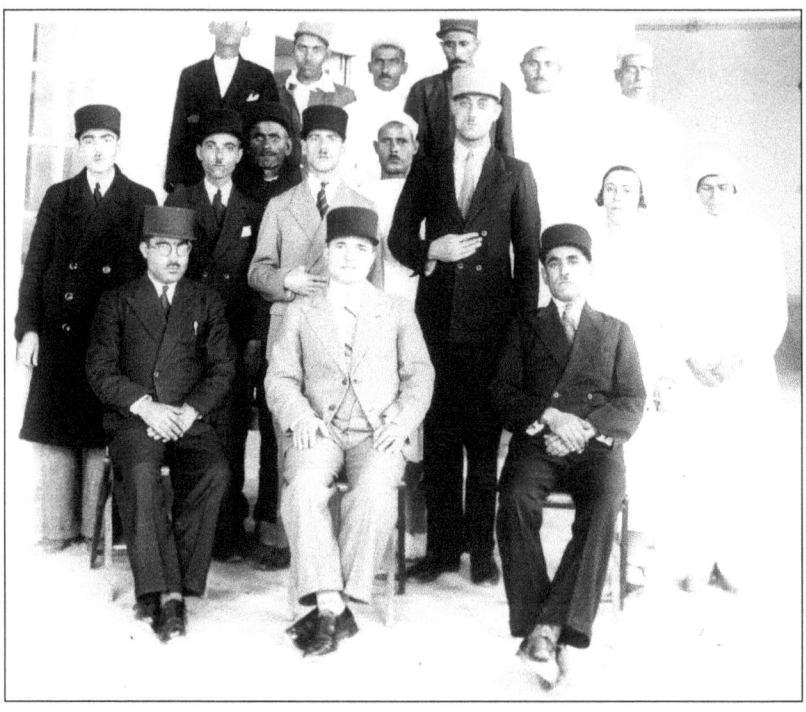

Medical staff of the government hospital of Bushehr, 1933

was well situated it "was poorly adapted for taking-in patients," which made the work for the medical staff difficult. Also, after complaints about subordinate staff these were all changed. Such a move was also important as the number of Moslem and Jewish women coming to the dispensary was large.[232] In 1917, Cursetjee visited "Dr. Hudson

---

232. Administration Report 1913, p. 34; Trade Report 1921-22, p. 1. In July 1911, Moses Khan, the Armenian deputy-chief of Customs in Bushehr proposed to the governor, with the support of the local merchants, to levy two *shahi*s per imported package. He estimated that this would yield 300 *tuman*s per month, which amount was to be used for the maintainance of a hospital which Sayyed Mohammad Reza, a wealthy local merchant, had promised to build. Moses Khan also suggested to buy a condensor for the quarantine service, which responsibility this Persian hospital also could assume. The governor collected 9,000 *tuman*s to that end and the municipality borrowed 16,000 *tuman*s from the Imperial Bank of Persia on condition that local merchants would guarantee the balance needed. The hospital was not built, but the financing arrangement was retained and used to support the British

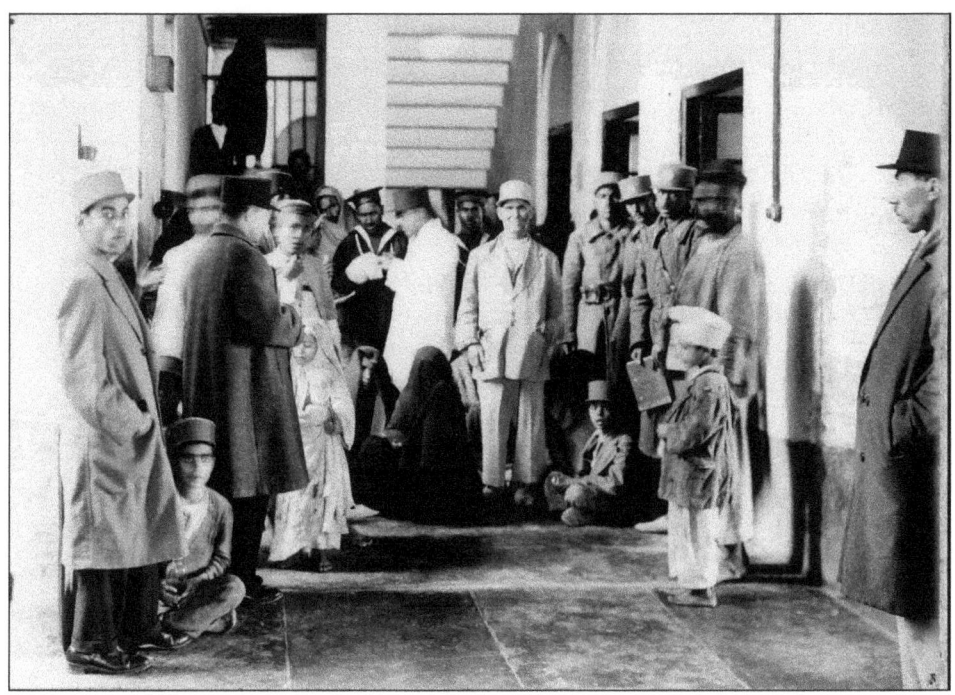

Patients waiting at the government hospital of Bushehr, 1933

in his dispensary which is located on the first floor of a rickety house on the sea-face, and which we had to climb up over a flight of narrow, portentously steep and dirty steps."[233] Given this description of the dispensary, it is understandable that the British Resident wrote: "The provision for a decent hospital for Bushire is much to be desired and had been mooted by a few leading members of the community, but it seems desirable it take the form of a development of the existing Residency Dispensary rather than that the latter should suffer or be eclipsed in any way by an independently conducted institution."[234] One of the main problems of the new location was that the building, located next to the Residency, was owned by Mo`in al-Tojjar, who did not maintain it and therefore, it being old, dirty and in disrepair

---

dispensary. Political Diaries vol. 4, p. 410.
233. Cursetjee 2001, p. 114.
234. Administration Report 1913, p. 34.

and only having small rooms, which made operations difficult, the medical staff considered that they needed better housing soon.

> A small fund, accumulated by contributions of some of the chief habitants of Bushire, has for some time been destined by them to go towards the provision of a good hospital, and until recently it appeared as if the intention was that the new hospital should be run by Persians. A counter-proposal with some considerable authority to back it is to effect that funds raised locally to assist in the building of a new hospital on a site to be granted free by its proprietor. The hope has been expressed that the Government of India would be good enough to permit the Staff of the Residency Dispensary to run the new Hospital intended to replace it, and that further the Government of India might possibly assist in the expense of building the hospital. There is little doubt that it will be a considerable time before the local efforts, if united, will suffice to build and maintain a good hospital.[235]

Dispensary Becomes Charitable Hospital

According to Denis Wright, a new hospital was established in 1916 with financial help from local merchants,[236] which is incorrect. Indeed such a plan for a hospital and a free dispensary was initiated many years ago, but its realization was delayed by the Great War.[237] He may have referred to the activities in that year by Mr. Chick, vice-consul and Major McPherson, the Residency Surgeon to start collecting funds from Persian and British sources for the construction of the hospital.

---

235. Administration Report 1914, p. 12.
236. Wright 2001, p. 127. Merchants had already started to contribute from May/June 1913 by collecting from all goods coming from the interior 1 *shahi* per package (*naqleh*) and 1 *qran* per weight difference. By October they had already collected 1,000 *tuman*s. Sadid al-Saltaneh 1371, p. 113.
237. In 1915, a house was rented and transformed into a British General Hospital with 66 beds (officers 23; ranks 41); another house was rented and and turned into an Indian General Hospital with 182 beds. Huts and tents were erected nearby to accommodate resp. 50 and 404 patients. Two additional houses accommodated physicians and nurses. Government of India 1924, p. 51.

Major McPherson proposed to buy the building from Mo'in al-Tojjar and to build a proper hospital, where he could safely operate patients and keep them in wards. Chick then proposed to collect money from British companies trading with Persia and from Persian merchants, because the main beneficiaries would be the people of Bushehr. He drafted an appeal which had the following result:

Table 10: Contributors to the cost of the construction of the hospital in Bushehr (1918)

Name contributor	Tumans	£	Rupees
BISNC, Bombay	-	-	4,500
Turner, Morrison & Co. Bombay-Persia Line	-	-	1,500
Turner, Morrison & Co. Arabian Steamers Company	-	-	1,000
Persian Gulf Steam Navigation Company, Bombay	-	-	1,000
Sir P. Z. Cox, Political Resident	-	-	500
Colonel Trevor, Deputy Political Resident	-	-	500
Sir P. M. Sykes	-	-	400
Some 20 other British individuals, Bushehr, India	-	-	1,826
Ziegler and Company, Manchester	-	-	1,000
E.D. Sassoon and Company, Bombay	-	-	1,000
Gray Paul and Company, Basra and Bushehr	-	-	1,000
Haji 'Ali Akbar and Sons, Manchester	-	-	1,000
A. A. and A. Gorji, Bombay	-	-	1,000
Other merchants in India, Indians and Iraqis	470	-	1,200
H.C. Dixon, Manchester	-	200	-
Anglo-Persian Oil Company, London	-	100	-
David Sassoon and Company, London	-	50	-
Imperial Bank of Persia	750	-	-
Assigned by the dept. Pol. Resident with approval of Govt. of India	-	-	11,700
Total	1,220	350	29,126

Source: IOR/L/PS/11/182.

From Persian merchants 7,793 *tuman*s were collected by Messrs. Chick, McPherson, the Residency's dragoman and the chief of the Municipality, who, night after night, called on the merchants to ask them to contribute. Daryabegi supported the activity, called several meetings and sent out a circular appeal asking merchants to give money to this initiative. Sheikh Khaz`al of Mohammerah donated 1,000 *tuman*s and two Persian notables from Bandar Abbas and Lengeh gave Rs2,000. The merchant community of Bushehr further contributed 429 *tuman*s and Rs13,500, the total collected by the voluntary 1 *shahi* fee per package imported between 1913 and 1915 with a view to build a hospital with the proceeds. By the end of 1918, an additional amount of 1,075 *tuman*s and Rs200 had been collected, so that total sum collected from local Persian sources amounted to 10,297 *tuman*s and Rs15,700. The Rs11,700 contributed by the government of India was a fund made available to the deputy Resident for charitable purposes.[238]

In 1917/18, a founding committee was established, which bought the land and premises from Mo`in al-Tojjar for 5,000 *tuman*s, of which he donated 1,000 *tuman*s for the construction of the hospital. On 30 January 1918, both Persian and British founders and contributors had a general meeting, which decided that the deed of sale of the land bought for the hospital would be transferred to a committee of two Persians and two Brits, as follows:

> In accordance with a Power of Attorney executed by Haji Mu`in-ut-Tujjar, Haji Muhammad Baqir Behbehani is to draw up a legal deed of sale of the two houses known as 'Kuzeh-Kanani' in the name of sale of the founders of the hospital, and the founders of the hospital are then to transfer the deed of sale to four persons, of whom is one the British Consul-General and the second the Residency Surgeon and (the other) two chosen from two of the founders deemed suitable (by the founders).

The four-man committee (two Persians, two Brits) formally was in charge of the construction and management of the hospital, although

---

238. IOR/L/PS/11/182. Rs or Indian Rupees.

it hardly functioned after the completion of the hospital, while the IBP was appointed honorary treasurer of the hospital.[239]

The deputy Resident further asked the government of India to give a grant of Rs30,000 for the hospital building and a grant of medical equipment of Rs16,000. In January 1920, already some Rs97,000 had been collected in Bushehr to finance the initial cost, while a continuation of a voluntary 1-*shahi* fee per imported package, paid by Persian and British merchants, was expected to yield Rs500/month. With these funds it was proposed to build a hospital with two small rooms for European patients, 35 beds for Persian male patients, a good operating theater, a good dispensary, and quarters for a nurse. It was suggested to start construction with the available funds and to add the upper storey when additional funds came available. Funds permitting, it was also intended to build "a separate women's ward under strict purdah conditions." Further that the existing dispensary and its staff would form the nucleus of the new hospital and that the annual grant of Rs3,400 to the Bushehr dispensary would be continued, given rising cost. On 9 September 1920, the government of India decided to give a grant of Rs15,000 to the building fund, a Rs15,000 grant for medical equipment and an annual grant of Rs1,500 for the hospital's maintenance, provided that the remaining funds to build the hospital were raised locally within a reasonable time. Also, it was expected that the hospital accommodation would be made available to its servants. The annual grant of Rs3,400 for the separately operating dispensary was continued. The funding was not without self-interest, for the government of India saw the hospital as a means to maintain influence among the population, while the annual maintenance grant gave it the means to ensure that the Residency Surgeon would be in charge of the hospital.[240]

It was only by the end of 1920 that "work had started by the residency mason and under the supervision of the British Executive

---

239. IOR/L/PS/11/182; Elgood 1951, p. 548.
240. IOR/L/PS/11/182, Finance Department to Secretary of State for India, Simla, 09/09/1921.

Engineer for the Gulf Ports."²⁴¹ It was expected that in 1922, the dispensary would move to better place; therefore, the old place was "demolished and is being reconstructed on a better and more sanitary basis."²⁴² The first storey was almost complete by September 1921.²⁴³ It was quite an improvement on the present building where the Residency surgeon carried on his work under adverse conditions.²⁴⁴ In 1922 it was reported that "The work on the new Charitable Hospital, built by public subscription, was practically complete by the end of the year. The equipment still remains to be purchased. It is hoped that it may be opened during the next year,"²⁴⁵ which indeed it was.

> The new hospital was occupied in April 1923. Its design is a compromise between what is needed for a hospital on the one hand and local Persian ideas of architecture coupled with insufficiency of funds on the other. As a result, when occupied, it lacked electric light, a water-supply, cookhouses, quarters for staff, and a sanitary and drainage system. Electric light has been installed, two engines purchased and, thanks to the Anglo-Persian Oil Company, a free supply of kerosene oil and petrol for power. A proper drain has been made into the sea, latrines constructed and a water-tank on the roof for finishing purposes supplied by an automatic electric pump from a well, is in course of erection. A large 'Ab-ambar' has been constructed to be connected by a semi-rotary hand pump to another tank on the roof for the supply of water to the operation theatre and dispensary. But until the quarters of the staff have been built the hospital can only be considered to be an 'outdoor' dispensary.²⁴⁶

---

241. Trade Report 1920-21, p. 1.
242. Administration Report 1920, p. 7.
243. Trade Report 1920-21, p. ii.
244. Trade Report 1921-22, p. 1; also Trade Report 1922-23, p. 3.
245. Administration Report 1922, p. 9.
246. Administration Report 1923, p. 14. It was nevertheless, considered to be "quite an improvement on the present building where the residency surgeon carried on his work under adverse conditions." Trade Report 1921-22, p. 1.

The facilities were still insufficient to receive in-patients. The hospital, therefore, continued to operate as dispensary, because much equipment was still lacking as was the chief medical officer.[247] By the end of 1925, shortages were overcome and the Bushehr Residency Dispensary and Charitable Hospital was fully operational. Nevertheless, there were still problems, because the great demand by outpatients hampered the extension of in-patient work.[248] The work was still not optimal, because facilities for proper in-patient care were lacking, in particular suitable accommodation for nursing staff, if such personnel were available, which they were not.[249]

It was not easy to run a hospital, for apart from the medical problems there were financial ones, because expenses tended to be higher than receipts, at least for the years that published data are available. In 1926, the budget deficit was due to the expansion of the out-patient attendances, despite the fact that in that March the hospital benefited from the stores transferred from the Indian Military Hospital that was closed when the Punjab regiment departed from Bushehr and was not replaced. This was not the only subsidy that the hospital received, for what is not shown in the tables is "the Contract Block Grant of the Residency Budget, being accounted for by the Residency and expended on salaries, and medicines and dressings received from the Medical Store Depot Bombay."[250]

---

247. Administration Report 1924, p. 8.
248. Administration Report 1925, p. 10.
249. Administration Report 1926, p. 5.
250. Administration Report 1926, p. 5.

Table 11: British Bushehr Hospital Receipts (1925-28)

	1925		1926		1927	1928
	Qrans	Rupees	Qrans	Rupees	Qrans	Qrans
Contributions from Govt. of India and Residency	-	1,485	2,015	1,860	7,801	5,698
Contribution of APOC and Customs Dept.	4,750	-	6,600	-	6,500	5,999
Proceeds of voluntary one *shahi* tax	16,098	-	14,587	-	12,798	10,339
Sale of medicines	550	152	545	9	1,229	66
Miscellaneous	1,946	500	2,574	-	2,042	-
Total	23,324	2,137	26,321	1,669	30,730	22,302

Source: Administration Report 1926, p. 5; Administration Report 1927, p. 6; Administration Report 1928, p. 11.

The most important source of income was that of the voluntary 1-*shahi* fee, which was an uncertain source of income, because this not only depended on the goodwill of the merchants, but also on how well their business and trade in general performed. This is clear from the downward trend of this revenue, which in 1925 still represented some 69% of total receipts, but only 46% in 1928 (Table 12). Most of the expenditures was represented by the salaries of the European medical staff (ca. 30-40%) and medicines (ca. 30%), which were imported from Europe and bought in the bazaar.[251] It was the hospital's intention to have a balanced budget in the future.

---

251. Administration Report 1899-1900, p. 15.

Table 12: British Bushehr Hospital Expenditures (1925-28)

	1925		1926		1927	1928
	*Qran*s	Rupees	*Qran*s	Rupees	*Qran*s	*Qran*s
On medicine and dressings	21,744	402	22,029	28	15,210	11,512
On equipment	12,702	2,020	623	-	-	-
On electric light and telephone	2,092	206	952	556	1,903	3,246
Petty expenses	7,065	228	5,357	-	3,872	-
On stationary	1,092	-	463	-	45	-
On salaries	2,878	1,750	4,159	1680	12,918	13,202
Miscellaneous	1,944	-	389	-	1,023	1,887
Dieting of patients	2,371	-	5,985	-	2,432	1,644
Repairs and maintenance	50	-	263	-	394	1,529
Contingencies	-	-	-	-	-	2,971
Total	51,938	4,606	40,220	2,264	37,797	35,991

Source: Administration Report 1926, p. 5; Administration Report 1927, p. 6; Administration Report 1928, p. 11.

In 1927, the hospital faced a larger number of in-patients, but it was still constrained by inadequate facilities. Expenditures (37,797 *qran*s) were still higher than receipts (30,370 *qran*s), but the objective remained to cut cost and assure a stable financial position.[252] In 1929, expenditures again exceeded receipts which was due to the fact that in September the Customs Department canceled its contribution, the 1-*shahi* voluntary tax, which was three months in arrears, averaging about 110 *tuman*s per month. Also, there was a slight drop in the number of patients treated, because as of September the medical care of the Customs Department, Post & Telegraph Department, and the Finance Department was taken over by the Persian chief quarantine medical officer.[253]

---

252. Administration Report 1927, p. 6.
253. Administration Report 1928, pp. 10-11.

Hospital Becomes Persian

In 1929, as indicated above, significant changes took place as to the status of the Charitable Hospital. On 9 February the British Residency Dispensary was removed from the hospital to the Residency compound. This move was due to the fact that in September 1928, 'Abdollah Khan Monajjami, the head of the finance department (*ra'is-e maliyeh*), who was acting governor of Bushehr at that time, informed the Residency Surgeon that the Charitable Hospital had to be handed over to the Persian authorities.[254] The British authorities pointed out that the funding for the establishment and maintenance of the hospital had mainly come from British sources, while "in addition to this contribution the Government of India allows the hospital to benefit gratis by the services of the Residency Surgeon, the Sub-assistant surgeon, compounder, dressers, sweepers, etc. whose salaries are all paid by that Government." At the same time the Persian government had contributed nothing. Also, the deed of the hospital was held in trust by the 4-man committee created by the hospital founders, so that legally the British government could not change the status of the hospital.[255] On 2 December 1928, the Resident reported to New Delhi that according to the Residency Surgeon continuation of the hospital was unimportant from a professional point of view. The cases he and his staff saw were insufficient to keep their professional know-how up-to-date. Also, 90% of the patients were Persians, while the remaining 10% (mostly Indians) would be better served by the re-establishment of a small hospital in the old Residency building. Because the cavalry guard had left their barracks were empty where at little cost a dispensary and a 4-bed ward could be prepared. Moreover, with the expected withdrawal of the contributions of the various Persian government institutions the hospital would be unable to continue to function anyway. Therefore, it was better to each party go separate ways, which was a better and financially viable alternative. Therefore, the Resident proposed to inform the Persian government immediately of the British withdrawal from the hospital.[256]

---

254. Administration Report 1929, p. 8.
255. IOR/L/PS/11/182, R.C. Parr, British Legation to Taqi Esfandiary, Tehran, 12/10/1923.
256. IOR/L/PS/11/182. Johnston to New Delhi, 02/12/1928.

And indeed, the Persian authorities were not interested in legalistic and other arguments to maintain the status quo. After all, the decision to demand the transfer of the hospital was a political one, based on national pride and the desire to rely as little as possible on foreigners, in particular the British. As the Resident expected, to put some pressure behind Persian government's 'suggestion', the Customs Department shortly thereafter withdrew its financial contribution to the hospital. It further instructed its employees henceforth to go to a dispensary that had been opened within the Customs Department and which was operated by Persian physicians. Soon thereafter the Post Office and the Finance Department likewise withdrew their financial contributions and their sick. The collection of the so-called one *shahi* voluntary fee, which represented some 50 per cent. of the Hospital's income (see above), had systematically been underperforming for some time and it was not paid at all during the last quarter of 1928. It was clear to the British authorities that all these measures were aimed at bankrupting the hospital and thus embarrass the British. As a result, the British government decided to sever its relationship with the Charitable Hospital on 9 February 1929, a relationship that had lasted some 60 years. The medical responsibility was immediately transferred to Dr. Bahrami, the Persian chief quarantine medical officer, who, assisted by Dr. Ali Khan carried out the medical work. The British government divided all medical supplies and surgical equipment in half, one part of which was moved to the Residency dispensary. As a result the dispensary's operating room equipment was incomplete and serious cases could not be dealt with.[257]

Despite the separation of the two medical establishments, there was a concern among the Persian authorities about the capacity of the now Persian hospital to sustain its level of previous quality service. During a visit made in January 1930 at the request of the governor of Bushehr, the British Residency surgeon noted that "the Hospital was not conspicuously clean and that Dr. Ali Khan's learning was not of a very high order, in fact not even of mediocre standards."[258] The same

---

257. Administration Report 1929, p. 8; IOR/L/PS/11/182.
258. Administration Report 1929, p. 8.

held for his chief, Dr. Abol-Qasem Bahrami, who was described as a pleasant person, but his medical qualifications were not immediately apparent. He was more interested in bacteriology than in operations, which he seldom did, and in serious cases he referred people to the British Residency or the IETD doctors.[259]

Despite this reduced level of service at the hospital, the Persian authorities expanded the capacity of medical services at Bushehr via the Red Lion and Rising Sun Society, which had been established in 1928 by the governor and was managed by Dr. Bahrami, the Health and Chief Quarantine Medical Officer. In 1930, the Society bought the old Turkish consulate and turned it into a maternity hospital. It was also active outside Bushehr in that the Society gave 5,000 francs to France for people in the inundated areas of the Seine and another sum to earthquake victims of the ruined Demavand villages.[260]

Meanwhile, the British received negative reports about the medical service offered at the hospital. A Persian patient, who came to the British Residency Dispensary, who had been to the hospital for treatment, "reported that there are no medicines available with the exception of Eno's fruit salts locally purchased which is issued to all and sundry, one teaspoonful at a time."[261] Another reported that if any more elaborate treatment was required, "a prescription is written which, on presentation at a local pharmacy, is made up on payment of a sum of money. It is also stated that Bahrami, the head of the Charitable dispensary staff, is more than part owner of this pharmacy. He and his staff are genuine apostles of the hypodermic syringe and cheap German ampoule, with which the bazaar is flooded." This led to misuse where patients even died (after repeated injections with

---

259. Administration Report 1929, p. 3.
260. Administration Report 1930, p. 4.
261. Invented in the 1850s by James Crossley Eno of Newcastle, Fruit Salt sold like hotcakes to sailors looking for something to keep them healthy on long journeys. The product is still available today; it sells in vast quantities worldwide as a popular anti-acid and a reliever of bloatedness, upset stomach, indigestion and heartburn that provides immediate relief from gas and acidity and is without known side effects. It is much used in Indian cooking. It contains sodium bicarbonate, citric acid and sodium carbonate.

strychnine and caffeine) or suffered bad side effects (ruptured spleen, acute arthritis).[262] In 1931 there were persistent complaints about the hospital, and the inadequacy of treatment by the new physician, Dr. Muniri and his staff. "The municipality are so dissatisfied that they have debated opening a municipal dispensary on the grounds that no medicines are to be had at the Charitable Hospital." The municipality also considered hiring part-time "Sub-Assistant Surgeon Jemadar Mohammad `Ali Najmi, I.M.D. (Retired)," who had begun a private practice in Bushehr. However, the anti-foreign elements in the municipal council were against hiring a foreigner. "Considering the present conditions of medical education in Persia it is not understood from where the nationalist elements in the Baladieh [municipality] consider they would get anyone more satisfactory than Muniri and it is probable that the proposal will come to nought."[263]

The replacement of Dr. Bahrami by Dr. Muniri as Quarantine and Health officer on 18 February 1931 did not bring the hoped for change in the hospital's performance. One potentially positive change was that Dr. Muniri's wife held a French diploma in midwifery. She took charge of the Shahdokht Maternity Hospital for some time at 80 *tuman*s per month. In April 1931, she began a glass of ten girls with an elementary school diploma training them in "midwivery and treatment of female cases."[264] However, in 1932, "General Coulonger, the French Director-General of the Persian Medical Service, visited Bushire in the early summer and was shewn around the Dispensary. For the period of his visit, the twenty beds of the Bushire Charitable Hospital were filled by twenty reluctant 'patients' who were paid Rials 3 per diem. It has been reported that after one or two days incarceration the 'patients' struck and demand Rials 5 per diem and were paid their demands. Normally the beds are empty, or occupied

---

262. Administration Report 1930, p. 12.
263. Administration Report 1931, p. 14. In January 1930, Dr. Habib Rezapour was appointed health officer. He condemned some meat and threw it into the sea. The butchers went on a strike and no meat could be had for a week." Political Diaries, vol. 9, p. 4.
264. Administration Report 1931, p. 5; Political Diaries, vol. 9, p. 483.

by members of the hospital staff."[265] Following the shah's visit and the report of General Coulonger, the Bushehr hospital began "to give free treatment and also actually to admit patients and treat them."[266] However, it would seem that these changes did not last long, because in 1933 the municipal council considered the services offered at the hospital inadequate. Therefore, in April 1933 new municipal taxes were levied with a view to provide 10 beds for a lying-in ward for poor persons in the municipal infirmary. Moreover, the municipality also funded a local physician "to look after them and to treat other poor patients free of charge."[267] It seems that thereafter the situation changed somewhat for the better, although problems remained. In 1934, when Merritt-Hawkes visited to hospital, she reported:

> Although it was scrupulously clean-there were even puddles on the floor after the morning wash-up – there were very few patients, and much of the apparatus and the instruments looked as if they were more ornamental than useful. There was so much obvious illness that the empty beds seemed odd; the doctor said no one would come into the hospital at No-Ruz, the great yearly holiday which was just due, but the out-patient department was very busy. There was a small maternity hospital in a good position on the front, but after a year of being in the hands of an entirely unqualified person, it had been shut up.[268]

In 1936, the municipality continued to fund the same medical service initiated in 1933, while as of that year it also provided funds for "a small asylum for a few lunatics and an isolated house for accommodating some 20 lepers."[269] The same municipal medical service was funded during 1937-1939 with the difference that the number of beds for the infirmary had been reduced to eight. In October 1938, the municipal infirmary was merged with the hospital to reduce the

---

265. Administration Report 1932, p. 11.
266. Administration Report 1932, p. 4.
267. Administration Report 1933, p. 4; Idem, 1935, p. 5; Political Diaries, vol. 11, p. 280.
268. Merritt-Hawkes 1935, p. 6.
269. Administration Report 1936, p. 5.

latter's deficit.[270] In October 1938, the existence of a military hospital in Bushehr is mentioned, without stating when it was established and where it was located, although presumably at Bahmani, where the barracks were.[271] In 1940, there is no information about the municipal-funded medical infrastructure. However, it seems that Bushehr hospital still existed, because it was reported that it maintained 20 beds for indoor patients.[272] In December 1941, there was a small pox epidemic. Only in Bushehr and in accessible villages vaccinations took place. The only hospital with room for 20 in-patients, was miserably equipped and had insufficient medicines even for the needs of the town. A small hospital was built in Borazjan, but so far it was used by the Head of Economics Department as his residence.[273] In September 1943, Dr. Siadat, the public health officer, opened a sanatorium outside town at Shekeri, where poor people suffering from malnutrition and tropical ulcers were received. The Anglo-Persian Reconstruction Relief Fund (APRRF) contributed with medicines and dressings. However, Dr. Siadat had difficulty finding money to keep his patients there. Merchants had promised to contribute 2,000 *tuman*s, but the money had not been given to him so far. Fortunately, the APRRF helped by assuming the responsibility for the patients' food, while the Health Department promised to provide adequate staff and maintain quality of medical service in the sanatorium.[274]

In 1947, the hospital had a nominal capacity of 40 in-patients, but due to a shortage of linen, nurses, etc. the actual capacity was only 15-20 in-patients. Its staff was able to perform minor surgeries, but the standard of medical care was low, which also held for the two dispensaries that existed in Bushehr at that time. This was partly due to the climate, which made it "very difficult to keep hospital equipment and surgical instruments in good condition; the latter seem to be only fit for post-mortem needs." Moreover, although the hospital

---

270. Administration Report 1937, p. 11; Administration Report 1938, p. 3; Administration Report 1939, p. 3; Political Diaries, vol. 13, p. 180.
271. Political Diaries, vol. 12, p. 179,
272. Administration Report 1940, p. 3.
273. Administration Report 1941, p. 7.
274. Political Diaries, vol. 15, pp. 586-87, 615; vol. 16, p. 224.

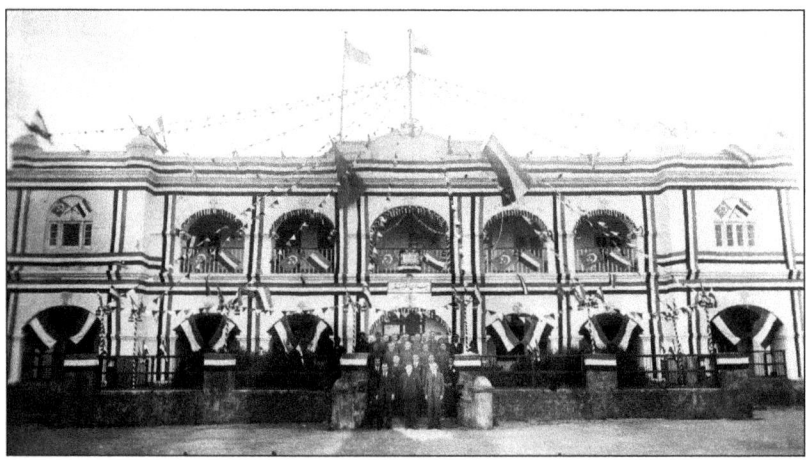

The quarantine and hospital building in 1939.
Now the Abu'l-Fazl private health clinic.

was given a good supply of medicines and food for patients, much of these were sold on the black market. By 1947, in addition to the ailments mentioned above, VD and TB were on the rise; 7% of the population had VD and the incidence of TB was even higher.

However, the public health situation of Bushehr was not as gloomy as in the past, for progress had been made. For example, between 1945-47, Dr. `Ataollah, the Medical Officer (MO) for the governorate, was able to practically eliminate malaria from the Bushehr peninsula and Borazjan Town. He was assisted by three physicians, one of whom was a dentist. Outside Bushehr there were six dispensaries in Khormuj, Ahram, Borazjan, Delam, Ganaveh and Kangan. In each of them a medical aid, trained in the Bushehr hospital, ran the dispensary. The MO or his assistants regularly visited these dispensaries to supervise their work.

Moreover, mortality of mothers or children in child birth was lower in Bushehr than in the rest of the governorate due to the presence of these physicians, who could take care of complicated cases. Outside Bushehr traditional midwives still performed this task, with often dire consequences. However, mortality of children up to 1 year in Bushehr was higher than elsewhere in Persia, probably due to the climate, when for part of the year goat and cow milk were not available.

Also, the government wanted to further improve the public health situation in the governorate. Thus, in 1947, the Ministry of Health purchased the old British Persian Gulf Residency at Sabzabad, 10 km from the town. There, in 1947, it intended to open a new hospital with 100 beds. However, given the supply-demand situation for health care workers and better living conditions elsewhere, it was expected to be very difficult to find sufficient qualified staff, thus endangering the opening of the hospital. The Health Department further considered developing the hot springs at Ahram and Khormuj for the treatment of rheumatism and related ailments.[275]

British Residency Dispensary Continues

After the transfer of the Charitable Hospital to the Persian authorities in February 1929, the British Residency Dispensary continued its work as before. It served "Residency Staff and the families, the employees and their families of the Imperial Bank of Persia and the three European firms, the Mesopotamia Persia Corporation, Messrs. Ziegler and Company and Messrs. A. and T. J. Malcolm."[276] However, because of rising cost of medical supplies the British Residency Dispensary ran into financial difficulties. Therefore, the Resident requested the government of India to continue to fund the annual grant of Rs4,000. Originally, since 1912, this amount was divided over Bushehr (3,050), Lengeh (650) and Jask (300). In 1921, an additional Rs200 was made available for the Lengeh dispensary, which, however, was closed in 1929. Because the Rs3,050 were insufficient the Resident asked New Delhi to continue to finance the annual grant of Rs1,500, which had been assigned to the Charitable Hospital. With these two amounts plus the Rs850 for Lengeh the Bushehr Residency Dispensary would have sufficient funds to cover its cost.[277]

Despite the reduced number of organizations whose sick the British had treated until 1929 the number of out-patients increased, but stabilized at between ten and eleven thousand per year until 1940, then it increased substantially, reaching over 38,000 in 1945 as discussed below. Initially, the number of in-patients also grew, but

---

275. NA, FO 371/15473.
276. Administration Report 1929, p. 8.
277. IOR/L/PS/11/182, Foreign Secretary India, New Delhi to Undersecretary for India, London. 07/01/1930.

dropped by 50% in 1932 and by 90% in 1935 compared to 1929. (see Table 1.16). The initial increase in operations was made possible by the purchase of new instruments imported from Great Britain so that most emergencies could be dealt with. "However, the waiting list is long as capacity is limited. In fact, anybody that needed an operation either has to come to the Dispensary or go to Basra, Bahrain or India."[278] Probably, the drop in operations after 1932 was due to the reduced number of Europeans living in Bushehr as a result of the worldwide economic depression.

Table 13: Number of patients and operations in the British Bushehr Residency dispensary (1929-1940)

Year/Activities	In-patients	Out-patients	Operations
1929	54	9,320	86
1930	67	9,346	235
1931	49	13,136	279
1932	27	10,119	127
1933	24	10,873	181
1934	22	11,353	214
1935	6	11,580	245
1936	1	10,990	168
1937	6	11,339	207
1938	15	13,069	261
1939	5	10,104	198
1940	8	11,237	117
1941	14	16,754	361
1942	18	35,486	385
1943	14	37,455	407
1944	7	35,876	369
1945	-	38,122	391
1946	-	35,166	323

Source: Administration Report 1929, p. 8; Idem, 1931, p. 14; Idem, 1932, p. 11; Idem, 1933, p. 11; Idem, 1934, p. 11; Idem, 1935, p. 13; Idem, 1936, p. 11; Idem, 1937, p. 11; Idem, 1938, p. 11; Idem, 1939, p. 11; Idem, 1940, p. 11; Idem 1941, p. 15; Idem 1942, p. 22; Idem 1945, p. 18; Idem 1946, appendix I.

---

278. Administration Report 1929, p. 8.

Malaria remained the main illness seen. In 1931, there was an increase in patients, due to the increase in malaria and non-malaria fever patients, in particular the influenza outbreak during the last six weeks of the year. Further, this was also due to attending the staff and families of the Public Works Department, E&M Section at Dastak. Prior to March 1931 they attended the IETD dispensary at Rishar, but from then on, they were seen to by the Residency surgeon. The number of operations had dropped because the surgeon was absent for two months. In November and December 1931 there were no winter rains, but instead very cold weather for a few days with a biting north wind. This contributed to an influenza outbreak with attendant cases of pneumonia that lasted till February 1932. This caused alarm in Bushehr as several hundreds of the aged and infirm died of pneumonia, due to weakness from endemic malaria and were not properly warmly dressed, while they lived "in buildings more fitted to let in air than to keep out piercing north winds." Because there was less rain in 1932, there was less malaria, which also applied to other ailments, because in general there was lower attendance in milder weather. This was the case in 1932, when "The autumn and early winter were remarkable for the paucity of attendances. In normal years this season is a 'rush' one for hospital staff."[279] In 1933, the weather was mild and the rains were good and well distributed. Moreover, they were not followed by the north wind that caused so many respiratory diseases. In addition, the hot season was one of the mildest. Because the water cisterns in each house were filled up this meant an increase in malaria cases (a rise from 1,200 to 3,619).[280] The same weather type prevailed in 1934, and as in the previous year it caused malaria to increase (1/3 of all cases). Despite this worrying trend, "The Health Authorities [did] not undertake any anti-malarial work, and it would be difficult to deal with the private reservoirs, as the inhabitants depend almost entirely on these for drinking water."[281] In 1935, the weather was mild

---

279. Administration Report 1931, p. 14; Administration Report 1932, p. 11. E&M means 'electrical and mechanical.'

280. Administration Report 1933, p. 11.

281. Administration Report 1934, p. 11.

and rains average, but the summer was one of the hottest and longest, and natives suffered almost as much as foreigners. Malaria cases continued to represent 1/3 of total cases seen.[282] In 1936, there was a slight fall in attendances due to the dwindling of Bushehr's population, but malaria continued to maintain its position, representing 1/3 of all patients, a situation that also held for 1937.[283] In December 1938 there was a mild epidemic of measles, while the summer was one of the hottest on record. There were 26 heat-strokes deaths among the local population, a cause of death that prior to 1938 was very rare. The share of malaria in total cases seen dropped to somewhat more than 25%.[284] In 1939, the hot season was mild, in fact, one of the best on record. There was also a decrease in attendances, not due to the mild weather, but because the British Residency assistant-surgeon was forbidden to engage in private practice. "Since the end of 1937, the Persian Government have refused the issue of further licenses to practice to foreign practitioners, but the Assistant-Surgeon was unofficially permitted to practice until June." Malaria continued to hold its position at higher than 25% of total cases seen.[285]

In March-April 1940, there was a severe epidemic of small-pox at Borazjan, and consequently there were some imported cases in Bushehr. General vaccination was carried out and the town escaped the threat. "A small branch dispensary was opened at Sabzabad in April 1940. This is attended by the Residency employees, their families and others from the nearby villages. The Assistant Surgeon sees cases there daily."[286] Malaria remained the main disease throughout the 1940s, while in 1942 dysentery, due to water supply problems was on the increase.[287] In December 1944, the British Residency went

---

282. Administration Report 1935, p. 13.
283. Administration Report 1936, p. 11; Administration Report 1937, p. 11.
284. Administration Report 1938, p. 11.
285. Administration Report 1939, p. 11.
286. Administration Report 1940, pp. 3, 11; Administration Report 1942, p. 15; Mahrad 1979, p. 89.
287. Administration Report 1941, p. 15; Administration Report 1942, p. 22.

> The Law relating to Foreign Physicians (August 30, 1933) provides that all foreign physicians, dispensers, dentists and midwives wishing to practise in Persia must, in addition to producing their diplomas, produce evidence that they have been in independent practise for at least five years before coming to Persia. An exception is made for doctors and others already in the country. The General Department of Health is authorized, when issuing licences, to specify the locality in which the applicant may practise, and the Council of Ministers is authorized to suspend the issue of licences altogether whenever it is considered that the numbers of foreign doctors is sufficient. Foreign physicians must pay a fee of 2,000 rials when receiving their licences and foreign dispensers, dentists and midwives a fee of 1,000 rials. These fees are additional to the taxes levied on all physicians in Persia, whether Persian or foreign.
> Source: IOR/L/PS/12/3472A, Annual Report 1937, p. 26.

to Choghadak with a new mobile dispensary. Because no Persian physician had ever been there, the people flocked to the dispensary to have their festering sores, ulcers and burns treated. The village had suffered terribly during the drought and many men had left to Abadan for work. Because of heavy rains the mobile dispensary only visited Khoshab and Halileh in early January 1945. In the second half of that month the dispensary visited Khisht and Konartakhteh and treated 300 patients. In February the mobile dispensary went to Borazjan, Ahmadi and Choghadak where in total some 400 patients were treated. In February the British dispensary visited Hoseyniki, Sural, Choghadak and Khark island. In March 1945, Ahram was visited, where many children were affected by trachoma. It was arranged that for two weeks a trained practitioner would be lent to the village chief to give free eye-drops to those affected. Also, follow-up visits were made to villages previously visited.[288] Again, there were many malaria cases in the fall and winter of 1945. In that year, the APRRF supported the Caravanserai Shakeran containing 85 paupers; distributed free medicines to the poor in Bushehr and villages, where neither government nor private persons provided medical services. In 1945, the mobile dispensary treated a total of 9,000 patients.[289] It is likely that the Residency Dispensary ceased its activities at the end of 1946 or in mid-1947, when the British consulate was closed down

> The Persian government also started a mobile dispensary, which arrived on 2 February 1945. It was led by Drs. Nur al-Din Pezeshki and Basirian, who had two assistants. Its purpose was to visit all parts of the governorate. The unit was to stay in the Bushehr area for four months, and was one of the six that had been established to tour the country. It was financed by the Public Health Department and by a gift from the Shah.[290]

DAMGHAN

In 1915, US missionaries explored the possibility of opening a hospital in Damghan, where ground for a hospital and 1,000 *tuman*s (ca. $9,000) were ready for the construction of a branch hospital. During the eight days they were there, the US team performed 8 cataract operations and 6 major operations, and each day 200 patients were seen. In Semnan, during 12 days, 21 operations were performed.[291]

---

288. Political Diaries, vol. 16, p. 271, 292, 295, 329, 349, 352-53, 375; vol. 17, p. 5.
289. Administration Report 1945, pp. 15, 18; see also IOR/L/PS/12/3542.
290. Political Diaries, vol. 16, p. 323.
291. Presbyterian Church 1916, p. 294.

ENZELI

In the summer of 1897 a group of Russian physicians arrived in Enzeli and established a dispensary, according to a report in the newspaper *Habl al-Matin*. They made use of a kind of prefabricated house, which allegedly was made of cardboard (*moqava-ye qardun*) and that could be disassembled and re-assembled. The Russian physicians provided medical care free-of-charge to the poor and gave their patients quinine as well as a kind of greasy oil (*rowghan-e zamat*). They also carried out operations and therefore, had many patients. Wealthy patients had to pay for the medical service and were given a prescription made out to the new pharmacy in Enzeli.[292] It is unknown for how long this group of Russian physicians remained in Enzeli and if they had anything to do with the establishment of a hospital there, which was established in 1905 or thereabouts. At that time, the town had some 8,000 inhabitants.

In 1908 people in Enzeli complained about the shortages at the hospital, which means that it must have been established prior to that date. There certainly was a hospital in 1907 as the newspaper *Habl al-Matin* published data on its income and expenditures. In 1911 the hospital still existed, because a newspaper article mentions that a victim of an attack was treated at the hospital. In 1924, the by then municipal hospital had 15 beds, 10 for men and five for women. It had further a dispensary and a pharmacy. Despite its limited capacity (one physician, two Russian nurses and one male nurse) Gilmour had the impression that the hospital was rendering excellent services. From March 1923 until March 1924 the hospital treated 375 in-patients, most of them suffering from malaria, and 3,000 out-patients. The hospital was still functional in 1926. By that time, there also was a hospital for women, which continued to exist in the years there after. Apparently it was a two-storey building with a few rooms, located just behind the municipality.[293] In 1949 Dr. Hoffman reported that, "an imposing

---

292. Tavili 1371, vol. 2, pp. 210-211 quoting *Habl al-Matin*, nr. 8, Calcutta, 2 Sha`ban 1315/27 December 1897, p. 90 and no. 36, 15 Rabi` I 1318/24 July 1899. Andreeva 2007, p. 193.

293. Ṭavili 1371, vol. 2, pp. 218-220, 223-224, quoting *Habl al-Matin*, nr.

government hospital was built at Pahlavi, to be centrally heated and with air-conditioning; it already has cost 10 million rials ($175,000)."[294]

Golpeygan

When in 1915 all British subjects were ordered to leave Iran many returned to Great Britain. J.R. Garland, a young clergyman, who in 1915 worked in Isfahan, went to Ahvaz and when in 1916 the situation in Iran had become less volatile he returned to Isfahan. He then opened among other things a dispensary at Golpeygan, a town of some 15,000 inhabitants. His work was supervised by Mirza Yusof Hakim and Mirza Ayub Hakim. It is not known to me how long this dispensary lasted, but probably only for a short period given the demand on medical manpower to deal with the famine of 1917-18 followed by the outbreaks of influenza, cholera and typhus in Iran.[295]

Hamadan

Around 1900, Hamadan had a population of about 60,000 for which hardly any medical assistance was available. As of 1882, American missionaries, including a medical missionary, Dr. E. W. Alexander, were active in Hamadan. However no information is available on any medical work during the first year of his residence in this city.[296] Initially, the activities of the American missionaries were opposed not only by the local government, but also by various ethnic-religious (Armenian and Jewish) communities.[297] The leaders of the Jewish and Christian community, fearing a reduced flock as a result of conversion by the

---

225, Tehran, 5 *Moharram* 1326/8 February 1908; Zahir al-Dowleh 1351, p. 319; Gilmour 1924, p. 29. However, in 1909, the *Diplomatic and Consular Reports* (henceforth *DCR*) 4828, pp. 11, 14 under the heading 'Public Health' makes no mention of a hospital in either Rasht or Astarabad.

294. RG 231-1-5, Personal Report 1949 and Rasht Hospital Report.

295. Waterfield 1973, p. 121. Eshraqi 1383, p. 886 does not mention this dispensary when he deals with the subject of health in Golpeygan.

296. Presbyterian Church 1883, p. 90.

297. Presbyterian Church 1884, p. 71.

missionaries, and the local medical professionals, fearing competition and loss of income, induced the local authorities to hamper the activities by the American missionaries. Dr. Alexander treated many Iranians who sought his help in spite of in particular the violent opposition of traditional Iranian doctors, "who, while secretly admitting the virtue of foreign medicines, say that they must shut out the foreigners as long as possible."[298] In 1885, Dr. Alexander had to discontinue his medical activities, because he had to return to the USA due to his wife's illness.[299] The following year Dr. and Mrs. Alexander returned and he began a dispensary, but he was convinced that what the city really needed was a hospital.[300] In 1887, Dr. Alexander constructed what he called "a substantial building" with funds earned from his own private practice and gifts from friends. As a result, medical work increased, in which he was assisted by a Mr. Terrill and Mirza Sa`id, one of Dr. Alexander's medical students. He had erected the new building, because all patients, including contagious ones, had to be treated in his own house, which was not an ideal situation. In the new premises provision had been made for a few beds, for special cases. Given the growing number of patients treated it was evident that the deep-seated prejudice against foreign medical practice was abating.[301] Although in 1888, Dr. Alexander worked part of the year in Urmiyeh and Tabriz, he and his assistant saw thousands of patients, made house calls and performed operations.[302] In 1889, Dr. Alexander treated 6,000 patients. Their number varied per month (in May 1,000). The dispensary was crowded in spring and summer, while in winter they came when they could. Half of them came from villages at 4-5 hours travel from the city. Therefore, he kept no regular hours, and when at home, he received them whenever they came at the dispensary. In

---

298. Presbyterian Church 1885, pp. 78-79.
299. Presbyterian Church 1886, p. 90.
300. Presbyterian Church 1887, p. 87.
301. Presbyterian Church 1888, pp. 91-92. On Mirza Sa`id and his decision to study medicine and Dr. Alexander agreeing to this, see Rasooli and Allen 1958, p. 60.
302. Presbyterian Church 1889, p. 94.

that same year, the 'substantial' medical building was found to be too small, because people had to stand in the yard awaiting their turn to be seen by the doctor. In the summer of 1889, beds were placed in the yard and, thus, there was a beginning of a hospital. Therefore, Dr. Alexander reiterated that a hospital was really needed. He intended to convert the houses and the enjoining dispensary into a hospital ($1,200) and build a house ($800). Such a modest hospital would enable the medical staff (which included his students Mirza Sa`id and Mirza Ya`qub) to better care for serious cases. He also needed an additional physician. In the interim, the former residence of the physician was connected with the dispensary, and an additional ward was added, so that Dr. Alexander thought that he had accommodation for thirty patients. In that year he not only worked in the Hamadan dispensary, which was open every day from 7 a.m. till midnight, but he also had opened a dispensary in Sheverin, a large Armenian village with beautiful gardens, 7 km from the city, where he spent two afternoons each week. In 1890, he only worked there Thursday afternoons. He also made tours to smaller towns near Hamadan, such as Bahar, a town of 6,000 and worked there among the poor. Dr. Alexander hoped to get a house there and open a dispensary once a week. This would enable patients from neighboring villages to come to Bahar instead of having to go to Hamadan. He observed that villagers listened better to his advice and instructions, and, therefore, took their medicine with less trouble. As a result of his outreach, Dr. Alexander felt that the suspicion and opposition against modern medicine had diminished. In fact, he wrote: "In the early years loss of a patient were interpreted as lack of skill resulting in loss of confidence, but now there is a willingness to accept what can be done to alleviate pain and even when death is inevitable." [303]

---

303. Presbyterian Church 1890, pp. 182-84 (Dr. and Mrs. Alexander also made visits to Bahar, Kurzara and Soltanabad; his assistant made medical tours in the villages around Hamadan); Presbyterian Church 1891, pp. 161-62; Alexander 1890, pp. 404-06 ("helps are Mirza Saeed and Yakoob, who often go for weeks to work in the villages with bibles and medicines").

In 1891, due to the absence and then resignation of Dr. Alexander, medical work suffered. Much dispensary work was done by Mirza Sa`id and Mirza Ya`qub, the Iranian assistant-doctors trained by him, as well as by Dr. Mary Smith who had come from Tehran to provide temporary assistance. She did much work in the dispensary and visited homes during her brief sojourn. To replace Dr. Alexander, Dr. George W. Holmes from Tabriz was appointed to Hamadan, who, however, suffered from bad health.[304] Dr. Jessie C. Wilson, who had arrived in the fall of 1891, temporarily was in charge of the dispensary. She was assisted by Mirza Sa`id and Mirza Ya`qub. The latter two looked after the male patients and Dr. Jessie Wilson after the female patients. Dr. Wilson reported that the hospital could only admit up to 12 patients and with Dr. Holmes also being there a start would be made.[305] Dr. Holmes was in charge of the men's and Dr. Wilson did the women's medical work. Two Jewish assistants, Khatoun and Tavus (also found as Tatevos) helped her by receiving the fees and giving directions as to diet and the use of the prescribed medicines. This required much time and work and, therefore, the national assistants were an essential part of the medical care.[306] Dr. Holmes also made many social calls, because this was important to gain and maintain the support of influential notables for the medical-missionary work.[307] In 1898, medical work for men was discontinued due to Dr. Holmes' absence. Dr. Wilson reported that the women's dispensary was open nine months, because she spent one month in Kermanshah and, as usual, dispensary was closed in July and August.[308]

---

304. Presbyterian Church 1892, p. 198.
305. Presbyterian Church 1893, pp. 164-65. In April 1893, Mirza Sa`id's "period of contract having ended, he wished to terminate his service with the Mission and so tendered his resignation. He had served faithfully for twelve years as language teacher, doctor's assistant, and then physician." Rasooli and Allen 1958, p. 70.
306. Presbyterian Church 1896, p. 185.
307. Presbyterian Church 1897, p. 159.
308. Presbyterian Church 1899, pp. 191-92.

In 1900, there was no American medical missionary at all, but the young men trained by Dr. Holmes and Dr. Jessie Wilson proved equal to the challenge. Some of them attended cases in distant towns and districts; one, Mirza Sa'id, even served as chief physician of the governor.[309] In 1901, Dr. Blanche Wilson arrived, who had intended not to do any medical work the first year, but study the language. However, demand was so great that she opened the dispensary on the first of December, putting Dr. Meyer, another Iranian physician trained by Dr. Alexander, Dr. Holmes and Dr. Jessie Wilson, in charge to treat all easy cases and those he did not understand to reserve for Monday and Wednesday mornings, when she would be present, and otherwise to only send her emergency cases. These two working days were so filled with medical and surgical cases that Dr. Blanche Wilson decided to devote one additional afternoon to surgical and gynecological cases. As a result, she was almost all the time in the dispensary. Like her predecessors she wrote that the Hamadan station really needed a hospital. "Patients lie now on the floor; we have no place for in-patients."[310] Medical work was crippled by the non-arrival of a male doctor for the men's department. Mirza Meyer and Mirza Tatevos took care of the male patients, while Mirza Meyer also did 14 major operations.[311]

In 1905, Dr. Clara H. Field began women's medical work. Because of her lack of language skills, in addition to language study, she mainly did consultation work for Iranian doctors trained by the American missionary physicians, because "I could do work with women that they could not." She also did 10 operations in people's homes and

---

309. Presbyterian Church 1901, p. 242. Mirza Sa'id served 'Eyn al-Dowleh for one year as his physician and that of his retinue, see Rasooli and Allen 1958, p. 88.

310. Presbyterian Church 1902, pp. 224, 231. In 1902, Dr. Blanche Wilson married the Rev. F. M. Stead. Presbyterian Church 1903, p. 246. In 1902, Dr. Jessie Wilson was transferred to Qazvin; one year later she married Dr. E.T. Lawrence, who was transferred from Rasht to Qazvin. Presbyterian Church 1904, p. 233.

311. Presbyterian Church 1904, p. 245.

the hospital under chloroform.[312] In 1909, Dr. Field married and left Hamadan, so that the hospital had no female doctor any longer. In November 1912, Dr. Mary Allen reinforced the staff, who took up again the work with women. Although she was still learning Persian, she also saw many women in the dispensary and in house calls. In the fall and winter the number of patients fell due to the disturbed condition of the country, but it picked up in spring. Also, the number of in-patients was down in winter, but increased in the fall and spring, when the hospital was pretty full with wounded government soldiers.[313]

Table 14: Patients treated and operations performed American hospital in Hamadan (1887-1915)

Year	Female			Male		
	Outpatients	Inpatients	Operations	Outpatients	Inpatients	Operations
1887	-	-	-	5,000	-	-
1889	-	-	-	6,000	-	-
1892	3,000	12	-	-	-	-
1896	6,000	-	-	4,549	-	some
1897	-	-	-	5,556	-	43
1901				2,000	-	27
1902	2,797	-	20	-	-	-
1903	2,766	-	14	-	-	
1904	3,566	22	19	-	-	-
1905	-	-	-	7,576	39	139
1906	-	-	10	12,521	53	90
1907	-	-	-	5,492	38	54
1908	-	-	-	8,249	44	66
1912	-	-	-	3,100	72	-
1913	1,073	-	-	3,285	-	>22

---

312. Presbyterian Church 1907, p. 299, 313-14. In 1905, Dr. Wilson-Stead was itinerating. Presbyterian Church 1906, p. 300.

313. Presbyterian Church 1913, p. 317 (Dr. Funk also made medical tours to Kermanshah, Soltanabad, Bijar and Senneh, see, e.g., Joseph Wright Cook, "In the Heart of Kurdistan," *The Princeton Alumni Weekly* vol. 32/20 (26 February 1932), pp. 458-59).

	Female			Male		
1914	1,529	-	-	-	97	49
1915	-	-	-	3,661	43	45

Source: Presbyterian Church, 1888, pp. 91-92; Idem 1890, pp. 183; Idem 1893, p. 165; Idem 1896, p. 185; Idem 1897, p. 159; Idem 1898, p. 183; Idem 1902, p. 224; Idem 1903, p. 256; Idem 1904, p. 245; Idem 1905, p. 282; Idem 1906, p. 300; Idem 1907, pp. 313-14; Idem 1908, p. 353; Idem 1909, p. 343; Idem 1913, p. 317; Idem 1914, pp. 329-30; Idem 1916, p. 295;

Dispensary Work

The dispensary started by Dr. Alexander was open 9-10 months per year, because the dispensary was closed in July and August, and some doctors also absented themselves for one month to go on missionary itineration.[314] The dispensary was located in the Kababian quarter, because in 1936 it was reported that, "The downtown dispensary has been for the last 53 years in the same location, and is well known to city people and villagers."[315] Since the dispensary at Sheverin is not mentioned any longer after Dr. Alexander's departure, it seems likely it was discontinued after 1890. In 1903, some money donated by Mrs. Whipple was used to fit up rooms for women in the Kakabian dispensary.[316] At that time, the Whipple Memorial Hospital, constructed in 1904, "consisted of two large rooms and a couple of smaller ones, which were fitted up over the dispensary." However, that intended location of the hospital dispensary was not used until 20 years later (see below).[317] In the 20th century, the Kababian dispensary was practically open all year, except Sundays. Until 24 April 1907, men and women were treated in the men's rooms; thereafter Dr. Field opened her women's dispensary.[318] In October 1913, Dr. Mary Allen opened the new dispensary in the Whipple Memorial Hospital, built with a donation from the ladies of the Utica Presbyterian Society in memory of Mrs. Bussey. Patients were seen three days/week in town

---

314. Presbyterian Church 1899, pp. 191-92.
315. RG 91-19-27, Healing in the Home of Avicenna 1936.
316. Presbyterian Church 1904, p. 245.
317. Presbyterian Church 1905, p. 282.
318. Presbyterian Church 1908, pp. 352-54.

and two days/week in the hospital. Dr. Mary Allen, who meanwhile had married the Rev. Geo. Zoeckler, was assisted by Dr. Khachatur, an Armenian graduate of the missionary medical school, who had assisted before. A graduate of the missionaries' Girls' School, who wanted to study at the medical school, also assisted in the dispensary.[319] Although in 1918, Dr. Funk had been called to Hamadan, Soltanabad and Tehran (in all more than two months absence), the work at the dispensary continued, but at a lower attendance than before,[320] Dr. Funk left on furlough in March 1918, but the dispensary remained open five days/week until his departure.[321]

In 1920, with the hospital closed (see below), the burden for medical work rested entirely on the dispensary, which, since October 1919, had been open five days/week. Dr. Zoeckler, who had given birth to her daughter Frances in Hamadan in 1919, was unable to spend much time at the dispensary. Consequently, most of the work was done by Dr. Khachatur, Dr. Funk's assistant. Dr. Zoeckler only came for special examinations and for cases where she was really needed. Most patients were women, and the majority was Nestorian refugees (of 3,034 patients 2,786 were Nestorians). Other patients mostly were patients referred by local physicians. Because Dr. Khachatur also was the physician for the American-Persian Relief Committee it was arranged that Nestorian women would come to the dispensary in the morning and Nestorian men to his office in the afternoon. The dispensary also received assistance, when needed, from Dr. Col. Belt and Dr. Capt. Campbell, of the British military hospital in Hamadan.[322]

Probably in 1929, when Dr. Cook joined the Hamadan medical team, a second dispensary was opened at Pay-e Mosalla. Dr. Cook usually spent there six mornings per week. He felt he had to do more

---

319. Presbyterian Church 1914, pp. 329-30; RG 280-1-10, Report of the Women's Medical Work. Hamadan, July, 1914.
320. Presbyterian Church 1919, p. 263.
321. Presbyterian Church 1920, p. 313.
322. Presbyterian Church 1920, p. 313; Idem 1921, pp. 332; RG 280-1-10, M. A. Zoeckler, Report of the Medical Department, Hamadan Station, July 1, 1920.

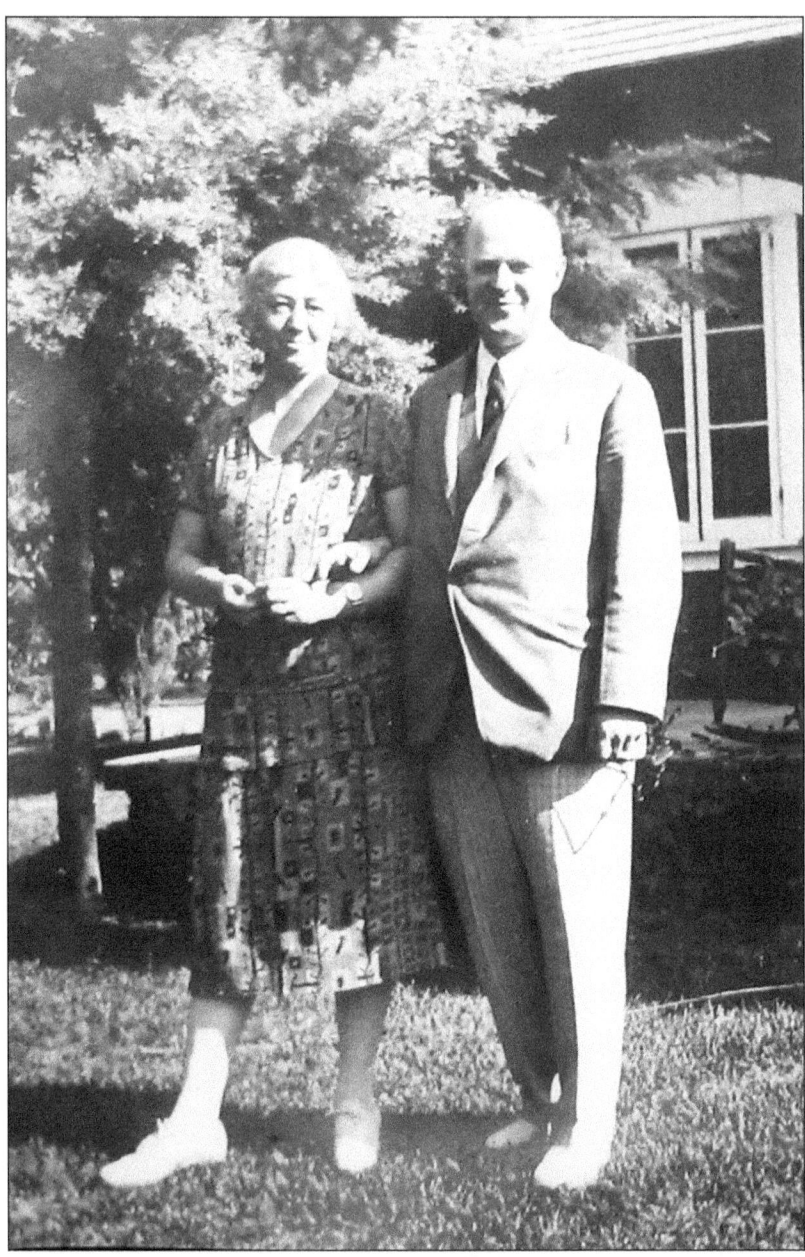

Mrs. and Dr. Joe Cook, 1915

and therefore, opened another dispensary in the Bun-e Bazar quarter three afternoons per week, when the physicians were not operating. After his death in 1932, the mission decided to continue the Pay-e Mosalla dispensary practically as before, but, instead of six, only three mornings, while the Kababian dispensary was continued five mornings. Dr. Funk went to Pay-e Mosalla on Mondays and Fridays and Dr. Andreas[323] on Wednesdays, who also was on Mondays at the Kababian dispensary. The number of patients fell off at the Pay-e Mosalla dispensary, because most were return patients. Therefore, it was first considered to discontinue the new dispensary Dr. Cook had opened, but Dr. Andreas later agreed to work there 3-4 afternoons, if he was released from hospital attendance, except for operations. The Bun-e Bazar and Pay-e Mosalla dispensaries were established as free clinics, but a few of the better class patients also attended. Although Kababian was a paying dispensary, not more than one-third of the patients paid the consultation fee, and many also received free medicines.[324] In 1933, the same dispensary work schedule was continued. For a time, Dr. Andreas also continued the Bun-e Bazar dispensary, in the poorer section of the city, but he found it so unsatisfactory that he gave it up entirely, being "unable to care for the crowds that came." Sometimes people came too late to be cured and died.[325]

In 1934, only the two dispensaries at Kababian and Pay-e Mosalla were continued, the former year round, the latter until 1 December. Dr. Lichtwardt on arrival (September 1934) from his previous post in the Mashhad hospital, took over Pay-e Mosalla, but he concluded that it would work better if the dispensary was part of the hospital. Therefore, rooms in the lower floor of the men's hospital, as originally intended, were made suitable for dispensary work and Dr.

---

323. He probably was: "Our Armenian assistant Dr. Andreos Hovanissian." RG 91-19-27, Hamadan, Healing in Hamadan 1939-40.

324. RG 91-19-27, Medical Work Hamadan 1932. The British soldiers formed part of the so-called Dunsterforce, which had arrived in Hamadan on 11 February 1918, see Dunsterville1920, p. 24.

325. RG 91-19-27, Hamadan Medical Report 1933; Presbyterian Church 1933, p. 179.

Lichtwardt saw patients there every weekday morning. It took some time for people to get to know the new location, also it was far from their homes, "while many who were attracted to that [old] location because of its being on a much-traveled street coming into the city failed to discover the new location." This meant less outpatients, but the advantage of the hospital dispensary was that patients were seen at once and, if need be, were immediately put in bed or operated. In 1935, attendance at the downtown Kababian dispensary was the same as the previous year, which was the largest in the mission's history. Having dispensaries away from the hospital meant practically doubling of the staff and requiring double supplies of drugs and equipment. But keeping the other dispensary there had a big advantage, because it was long-established in the center of the city and was easy accessible to many potential patients. Therefore, one extra attendant was hired, who had some experience in compounding drugs and took especially care of filling prescriptions.[326]

In 1935, the work at the downtown Kababian dispensary kept Drs. Funk and Andreas very busy. Attendance at the new dispensary established at the hospital by Dr. Lichtwardt grew steadily. Also, it was very convenient to have a doctor on duty at the hospital the entire day.[327] Dr. Andreas looked after the daily patients at the hospital when Drs. Funk and Lichtwardt were away. In 1936-37, the hospital dispensary was open six workday mornings, while the old one was open five mornings; attendance grew at both.[328] In 1937-38, there were three dispensaries open six mornings per week. The Kababian, so long run by Dr. Funk (who died in 1939) was in charge of Dr. Lichtwardt. Dr. Mary Zoeckler took over the hospital dispensary, while the Pay-e Musalla dispensary, which had been discontinued, was re-opened that winter and was in charge of Dr. Andreas. Clients of the Kababian were mostly paying patients, while the others treated mostly free patients. As the hospital dispensary was outside the city

---

326. RG 91-19-27, Medical Report Hamadan Station 1935.
327. RG 91-19-27, Healing in the Home of Avicenna 1936.
328. RG 91-19-27, Hamadan Medical Report 1937.

it had the smallest number of patients.[329] The year 1939 was the busiest in the dispensaries' history. Two dispensaries were open six mornings per week and during part of the year a third one was open. All three were crowded, more than 24,000 treatments were given, an increase of 35% over previous years. Much of the increase was due to the presence of >2,000 Assyrian refugees, who had been deported from Russia and were sent to Hamadan. They had neither work nor support and thus, there was much disease among them. They came to the Christian dispensary for treatment; more serious cases were admitted to the hospital.[330]

In 1939, the Pay-e Mosalla dispensary was finally closed down. Henceforth, for 6 mornings, there were two outpatient dispensaries with large attendance, except in winter, when roads were blocked by snow and mud. Dr. Andreos Hovanissian was in charge of the all-daily clinic at the hospital, while Dr. Lichtwardt did the city dispensary after hospital morning rounds and staff prayers.[331] In 1940, the two city dispensaries were consolidated; all outpatients were seen at the Kebabian dispensary. Until then Hamadan had been the only American hospital that conducted two daily dispensaries, one in the hospital and one in the city. Other US physicians felt that they could do their best work by restricting the number of patients daily at one dispensary each day. However, the hospital dispensary was never full, except when Dr. Andreas was looking after the Assyrian refugees there. Therefore, it seemed better to have all clinic work in the city. However, the only problem was that the Kababian dispensary had never been planned for two doctors and, as a result, it was very difficult to run things smoothly without confusion. Also, they had no record clerk. Dr. Lichtwardt did that always himself, and during Dr. Packard's stay (March 1941-42) it was Dr. Andreas who did it. For some time Ms Murray, the evangelist, helped out doing it, but this was not a good use of her time, so Dr. Zoeckler did it for some time, but soon one of the nurses spent mornings in the dispensary to keep

---

329. RG 91-19-27, Report Medical Work Hamadan 1937-1938.
330. RG 91-19-27, Christian Healing in Hamadan 1939.
331. RG 91-19-27, Healing in Hamadan 1940.

the records. Until 1943, the schedule had been: dispensary six days of the week and operations two afternoons/week. This was too great a burden for Dr. Packard. Therefore, the schedule was changed to: dispensary in the downtown office Monday, Wednesdays and Fridays and Saturdays with Tuesdays and Thursdays mornings for operations at the hospital. This schedule was not changed thereafter, because it was convenient for the doctors given heavy workload.[332]

Hospital Work

In 1901, Dr. Blanche Wilson wrote: "We really need a hospital; patients lie now on the floor; we have no place for in-patients," reverberating Dr. Alexander's earlier plea for a hospital in 1886.[333] In 1904, with funds made available by Mrs. Whipple, the Whipple Memorial Hospital for Women was built. It consisted of two large rooms and a couple of smaller ones, which were constructed over the dispensary. They were to be used for women patients, but, as Dr. Blanche Wilson-Stead was itinerating, they were used for men, until the time that a men's hospital would be built. The hospital was closed in summer, while cholera began on May 23 and lasted till 1 September.[334] In 1907, land had been acquired for the Reid Memorial Hospital and the building was almost complete by year's end. During the winter and spring 10 hospital beds were filled and sometimes patients had to be turned away. Mrs. Reid financed the hospital in memory of her daughter Lily Reid-Holt. The NW Women's' Board provided furnishings and the residence for the medical missionary. Until 24 April 1907, men and women were treated in the men's rooms; thereafter Dr. Field opened her women's dispensary. One of the leading men of Hamadan promised to erect an entrance to the hospital, a gate and gate-house, as recognition of the treatment of his wife, a sister of the shah.[335]

---

332. RG 91-19-27, Medical Report Hamadan 1941; Idem, Report of Medical Work Hamadan 1943; Presbyterian Church 1943, p. 83.
333. Presbyterian Church 1902, pp. 224, 231.
334. Presbyterian Church 1905, p. 282.
335. Presbyterian Church 1908, pp. 352-54. Idem 1906, p. 299-300. (In 1905, it had not yet possible to get land for the Reed Memorial Hospital)

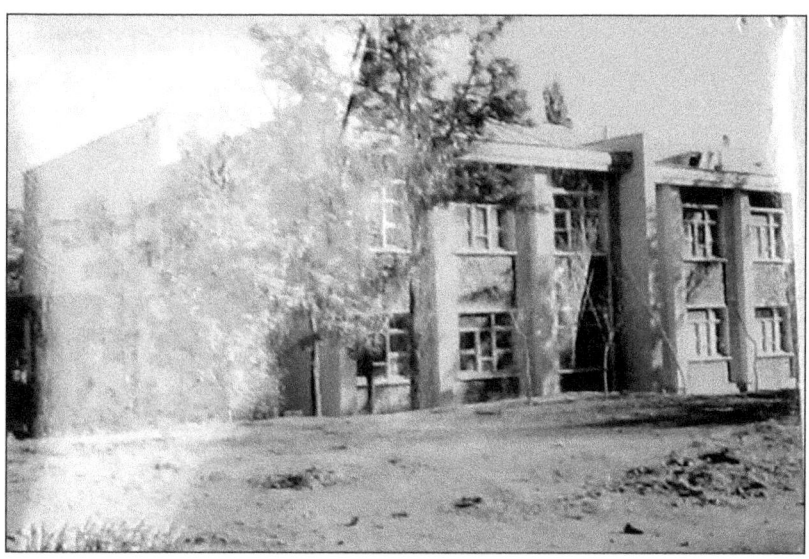

New American hospital in Hamadan

In 1908, it looked as if a new bright and promising era would begin. Dr. Funk arrived in 1903 and thereafter men's work received more attention. Also, on 29 November 1907 the new Reid-Holt Hospital for Men received its first patients, while on 31 January 1908 the new Whipple Memorial Hospital for Women was opened and its first patients were received. However, the hospital did not fill up immediately, probably due to disturbed condition of the country. Most hospital patients were villagers, who were too poor to find other lodgings in the city.[336] The period from 1909 to 1919 was a decade of political turmoil, in particular, the Salar al-Dowleh rebellion (1910-13), which was followed by military operations by the Russians and Turks (1915-17).[337] During that period, Hamadan itself was sometimes occupied by the rebels or by one of the warring parties, but even when it was not, its environs were the scene of looting and killing, which greatly impacted the rural population, many of whom were among the patients of the American doctors. In November 1912, Dr. Mary Allen reinforced the staff, who

---

336. Presbyterian Church 1910, p. 327; Idem 1909, p. 343.
337. On these events, see Floor 2018 b, pp. 336-65 and Idem 2018 c, pp. 34-68.

took up again the work with women, although the Women's hospital was closed, because she had to learn Persian.[338] The following year, women's medical work began by cleaning and renovating the Whipple Memorial Hospital and dispensary, which was made possible thanks to a gift from the ladies of the Utica Presbyterian Society.

> The low French windows in the main ward were removed and close fitting windows with tile-covered-window-seats were put in. An extra large window was placed in the middle of the ward, and it was surprising that a difference these simple changes made. Another large room over the dispensary which had not been used recently and was in very bad condition was quite transformed by a new floor and ceiling; the kitchen was plastered and a good stove built in the place of smoke Persian ojaks (charcoal stove); the hallways were plastered; the stairway leading to the dispensary was renewed; the whole building was freshly painted on the inside, and the walls were tinted a restful green in the place of the staring white. The hospital was further enriched by a gift of twelve iron beds from the Lily Reid Memorial Hospital, these beds having proved to be too short for the men patients, and some more of our money was spent in making new mattresses for these beds as well as renovating the old ones. When the work was done, we found ourselves in possession of a hospital which, in no way elegant or expensive, was, nevertheless, neat, clean, and fairly well equipped, comprising two wards, two private rooms, operating room, kitchen, bathroom, store-room, with beds for eighteen patients.[339]

Dr. Mary Allen-Zoeckler opened the women's dispensary and women's hospital in October 1913, although she had already seen many patients before in the men's dispensary. She lost her single nurse, who had fallen ill with tuberculosis. Fortunately, an older woman was hired, who was looking for work, had the right attitude, was hard-working,

---

338. Presbyterian Church 1913, p. 317.
339. RG 280-1-10, Report of the Women's Medical Work. Hamadan, July, 1914; Presbyterian Church 1915, p. 316-17.

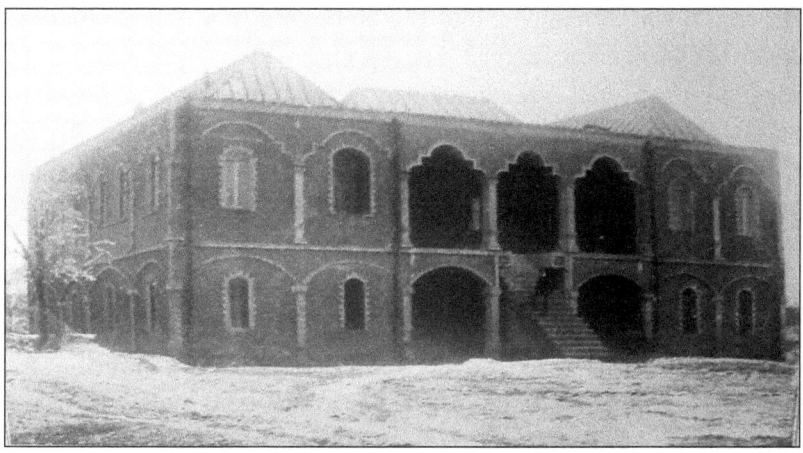

Lily-Reid Memorial Hospital, Hamadan, 1909

and quickly learned the hospital ways and fit in nicely.[340] In 1915, the Women's hospital was closed (but not the women's dispensary), because Dr. Zoeckler moved to Dowlatabad. Nevertheless, four women were received and operated in the Men's hospital.[341]

In 1917 and the beginning of 1918, the Russian Red Cross occupied the Lily Reid-Holt hospital, so male patients were sent to the Whipple women's hospital, which was unsatisfactory. Dr. Funk was unable to attend medical work for two months and the work was done by students, because Dr. Funk's Armenian chief assistant had left with the Armenians (who had fled rightly fearing the Turkish killing rage). When the Russian Red Cross left, the hospital was like a pigsty and had to be thoroughly cleaned. Because all the bedding had been destroyed or lost, new mattresses, quilts, pillows, sheets, etc. had to be made, but when the hospital was about to be cleaned "unrestrained Russian soldiers" occupied the hospital for six weeks, causing damage to the building estimated at 200 *tuman*s. A Commission decided that the American mission was owed this amount in damages, but they did not expect to see a penny of it. In February 1918 the British arrived

---

340. Presbyterian Church 1914, pp. 329-30.
341. Presbyterian Church 1916, p. 295. Mary Zoeckler wrote that it had been intended to continue "the present work through a new missionary with the help of Dr. Khachatour." RG 280-1-10, Report of the Women's Medical Work. Hamadan, July, 1914.

and asked whether they could use the building for their soldiers to which the missionaries agreed. The dispensary at the Whipple Hospital carried on as usual; attendance was good, although the number of patients was not higher than in previous years. Before the British took over the hospital the missionaries cleaned it. The place was filthy and it took 10 days to dig out the dirt. The British asked constantly for cooks, washerwomen, tailors, carpenters, servants and bedding for patients.[342] Hamadan medical work was less than usual, due to British army's occupation of the hospital and Dr. Funk's departure on furlough in March 1919. Only a few patients were admitted to the Whipple Hospital for Women. Dr. Funk continued his work for the British Army Medical Corps until sufficient British doctors arrived.[343]

As of March 1919, the hospital was closed, because Dr. Funk was on furlough, but the dispensary was operated by his assistant, Dr. Khachatur. Most of the patients were women. However, because the British military still occupied the Hospital for Men a reduced number of male patients had to be received in the Hospital for Women. Despite these setbacks the four medical trainees all graduated on Dr. Funk's departure and were given their MD certificate. The government of Iran issued them all a license to practice as physicians.[344] Dr. Mary Zoeckler, who had returned from Malayer to take charge of the medical mission in Hamadan, had not much to report, because, due to Dr. Funk's absence the hospital was closed. With the departure of the soldiers the hospital again became a relief institution. Dr. Zoeckler could not give much time to private practice, which meant less income for the medical mission. However, the US missionaries received helped from the American-Persian Relief Committee in the form of a large shipment of sugar and condensed milk, and friends in town gave rice. In the fall of 1920, Dr. Zoeckler had help from Ms Taillie, a newly arrived

---

342. Presbyterian Church 1918, pp. 283-84; Idem 1919, p. 263. On 24 March 1916, the Americans moved to Hamadan and set up a hospital in a carpet factory. Later they withdrew to Qazvin. History of American Red Cross Nursing. American National Red Cross. Nursing Service–1922, pp. 159-60.

343. Presbyterian Church 1920, p. 313.

344. Presbyterian Church 1921, p. 332; Idem 1920, p. 313.

trained nurse, who was temping in Rasht. A graduate of the mission's own school worked as matron nurse. However, her special charge was the operating room and preparation of sterilized dressings. She was good, so that the physicians were able to do emergency operations in one hour. The assistant matron, a girl of 17, was in charge of housekeeping. At the beginning of the year, Dr. Zoeckler and her matron reviewed the food available and the dishes Persians generally used, and worked out a diet together.[345]

In 1920-21, Dr. Khachatur continued the dispensary, while Dr. Zoeckler regularly assisted with examinations and treated special cases. In late December 1920, news arrived of the exodus from Tabriz and the flight of thousands of Nestorian refugees. As the Whipple Memorial Women's Hospital had not been used for some time one of the dispensary rooms was turned in a hospital ward for men, while the hospital was being readied to receive women. With the arrival of Dr. Dodd (Urmiyeh) and Ms Wells (Tabriz), who took charge of the hospital, as well as three Iranian nurses (Urmiyeh) the Hamadan hospital had never known such medical efficiency, Dr. Zoeckler remarked. After one month Dr. Dodd left for the USA, so that Dr. Zoeckler took charge of the hospital. On 1 April 1921, Dr. Funk, who had returned two days earlier, took over. However, he was unable to open the Lily Reid Memorial Hospital, which still required major repairs due to its use by the Russian military as well as having been used as an orphanage for Assyrian children. However, he received a few special cases in the Women's Hospital and intended to open the Men's Hospital as soon as the repairs were completed.[346] There is a hiatus of ten years in medical reports from Hamadan. During this entire period Dr. Funk was in charge of the hospital, who was joined by Dr. Zoeckler (who returned to Malayer in 1923) and Ms Jeanette Jones R.N. in 1922.

In 1931, the hospital was given a new name, American Christian Hospital, which did not arouse any adverse criticism. In 1930, Dr.

---

345. Presbyterian Church 1921, pp. 332-33.
346. Presbyterian Church 1922, pp. 366-67; RG 280-1-10, Report of Medical Work. Hamadan Station. 1920-21.

and Mrs. Joseph W. Cook returned to Hamadan, after having been for many years in the USA, making it again a two-doctor hospital.[347] However, six months later the hospital was again a one-doctor affair, because Dr. Cook died. The nursing staff lost Ms Jones, who went on furlough. Fortunately, Ms Kelley of the Friends of Arabia Mission in Hillah, Iraq, who was in Hamadan for the summer, agreed to stay until Ms Jones' return. However, Ms Jones resigned, but fortunately, Ms Kelley agreed to stay for another year. Dr. Packard relieved Dr. Funk during a 3-week vacation.[348] The next year, there still was only one doctor and one US nurse. Fortunately, the number of in-patients increased slightly only. Work among women continued to grow in the dispensary and the hospital "showing greater confidence in male doctors and increasing freedom from bigotry and oriental reserve," Dr. Funk observed.[349] In early September 1934, Dr. and Mrs. Lichtwardt R.N. arrived; he became the second doctor, while she assisted in nursing. This was a most welcome moment for Dr. Funk, because Hamadan had been a one-doctor operation for the last three years. This was technically not entirely true, because the hospital also employed Dr. Andreas, the Iranian assistant-physician. There was no doubt about his competency, because when in 1937 Drs Lichtwardt and Funk were away, he looked after the daily patients at the hospital. Although in 1934 Ms Kelley left, Ms Pease from Urmiyeh came to take over the supervision of the hospital and nursing.[350] The new law that foreign doctors must have five years experience before receiving a license to practice and must service in a location assigned by the government of Iran had the result that only two foreign doctors worked in Hamadan.[351]

In August 1937, Dr. Funk left on furlough leaving Dr. Lichtwardt in charge; he worked alone until October 1939. Fortunately, Dr. Zoeckler came to take over part of the work. She stayed until Dr.

---

347. Presbyterian Church 1932, p. 169.
348. RG 91-19-27, Medical Report Hamadan 1933.
349. RG 91-19-27, Medical Report Hamadan 1934.
350. RG 91-19-27, Medical Report Hamadan 1935; Idem, Hamadan Medical Report 1937.
351. RG 91-19-27, Medical Report Hamadan 1934-1935.

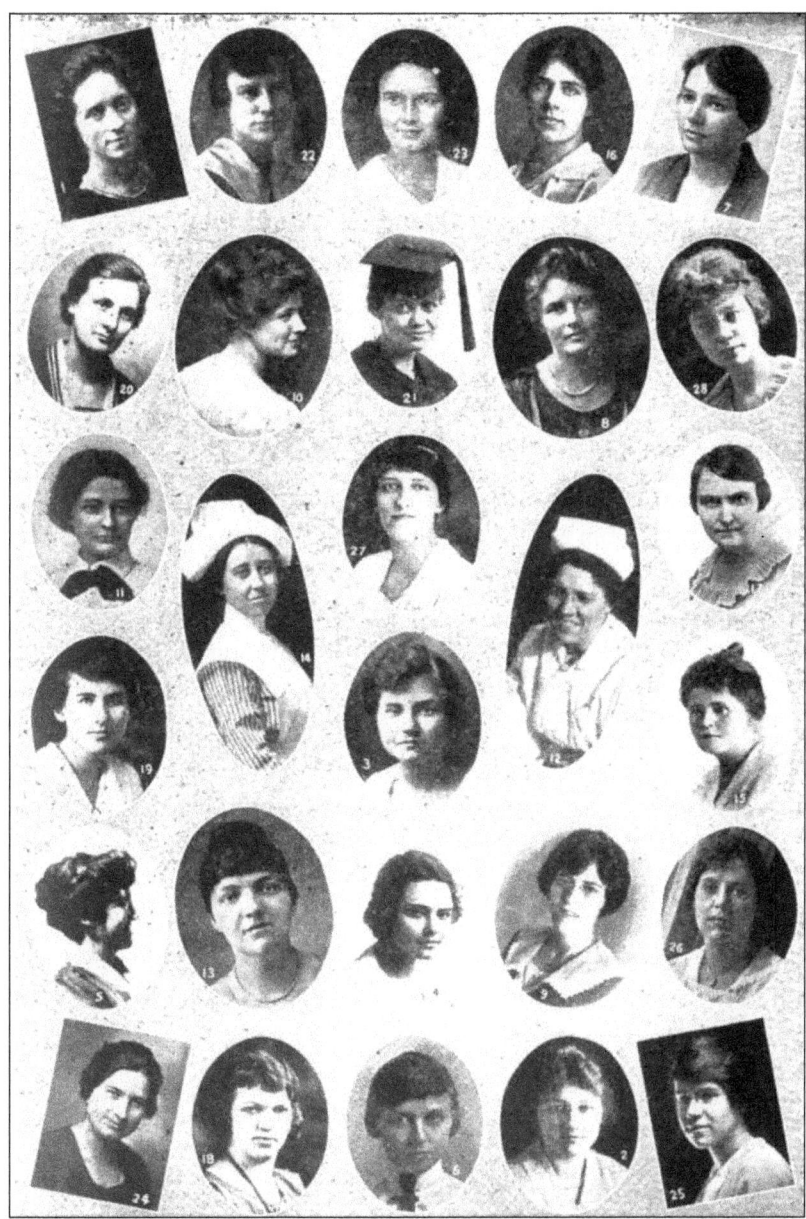

American missionaries in Hamadan, 1921

Funk returned, and then returned to Malayer. On 5 March 1939, Dr. Funk died after 37 years of service in Hamadan. He had returned from his furlough in the last week of December 1938. In the US he had been warned about his heart condition and told to take it slowly, but he immediately dove into the routine of work. Hundreds, Moslems, Jews and Christians came to the chapel to say farewell. This was a blow for the medical mission. It lost a long-time fixture and locally much respected physician, but it also was having a nursing shortage. Dr. Lichtwardt made an appeal to send him a US nurse, because Ms Harvey had gone to Mashhad, while Mrs. Lichtwardt supervised nursing. The hospital had only one graduate Iranian nurse, from the Tabriz hospital.[352]

Because Dr. Lichtwardt returned to the US on 12 April 1940, Dr. Zoeckler came from Malayer to replace him until Dr. Packard arrived. Mrs. Packard took over from Mrs. Lichtwardt in supervising nursing and housekeeping.[353] In September 1942, Dr. Packard and family (his wife was treasurer and superintendent of nursing) returned to the USA, which forced the Iran mission to close down the Dowlatabad dispensary and have Dr. Zoeckler take over the management of the Hamadan hospital. For a moment in mid-1942, it looked as if the hospital had to be closed, due to a lack of US missionary doctors, but finally it was the Tehran hospital that was closed down. Fortunately, the services of Dr. Alfred Cohn, a Jewish-German graduate of Leipzig University and an experienced surgeon, came available. He had been surgeon in the Shah's Hospital in Mazandaran, but the Russians had not allowed him to remain there. He started in September as chief surgeon and took charge of the male patients, while Dr. Zoeckler took the female ones, obstetrics and the administration. At that time, Dr. Andreas left, who had been with the hospital for many years. Part

---

352. RG 91-19-27, Report Medical Work Hamadan 1937-1938; Idem, Christian Healing in Hamadan 1938-1939. Mrs. Funk returned to the USA, after 48 years of service, many of which as matron of the hospital. Presbyterian Church 1940, pp. 70, 72.

353. RG 91-19-27, Healing in Hamadan 1939-40; Idem, Medical Report Hamadan 1940-1941.

of his work was assumed by two men, who worked as druggist and assistants. In October 1941, Ms Gertrude Winkelman R.N. arrived from India. Although she started language lessons, her impact on nursing practice was also felt. In December 1942, an Iranian graduate nurse trained in Kermanshah joined the nursing staff, which now consisted of two graduate nurses and five practical nurses.[354] Nurse Winkelman completed her 1-year language study and took more responsibility in supervising the nursing staff, which had not changed. What changed was the hiring of a new lab assistant, who had worked for years as lab technician for AIOC in Abadan, who returned to his home town of Hamadan. Although the hospital didn't have all the necessary equipment his work was an asset.[355]

Since Dr. Lichtward's departure in 1940 the hospital had a precarious existence, an uncertain future, and faced possible closing. Although with the closure of the Tehran hospital in September 1942 the situation of the Hamadan hospital seemed secure, nevertheless two years later its future was again in jeopardy. It was hoped, but uncertain, that Dr. and Mrs. Lichtwardt would return before Dr. Zoeckler would leave on furlough. Also, in mid-1945, Ms Winkelman would be transferred to Mashhad to continue the Nursing School. It looked as if the hospital had to be closed altogether. Fortunately, with some staff re-arrangements, the hospital was kept open with Dr. Cohn in charge of medical and surgical work, while Mrs. Arthur Muller R.N. would be looking after the nurses and Ms Enderson as general superintendent.[356] In 1942, Dr. Mary Zoeckler, without any professional assistance, performed 29 major operations, 27 obstetrical cases, and 14 obstetrical consultations.[357] Dr. Zoeckler went on furlough in September 1945 and on 1 July 1945 Mrs. Enderson took over the management of the hospital. Ms Winkelman had left in June for Mashhad. This made it necessary to make a few changes on the women's side, because the head of nursing there was acting as recording clerk four days/week.

---

354. RG 280-1-10, Report Medical Work Hamadan 1942-1943.
355. RG 280-1-10, Report Medical Work Hamadan 1943-1944.
356. RG 91-19-27, Report of Medical Work Hamadan 1944-1945.
357. Presbyterian Church 1943, p. 84.

Also, one of the practical nurses left, for whom in December 1945 a replacement was hired. Of course, the number of female patients decreased after Dr. Zoeckler left. Many women refused to be examined by Dr. Cohn, but after the governor's wife had been confined in the hospital there was an upsurge in confinement cases. She was delivered by one of the graduate nurses with Dr. Cohn standing by outside the delivery room in case of need. Because, as was feared, Dr. Lichtwardt resigned, the future of Hamadan's Christian hospital was again topic of discussion.[358] Dr. Zoeckler returned to Hamadan in February 1947, and found that the hospital was running smoothly. She took over as superintendent of the hospital from Ms Anderson, who continued as business manager. In January 1947, Ms Pease arrived to take over the nursing superintendence from Mrs. Muller. Dr. Cohn remained as chief surgeon and in charge of the male patients and Dr. Zoeckler of the women, maternity ward, administration, and assisted in the OR. In March 1947, Ms Evert Harutunian left to the USA. She had been head nurse on the men's side and in the OR for the last 12 years. Thereafter, the hospital had only one Iranian graduate nurse and two practical nurses, who had been there for many years. However, one was about to marry, while two other nurses were just beginning.[359]

In December 1947, Dr. John Davidson Frame Jr., son of Dr. John D. Frame Sr. of Rasht, arrived, while in February 1947, Dr. Cohn left and opened a private practice in the city. The arrival of Dr. Frame Jr. at the end of 1946, who knew Persian having spent his youth in Rasht, not only seemed to put the future of the hospital on a solid foundation.[360] However, this hope soon failed to have the desired result, because the hospital was closed in 1953, due to lack

---

358. RG 91-19-27, Hamadan Hospital Report 1945-1946.
359. RG 280-1-10, Report Medical Work Hamadan 1946-1947. The employment of Dr. Cohn was made possible from the Presbyterian Board's fund for employment of national doctors. Presbyterian Church 1948, p. 53.
360. RG 91-19-27, Christian Healing in Hamadan 1938-1939 (gift of $3,000 for X-ray etc. in 1928).

of medical staff.³⁶¹ In December 1955 the hospital was reopened, although Dr. Homer Rice commented that the hospital would be unable to function properly without a school of nursing, indicating the chronic shortage of qualified nurses in Iran. Therefore, he asked the Board to send him a short-term nurse. "All depends on this! This isn't simply making it sound easy, but honestly and truly stating the key to the whole problem."³⁶² Although the Board promised to send such a nurse, Dr. Rice insisted that he needed four of them, because the two American nurses (Ms Wheeler and Ms Pease) worked very long days. He feared that when Ms Wheeler would leave of furlough in July 1956 the workload would become too much, also because Dr. Ira Walstrom was still learning Persian.³⁶³ The nursing problem was averted when two young graduate nurses from Rasht were willing to come to Hamadan after *Nowruz*, Ms Keller arrived on 6 March and Mrs. Stetner would arrive soon thereafter, and since she did not need any language training would be able to start working immediately.³⁶⁴ In May 1956, the situation had not improved much, because Mrs. Stetner (short-term), three Iranian nurses and one who had not done any nursing for years constituted the entire nursing staff.³⁶⁵ Despite this situation, in November 1956 the missionaries proposed to build a new Christian 50-bed hospital in Hamadan, because the government hospital was overloaded and the Christian hospital was the only one that trained *behyar*s or nurse-assistants. However, to get government recognition for this training the hospital and the school of nursing needed to improve its existing facilities. Dr. Rice rejected the notion that the Hamadan hospital be closed and that the staff moved to

---

361. Presbyterian Church 1955, p. 50. Dr. Mary Zoeckler died in 1948.
362. RG 161-3-44, Ms Francis Gray to Dr. Rice, 26/01/1956; Rice to Ms Francis Gray, 12/02/1956.
363. RG 161-3-44, Rice to Ms Francis Gray, 12/02/1956.
364. RG 161-3-44, [Extract of] Action taken at the Meeting of the Executive Committee of the Iran Mission on 6-8 March, 1956.
365. RG 161-3-44, Walstrom to Dr. Dodd and Dr. Stevenson, 15/04/1956; Idem, Walstrom to Ms Francis Gray and Dr. Romig, 29/04/1956 (mentions the departure of Dr. Theodore F. Romig who had been in Hamadan for one month).

Kermanshah, which would make the missionaries look foolish in the eyes of the Iranians after having left there. Also, Dr. Muradian was quite able to competently run that hospital.[366] Despite all kinds of difficulties, Dr. Rice was able to get sufficient funds to start building a new hospital in mid-1959.[367] By that time the 30-bed hospital had a men's wing built in 1906 and a female wing built in 1927. In 1959, the hospital had electricity, running cold water and European-style flush toilets. Samovars were used to heat water. As sterilizer an Army portable kerosene burner was used, but a Wilmot Castle electric unit had been ordered. Its laboratory could perform simple tests such as urine analysis, blood count, stools, sputum, and Kahn or Kline tests. Its staff consisted of two American physicians and two American nurses, five Iranian nurses and one Iranian technician.[368] Despite the faith and perseverance of the missionaries their joy in the continuation of the hospital did not last long, because in 1970 the American missionaries ceased their activities in Hamadan.

Hospital Renovation

To better serve patients there were regular repairs and additions to the hospital. In 1927, a women's annex was added to the hospital.[369] In 1935 new toilets were constructed in the women's and men's hospitals, with a new septic tank in the men's department. An isolated sleeping room for the night nurse was built. On the east verandah of the women's hospital a new bathroom was constructed and the old one remodeled into a nursery; this was useful as there were 40% more obstetrical cases than in 1934. In 1935-36, new toilets in women's and men's hospitals were installed, with a new septic tank in the men's department. An

---

366. RG 161-3-44, Rice to Sundberg, 18/11/1956. Later the school of nursing was discontinued.
367. RG 161-3-44, Memo Sundberg to Cochran, 30/11/1959.
368. RG 161-3-44, Questionnaire for the medical office 1958. 30/01/1959.
369. Presbyterian Church 1928, p. 188; RG 91-19-27, Tower to Speer, 29/12/1925 (gift from Chicago First Church for women's annex and nurses' home).

isolated sleeping room for the night nurse was also built. On the east verandah of the women's hospital a new bathroom was constructed and the old one remodeled into a nursery; this was useful as there were 40% more obstetrical cases than in the previous year.[370]

Thanks to gifts from various church organizations in the US, a two-story addition was constructed. In this way a second OR was obtained by adjoining to the old one; under it a dining room for the nurses was built. Also, the former store room in the men's building was converted into an X-ray room, thus releasing an upstairs room for the use as a private room. Furthermore, a new septic tank was constructed for the US nurse quarters as well as a new outbuilding for the storage of firewood.[371] In 1938, the men's ward walls were whitened and floors in the kitchen and corridor leading to the OR suite were cemented.[372] In 1939, a cement floor was laid in the large main ward of the men's building; it was hoped to gradually cement the whole hospital, because cement work was very expensive in Iran. In addition to these changes, the interior walls were all re-calsomined and all beds, bedside tables and other ward and OR furniture received a new coat of white enamel. Because electricity was becoming reasonable in price, due to a hydro-station in the mountains, the medical staff used their electric equipment more than before. Small electric stoves in the men's and women's hospitals were very convenient.[373] In 1940, under the verandah on the south side of the Men's Hospital a dining room for the male orderlies had been constructed. It opened directly into the kitchen and was very convenient as they liked to have a place to eat in private. The piped water system was extended to the Iranian nurses' apartments, while other repairs were done throughout the hospital.[374] This piped water system needed repairs in 1946, so that the nurses' quarters and service rooms had piped water

---

370. RG 91-19-27, Healing in the Home of Avicenna 1935-1936.
371. RG 91-19-27, Hamadan Medical Report 1936-1937.
372. RG 91-19-27, Report Medical Work Hamadan 1937-1938.
373. RG 91-19-27, Christian Healing in Hamadan 1938-1939.
374. RG 91-19-27, Healing in Hamadan 1939-1940.

again.[375] According to Dr. Morton, the building was "a three-story, up-to-date hospital, which he [Dr. Funk] designed and supervised in every detail so that he was in fact architect, contractor, and builder."[376] Nevertheless, despite this praise, in 1947, Dr. Zoeckler opined that the "hospital is still inconvenient and inadequate."[377]

OTHER LOCAL HOSPITALS

There was a 12-bed municipal hospital in Hamadan, housed in part of the Municipality building. It had been established around 1920 and was financed by a tax on transportation. Although it was a bare-bones operation it provided better treatment to patients than they would have received at home. However, there was no surgical service, even of the most elementary kind.[378] This situation had not changed ten years later. At that time, the municipal hospital still had a small bed capacity, the patients were all very poor, and only very minor surgery was done.[379] The new Pahlavi hospital, built around 1935, was taking care of a number of poor patients, both in their dispensary and in-patient department, thus relieving the Christian hospital somewhat.[380] Nevertheless, even as late as 1940, Dr. Lichtwardt opined that, "there is still a need for mission hospitals, although the Persian government is doing a lot now." For, although there was a small free government hospital and a free dispensary in the city, people preferred to come to the Christian hospital, because "50 years of experience gives you a reputation." Also, neither the small government hospital with a minimum of equipment nor the local municipal hospital was doing any surgery. They had no surgeon and, therefore, the health department asked the Christian to their surgery for them. In spite of this and the

---

375. RG 280-1-10, Report Medical Work Hamadan 1946-1947.
376. Morton 1940, pp. 262, 268 (training of Iranian staff).
377. RG 280-1-10, Report Medical Work Hamadan Station 1946-1947.
378. Gilmour 1924, p. 29. It is sad that Hamadani 1382, p. 176 does not even mention these earlier hospitals, thus relegating the endeavors of these physicians, both American and Iranian, to the dustbin of history.
379. RG 91-19-27, Medical Report Hamadan 1934-1935.
380. RG 91-19-27, Healing in the Home of Avicenna 1935-1936.

two free government dispensaries the work of the missionary doctors was increasing.[381] Occasionally, there was some friction, such as in 1941, when a patient was discourteously removed to Pahlavi Hospital in the city, where he died. The family then lodged complaint against Dr. Lichtwardt.[382] In November 1956 the American missionaries proposed to build a new Christian 50-bed hospital in Hamadan, because the city had only one government hospital (100 beds), but this was sometimes so full that patients had to sleep on the floor.[383] By 1959, there was a second government hospital; the missionaries considered the quality of service in one of them good and average in the other.[384]

Hesar

In March 1905, Hajj Dhu'l Faqr Khan Bayat Samsam al-Molk Amir Tuman made funds funds available for the construction of a hospital in the village of Hesar, at 35 km from Arak. The hospital was called Samsamiyeh and the revenues of several villages were deeded to it for its operational expenditure.[385] These were detailed as follows in the endowment document:

Table 15: Expenditures of the Samsamiyeh hospital in Hesar according to the endowment document

Administration rights	Expenditures	Annual total in *tumans*
		1 `oshr (346.25)
	Honorarium physician	600
	Wages of staff and laundry cost	50

---

381. RG 91-19-27, Christian Healing in Hamadan 1938-1939; Idem, Healing in Hamadan 1939-1940.
382. RG 91-19-27, Medical Report Hamadan 1940-1941. Although the American missionaries don't mention another hospital, it seems that in 1939, "the Hamadan Municipality are building a hospital of fifty beds." Jarman 1997, vol. 1, p. 184.
383. RG 161-3-44, Rice to Sundberg, 18/11/1956.
384. RG 161-3-44, Questionnaire for the medical office 1958. 30/01/1959.
385. Rezai 2012, pp. 120-21.

Administration rights	Expenditures	Annual total in *tumans*
	Wages of the cook	15 (4 `oshr*)
Hospital expenditures		
	Medicines, food, physician's things	700
	Guard	20
Total		1.732,25

Source: Rezai 2012, p. 121.

There are no further details available about this hospital, which may not have survived after the legator's death.

ISFAHAN

Around 1900, Isfahan was a city with 60,000 inhabitants, which did not even seem to have had a *dar al-shafa* any longer. In Safavid times (see above), there had been such an institution, but it had been turned into a mosque (*masjed-e dar al-shafa*). There also was a *madraseh-ye dar al-shafa*, a reminder that this institution traditionally had been part of an Islamic religious complex. Another sign of its past presence was the existence of a Dar al-Shafa avenue (*khiyaban-e dar al-shafa*).[386] However, as of 1883, a modern dispensary with waiting rooms for either sex was opened in Jolfa-Isfahan, which had been established and as of 1880 was managed by Dr. E. F. Hoernle of the British Church Missionary Society. "Another room had been set apart as a hospital where the more serious cases are treated surgically."[387] When Dr. Collins visited Isfahan performed eye operations at the Jolfa hospital.[388] According to Janab, the Missionaries' Hospital (*mariz-khaneh-ye morselin*) only had some surgical instruments, some wooden beds, and some new medicines that people in Isfahan had not used before.[389]

---

386. Jaberi-Ansari 1373, pp. 137, 147, 287, 341.
387. Wills 1893, p. 164; Elgood 1951, p. 534; Waterfield 1973, p. 150. According to Janab, in 1305/1887-88, the CMS bought a piece of land in `Abbasabad and built there a new hospital. Janab 1303, p. 66.
388. Anonymous 1895, pp. 264.
389. Janab 1303, p. 66.

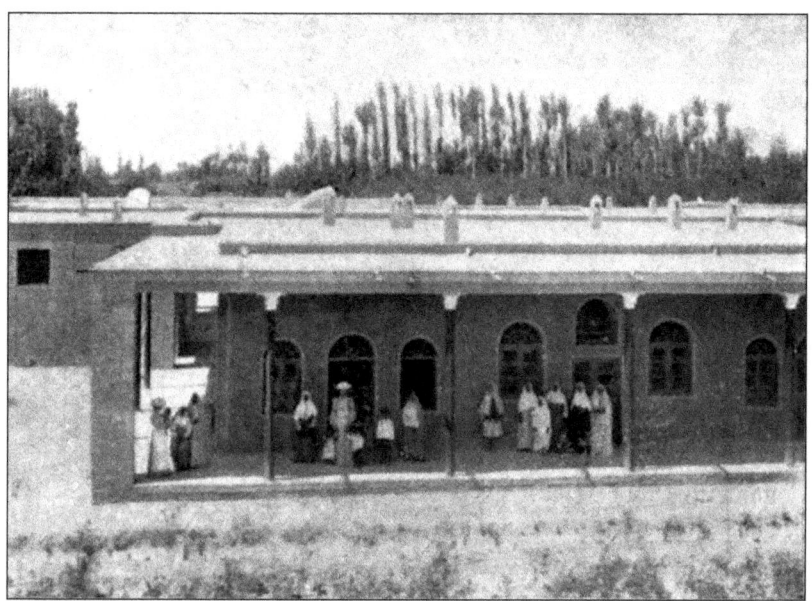

The new women's hospital, 1905

In 1891, Mary Bird of the CMS opened a dispensary for Moslem women in the Isfahan bazaar, which remained open due to popular support from her patients, despite the opposition by the ulama, who, during 1894-97, forcibly shut it down no fewer than five times.[390] The first time this happened was on 4 January 1891, when Ms Mary Bird opened a women's dispensary in the Bidabad quarter of Isfahan. On 15 February it was closed down by the mullahs; during that time she had seen 537 people. Ms Bird then moved to the Dar Dasht quarter and opened a dispensary there to work among Jewish people. The mullahs also opposed this saying that the women would be converted to Christianity and the governor, Rokn al-Dowleh, put armed men at the door to prevent women from entering. Many came anyway before dawn and over the roofs. On 14 November, religious students incited by mullahs surrounded Ms Bird when she wanted to enter the dispensary and forced here to return to Jolfa.[391]

---

390. For the story of the clerical opposition, see Rice 1916, pp. 70-77; Waterfield 1973, pp. 155-156.

391. Anonymous 1895, pp. 264 (April 1895). For the story of the clerical opposition, see Rice 1916, pp. 70-77; Waterfield 1973, pp. 155-156.

It was not the only anti-CMS activity in the Isfahan region. In March 1891, the CMS began activities in Najafabad with a catechist and dispenser in a house it had rented there. Attendance reached 450 patients per month. On 5 September 1891 the prince-governor had the house forcibly closed and the medicines, books etc. removed to a caravanserai. The *zabet* or chief of the town was forbidden to allow the CMS agents to return. The owner of the rented house was bastinadoed.[392]

In 1894, Dr. Donald Carr took over medical operations, and in 1896 the CMS opened a hospital with dispensary in Jolfa-Isfahan and made great progress in improving its facilities. The hospital was located in a house rented from an Armenian, which, in 1889, Carr had bought.[393] Dr. Carr had two days in the week to receive out-patients at his house. Bishop Stuart's niece, Dr. Emmeline Stuart and her sister saw female patients on Saturday.[394] At the beginning of 1899, Dr. Stuart performed her first two ovariotomies with success. The result was that more patients were willing to undergo surgery.[395] The men's hospital at Jolfa was closed for a few months due to absence Dr. Carr, but was reopened when Dr. Griffith arrived.[396] In 1901 Dr. Carr observed:

> When he came he found the hospital in a very bad state of repair, more like a caravanserai than a hospital, with only three wards accommodating six men and seven women. In 1901 there was an entire wing for women and beds for twenty-three men. In 1894 there was no nursing staff, each patient being looked after by a friend or relative. In 1901 nursing care had been revolutionised by the Canadian sister, Helen McKin. In 1894 there was a minimum of hygiene and cleanliness and the patients

---

392. Anonymous 1895, p. 264 (April 1895).
393. Janab 1303, p. 66.
394. *Mercy and Truth* 1900, vol.4, p. 188.
395. Stuart 1902, vol. 6, p. 116.
396. *Mercy and Truth* 1900, vol. 4, p. 188. Dr. Griffith probably is the Dr. Krit/Krist mentioned by Janab 1303, p. 66. One of Dr. Griffith's Isfahani graduates was Dr. `Isa `Ali. Dr. Carr also taught medical classes.

remained in their own clothes, which were often torn and filthy. In 1901 they had clean linen and clean hospital garments and there was a high standard of antisepsis in the hospital. Between 500 and 600 patients passed through the hospital during the year 1900, with an average stay of fourteen days.[397]

In 1902, CMS opened a clinic in Isfahan itself, and in 1904 a hospital was built on the Isfahan side of the river helped by a land gift from a local rich merchant. Subsequently, a women's hospital was founded and placed under the supervision of Dr. Emmeline Stuart. The hospital could accommodate 200 in-patients, with a male (110 beds) and female wing (80 beds).[398]

In 1904 the men's hospital moved from Jolfa to Isfahan and in the third week of April this year the women's hospital did, adjoining the men's. Six weeks later 40 beds arrived, by begin June the hospital had 60 beds. Everything was moved on donkeys, including the patients. In total 200 loads were moved. The CMS had three house-warming parties: European, Armenian and Persian.

> On the photo you see at the left the assistants' room, i.e. three bed rooms and on sitting room on the upper-storey. Our four Armenian nurses have pink uniforms with white aprons. Underneath are four rooms, one of which is their kitchen, one the

---

397. Waterfield 1973, p. 158. "The cost of supporting a bed in Persia is £10/ year". *Mercy and Truth* 1906, vol. 10, p. 375. People could also support CMS hospital with non-cash donations. "The flanel bed-jackets very useful, in particular for hernia cases of which there were 60 before June. The pillows in the men's hospital are large 42 x 22 inches, needed are fitting pillow cases. Blankets are needed; native padded quilts are used but are heavy and unsatisfactory. Their block of the hospital has just been opened. Ms Phillips writes on 2 June, 1906 that there are private wards; wide bandages had run out and she had to buy native stuff and make some. The nice English ones brought smiles to the faces of the physicians in the operating room." *Mercy and Truth* 1906, vol. 10, pp. 253-54.

398. Wright 2001, pp. 118, 122; Stead 1906, pp. 13-14 (18 October, 1906). Therefore, the British noted that "there are two British hospitals in the city." Adamec 1981, vol. 1, p. 251. It was in this hospital the late Queen Soraya was born in 1936.

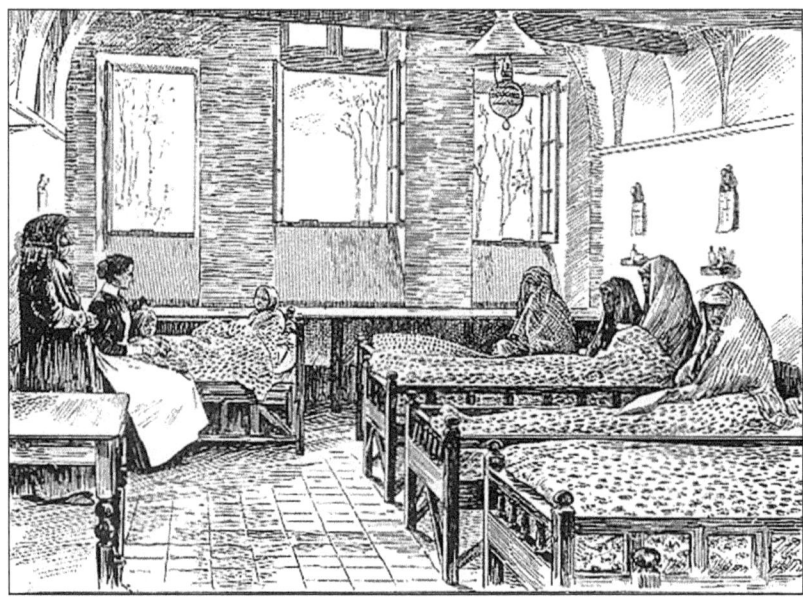

A women's ward at the hospital in Jolfa, Isfahan

room of the Armenian woman who cooks for them and acts as 'chaperone.' Two are little wards for private Armenian patients. In front is a little garden, which makes this 'Armenian quarter' private. Beyond the assistants quarters one sees the hospital well and kitchens, and the jutting-out room is part of the out-patients' department. The door is into the drug store-room and the corner room is the sitting room for the dispensary assistants when on duty. The entrance is at the poplar trees. At the south wall the small operating room with 2 windows, where we do small operations and attend septic cases. The big room is beyond that. The south wing has had the Clifton and Bradford wards, the matron's room, the servants' room, and inquirer room (far right). The hedge divided our garden from that of the hospital. Beyond the main building are some store-room, the hammam, and the door leading to the men's hospital. Not shown are three isolation wards, four private wards, and a mortuary situated along the north wall. The OR faces a garden, which separates the north from the south wing of the hospital. In the north wing are two large wards, the Memorial and the Rawtenstall, or children and cataract wards, apart from one or two single bed wards for bad cases. In this wing also a battery-room and a

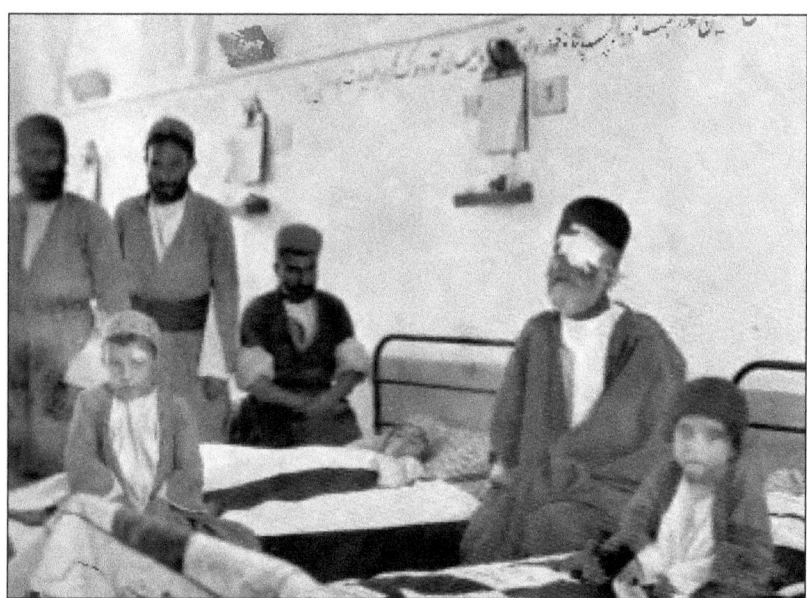

A ward at the hospital in Jolfa, Isfahan

sitting-room for the assistant when on duty. The Memorial has a plaque in memory of my father, and 12 beds and so do the other large three wards. On Sunday I preach here, while Dr. Ironside and Ms Proctor give scripture elsewhere for the children.[399]

In 1915, the hospital was temporarily closed, because British subjects were ordered to leave, but they returned in 1916 after the Russians had occupied the city in May of that year.[400] Dr. Carr remained in charge of the hospital until 1922, when he died, after he had returned from furlough in Europe. He was succeeded by Dr. H.T. Marabelle, who, at least since 1905, had been his assistant.[401]

---

399. Stuart 1906, pp. 368-70.
400. Waterfield 1973, p. 162; Rice 1916, p. 189.
401. Janab 1303, pp. 66-67. CMS staff present in Isfahan in 1905: Drs. D.W. Car and H.T. Marrable in Isfahan; Ms H, McKim, Ms E.F. Phillips; Mr. S.H. Biddlecombe (evangelist); Dr. Ms M.E. Stuart; Ms C.M. Ironside MB; Ms E. Proctor, Ms P. Braine-Hartnell (evangelist) *Mercy and Truth* 1906, volume 10, p. 378.

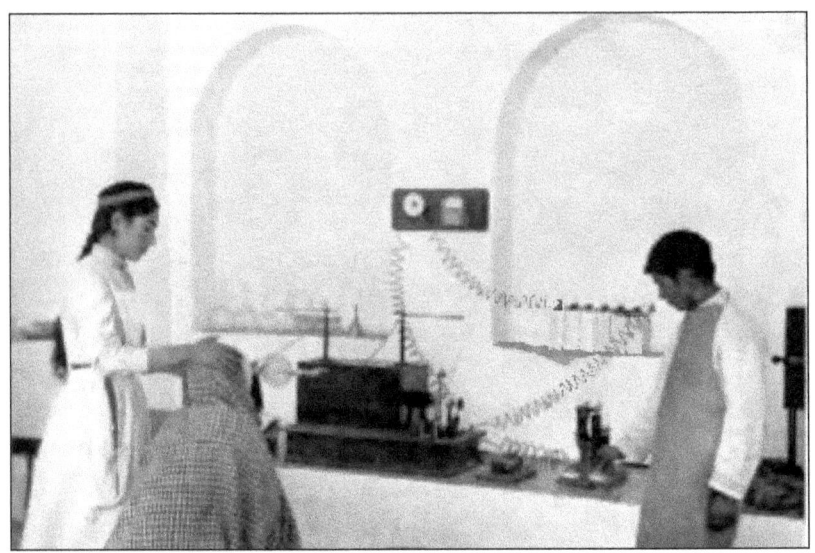

Patient being x-rayed at the hospital in Jolfa, Isfahan

Already soon after Dr. Hoernle had started his medical activities in Jolfa, two graduates of the Dar al-Fonun, established a medical practice in Isfahan. These were Eskandar Mirza and Mirza Musa Khan Hafez al-Sehheh, who was from a family of traditional physicians, the Mohammad Hoseyn Saheb al-Qarabadin Kabir family. Musa Khan's son, Masih Khan, also was a physician and became chief of the public health office (*ra'is-e edareh-ye hefz al-sehheh*). These were the first Iranians who began practicing modern medicine in Isfahan. As a result, many traditional physicians came from other cities to be trained by these two physicians knowledgeable about modern medicine. Among them were Mirza Mohammad Baqer Hakim-bashi Sadr al-Atteba, Mirza Habib, Mirza Abdol-Karim, Mirza Abdol-Baqi and others. Soon also from among the new students also came to be trained such as Mirza Ali Akbar Khan Nazem al-Atteba, Mirza Habib Tabib-e Fowj, Mirza Sheikh Mohammad Khan, Mirza Hoseyn Khan etc. By 1886 some 10 physicians who used modern medicine practiced in Isfahan and were graduates of the Dar al-Fonun. There also still were more than 20 traditional physicians who had received a certificate to practice.

The consequence was that by the 1920s, the training of traditional physicians in Isfahan had completely been discontinued.[402]

OTHER HOSPITALS

In 1908, Dr. `Isa Qoli established a small hospital with a few beds, which four years later was closed, when he left to Europe. In 1913, a hospital was founded with the help and financing of the people of Isfahan, which was placed under Dr. Mozayyan al-Soltan. It had sufficient equipment and 20 beds, but in its third year it was closed down when the Russians entered the city. For some time, the Islamic Hospital (*bimarestan-e eslami*) was under Mirza Masih Khan, Ehtesham al-Atteba and Mohammad Hasan Mirza, but it was closed.[403] Probably in the late 1920s or the early 1930s, a military hospital (*bimarestan-e qoshuni*) was built next to the barracks in Isfahan.[404] In 1939, a *civil hospital* of 100 beds was constructed in the Avenue Shahpur, Isfahan.[405]

KERMAN

In September 1897, the governor of Kerman, Bahjat al-Molk, opened a hospital for the poor inside the citadel of Kerman, which had 20 beds as well as a nursing staff. The medical director was Hajj Mahmud Khan Kermani.[406] Probably for this reason, when in 1897, Dr. Carr of Isfahan came to Kerman for 6 months hoping to get permission to stay, he did not get it and he returned.[407] Whether this hospital lasted beyond the governor's time in office is not known, but seems unlikely (see below).

In the spring of 1902, Dr. White in Yazd received a telegam from the governor of Kerman asking him to come and treat his wife. Dr and Mrs. White came and stayed for 2 weeks treating many people.

---

402. Janab 1303, pp. 66-68.
403. Janab 1303, pp. 67-68.
404. Jaberi-Ansari 1373, p. 150.
405. Jarman 1997, vol. 1, p. 184.
406. Sepehr 1368, pp. 169-170.
407. Griffith 1902 a, p. 12.

Soon thereafter CMS received permission to start its activities in Kerman and then the medical mission was opened by Dr. Griffith. However, Dr. Griffith had limited supplies (lent by Dr. White) and hardly any instruments, which was a great handicap, especially for eye cases such as cataract. He had to tell patients come back in three months, which was understood as: "I cannot don't do anything for you, because that is what their own doctors tell them." Meanwhile, instruments had arrived at Bushehr and he hoped to receive them end of August. Another handicap was the lack of language skills, because they had too little time. Therefore, he opined that it would be nice if missionaries would be given ample time to learn the language. Ms Bird and Ms Willmott were supposed to come, but when Dr. Mrs. Malcolm fell ill in Yazd they remained there, as they were needed. "I had taken two Armenians one as dispenser the other as senior assistant, but the latter fell ill and returned to Jolfa. Only the educated class believe in superiority of modern medicine; the others only come when all else has failed. Also, they consult their beads tod ecide whether to take their medicine or not. For fractures and dislocations they go the the bone setters or butchers, and if things go wrong, in most cases, they get gangrene and come to me."[408] Despite its small size, it certainly satisfied a great unmet need in the town of 50,000 inhabitants, for some 28 in-patients were treated in a small Persian house, with a male and a female section.[409]

In the first three months of 1901, Dr. Griffith saw >2,000 patients of which 500 house calls and had three in-patients. He reported that the local officials and mullahs were friendly and that he used the house of the late Rev. Carless as dispensary. He believed that he might change it into a hospital of 15 beds, because the owner was in debt and would be willing to sell the house for £300. It could also be used as a doctor's house, in which case he had to buy the adjacent land to build a hospital for all this, which in total would cost £1,000. Dr. Griffith was very glad for his four in-patients, because a local Iranian doctor (presumably Hajj Mahmud Khan Kermani) had told him that a previous governor

---

408. Griffith 1902 a, pp. 12-15.
409. Administration Report 1933, p. 31.

(presumably Bahjat al-Molk) had established a hospital of which he was put in charge, but nobody wanted to come, "for they said he was in league with the English doctors, who wanted to take the fat from their bodies for the compounding of strange medicines." There was still a garden in Kerman belonging to Iranian doctors, a remnant of olden and better days. Dr. Griffith lived a few yards from the dispensary and the Armenian assistants in the dispensary. In the morning, the doctor first checked whether there were new cases, the assistants took care of the dressings. Monday was operating day, but due to lack of instruments only minor operations were performed. Tuesday and Friday were proper dispensary days. There was reading and prayer as well. Eye diseases prevailed. Dr. Griffith had the diphtheritic antitoxin (Behring's) apparatus, but lacked the serum for which he needed an annual grant. He needed many other things, such as a microscope and medical books (surgery, eye diseases, and ear and throat diseases).[410]

Initially though, its prospects and reception did not look very propitious. In 1908, the British consul reported that the CMS hospital work was "neither judicious nor popular and in place of being a help to my work has become a source of anxiety." Contrariwise its small school was very popular.[411] The reason for the problem was personal as well as professional. Dr. Dodson, who had been given the task to run the hospital in Kerman in 1906 (replacing Dr. Griffith),[412] apparently had behaved in a way that raised the eyebrows of the British consul. He wrote to the CMS committee in London asking it to remove Dr.

---

410. Griffith 1902 b, pp. 48-52.
411. Administration Report 1907-08, p. 69. In 1905, CMS staff at Kerman consisted of: Ms W.A. Westlake; G.E. Dodson and Mrs. Dodson, Ms E.M. Seton-Adamson. *Mercy and Truth* 1906, vol. 10, p. 378.
412. In Kerman, soon after her arrival, "Mrs. Dodson asks for: knitted caps, curtains (red twill) 2.5 x 2.25 yards; handkerchiefs, flannel red bed jackets; flannel and flannelette (12 yards of each), long stockings, socks, doctor's overalls, aprons for male assistant with pockets, eye shades, sheets, draw sheets, towels (not fringed), trousers for men and boys; the last 4 items are most urgently needed." *Mercy and Truth* 1906, vol. 10, p. 93.

Dodson from Kerman. Because Dr. White of the CMS hospital in Yazd refused to have Dr. Dodson near him, CMS London decided to close the hospital in Kerman and told Dr. Dodson to move to Isfahan to go "through the course of training under the doctor there." However, by that time the political situation in Kerman had changed. Also, finally Dr. Dodson had realized that the British consul's observations had to be taken into consideration and, as a result, he "had left off performing operations recklessly." Therefore, the consul informed the London committee that Dr. Dodson's removal was no longer necessary. Also, the considerable European community in Kerman had begun to rely on the services of the CMS physician. The consul's request was supported by the local community at large, "whom the Mission had educated to appreciate European medicine and surgery within reason." This only allowed the delay of the hospital's closure, because initially the hospital had relied on fees and local contributions to pay for its cost, which had fallen off in recent times, and therefore, it was unable to support itself. Therefore, the London committee decided that the hospital would be closed in early 1909.[413]

Apparently, the local wishes were heard, because the CMS continued supporting the hospital in Kerman under Dr. Dodson. The average in-door and out-door patients numbered 60 per day in 1909.[414] In 1910, the hospital's medical staff was reinforced by Dr. Westlake, a female physician and two female nurses. On 21 November 1910, cholera broke out of a very mild type. Dr. Dodson and Dr. Westlake and asst. surgeon Salt provided medical assistance, while the governor took some primitive preventive measures. The outbreak led to an exodus of the population, but most people returned by the end of December.[415] In 1912, there was the usual spring epidemic of small-pox and people were ready and anxious for vaccination. Typhoid, small-pox and whooping cough were endemic. The prevailing diseases were genital

---

413. Administration Report 1908, p. 58.
414. Administration Report 1909, p. 33.
415. Administration Report 1910, p. 33-34.

and ocular. There also was an IETD dispensary run by assistant-surgeon Steinhoff, who also had the medical charge of the British Consulate.[416]

Table 16: Patients seen and operated at the CMS Kerman hospital (1912)

	Male	Female
Fresh cases	620	316
Repeated visits	Unknown	-
Operations - major	97	15
Operations - minor	-	25

Source: Administration Report 1912, p. 56

In 1913 a bigger hospital was completed, mostly with funds and land gifts from the local Kermani community.[417] In 1914, the hospital was kept busy as ever and the stream of patients taxed the capacity of the staff.[418] The political situation in Iran became tense during WW I, in particular because the warring parties ignored Iran's neutral position. As a result, in some cities, among which Kerman, members of the fierce nationalist Democrats, who opposed foreign interference in the internal affairs of Iran, grabbed power towards the end of 1915. As a result, all British subject left Kerman on 17 December 1915. Although the Democrats only remained in power until May 1916, when they were ousted by the British-officered South Persia Rifles, the hospital remained closed until the end of 1917. This was because there was an embargo on superfluous British subjects, which CMS staff was considered to be. However, when Dr. G. E. Dodson and Dr. Gertrude Westlake returned in December 1917 they immediately began collecting staff, furniture and material for respectively, the men's and the women's hospital. Most of the hospital equipment had been looted either by the Democrats or the Persian staff after the Democrats takeover in 1915. Because all the Iranian male staff had taken service with the South-Persian Rifles (SPR) the two physicians

---

416. Administration Report 1912, p. 56; Administration Report 1914, p. 20.
417. Rice 1916, pp. 133-134.
418. Administration Report 1914, p. 25.

had a thankless task to retrieve equipment. However, they were able to open the hospitals to patients. This development was greatly welcomed by the population, which had regularly queried the consul about the doctors' return.[419] Starting anew had also its advantages, for the old building was cramped and inadequate, and thus plans to have a new building were initiated. Dr. Dodson and Dr. Westlake made much progress with the construction and equiping of the new hospital.[420] In 1919, Dr. Dodson and Mrs. Dodson managed the hospital assisted by the Iranian nursing staff. Attendence was lower that year, because the first three months of the year the European staff were ill. Medical work continued in the old, cramped and inadequate building, while "building work has been continued on the new site, where the men's new out-patient department, one new ward block for 28 men's beds, the new kitchen and store rooms, and part of the new Doctor's house have been put up."[421] In the 1920s the hospital was further enlarged and modernized.[422]

Dr. Dodson put his stamp on the CMS hospital in Kerman that he had founded. He served it for 34 years and was well liked and respected in the city. In Kerman, as of 1910, he was joined by a female physician, Dr. Getrude Westlake and two nurses (Ms Parry and Ms Carrick), who together with Dr. and Mrs. Dodson formed the medical team until 1922. Thereafter several physicians from other CMS hospitals provided back-stopping or new ones came for only one or two years. What was encouraging that there usually always was a female physician to head the Women's Hospital, at one time (1942) there were even two female physicians. The British medical staff were assisted by Iranians, both male and female, some of whom through on-the-job training and study obtained their medical license to practice.

---

419. Administration Report 1915, p. 23; Administration Report 1916, pp. 19, 24, 42; Administration Report 1917, p. 26.
420. Administration Report 1918, p. 31.
421. Administration Report 1919, p. 31; Cash 1930, p. 40.
422. A Friend of Iran 1940, pp. 27, 34, 54-56, 58-59, 63. For a description of the modern equipment the Isfahan hospital had acquired by around 1920, see Stuart n.d., pp. 17-19.

Table 17: List of Medical Staff of the CMS Hospital Kerman (1902-46)

Year	Physician in charge	Physician on furlough	Physicians assisting	Nurses, female	Iranian staff male	Iranian staff female
1902-1909	Dodson	-	-	-	-	-
1910	Dodson-Westlake	-	-	Ms Parry and Ms Carrick	-	-
1911	Dodson-Westlake	Dodson per 28/10/1911	-	Ms Parry and Ms Carrick	-	-
1912	Westlake	Idem	Dr. Carr (July-Oct); Dr. Schafter (Nov-Dec)	Ms Parry and Ms Carrick	-	-
1913	Westlake - Schafter	Dodson returned 11/1913	Schafter left in October	Ms Parry and Ms Carrick (left December)		
1914	Dodson-Westlake	-	-			
1915	Dodson-Westlake					
1916-17	hospital	was	closed			
1918	Dodson-Westlake	-	-			
1919	Dodson	Westlake	-		7	4
1920	Dodson	Idem	Dr. Ironside (April-December)	Petley; Seagrave (as of July)	6	3
1921	Westlake	Dodson	-	Petley; Seagrave	3	5
1922	Schafter; Westlake	Idem	-	Petley; Seagrave	5	3
1923	Schafter	Idem	-	Petley; Seagrave	5	-
1924	Schafter (till May); Dodson; Mary Price	-	-	Petley; Seagrave	-	-

Year	Physician in charge	Physician on furlough	Physicians assisting	Nurses, female	Iranian staff male	Iranian staff female
1925	Dodson; Price	-	-	Petley; Seagrave	-	-
1926 - 27	Dodson; Price	-	-	-	-	-
1928	Dodson; Price	Dodson per October	Dr. Moloney from November	-	-	-
1929	Price; Moloney †	-	-	-	-	-
1930 -31	Dodson; Pigott	-	-	-	-	-
1932	Dodson- E.E. G. Baillie (2nd half year)	Ms Dr. Pigott	-	-	-	-
1933	Dodson- Baillie	Idem	-	-	-	-
1934	Dodson; Pigott; Ms Pigott (as of May); Baillie (left March)	Dodson as of September	-	Petley; James	-	-
1935	Pigott; Dodson; Ms Pigott, Ms Enriques	Pigott per August; Dodson until October	Robertson, pathologist; Oddy, electrician; one Iranian doctor part-time	Petley; James	7	7
1936	Dodson; Enriques	-	-	James; Petley	-	-
1937	Dodson † 9 May; Enriques; Carpenter per November	-	Dr. Martin (July-October)	James; Petley	-	-

Year	Physician in charge	Physician on furlough	Physicians assisting	Nurses, female	Iranian staff male	Iranian staff female
1938	Carpenter; Enriques	Enriques per October	-	James; Petley	-	-
1939	Carpenter; Dr. Ms Howgate	Carpenter per October	-	-	-	-
1940	Howgate	Idem	-	-	-	-
1942	Howgate; Enriques	Idem	-	-	-	-
1944-45	Dr. Wild; Dr. Ms Blackwood	-	-	0	12	11
1946	Wild; Blackwood	Blackwood per April	-	-	-	-

Source: Administration Report 1908, p. 58; Idem 1909, p. 44; Idem 1910, p. 33; Idem 1912, p. 56; Idem 1913, p. 70; Idem 1917, p. 26; Idem, 1920, p. 30; Idem 1921, p. 29;Idem 1922, p. 31;Idem 1923, p. 49; Idem 1924, p. 32; Idem 1925, p. 39; Idem 1926, p. 22; Idem 1927, p. 19; Idem 1928, p. 32; Iem 1929, p. 28; Idem 1930, p. 25; Idem 1931, p. 30; Idem 1932, p. 26; Idem 1933, p. 31; Idem 1934, p. 34; Idem 1935, p. 38; Idem 1937, p. 27; Idem 1938, p. 20; Idem 1939, p. 18; Idem 1940, p. 20; Administration Report for 1944, Administration Report 1945, p. 4; Administration Reports of the Persian Gulf, 1946, p. 3.

Mr. Robertson, the pathologist retired and returned to Great Britain in April 1936. IOR/L/PS/12/3413, 'Persia; Diaries; Kerman Consular 1931–1939', f. 279.

In 1924, hospital beds were in constant demand, and patients came from a 160 km radius throughout the year. Some medical work was also done in Bam and Kerman by a former assistant of the men's hospital. Work on the new hospital was progressing and it was expected to be ready in 1925 and would have a capacity of 70-80 in-patients.[423]

By the end of 1925 the new hospital was almost ready for use. "The compound is about eight acres in size and the most modern types of building have been erected." Another positive development was the acquisition of a car in 1925, which made rural visits more efficient. Four visits of rural patients on mule or horse back in the

---

423. Administration Report 1924, p. 32.

Table 18: Number of patients seen, operations performed in Kerman CMS hopital and house calls made (1910-1925).

Type/Year	1910	1912	1913	1919	1920	1921	1924	1925
Total								
Male		8,442						
Female		12,647						
New patients			4,981					
male	2,933	2,040	-	1,466	1,502	217	-	
female	2,705	2,669	-	1,615	2,094	2,078	-	
Repeat patients			12,042					
male	7,080	6,025	-	4,394	3,109	1,035	-	
female	9,038	9,555	-	3,267	8,203	6,535	-	
Out-patients/new			4,982					
male	2,311	-	-	-	-	-	-	
female	1,417	-	-	-	-	86	2,144	-
In-patients			469			447	565	581
male	224	208	-	169	155	30	-	
female	214	166	-	155	148	111		
Operations	204							
major	-	175 Men	377	287	144 Men	80/201	540	522
minor	Not recorded	157 Female	not recorded	-				
Urban house calls	-	-	1,537	2,427	803	2,103	incr.	2,150
Rural visits	-	-	475	505	-	-		70
Pathological examinations	-	-	-	-	-	-	-	
New gyanecological examinations	-	-	-	-	-	-	-	

Source: Administration Report 1910, p. 33; Ibid., 1912, p. 56; Ibid., 1913, p. 70; Ibid., 1919, p. 31; Ibid., 1920, p. 30; Ibid., 1921, p. 29; Ibid., 1924, p. 32; Ibid., 1925, p. 39 (581 in-patients compared with 565 last year [1924] and 447 the year before [1923]; 522 operations as compared with 540 in 1924.). Administration Report 1926, p. 22; Administration Report 1928, p. 32; Administration Report 1929, p. 27; Ibid, 1930, p. 25; Ibid, 1931, p. 26; Idid. 1932, p. 31; Ibid, 1934, p. 34; Ibid 1935, p. 38; Ibid., 1939, p. 18; Ibid., 1940, p. 20.

past required 27 days, now the same trip lasted only 42 hours; 700 patients were treated.[424] In 1926, Dr. Dodson and Dr. Mary Price made another itineration during the summer and saw 1,755 patients. In the same year the new men's hospital was opened.[425] During Dr.

---

424. Administration Report 1925, p. 39.
425. Administration Report 1926, p. 22.

	1926	1928	1929	1930	1931	1932	1933	1934	1935	1939	1940
		5,230									
		18,922	12,280	25,942	16,680	21,981	19,767	18,554	16,768		
		5,320	8,128	7,340	5,968	6,429	6,326	6706	4616	29,000	15,994
	621	792	632	1,104	805	699	782	728	550	774	697
		500	311	737	529	529	642	638	507	272	
										2103	
					2,125	4,589	2,701	2,347	829		
								247			
		.	.	.	.	.	.	770	1129		
		.	.	.	.	.	.	190	54		

Dodson's absence, Dr. Price also supervised the men's hospital until Dr. E.F. Moloney arrived in November. At that time, the hospital had a normal staff of 12 trained Persian asisstants, two of whom obtained Iranian licenses to practice medicine. One of them became medical officer of the *Amniyeh* (gendarmerie).[426] In 1929 there was a decrease

---

426. Administration Report 1928, p. 32, 39 (Dr. Hasan Zamani was

of patients treated due to the death of Dr. Moloney, who died of typhus. Dr. Ms Hodgkinson refused to attend the male patients. This difficult situation was proposed to be resolved by the appointment of an Assistant Surgeon of the IMD as consular surgeon, but finally Dr. D. Carr, a CMS veteran and living in Great Britain in retirement after 30 years of service filled the gap and came in June 1929 and stayed till Dodson's return in November. The capacity of the hospital had been enlarged to a 70 beds men's hospital and 35 beds in the women's. Whereas the male beds were double that of female beds, in 1929 the number of female out-patients was double that of the male ones.[427] In 1930, there was no change in the medical staff, although new Iranian assistants were hired to replace those who had left the previous year.[428] Like everybody else managing a private hospital, Dodson also had to spend much extra money on customs fees and other charges on import of medical goods due to new regulations. Some 2,000 visits were made free of charge to over 600 typhus patients between January-July 1932, when there was an epidemic.[429] An electrically driven centrifugal pump was installed in the medical officers' quarters and both hospitals were wired for electric lighting. Without batteries there was only light when the engin was drawing water. Pathology work was much improved due to the arrival of Mr. A. Robertson, who formerly worked fo IETD in that function.[430]

Table 18 shows that the Kerman hospital-dispensary was well attended even during the years for which no quantitative data are available, such as in 1914.[431] In 1915, the CMS hospital-dispensary, which was doing well, unexpectedly suffered a major setback due to the local 'coup-d'etat' by the Democrats, which led to a temporary

---

Ra'is-e Sehhiyeh, but had no funds to improve the sanitation of town. General health was fair, but the standard of living very low, while extreme poverty and under-noursihment were noticeable.)
427. Administration Report 1929, p. 27.
428. Administration Report 1930, p. 25.
429. Administration Report 1932, p. 26.
430. Administration Report 1933, p. 31.
431. Administration Report 1914, p. 25.

departure of staff.⁴³² In 1916, the Kerman hospital-dispensary was not operational.⁴³³ In 1917, the political situation became favorable again and the CMS staff returned to Kerman. However, CMS Kerman had to start almost anew as most of its medical equipment had been looted by the Democrats during the staff's absence.⁴³⁴ As of 1918, attendance grew, as expected. A positive development was the acquisition of a car in 1925, which made rural visits more efficient. "Visiting rural patients on mule or horse back in the past required 27 days, now the same trip lasted only 42 hours."⁴³⁵

When Dodson went on leave in September 1934, he was replaced by Dr. I.W. Piggott. Dr. Ms Baillie was transferred to Yazd in March and Dr. Ms Charis Pigott returned from furlough in May and took charge of women's hospital. Ms E.J. Petley and Ms M. James were respectively, matron of the men's and women's hospital. Mr. G.N. Oddy, the hospital's electrician went on furlough in November and Mr. Robertson continued to assist the hospital as pathologist and accountant in 1934. When Dr. Pigott began working in September he opened a weekly ear, nose, throat department, which was well-attended and appreciated. Pathological examinations increased and Dr. Charis Pigott started the Kahn test for syphilis since her return from furlough, which was a very useful aid in diagnosis. Despite Dodson's absence, the number of patients and receipts went up.⁴³⁶ When in 1936, Dr. Dodson returned from furlough, there was a marked increase in work, a sure indication of his local popularity.⁴³⁷ Therefore, the hospital suffered a severe loss when Dr. Dodson died on 9 May after 34 years of work in Kerman. His funeral was attended by all classes. In July 1937, the men's hospital was temporarily in charge of Dr. Martin from Shiraz, but due to the absence of a permanent physician there was a

---

432. Administration Report 1915, p. 23. The hospital was also visited by German soldiers. Waterfield 1973, p. 162.
433. Administration Report 1916, p. 42.
434. Administration Report 1917, p. 26.
435. Administration Report 1925, p. 39.
436. Administration Report 1934, pp. 34-35.
437. Administration Report 1936, p. 26.

drop in attendance. Dr. R.H. Carpenter arrived end October 1937 and took charge of men's hospital and dispensary. Dr. Ms G. A. (Stella) Henriques was in charge of the women's hospital.[438] Since October 1939 until 1941, Dr. Ms D. M. Howgate was in charge (Carpenter and Enriques were on furlough); she also was medical officer to consulate.[439] In 1942, the hospital was in charge of two lady doctors, presumably Howgate and Henriques, with a local Iranian male and female nursing staff and a capacity of 150 beds.[440] During 1943-46, Dr. E. B. Wild was in charge of hospital, which at that time had only 110 beds. On 3 February 1944, he was joined by Dr. Ms K. Blackwood from Australia to take charge of women's hospital. Despite shortage of funds and European nursing staff it continued to perform well. Treatment of the poor, who represented 75% of the hospital's patients, was rendered difficult by the high cost of drugs and medicines. Fortunately, the AIRF provided the hospital with them. "With the introduction of penicillin treatment many remarkable cures were affected."[441] In 1952 all CMS hospital and school work had closed in Kerman.[442]

A novelty in medical care, Women's Welfare Work (WWW), was pioneered by the CMS in Kerman in 1922. Later similar work was also begun by the American missionary hospitals in Mashhad and Rasht. According to Ms E. C.H. Stratton, who was in charge of WWW, the main objective of social work was "to get in touch with deformed carpet weavers so that expectant mothers may be taken to the hospital to receive medical attention they so sorely need."[443] This situation was

---

438. Administration Report 1937, p. 27; Administration Report 1938, p. 20.
439. Administration Report 1940, p. 20.
440. IOR/L/MIL/17/15/13, M.T. Routes in Persia, p. 269. According to Waterfield 1973, p. 171 Dr. E. B. (Peter) Wild arrived in 1941 in Kerman.
441. Administration Report 1944, p. 5 (Kerman and Yazd); CMS Kerman received a cinema van from the British embassy in November 1945. Administration Report 1945, p. 11.
442. Waterfield 1973, p. 174.
443. Administration Report 1924, p. 32.

caused by abominable working conditions of the mainly child and female labor in the carpet factories in Kerman. Conditions were such that many children and women (girls rather) often became crippled for life. Apart from having to work in subterraneous, often cave-like, badly-lit, cold, humid, unventilated areas, the workers were seated in such a way that they always were sitting stooped. This position was often conducive to "permanent deformities of the arms and legs, and irreparable damage to general health."[444] In Kerman the girl workers were often afflicted by ankylosis of the lower abdomen. When these girls became pregnant they often died in childbirth. When a hospital was available, a craniotomy operation could be done, in up to 50 per cent of births. In the streets of Kerman the Reverend Boyland observed "one is constantly reminded of the iniquity of this child-labor by seeing deformed and stunted women, and occasionally men who are no longer able to work, as their hands are often deformed as well, and are reduced to beggary."[445]

In 1924, in all 59 confinement cases were undertaken; mostly Moslem women. As a result of this health outreach program, the British consul reported that, "the health of the carpet workers is now better than 15-20 years ago."[446] There was close cooperation between the Women's Hospital, which was under a female physician, and the WWW Center. All doubtful pre-natal cases were seen by the doctor.

---

444. Chaqueri 1978, pp. 210-12 quoting British missionaries such as Reverend Boyland (FO 248/1343) Kirman 1921; Bishop Linton (1924). It is noteworthy that similar problems were not reported from other areas in Iran, see for example Chaqueri 1978, p. 205 reproducing a letter from the British consul at Soltanabad (FO 371/10131, f.140, f.14) and also the British consul at Tabriz, FO 371/9030, f.215 "At the commencement of the weaving of a carpet the operatives squat on the floor, as the work gradually rises from the ground they rise with it and sit cross-legged on planks. This is not considered a hardship for Persians as it is the posture they usually adopt when resting in their own homes. It they had chairs provided (or any other sort of comfortable seat) I doubt whether they would appreciate the innovation."
445. Chaqueri 1978, p. 210.
446. Administration Report 1924, p. 32.

Two combined pre-natal and post-natal clinics were held weekly, one of which was especially for carpet weavers and children of all ages came. Pregnant women were seen and advice was given to mothers.[447] In 1928, the WWW's staff consisted of one European (Ms Stratton), one part-time European, and two trained Armenian women. WWW focused on child-welfare and maternity care, both pre- and post-natal as well as midwifery work. In 1928, the total number of visits was 3,998 and 2,055 cases treated at the WWW center.[448] The WWW center under Ms E.M. Robinson continued strongly despite Ms Stratton's absence due to leave in October 1932, returning in December 1933.[449] In 1934, the WWW center had two senior and three junior workers; the latter had started midwifery training. Two workers passed the CMS doctor's examination (equivalent to CMB = Central Midwives Board) in September 1934 and another was to retake it in January 1935. The result of WWW's activities was that the number of abnormal midwifery was decreasing; partly due to improved weaving conditions and partly because the native midwives were "afraid to perform the awful deeds which they formerly performed. Public opinion had also been raised as a fruit of the years of midwifery and welfare work by the C.M.S. workers."[450] In 1935, Ms Robertson was in charge of the WWW center in town assisted by three Iranian women midwives. They continued their standard program of regular prenatal instruction and further teaching during convalescence.[451] In 1936, the level of WWW's activities dropped, because Ms Robinson went on furlough in April, while Ms Stratton only returned in October.[452] In the following period Ms Stratton remained in charge of WWW until mid-1945 when she went on furlough. On 6 June, Ms Woodruff arrived to relieve her.[453]

---

447. Administration Report 1925, p. 39.
448. Administration Report 1928, p. 32.
449. Administration Report 1933, p. 31.
450. Administration Report 1934, pp. 34-35, 45.
451. Administration Report 1935, p. 38.
452. Administration Report 1936, p. 26.
453. Administration Report 1945, p. 4.

Table 19: Women's Welfare Center Activities - CMS Kerman 1924-1935

	1924	1925	1929	1931	1932	1933	1934	1935
No. of confinements	59	97	?	76	92	89	68	75
Visits to patients' homes	-	-	3,972	1614	1936	2049	1251	1322
Patients attending center	-	-	-	347	321	274	284	376
Repeat visits	-	-	1125	1125	1125	867	793	644
No. of cases referred to hospital	-	-	-	126	-	-	-	-

Source: Administration Report 1924, p. 32; Idem 1925, p. 39; Idem 1929, p. 28; Idem 1931, p. 30; Idem 1932, p. 26; Idem 1933, p. 31; Ibid 1934, p. 35; Ibid, 1935, p. 38.

In addition to the CMS or the so-called *Morselin* (i.e., Missionaries) hospital, there were two other medical establishments in Kerman. In 1912, the IETD's dispensary was operating in Kerman, but it is unknown from and until when. The dispensary was managed by assistant surgeon Mr. Steinhoff, who also had the medical charge of the staff of the British Consulate.[454]

Table 20: Patients seen and operations performed at the Indo-European Telegraph Department Dispensary at Kerman (1912)

	Male	Female
Fresh cases	620	316
Repeated visits	Unknown	-
Operations - major	97	15
Operations - minor	-	25

Source: Administration Report 1912, p. 56

Finally, there was the so-called *Nuriyeh* Hospital, which was a *vaqf* or endowed medical institution set up by Nurollah Khan Zahir al-Mamalek, which had been established in 1917. The endowment deed stipulated that two officially licensed physicians trained (preferably in

---

454. Administration Report 1912, p. 56.

Europe) in Western medicine and one trained in traditional medicine as well as one midwife had to employed by the hospital. The hospital also was to have a medical training program. In 1924, Dr. Musa Khan, an Iranian physician with French qualifications and English experience, had come to Kerman to take charge of this hospital as well as to act as ex-officio Health Officer for the town. After a few months he resigned and left Kerman "as he was unable to obtain either his pay or medicines from the Mutawalli."[455] In 1925, he was succeeded by Dr. Aristu Khan.[456] In April 1932, Dr. Mirza Ali Khan Irani was in charge of the Nuriyeh Charitable Hospital, who temporarily also took charge as Health Officer, when Dr. Ahmad Khan Philosopher and Health Officer resigned and left.[457]

Given this much private activity the government could not remain behind. In December 1931 the governor-general of Kerman intended to collect 20,000 *tuman*s to establish a charitable hospital in the city. He expected help from the *Owqaf* and *Baladiyeh* Department.[458] This had the required result, because in November 1933, the British consul reported that "The orphanage and a charitable hospital have been placed under the direct management of the Department of Education as the result of complaints about these two institutions and the Commission of Enquiry."[459]

Whether due to the presence of these various medical institutions or not, after 1925 there was no epidemic, nor an outbreak of the endemic diseases greater than usual. In fact, despite the appalling filth of the town "the general health of the place kept fairly good." In 1929, the

---

455. Rezai 2012, pp. 127-28; Ebrahimnejad 2014, pp. 152-53; Administration Report 1924, p. 36.

456. Rosta'i 1382, vol. 2, p. 45.

457. IOR/L/PS/12/3413, Diary of HBM's Consulate, Kerman, no. 4, for the month of April 1932, p. 1. There was a Russian doctor (both husband and wife were) in the Russian Consulate in Kerman, but they were called to Tehran on 19 April. It is not known whether they treated any patients. Administration Report 1928, p. 39.

458. IOR/L/PS/12/3413, Diary of HBM's consul, Kerman, no. 10, for the month of December 1931, p. 1.

459. IOR/L/PS/12/3413, Diary of HBM's consul, Kerman, no. 11, for the month of November 1933, p. 1

post of Health Officer (*ra'is-e sehhiyeh*) changed hands on several occasions, but without any effect on the city's sanitation or public health, for which there were no funds available. Because people were extremely poor and undernourished, "It is encouraging to learn that the prevalent occupational diseases of rickets and tuberculous joint disease (which claims child weavers for their victims) are definitely less common than they were a decade ago."[460] Despite the lack of funds, health officials in Kerman nevertheless tried to improve the sanitation of city and to a certain extent unhealthy practices were held in check. Dr. Sohrab Barkhordar was the health officer at the end of 1932. In January 1932 there was an outbreak of a typhus epidemic that only died down in July. It mostly hit the poor, "where it ran through whole families taking all members together, or one after another in turn. Despite frequent cases of marked hyperpyrexia, the disease had a low mortality, broadly speaking only weaklings and aged folk succumbing to it." The CMS staff treated >600 patients.[461] One positive step by the governor-general was the closing in mid-1933 of bathing tanks in public baths and the affixing of taps. Orthodox Moslem groups complained to Tehran saying that religious ablutions could not be performed, so that by the end of 1933 orders came to have the taps removed. "Most of the baths, however, retain the newly introduced shower bath arrangement." In November 1933, the governor-general of the province was informed that the funds for the health departments was cut from the general budget per 1 November and that the respective municipalities had to make arrangements for the payment of the health services in their area as of that date. Given the impoverished condition of the Kerman municipality the authorities feared that health arrangements there would suffer.[462]

In early 1935 some type of flue passed through the city causing a number of deaths. There was also a small typhus epidemic in summer, mainly in the Jewish quarter, in another part of town. There was

---

460. Administration Report 1926, p. 24-25; Administration Report 1929, p. 35; Administration Report 1930, p. 25.
461. Administration Report 1932, p. 26, 31 (At year's end mild influenza).
462. Administration Report 1933, pp. 31, 39.

also much tuberculosis of every variety in the city. "The Tubercular Ward in each of the two Mission Hospitals is always full, mainly of bone cases. These patients receive daily sun-treatment all the year round, which, combined with Cod Liver Oil, good food and constant 'scraping', produces slow, but good results in most cases." [463]

In 1939, Dr. Vakili became the new Health Officer or *Ra'is-e Behdasht* as he was called since 1936. Dr. Vakili was educated in Germany and was married to a German wife. As the municipal medical officer he was in charge of the monthly inspection of butchers, bakers, fruit sellers and prostitutes twice a week. "It is said that a 'clean' certificate is granted on suitable payment." The Health Department provided vaccinations and inoculations without charge.[464] By the 1940s, Kerman had acquired more than one government hospital. In fact, in 1944, Dr. Vakili was in charge of two dispensaries and one hospital: the *Behdari Ostan*, the *Behdari Shahrdari* and the *Bimarestan-e Mobarezeh* (epidemics hospital). The expense of the latter was met by public contribution. To check the outbreak of serious epidemics the doctors of the Health Department were regularly sent into various parts of town, especially where the poor lived, to round up all destitutes and beggars. The medically fit were sent to the asylum where they were housed and fed. The sick were treated in the *Mobarezeh* and later sent to the Kerman asylum. In this way 17 cases of typhus and 86 of dysentery that might have become epidemic were successfully treated. A Poor Relief Committee was also formed to assist the Health Department in collecting poor people for segregation in the asylum.[465] In 1945, the Shah contributed 170,000 *tuman*s for the construction of a 60-bed hospital, the foundations of which had been laid three years earlier.[466]

All hospitals showed an interest to treat the poor. 'Two new hospitals were opened in Kerman and Rafsanjan for them, and the

---

463. Administration Report 1934, pp. 34, 44-45.
464. Administration Report 1939, pp. 18, 20; Administration Report 1940, p. 20.
465. Administration Report for 1944, p. 9.
466. Administration Report for 1945, p. 6.

Ustandar [governor-general] made many attempts to raise the funds for their treatment."[467]

KERMANSHAH

In 1904, there was a positive change in the public health situation of Kermanshah (a city of 60,000 inhabitants), because two events brought medical care closer to many of its inhabitants. In that year on 27 December, Abdol-Hoseyn Mirza Farmanfarma, when governor of Kermanshah, opened a newly built hospital in the town for sick pilgrims and appointed Dr. Mahmud Mo`tamed, a Paris medical school graduate, as its director. However, when Farmanfarma was dismissed one year later the hospital was neglected and became dilapidated. When Farid al-Molk visited it in 1905 it had no patients, although its physician, Dr. `Abdollah Tabib and its director `Ali Reza were present. The physician told the new governor that Farmanfarma had given 70 *tuman*s per month, which was insufficient for the operating expenses of the hospital, which, excluding the physician's salary and the cost of charcoal, were 100 *tuman*s per month. Farmanfarma had wanted to secure funding for the hospital by allocating a certain percentage from the tax paid for the transport of the corpses going to Kerbela to be paid by the chief of the Customs Department, who wrote that this was a decision to be taken by Tehran.[468] According to the British, Farmanfarma's real objective in establishing the hospital "was to obtain a free gift of land for personal gains." He wanted to mount the same scheme two years later in Kerman.[469]

This medical gap was filled by the British Consulate and American missionaries. The British opened a charitable dispensary and Civil Hospital, at an unknown date, probably starting in 1904 when their Consulate was opened, because it had a British physician on its staff.[470]

---

467. Administration Report for 1945, p. 8.
468. Soltani 1370, vol. 1, pp. 533-534, quoted from Farid al-Molk Hamadani 1345, pp. 64-65, 228, 238, 223; Rusta'i 1382, vol. 1, pp. 333; Presbyterian Church 1904, p. 242; Ebrahimnejad 2014, p. 153.
469. Political Diaries, vol. 1, p. 379.
470. Administration Report 1905-06, p. 45; Administration Report 1908,

It is not known whether the Russian Consulate-general offered similar services, although a Russian physician was attached to it. Dr. Ost left in early December 1905, but it seems that there always was a physician attached to the Russian Consulate-general. In March 1913, there was a suspected outbreak of cholera in the Kalhor district, where the Russian consular physician was sent to investigate.[471] In 1905, the British Consulate dispensary has a daily average attendance of 60-80 out-patients, who received advice and medicine free.[472] In 1906-07, the dispensary saw an average of 100 patients per day. Most were Kurds, but the number of non-Kurdish patients was increasing.[473] In 1908, the British dispensary was transferred from the consulate to more commodious quarters in town, consisting of: a surgeon's office, a hospital assistant's office, a dispensing room, two dressing rooms, two small waiting rooms, one for male and one for female patients; an operating room, one small ward for emergency cases and hospital assistant's quarters. It was open for 174 days in that year, because for the remainder of the time, the medical staff accompanied the consul on tour. In 1908 it treated 20,981 patients of which 8,000 were males, 10,762 females and 5,942 children. At the Civil Hospital a total of 308 in-house patients were treated, of which 284 were men and 24 women. In the dispensary the physician performed also simple operations.[474] It is not known when the British dispensary was closed, but this must have been in or before 1911, when no physician was attached any longer to the consulate.

---

p. 49; Wilson 1941, p. 114.

471. Political Diaries, vol. 1, p. 237; Administration Report 1908, p. 45; January 1907 Russian physician Velonsky. Political Diaries, vol. 2, p. 29; Further Correspondence Persia no. 1 (1914), p. 60.

472. DCR 3683 (Kermanshah 1905-06), p. 5.

473. Administration Report 1906-07, p. 43.

474. The more serious operations included "removal of sequestrum of palatal process of upper jaw; excision of rodent ulcers in the inner angle of the eye, fistula *in ano*, lateral lithomy, cataract, iridectomy." Administration Report 1908, pp. 49-54.

Despite the British medical services offered to the population of Kermanshah, there was still room for more of the same. In 1907, after their arrival, the 35-year old American missionaries, Mr. B. W. Stead and Dr. Mrs. Stead, the latter, who was a physician, also known by her maiden name as Dr. Blanche Wilson, offered medical services in Kermanshah. That same year, she opened a small dispensary and for two years carried on active medical practice. She saw 20-35 patients/day in the forenoon. Very few left without hearing the gospel. She also made medical house calls to bind wounds etc. as well as did some minor operations, such as a compound fracture wound. She also turned her house in a temporary hospital for a poor Jewess who was living in a dirty dark room.[475] In 1907, Mrs. Stead enlarged her dispensary with a few rooms and henceforth also received in-patients. In 1909 or 1910, the Steads left for one year's furlough in the USA and returned to Kermanshah in 1911. The wounded of the street fights between royalists and constitutionalists in 1912-13, were the first in-patients in a hastily constructed first medical building by the Steads. It was built on property that the Steads had bougt for the permanent home of the Mission. This general clinic was usually attended by 50-70 Moslem women/day.[476] In 1914, a young widow helped Mrs. Stead since spring. During eight months she did dispensary work of three hours/day with a few house calls. She saw a total of 2,877 patients, of whom 1,139 received treatment and was able to pay the expenses from her receipts.[477]

There also was a Belgian physician, Dr. Bruneel, who was attached to the Customs administration and had been working in Iran for a

---

475. Stead 1907, p. 234; RG 91-19-28, Westminster Hospital Report no. 2, 1932. The Rev. Stead had arrived in 1902 in Tehran. Presbyterian Church 1903, p. 246.

476. RG 91-19-28, Westminster Hospital Report no. 2, 1932; `Eyn al-Saltaneh 1376, vol. 1, pp. 377, 865; UNESCO 1343, vol. 2, p. 1451; Elgood 1951, pp. 511-512, 534; Waterfield 1973, pp. 139-140; Presbyterian Church 1915, p. 313. For the turmoil in Kermanshah, see Floor 2018 b, pp. 306-16.

477. Presbyterian Church 1915, pp. 318-19 (Receipts for medicines and fees 2,969 *qran*s and expenses 2,300 *qran*s.)

number of years. He also provided medical care to the local population from his office, where he, among other things, performed many cataract operations. In January 1915, Dr. Bruneel offered to buy all medicines still stored in the British consulate. The British consul asked the Legation for permission to do so, as there was no physician any longer there and it this way the medicines would be put to good use. However, when the German occupation force came looking for him on 24 January 1916, Dr. Bruneel decided to flee to Basra, where he, be it seriously wounded due to treachery of his Kurdish guide, arrived in mid-February 1916.[478]

WW I brought other problems as well. Between 1915 and 1921 Kermanshah was held by three different foreign armies.[479] All three occupation forces, i.e. the Turks, Russians and the British had their own military hospital. The local Iranian administration and its Turkish allies in 1916 used a building in the heart of the city as a temporary hospital. However, this hospital seems to have had limited capacity, for when wounded from the fight at Bidsorkh were brought to Kermanshah in March 1915 there was no hospital where they might be treated.[480] In February 1916 Turks withdrew from Kermanshah leaving Dr. Stead in charge of a hospital full with Turkish sick and wounded.[481] With the Russian troops that took Kermanshah came a medical unit in May 1916 that was supported by an American Red Cross team. It decided not to use that hospital, because typhus had raged there. Moreover, it had not been fumigated. Because many wounded were expected the US-Russian medical team moved to Del-gosha, a deserted Kurdish village some 1.5 km outside town. In an Iranian Khan's palace with nice gardens the surgical hospital was set up. Because the capacity of the village was too small to put up the wounded, raised beds were built of boards, with an awning over them, along the walls of the gardens. Straw mattresses and pillows were made and all gauze

---

478. Guillaume 1994, pp. 11, 24-27; Laureys 1996, pp. 320-23; FO 248/1112, McDoual to Legation, 26/01/15; Soltani 1372, vol. 4, p. 794.
479. On this period, see Floor 2018 b, pp. 377-439.
480. Ezz al-Mamalek 1332, p. 84.
481. RG 91-19-28, Westminster Hospital Report no. 2, 1932.

available in the bazaar was bought. Each soldier was given such a covering as protection against mosquitos. Most of the work was done by American doctors, one Russian doctor and nurse, and two *felcher*s and two *sanitar*s. Hundreds of wounded each day came in. Medical staff from other places, the US missionary and the Imperial Bank of Persia (IBP) banker all helped. The operating room, though well-lighted had a mud floor. There was neither a sterilizer nor rubber gloves. Sterile supplies came in sterile paper packages; cotton was dipped in biochloride before it was sterilized. When carbolic acid and alcohol were finished they used arak, denatured alcohol and bichloride in mercury tablets. Potassium permanganate was used for all dressings. The US-Russian medical staff used granite plates and basins that were sterilized with alcohol. Clean water came from a spring at 3 km distance. Soiled dressings were burnt, but when wet they smoldered all day. Therefore, the staff tried burying them, but at night they were dug up and taken by enterprising Persians, who washed them in a stream nearby, dried them and then sold them in the bazaar. The Russian nurse handed everything with sterile forceps and handed all that was needed to the staff. The sanitars removed the bandages. Operating was done in the morning; light wounded were sent back when they had recovered; more serious cases remained in the hospital and then were sent in carts to Russia. The soldiers came in all kinds of conveyances from the front usually after 3-6 days travel. On 28 June 1916, the medical unit was told to leave Kermanshah. How this was done and arrived on 5 July in Hamadan, where there were three Russian hospitals (Red Cross, Military and Zemsky Zayust).[482]

> The patients were to be sent first, then household and hospital supplies, and lastly the sisters were to go; the doctors were to remain with the retreating army. All went to their various duties, some into the operating room, dressing the newly wounded, while others packed the supplies or prepared the sick and wounded for the trip back. We had an amputation case that evening, a patient who came to us with a tourniquet on his leg, which had been there, presumably, for two days.

---

482. McClintic 1917, pp. 34-40, 102-06.

The most important things were moved, although some had to be left behind and were loot for the Persians. The covered vans were piled high with articles and upon these the convalescent soldiers, who were too weak to walk, sat holding on. All sorts of conveyances were used to carry us back: two-wheeled carts; lineakas, carriages with low side seats; horses, donkeys, and camels. Each person was armed with a rifle, bayonet or revolver and all the cartridges he could carry.

As we rode slowly out of Kermanshah, the roofs were filled with townspeople to see us leave. Some were sad, others gay, due to the excitement which prevailed. Now for a long journey again, without food or water, in the scorching sun; but as I lookback, we were kept so busy with the dreadfully sick, delirious, and heavily wounded, that little thought was given to our own personal needs. Each evening when the tents were pitched, the dinners were cooked, medicines given out, and each soldier, lying on the ground or in the wagon, was made as comfortable as could be, in his heavy uniform and boots.

The "Zemsky Zayust," [Land Association] one of the foremost organizations in Russia, had wayside stations. What a treat to the half-sick, distressed soldiers who had to walk! With their boots off, they would struggle along, nothing to eat or drink all day, to these places, which would provide for them. About one o'clock in the morning, the second night out on the road, our mounted patients, who were in the front of this long march were attacked by a tribe of the fierce, wild Kurds. They removed all the dressings and bandages, thinking money was concealed under them. One sanitar was seriously injured, all the soldiers were in a state of collapse, and the march was delayed until the next afternoon. The sisters acted very bravely, working hard to quiet the soldiers, and because of this had the St. George's medal conferred upon them. A Russian soldier receives for bravery the St. George's Cross, with a black and orange striped ribbon.

The Turks returned on 29 June 1916, establishing 11 hospitals in Kermanshah. The Turkish commander asked Dr. Stead to help in these military hospitals. For a long time she had charge of the Russian wounded and sick.[483] The Turks also commandeered a house that they turned into a convalescent hospital. The Turkish troops cut down its big walnut trees, which were used as firewood.[484] When the Turks left in early March 1917, the Russians set up their own hospital structure. However, by October 1917, "the Russian Red Cross has closed its local hospital, but the Russian Land Association has two hospitals manned by women doctors and nurses, male orderlies, and one or two surgeons." There were no wounded, but many sick suffering from typhus and malaria and the wards were congested. The hospital was not optimally managed, but the women in charge, although worrying about the fate of their families back home, persevered and coped better than the Russian officers and soldiers. Among the last Russians to leave were the sisters at the one remaining hospital.[485] How long that hospital lasted I don't know, but not beyond February 1918 when the last Russian soldiers had left. The British built a hospital complex outside Kermanshah, which they used until April 1921 (see below), when they withdrew all their troops. In 1917, the wife of the Russian assistant-consul was a dentist, who had a flourishing practice during her short stay in Kermanshah.[486]

In July 1918, typhus and cholera was prevalent. Amir-e Koll, the acting governor took sanitary measures; although the city became cleaner, much needed still to be done.[487] In September 1918, following

---

483. RG 91-19-28, Westminster Hospital Report no. 2, 1932. One of those hopitals was established by the *Shir va Khorshid* organization that had been founded in Kazemeyn (Iraq) against the will of the Ottomans by Navvab al-Towliyeh Yazdi. With a few others (names given in the source) he established a hospital in the abandoned British Consulate. A group of gendarmes guarded the place and in the afternoon they played music for the sick. In the Consulate's garden were three small buildings, one of which was used for Iranian sick, the other for Ottoman sick, and the third as administrative office. The Ottomans did not like the *Shir va Khorshid* sign and sent an armed detachment that took over the hospital, tore down the Iranian signs and flag and replaced it with the Red Crescent, the Ottoman sign. Qodsi 1342, vol. 1, pp. 387-88.

484. Hale n.d., p. 225.

485. Hale n.d., pp. 212, 216; McClintic 1917, p. 40.

486. Hale n.d., p. 226.

487. FO 248/1204, Kermanshah report no. 6, 02/08/1918 by Lt. Col. Kennion.

the famine, Kermanshah was struck by the worldwide influenza pandemic, which caused many deaths, especially in the villages. By the end of October all villages in Mahidasht and Kermanshah valleys had 8-10 graves. Due to last year's famine people had no resistance.[488] Hale, the Imperial Bank manager wrote: "Pneunomia and malaria on top of it have caused many deaths, particularly among the Indians, and the hospitals here and in Hamadan are full of sick. ... Half the population seems to have suffered more or less."[489] In December 1918, Hall reported that "the hospitals are no longer congested, and the work of the doctors (and padres) is less onerous than it was."[490] Not only the local population suffered from the pandemic, but so did the British troops. Forbes-Leith wrote when he returned to Iran after WWI: "I lost many friends and my men from all kinds of foul disease, and under such conditions it is little wonder that many of my brother officers, especially those who until the war had never been out of England, regarded Persia as a veritable Hell on earth."[491] During the famine and the flue pandemic Dr. Stead worked tirelessly, providing famine relief, setting up an orphanage and caring the sick, both Iranian and British. Dr. Stead's work was much appreciated by everybody, even in the British Parliament.[492]

Her dispensary had suffered during the Great War. In fact, during 1917-18 the dispensary had to be closed due to the hostilities and the lack of medical supplies.[493] In 1919, Mrs. Stead was able to re-open

---

488. FO 248/1204, Kermanshah report no. 9, 01/11/1918 by Lt. Col. Kennion.

489. Hale n.d, p. 237. On the pandemic, see Floor 2018 a, pp. 96-103.

490. Hale n.d., p. 240.

491. Forbes-Leith 1927, p. 21.

492. Dr. Stead took care of the many orphans among the refugees and saved thousands of lives. Many of these orphans did well in our schools and some are now working as teachers and nurses. RG 91-19-28, Westminster Hospital Report no. 2, 1932.

493. Presbyterian Church 1919, p. 266. In 1921 the dispensary was closed due to the absence of Mrs. Stead. Presbyterian Church 1921, p. 335.

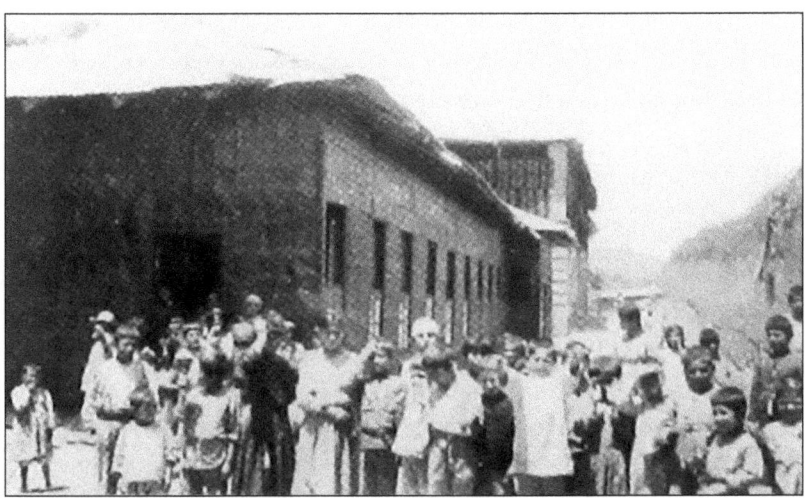
Orphanage in Kermanshah established by Dr. Stead

the dispensary, but she provided only medical care to out-patients. Meanwhile, some of her work was seen to by the British Medical Corps, although as of March of that year the latter received orders to no longer treat civilians.[494] On Dr. Stead's return in March 1920 she opened the dispensary in her sewing room, where she received 30 patients every day. Because the Assyrian school children had all malaria her out-door hospital covered most of her yard. She had 44 in-patients and no dispensary attendants. At that time, Dr. Stead received permission to build two wards, for which she had the materials. However, the Presbyterian mission committee of Kermanshah decided on the rule "that no station may have a hospital of more than forty till it has two male physicians and an X-ray machine." In 1921 the dispensary was closed due to her absence. When the British army left Kermanshah in April 1921, it offered the huts that had served as their military hospital for sale to the American missionaries. The 21 huts, 12 of which 80 feet long, were nicely located on a hill outside the city. Moreover, they were located at a distance from one another such that this made the establishment of a cottage-hospital possible. The Americans bought them for 3,350 *tuman*s, much below market

---

494. Presbyterian Church 1920, p. 318.

value, but they had to break down the 'ideal hospital' as they had neither the staff to guard them nor a doctor to work there, while looting of building materials had already occurred.[495]

THE WESTMINSTER OR AMERICAN HOSPITAL

It happened that when Dr. Harry Packard was returning to Iran (Urmiyeh) he found Dr. Stead very ill at Qasr-e Shirin, where she had been visiting friends. He took her to Kermanshah where she died on 21 February 1922 in Kermanshah, aged 52 years. The Eastern Mission asked that Dr. Packard stay in Kermanshah and finish the hospital building and remain there until the arrival of Dr. Bussdicker, the new physician. Dr. Packard not only built the hospital, but also a physician's residence and a chapel in memory of Dr. Stead, funds having been made available by her husband's supporting church in Kansas City. Dr. Packard constructed the building using materials from the British Rest Camp. It was not yet an adequate place, but it was the beginning of a hospital with new buildings for a dispensary and examining rooms. The old dispensary was renewed and a kitchen as well as a laundry were added, plus a ward above it. Because the waiting room capacity was inadequate as well as to provide more space for in-patients and a suitable operating room a second floor to the new medical building should be added immediately, Dr. Packard wrote. However, the immediate needs for medical work were met. If the second floor would be extended over the chapel-waiting room, the hospital could receive 65 patients and its capacity should not be less. Packard also argued that one doctor and nurse was not enough- a second doctor was needed. Demand for medical care from the city was such that it would tie down one physician, which would make touring in the districts impossible, which was needed. One man alone, if he would go on itineration, was detrimental to hospital care. Dr. Packard saw daily 160 patients of which 97 patients for treatment, while the room had only place for 25 people to wait in. While they

---

495. Presbyterian Church 1922, pp. 68, 368-369; RG 91-19-28, 30/08/1921, Mrs. Stead to [Mission HQ].

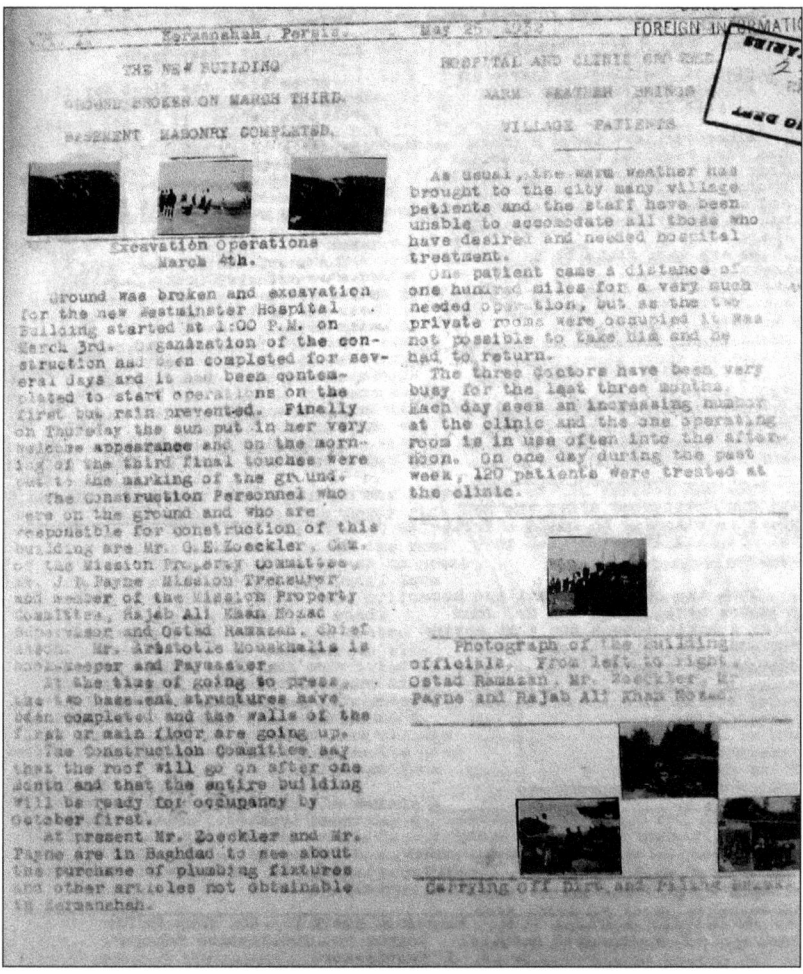

Breaking ground newsletter for the Westminster Hospital, Kermanshah, 1932

waited for the doctor, Rev. Stead took care of their spiritual needs. When Dr. Bussdicker and Mrs. Bussdicker R.N. arrived in Kermanshah at the end of October 1922, the hospital had been finished and the first patient had been admitted. Because Dr. Bussdicker did not yet speak Persian, the Eastern Mission asked Dr. Packard to stay for the winter. He left in the spring of 1923, and Dr. Bussdicker and Mrs. Bussdicker continued the medical work helped by some half-trained girls and ignorant boys. Their work was facilitated by the arrival of a nurse, Ms Mary Edna Burgess, who, in 1922, joined the medical team.[496]

In 1926, Dr. Packard returned to Kermanshah, while Dr. and Mrs. Bussdicker R.N. went to Rasht for 18 months to relieve Dr. Frame and returned to Kermanshah in 1928. Because the work load increased, they were able to convince a meeting of the US missionaries in 1928 of the need for a permanent second physician. That meeting decided to ask the missionaries of the Kermanshah station to draw up plans for the adequate housing of their medical work, while it went on record that a second physician was needed in Kermanshah.[497] Drs. Packard and Bussdicker (who were both formally permanently assigned to Kermanshah in 1930) were carrying out their medical work in very inadequate quarters. The chapel was the last building built by Dr. Stead; only a shell of the walls and roof remained when she died, for she had done all her work in inadequate buildings and for much of the time in rented places poorly adapted to her needs. This building was sufficiently finished to serve for the care of the in-patients and it also served as the operating room.[498]

---

496. Presbyterian Church 1922, no. 48, p. 27. "The Linwood Presbyterian Church (Kansas City, Mo) gave $4,000 as a memorial to Mrs. Stead which would be spent on the completion of the hospital and Medical Plant." RG 91-19-28, Trull to Speer, 21/12/1922; Idem, Letter for the Supporters of the Orphanage at Kermanshah, 1923; Idem, Harry Packard to Dr. Speer, 08/03/1923; Idem, Dr. Packard to [?]. (undated/rec. 15/03/1923) (Mrs. Stead had estimated 2,000 *tuman*s for completing the new medical building and the physician's residence at 7,500 *tuman*s. Packard estimated the cost of the second floor of the hospital, incl. operating room at $4,500; the second floor of the chapel at $2,500). A missionary described the hospital as "just building an addition to the old dispensary." RG 91-19-28, [?] to Mrs. Cyrus McCormick, 11/01/1923.

497. Elgood 1951, pp. 511-512, 534; Waterfield 1973, pp. 139-140; Presbyterian Church 1919, p. 266. Idem 1921, p. 335; Idem 1928 a, pp. 12, 17.

498. RG 91-19-28, Westminster Hospital Report no. 2, 1932. For "the enlargement of the hospital a total gift of $60,000 will be made available." RG 91-19-28, Note 14/04/28.

Dr. Packard, who had returned to the US in 1930, had been able to convince the Westminster church in Buffalo, N.Y. to build a new hospital in Kermanshah rather than in Urmiyeh, as had been the original plan (see Urmiyeh). Meanwhile, the Bushdickers, with one graduate nurse, continued their medical work in Kermanshah, later, in 1931, rejoined by Dr. Packard.[499] Before the doctors could start constructing their new hospital there were some problems to be resolved prior to the actual construction (expertise of the mason; collection of all materials). Also, although the supply of electricity would be enough for the X-ray machine and hospital lighting, it was only available for six hours. That did not fit the requirements of the new hospital, and, therefore, the doctors argued that they needed a small generator when they needed light in the OR or when city power was cut off.[500] The church in Buffalo made $30,000 available to build the Westminster Hospital in 1932 in Kermanshah. Ground was broken in March 1932 and on 15 October 1932 the hospital was completed. Rajab Ali Khan Nozar was the construction supervisor and Ostad Ramazan the supervising mason. The former physicians' residence was turned into a nurses home, both American and Iranian. The new physicians' residence was also completed on 15 October, although Dr. Packard and family lived for a while in the basement while the upper part was being finished.[501]

The missionaries considered the Westminster Hospital the finest in Iran. The building, which still exists, "faces a little west of north and in the midsection elevation is 102 feet. The wings sweep away for 70 feet at an angle of 135 degrees with the midsection. Because of the slope of the land the building is four stories high to the east of the

---

499. RG 61.3.46, Bushdicker/Kermanshah to Huntwork/New York, 29/09/1957. Earlier some donations were given for hospital equipment. A money gift of $450 for enlargement hopital and equipment, operating table and microscope. RG 91-19-28, Note 27/07/1927. Another gift of $1,812.62 was for an operating table, stretchers, a sterilizer, two wheeled chairs, instruments, and 25 bedside lockers. RG 91-19-28, Note 29/10/27.
500. RG 91-19-28, Packard/Kermanshah to Holmes/Buffalo, 15/11/1931.
501. RG 91-19-28, Speer to Butzer, 16/10/1933.

entrance and three stories high to the west. The elevator and dumb-waiter are on opposite sides of the wall on which they are indicated, in the room marked 'service'. In the sub-basement are: a very large water reservoir (*ab-anbar*), store rooms, toilet and morgue. In the basement the nurses class room, night nurses' sleeping rooms, bath, toilets, the X-ray department rooms, the lab, kitchen, store rooms, laundry & ironing and mending room, and a large drying room for bad weather." The room marked 'Diathermy' became the lab. People were impressed with the solidity of the construction and it was expected to serve the needy for generations. Male and female patients were separated by having men and private rooms on the first floor and the wards and private rooms for women and children on the second floor. The surgical department was on the top floor. Everywhere was running water, which made this hospital almost unique in Iran. The doctors rooms with lockers and comforts, including a shower, were a special delight. On this level there were 52 beds for adults, nine for children, one crib and five baskets for tiny babies. Further, 50 bedside tables and 50 stools without a backside had been made and painted and were in place. A carpenter, a former patient, had given six chairs; another Iranian completely furnished a private room. Other Iranians also had promised to donate various things. There was a fine scrub-basin for the surgeon as well as a flush toilet and shower in the surgical section. The running water in the building was perhaps the greatest boon. Electric light was great, but it was considered a luxury that the hospital as yet could ill afford. The dispensary was in the old hospital building. The new building also meant that both physicians were now housed under one roof, so that it was more comfortable to consult each other and treat about patients who come to the clinic through intercommunicating rooms, while their assistant could move between the consulting and dressing rooms. The waiting room was spacious, while the lab was the real show piece of the hospital. The evangelist helped with the patient records. This was no easy task, for he had to handle 75-100 patients, each one with 2-3 friends, between 9 a.m. and 1 p.m.[502] Others had also worked hard to make the hospital

---

502. RG 91-19-28, Westminster Hospital Report 07/03/1933; RG

an efficient institution. Five women were busy for weeks hemming sheets, making comforts, mattress, covers, pillows cases and a hundred other things. Two sewing women were still busy. Russian sheeting was very satisfactory, heavier and lasting than imported stuff and obtainable in Tehran. The hospital used native-made unbleached muslin for removable mattress covers and for the mattresses themselves. This material was better for the laundry than colored material.[503]

On 17 October 1932, the first patients were admitted to the 75 bed, 4-storeys hospital, although painting and carpenter work was still going on. One of the outstanding features of the new hospital was that there was running water everywhere it was needed, which made it almost unique in Iran.[504] The men's ward was on second and third floor. The second floor ward had 10 beds and two small private rooms. This floor was almost reserved for patients sent by the city health department and were all the poorest and hopeless patients. Many had chronic diseases and were mostly there to ease their last days and have them die in comfort. The third floor had two wards with 21 beds, an enclosed porch with four beds for TB patients and five private rooms. Most patients there were able to pay all or part of their expenses. Some were still full charity patients. The women's ward was on the top floor; here were also the operating rooms. There were three wards with respectively four and six beds, two general and one obstetrical with four beds. There were six private rooms of which two obstetrical. There also was a porch that was partly enclosed with glass windows with four beds; the open part had four to six beds, but was only used in summer.[505]

The nurses quarter was in the old residence adjoining the new building. The hospital was the finest building in Kermanshah and so many visitors came that the doctors had to put up a sign forbidding any one to enter without permission. To make the old dispensary suitable as a clinic and out-patient department they had to send out

---

91-19-28, Westminster Hospital 1933.
503. RG 91-19-28, Linens and Laundry [undated].
504. RG 91-19-28, Packard to Butzer 03/06/1933.
505. RG 91-19-28, Report Westminster Hospital Kermanshah 1938-39.

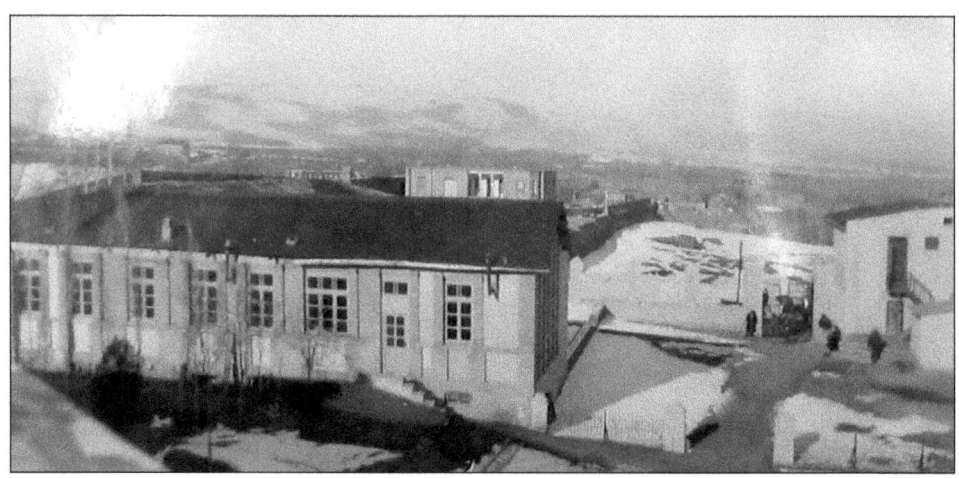

Above and opposite: New and old hospital building, Kermanshah

all patients and close the hospital on 1 July 1932. It was bad for both doctors and patients, but there was no alternative. Two rooms in the Stead Memorial Chapel were used as doctor's office and pharmacy. The corridor between them served as waiting room with overflow into the yard. The new clinic building had three consultation rooms, two large waiting rooms for men and women, and one small waiting room for private cases. There was also a dressing room for men and a treatment room for women. The pharmacy was in the newly built addition. It was not as roomy as a clinic building should be but it was a great improvement compared with the previous situation.[506] The new hospital was not a quiet place, and at times:

> One would think he were entering a High School during recess time rather than a hospital. Yes we have rules, rules to keep things as they ought to be, rules for visitors. Lots of rules, but people of Kermanshah do not believe in rules, anymore than people in other places, and there you are. Why, for generations, no patient ever goes through illness without

---

506. RG 91-19-30, Westminster Hospital News vol. 1/3 -15/09/1932 (Dr. Ibrahim is on vacation; Mr. David Sergis from Cairo General Hospital assisted the doctors. Ms Vartanush Minassian, the graduate nurse left to Tehran).

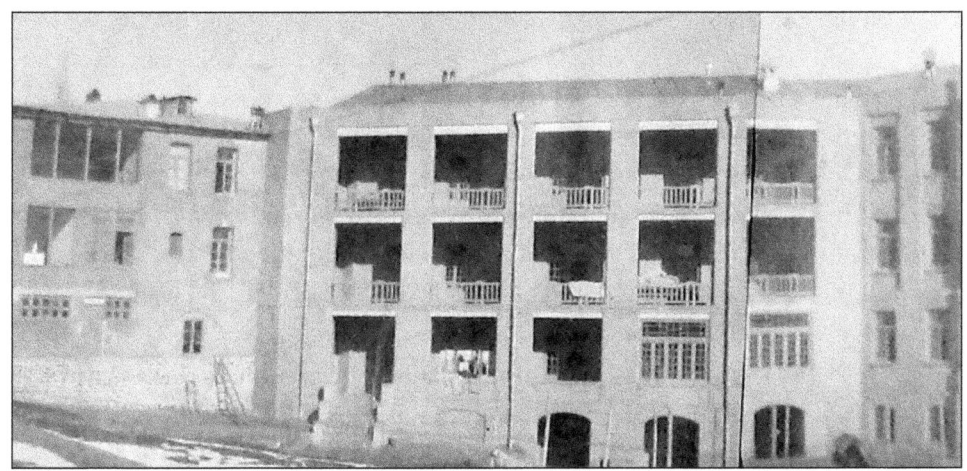

four or five people besides children in his room, should he forego these essentials when entering the hospital? Of course, we have lots of reasons why these things shouldn't be- but we've got to prove our reasons first and the proof will come after years of effort, perhaps. The friends of one patient tried to bring a sheep up the stairway to the patients room on the top floor so that the children visiting there might play with it.[507]

According to Dr. Packard, due to the construction delays, the hospital was even better than they had planned. However, he considered it unfortunate that work had to be done on Sundays in their compound, because the workers were Moslems. "Many Moslems have remarked about the work going on in our yards on our day of worship." The mission committee had allowed this, but he felt that it harmed their Christian mission.[508] The building withstood the winter of 1932-33, and although some water pipes were frozen they did not burst. There was no settles either, but there were still some minor items that need to be taken care of. In the spring of 1933, shrubs and flowers were planted before the entrance. The governor, the chief of police and many others urged the doctors to have an official dedication, which took place on 26 June 1933, when Col. Theodore Roosevelt as well as Rev. Stead spoke. The latter also wrote the obituary of Mrs. Stead that was placed

---

507. RG 91-19-30, Westminster Hospital 1933.
508. RG 91-19-28, Packard to Speer, 30/07/1932.

in the cornerstone of the hospital. Several hundred people attended the dedication.[509] The winter of 1936-37, was the coldest in year and all the hospital's water pipes froze. Fortunately, Mr. Zoeckler was in Kermanshah, who had helped build the hospital, and he could make the necessary repairs and alterations. After the repairs, all the pipes were placed under the roof of the upper floor and so unlikely to freeze again. It was planned to put in a hot water circulation system. The septic tanks also needed to be unclogged in which task the hospital received help from pipefitters lent by the APOC.[510]

The lack of an X-ray machine remained a problem. Patients had to travel 160 km or more to have one taken and treated by X-ray. Although instrument-wise the hospital was almost fully equipped, the doctors really hoped to get an X-ray in the near future.[511] In 1936, the doctors still could complain that theirs was the only US hospital in Iran that had no X-ray, which they really needed for better diagnosis and treatment. Fortunately, in 1937 they were promised one and, therefore, renovations were made to be able to receive the X-ray machine.[512] On 12 May 1938, the steam dressing sterilizer was used for the first time and on 20 May the first X-ray photo was taken. It and the electric generator were slightly damaged on arrival and needed repairs. On 21 May, the first treatment with the Diathermy was given.[513] The X-ray and Diathermy Department demanded more time from the doctors and, therefore, was mostly done in afternoons. It was the only apparatus in the province and, consequently, demand for its use was high, because people thought that it could be used to diagnose and treat any disease

---

509. RG 91-19-28, Speer to Butzer, 16/10/1933; RG 91-19-30, Westminster Hospital Report 07/03/1933; RG 91-19-28, Packard to Speer, 30/07/1932.
510. RG 91-19-30, Kermanshah Medical Report 1937.
511. RG 91-19-30, Report of Westminster Hospital 1933-1934.
512. RG 91-19-30, Kermanshah Medical Report 1936, statistics.; RG 91-19-28, Kermanshah Medical Report 1937.
513. RG 91-19-30, The Westminster Hospital Bulletin. vol/. 1/2. May 1938; Idem, Report Westminster Hospital Kermanshah 1938-39 (X-ray, Physio-therapy department and power plant thanks to Mr. Muncie from Indiana.).

or pathological condition.[514] Much diathermy treatment was done in the out-patient clinic to the benefit of many patients.[515]

The sterilizing and dress preparation room were two of the busiest places in the hospital. Here a graduate nurse and a student nurse worked. Usually all stock of sterilized gauze and goods was used and it required nimble fingers and hard work to fold and prepare linen for the sterilizer. On 12 May 1938, the hospital used a new electric steam dressing sterilizer for the first time, a gift from the Westminster church in Buffalo. The kerosene one blackened the room and tried the patience of the nurse, but nevertheless was kept as back up. These were not the only new and modern equipment items that the Westminster hospital introduced. A real novelty for Iran and the other hospitals was a radio program that in 1938 the Westminster Hospital Program broadcast at 10.30 PM EST through station WHK as well as broadcasts of 24 hours/day on various regular and irregular frequencies. The program aired on Monday, Wednesday, Friday mornings from the studio in the clinic. Tuesday, Thursday and Saturday mornings from the operating room. In the afternoons the programs varied; sometimes the microphone traveled with the doctor and reached the man in the street or in his home, sometimes the program was educational. There also was a nursing appreciation hour. At other times the other parts of the hospital presented their activities via WHK.[516] I have not been able to ascertain whether this radio program was continued in the years thereafter.

Hospital work

Although the hospital initially had two physicians, and at one time even three for a short time, this did not mean that this number of doctors was sufficient for the hospital's workload. Therefore, the help of other physicians or assistants was always welcome. Dr. Rustam Sarfeh (with 3-years of medical school in Beirut), who stayed during the summer

---

514. RG 91-19-30, Report Westminster Hospital Kermanshah 1937-1938.
515. RG 91-19-30, Report Westminster Hospital Kermanshah 1939-1940.
516. RG 91-19-30, Report Westminster Hospital Kermanshah 1937-1938.

of 1933, was a great assistant in the operating room, dispensary and lab and relieved the regular physicians from much routine work.[517] Therefore, when Dr. Sarfeh came again for the summer of 1934, his help was greatly appreciated.[518] In 1935-36, he continued to work for the hospital, but Dr. Sarfeh was only able to give half of his time and many things he could not do. This was unfortunate, because Dr. Bussdicker was leaving on furlough and, given that the staff was already overburdened, they could only hope for the best. In October 1936, Dr. Mary Zoeckler of Malayer came and immediately took over the care of women and children. Unfortunately, before Dr. Zoeckler's arrival, Dr. Sarfeh resigned and took employment with APOC. Fortunately, Dr. Jenny Stead gave a helping hand as she had done so often helped in the past in extremities.[519] This physician staffing situation did not change, for when Dr. Bussdicker returned, Dr. Packard left on furlough on 17 February 1937, Dr. Zoeckler left for Hamadan and Ms Estelle Chambers RN was temporarily absent in charge of the nursing school at Rasht. Fortunately, again Dr. Jenny Stead took over the entire women's and childrens department in both hospital and clinic part time. In mid-1938, the hospital's medical staff was at its top strength. Three physicians plus five nurses and four national staff (registration clerk; dresser on the man's side; practical nurse of women's side; pharmacist). Also, Dr. Rustam Sarfeh from the Beirut medical school, who had worked in the hospital during his vacations in the summers of 1936 and 1937, joined the medical team with his wife, who had been trained at the nursing school there.[520] Every day,

---

517. RG 91-19-30, Report Westminster Hospital 1932-1933.

518. RG 91-19-30, Report of Westminster Hospital 1933-1934.

519. RG 91-19-30, Kermanshah Medical Report 1935-1936; Idem, Kermanshah Medical Report 1936-1937. On 20 April 1933, Dr. Jenny Crozier, a former medical missonary in India, married the Rev. Francis M. Stead at Basra. He was the widower of Dr. Blanche Wilson-Stead. *The Michigan Alumnus*, 39 (September 1933), p. 638.

520. RG 91-19-30, Report Westminster Hospital Kermanshah 1937-1938; Idem, Report Westminster Hospital Kermanshah 1938-39. (Physicians: Harry P. Packard; Russel D. Bussdicker. Nurses: Ms Janet Fulton BA, RN, Mrs. H.P. Packard R.N.; Mrs R.D. Bussdicker R.N.; Ms Magdaleta

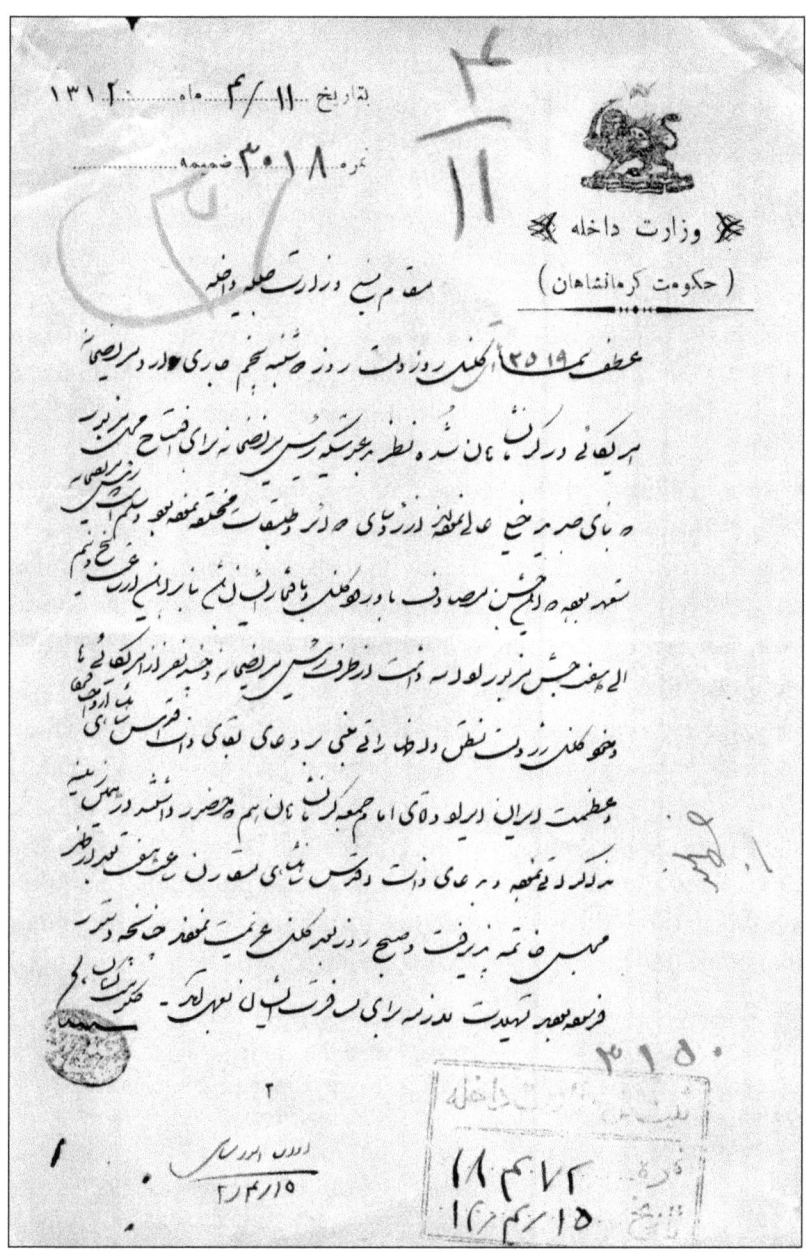

Report from Ministry of Interior mentions the presence of Colonel Theodore Roosevelt (son of the U.S. President) at the opening of the Westminster Hospital, Kermanshah.

before doing his rounds the doctor read the night report written by the night nurse. After the having made his rounds and having given instructions to the nurses, dispensary work began, if it was not a day for operations. During this period life was hectic. For example, during 1937-38, more than 3,000 persons made more than 9,000 visits in the out-patient clinic. Nearly 1,100 of them were treated in the hospital. The doctors treated 168 different diseases or injuries; 30% were infectious diseases; 14% eye diseases; 14% digestive or intestinal disorders; about 10% diseases of women, and the balance of 32% were wounds and injuries. There were 151 patients with some kind of TB, which required long time care for which the hospital had neither the place nor the funds. Therefore, there were only a few of them in the hospital. Trachoma and its complications represented 20% of the eye diseases.[521] When the general wards lacked space, empty private rooms were used with three beds; also with surgical and onbstretical patients; which additional income paid for the cost to treat poor patients. The porch was used continuously with TB patients, who stayed for a long time.[522]

Surgery formed a significant part of the hospital's work. Three alternate mornings of the week were set aside for operations, when most of the activity was on the upper floor of the building.[523] In 1932-33, operations were less numerous than before, but there were more emergencies and a greater variety of cases. For example, a policeman shot himself in the abdomen because his girl turned him down. A soldier shot himself in the head, because he believed his officer had wronged

---

Essa, graduate nurse, Ms Margaret Yohanna, graduate nurse. Clininal Records: Mr. Hoseyn Sohbati; Rabbi Yona Alie lab technician and pharmacist; Mahmud Muradi, dispensary assistant, Z. Bagherpur, information and telephone).

521. RG 91-19-30, Report Westminster Hospital Kermanshah 1937-1938. "Cars and bandits furnished several emergencies." RG 91-19-30, Report Westminster Hospital 1932-1933. "Fear and ignorance make that patients often come late." RG 91-19-30, Kermanshah Medical Report 1936-1937.
522. RG 91-19-30, Report Westminster Hospital Kermanshah 1938-39.
523. RG 91-19-30, Kermanshah Medical Report 1935-1936.

him; he lived and fully recovered. General anesthesia was given by Dr. Ibrahim and Ms Oozhenig Maliksayidian. As many operations as possible were done with novacaine field block and few with sacral block.[524] In 1937-38, the doctors did 962 operations, an average of six operation/day. The only help the doctors had was from staff, who had never seen another hospital and whose training was mostly by observation. The two operating rooms were often in use at the same time and the nurses had to work very hard to prepare the insufficient number of surgical instruments, prepare the patients and sometimes a grad nurse had to assist the physicians. The two white-tiled operating rooms on the top floor were on either side of a central preparation and sterilizing room. In the main room was the shadowless lamp operated by the electric generator given by a donor in Indiana, so that it could be used night and day.[525] A common disease in Kermanshah was intestinal obstruction. Unfortunately, often these cases were maltreated by themselves or relatives and in need of surgery they came too late, which was fatal. Accident cases were more common, cars in the narrow streets and roofs without railing contributed most cases.[526]

On 10 May 1940, when the Packards returned from furlough, Dr. Jenny Stead took a holiday.[527] Nevertheless, for one-third of 1939-40, it was a one-man mission hospital,[528] a situation that would become normal in the years thereafter. This was an unhealthy situation, because, until 1940, the Westminster Hospital was the only civil hospital in *Ostan* V, although there was a great need for it in several of its towns. There were some health officers working in Kermanshah, but they

---

524. RG 91-19-30, Report Westminster Hospital 1932-1933.
525. RG 91-19-30, Report Westminster Hospital Kermanshah 1937-1938. A Bostonian lady passing through saw the make-shift dust catching light and she gave them a modern shadowless light. RG 91-19-30, Report of Westminster Hospital 1933-1934.
526. RG 91-19-30, Report Westminster Hospital 1933-1934.
527. RG 91-19-30, The Westminster Hospital Bulletin. vol. 2/1. October 1939 (Col. Nicola of Imp. Russ. Army worked for 25 years as a mechanic and chauffeur; he owns two Ford trucks.).
528. RG 91-19-30, Report Westminster Hospital Kermanshah 1939-1940.

were unable to satisfy the needs of the population, while the existing military hospitals were not even able to care for major surgery of the troops in the region.[529] In fact, before the Westminster Hospital was even completed in 1932, the military authorities asked its physicians to perform 270 hernia operations on new conscripts as soon as possible. "This means that 30 beds are filled and refilled with 30 soldiers as fast as they can be dismissed."[530] Fortunately, there was a positive development that compensated for the loss of capacity of the Westminster hospital.

In 1940, later than was expected, a Red Lion and Sun state hospital was established in Kermanshah, which was able to care for the most distressing cases that before were all sent to the Westminster Hospital. Because the Department of Health required that the state hospital took care of all charity cases in the region this lightened the burden somewhat for the Westminster Hospital. This meant that it was able to focus on more highly specialized work for which it staff was qualified. During a visit by Dr. Packard to the Red Lion hospital he observed that three doctors, one druggist, one midwife and several helpers were caring for 27 patients quite satisfactorily and that a new grant enabled them to install another five beds. There were plans for a 20-bed isolation hospital for infectious diseases next to the current hospital; the land had already been purchased. People were getting more accustomed to hospitals and that they could be better taken care of there than at home. The Westminster Hospital collaborated with the staff of the state hospital in the area of the use of its X-ray machine and its superior facilities in obstetrics and surgery.[531] In 1943, when the 75-bed Westminster Hospital had only one physician, the Red Lion and Sun state hospital employed five doctors for 35 beds.[532]

---

529. RG 91-19-30, Westminster Hospital Report no. 2, 1932.

530. RG 91-19-30, Westminster Hospital Report no. 4, 1932.

531. RG 91-19-30, Report Westminster Hospital Kermanshah 1939-1940. The arrival of this civil state hospital was already expected in 1932. RG 91-19-28, Packard to Speer, 30/07/1932.

532. RG 91-19-30, Report Westminster Hospital Kermanshah 1943-44.

In 1940-41, the missionary physicians saw an increase in communicable diseases such as typhus fever and typhoid and they noted that hospital care made all the difference. New medicines such as sulfanilimide, sulfapyridine, albucid and prontosil made an enormous impact on the treatment of pneumonia, puerperal fever, erysipelas, mastoiditis and many other infections.[533] In January-February 1943, the public health situation in Kermanshah was disastrous. According to Dr. Mohammad Daftari, the Director of Public Health, there were 1,230 deaths due typhus alone.[534] The only institution that was able to provide effective help, and even that was not adequate, was the Westminster Hospital. Dr. Bussdicker reported that they saw the worst typhus epidemic in their history in Kermanshah. They treated 105 cases, of whom 14 died.[535] In 1941, Dr. Packard had been transferred to Hamadan, but fortunately he was back in 1943 to help battle the typhus outbreak. Shortly thereafter, he and Mrs. Packard retired after having worked for thirty-seven years as missionary physician in Iran. The common people as well as the local authorities paid exceptional tributes to him. To deal with eventual further outbreaks of typhus in Kermanshah the government opened a Typhus Hospital in that city, which probably was a temporary arrangement.[536] At Dr. Daftari's request, the British Army made a sample disinfector, which was handed

---

533. RG 91-19-30, Report Westminster Hospital Kermanshah 1939-1940; Idem, Report Westminster Hospital Kermanshah 1940-1941.

534. FO 371/40177, Kermanshah Diary February 1944; FO 371/40177, Kermanshah Diary March 1944.

535. RG 91-19-30, Report Westminster Hospital Kermanshah 1942-1943 (Increased traffic on the roads meant 145 accident cases; also many other cases. On Thursday evenings there were many stab wounds, while suicide by opium was also a regular weekly occurrence); Dr. Cohn substituted for one month so that the Bussdickers could have a holiday. RG 91-19-30, Report Westminster Hospital Kermanshah 1942-1943. In 1941, Dr. K.M. Cohn, a Jewish-German physician, who had fled and come to Kermanshah, where he set up practice with the help of Dr. Bussdicker. RG 91-19-30, Report Westminster Hospital Kermanshah 1940-41; for his further activities, see Hamadan section.

536. RG 61.3.46, Bushdicker/Kermanshah to Huntwork/New York, 29/09/1957.

to him in January 1944. At his follow-up request, the British Army emptied 12 bitumen drums to be turned into disinfectors. Dr. Daftari also became the chairman of the local committee of the Imperial Iranian Pharmaceutical Institute for the control of the sale of drugs by reputable pharmacists, which was formed in January 1944. Members of the committee included the Director of Finance and Dr. Bussdicker of the Westminster Hospital.[537]

After Dr. Packard's departure, Dr. Bussdicker was working alone and he found the workload overwhelming. He had to be administrator, surgeon, physician, intern, lab and X-ray technician, instructor for nurses, treasurer and accountant. The US nurse was not only instructor and nursing supervisor, but also anesthesist, floor nurse, and supply nurse. In short, everybody was overworked.[538]

In 1944 Dr. Mohammad A`zam Zanganeh, a graduate of Tehran and Bern Universities, joined the medical staff, attracted by a special financial arrangement. In 1945, the Bussdickers returned to the US on furlough.[539] The year 1944-45 was a busy one, which went through its usual cycle of endemic diseases. The greatest enemy were fevers thoughout the year, accounting for 14% of total in-patient days. "The year begins with typhys fever (for which the *korsi* is the ideal breeding place), when that is over then comes typhoid fever at the beginning of summer, malaria is most common casue of fever in summer and fall, and in winter the two main diseases are meningitis and pneumonia." In 1944-45, there was less malaria, because there had been a drought in the summer of 1944. Malaria, pneumonia and TB required expensive medicines, which due to the war were unobtainable. Sulfa drugs were great and shortened patients' stay; however, penicillin was only available to the military and the government. Also, in Kermanshah there was no cold storage, so even there the military and the government didn't have it. With the start of pilgrim traffic, relapsing or tick fever raised its head. This required a microscope examination of blood, then

---

537. FO 371/40177, Kermanshah Diary January 1944 (there was also a hospital at Shahabad).
538. RG 91-19-30, Report Westminster Hospital Kermanshah 1944-1945.
539. RG 91-19-30, Report Westminster Hospital Kermanshah 1944-1945.

two injections of neosalvaran healed it. Dr. Busddicker announced this finding to the other medical people in Kermanshah. He observed that education was still needed to have people come early to hospital rather than to wait when it is almost too late. In 1944-45, 25% of in-patient days were for patients suffering from accident and physical defects.[540]

Fortunately, Dr. Mohammad A`zam Zanganeh remained working in the hospital until the early 1950s and, thereafter, went in private practice. However, he continued to serve as otolargynologist consultant for the hospital. Dr. Zanganeh also referred his patients to the hospital. In 1946, Dr. Frances Zoeckler joined the medical staff and took over the women's ward and clinic. She left in 1953 on furlough and was replaced by Dr. Burton Dyson, who in 1955 returned to the USA. Dr. Zoeckler returned in September 1955, who wrote enthusiastically: "In 1952 a water piped system was a dream, now we have it with a purification system."[541] Dr. Zanganeh was replaced by Dr. Art Moradian, who was trained in the USA. Ms Estelle Chambers was still the head of nursing.[542] The Westminster hospital closed in 1958, coinciding with the retirement of Dr. Bussdicker, because the mission was unable to recruit and send doctors and nurses.[543] Because of their significant contribution to the health of so many patients, starting with Dr. Blanche Wilson-Stead, the Westminster Hospital or *bimarestan-e masihi* (the Christian Hospital) was known among the people of Kermanshah as *Bagh-e Hakim Khanom* or *bimarestan-e Amrika'i* (The Female Doctor's Garden or the American Hospital).[544]

---

540. RG 91-19-30, Report Westminster Hospital Kermanshah 1944-1945; Idem, Social and Education Project 1944-1945

541. RG 91-19-28, Frances Zoeckler to Board of Foreign Missions 08/02/1956.

542. RG 61.3.46, Bushdicker/Kermanshah to Huntwork/New York, 29/09/1957.

543. Miller 1989, pp. 328.

544. RG 61.3.46, Muradian to Bussdicker, 06/08/1959. Unfortunately, the hospital was destroyed by fire on 16 February 2020.

Dispensary

The out-patient clinic was open three mornings/week, when the doctors and their assistants, saw on average 50-100 patients.[545]

> Each patient, if seen for the first time, visits the record desk where his name, age, residence and chief complaints are recorded. This is done by Mr. Hancock the evangelist; he needs an assistant, as he also has to look for the patient's history in case of return visitors. The patients comes with his record; he can chose any of the 3 doctors, and the doctors writes his notes re history, examinations and treatment on it. A prescription is given or order for the dressing room. Most patients get medicines for 2-3 days or until the necxt clinic day. The record remains on file in the hospital and is great help for all; also for reports, statistics and research.[546]

Women of the best and the poorest families mingled on the women's floor share their stories and the poor appreciated the kind deeds by the well-to-do. In 1934, the hospital had to let go Dr. Ebrahim Aghajan, who had done much of the free work in the out-patient dispensary and saved the doctors much time, but the economy was necessary. It meant that sometimes the doctors left the dispensary after 2 p.m., because otherwise patients would have to wait another day to see them, if they closed at 12. When one of the physicians was absent, Dr. Jenny Crozier-Stead helped out in the hospital and dispensary. Having a lady physician was a great help and her male colleagues hoped that she would come more often to Kermanshah.[547] In the dispensary all the tooth aches were taken care of by extraction, abscesses were lanced by the scores and many intravenous medications

---

545. For example, in 1933-34, the outpatient clinic handled 4,517 new cases, 5,392 return visits, and 516 housecalls. The in-patient department had 14,397 in-patient days or a bed occupancy of 67%. RG 91-19-28, Speer to Butzer, 22/10/1934.
546. RG 91-19-30, The out-patient clinic.
547. RG 91-19-30, Report of Westminster Hospital 1933-1934. She and her husband worked in Faraman.

were given and many eye operations for trachoma done. In 1936-37, a total of 400-500 cases.⁵⁴⁸ In 1939-40, there were 48% more out-patients. Because of this the dispensary needed renovation, repairs and replacement to be able to take better care of patients.⁵⁴⁹

Local hospitals

In 1931, the municipality created a *Behdari* or public health section for the treatment of poor people by physicians such as Dr. Fakhr Pezeshkan and Dr. Ebrahim Khan Tizabi, who received 690 and 300 rials/month. In that same year, the municipality also established a mental asylum in the Bagh-e Hajj Aqa Mohammad Mehdi Feyz Mahdavi, who rented it. It employed some staff, and the institution was served in turns by Dr. Allah Khan Mo'ed, Dr. `Abdal`Ali Khan Aresta, Dr. Ahmad Khan and others. Furthermore, a house for invalids was created in the Shabestan of the Amir Nezam Garrusi Mosque, south of the Friday Mosque, which for years had been abandoned. It daily housed 82 men, 69 women and 11 children.⁵⁵⁰ However, this arrangement did not work so well, in fact, not at all. In 1934, the municipality had asked the Westminster Hospital to care for indigent patients, for which service it would pay less than one-third of cost of patients it would sent. However, by mid-1935 the Municipality was many months in arrears (see above).⁵⁵¹

Since 1919, physicians had to be licensed to be able to practice and Kermanshah was one of the cities where examinations took place to establish whether a doctor could get a license.⁵⁵² However, in 1936 the British consul concluded that "nor are the local doctors and dentists any better now than 20 years ago. The same filthy 'hammams'

---

548. RG 91-19-30, Kermanshah Medical Report 1936-1937.
549. RG 91-19-30, Report Westminster Hospital Kermanshah 1939-1940.
550. Soltani 1373, vol. 1, pp. 553-54.
551. RG 91-19-30, Westminster Hospital Annual Report 1934-1935.
552. Rusta'i 1382, vol. 1, pp. 32; See Soltani 1373, vol. 1, p. 535. If the health authorities believed that somebody was practicing without a license a notice was sent. Rusta'i 1382, vol. 1, pp. 94-95.

which were patronized twenty years ago are still used and germ-laden kanat-water is boiled over and over again for successive batches of bathers now, just as it was a century ago. Sanitation and public hygiene are as little understood now as they were before the present era of progress was ushered in."[553] In April 1944, there were only six reputable pharmacists, according to the local committee for the Imperial Pharmaceutical Institute.[554]

Khoy

A team of the American Red Cross was sent in November 1915, to establish a 200- bed hospital for Russian soldiers at Khoy. The Americans set up a hospital in low adobe building in which camel drivers had housed their caravans.[555]

Lahejan

As a result of Dr. Frame's itinerations it was decided to set up a drug room and a dispensary in Lahejan in 1911. This was left in charge of Baron Hagop, Dr. Frame's medical assistant. He knew the Bible, got along with Moslem Iranians and, although he had not had a full medical training, he probably was as well qualified as any practitioner at Lahejan, according to Frame. However, he was not to do medical work, but concentrate on the drug room, "where he would probably do the same kind of treating simple ailments that all druggists do throughout Persia. This undertaking has to be self-supporting but would involve an initial expense of four hundred tomans." Frame had hoped to pay for this activity from the Rasht medical fees, but his long absence made this impossible.[556] During the first year Dr. Frame made monthly 3-4 days visits to Lahejan, seeing more than 200 patients.[557] In 1916, work in Lahejan was abandoned, after one successful year, because

---

553. FO 371/21900, f. 113.
554. FO 371/40177, Kermanshah Diary April 1944.
555. Red Cross 1922, pp. 159-60.
556. RG 91-1-12, Report of Resht Station 1910-1911.
557. Presbyterian Church 1914, p. 332.

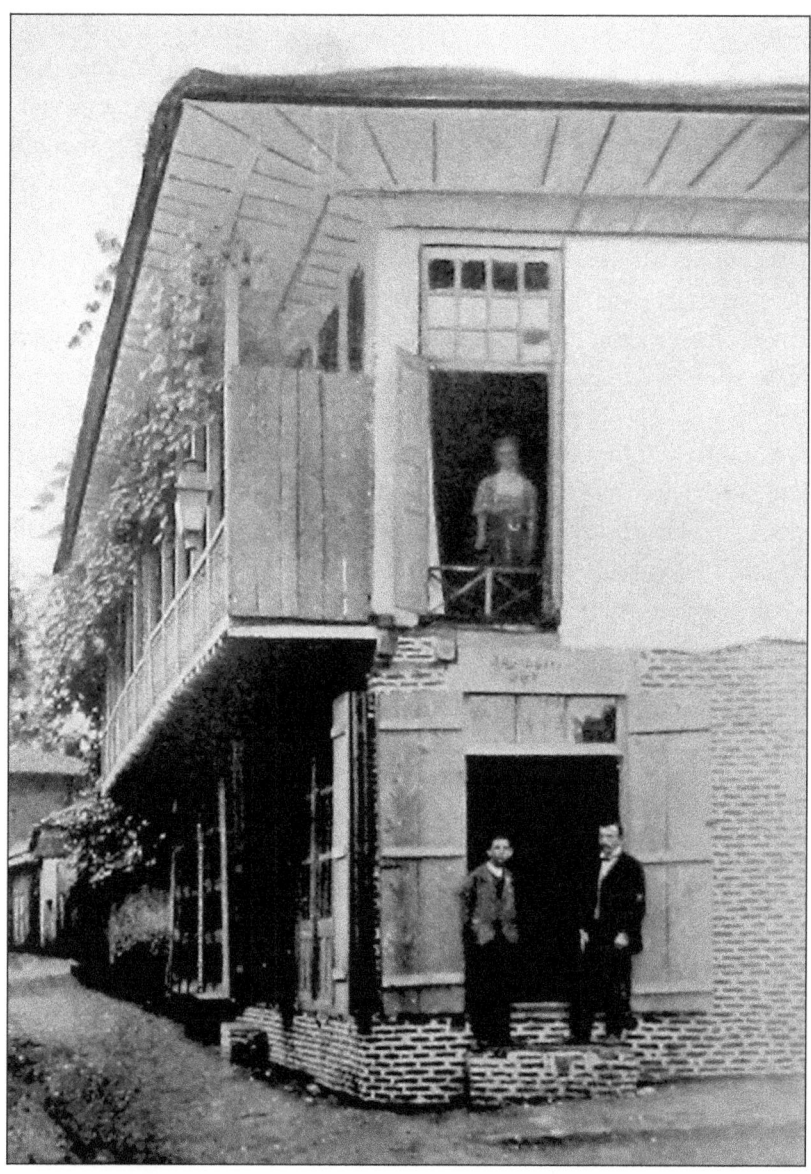

The American missionary drugstore at Lahejan opened in 1911. Baron Hagop (right), is the druggist and the evangelist, 1913.

the assistant had a nervous breakdown. An advantage was that drugs ordered for Lahejan were not available for Rasht and could be used there.[558] Although in 1920, the province was still much disturbed by the Jangali movement, Frame re-opened the station at Lahejan and intended to itinerate in some mountain districts in the summer.[559] Dr. Hagop Kachaturiants, Frame's former assistant, made this town his headquarters much of the time and established through visits etc. a wide group of friends. In the early 1930s, American doctors visited Lahejan one day each week, and from time to time they also visited neighboring towns.[560] In 1932, the Department of Education asked the American missionaries to begin working in Lahejan and they decided to do so with two doctors in Rasht (Frame, Brinkman). The more so, because usually the government curtailed "our liberty to educate, medicine etc." Frame rented a house where Dr. Hagop would reside and have a drug store and Dr. Brinkman would visit there every other week.[561] The weekly trips to Lahejan were maintained, which often resulted in patients coming to the hospital in Rasht.[562] The Lahejan visits were continued until Frame's departure on furlough in 1935. Dr. Hagop went into the mountains with a good supply of medicine, especially of quinine and he was able to alleviate much suffering and he continued to do so thereafter.[563]

LENGEH

Although similar in population size[564] as Bushehr and Bandar Abbas and having the same kind of diseases attendance at the charitable

---

558. Presbyterian Church 1917, pp. 299-300.
559. RG91-19-9, Report Medical Work 1919-1920.
560. RG 91-19-9, "History of Resht Station," p. 2.
561. RG 91-19-9, Rest Medical Report 1931-1932; Idem, Resht Medical Report 1932-1933.
562. RG 91-19-9, Resht Medical Report 1933-1934.
563. RG 91-19-9, Report Resht Medical Work 1934-1935; Idem, Medical Report Resht 1935-1936.
564. Lengeh had a population of some 20,000 in 1919. Administration Report 1919, p. 10. The doctor's house "is a very large straddling edifice very much out of repair. The Persian clearly has an aversion to repairing." Cursetjee 1918, p. 72.

dispensary was lower in Lengeh.⁵⁶⁵ This did not mean it was unpopular, for patients came from the outlying districts with the caravans as well as from the islands to receive treatment. Ass. surgeon E.M. Cuzen was both the quarantine officer as well as in charge of the charitable dispensary, which was housed in the British Consulate's annex. Although women patients remained in the minority, by 1925 it was noted that a "better class women now attend the dispensary."⁵⁶⁶

Table 21: Number of visits to the British charitable dispensary of Lengeh (1912-1925).

Year	Total	Men	Women	Boys	Girls
1912	947	-	-	-	-
1913	1,846	-	-	-	-
1914	2,072	-	-	-	-
1916	2,587	-	-	-	-
1917	2,023	-	-	-	-
1918	2,630	-	-	-	-
1919	2,318	-	-	-	-
1921	1,521	-	-	-	-
1922	1,630	-	-	-	-
1923	2,203	-	-	-	-
1925	2,095	1,284	476	190	145
1926	1,850	-	-	-	-
1927	1,838	-	-	-	-
1928	1,858	-	-	-	-

Source: *Administration Report* 1914, p. 16; Ibid., 1915, p. 15; Ibid., 1916, p. 15; Ibid., 1917, p. 14; Ibid., 1918, p. 14; Ibid., 1919, p. 14; Ibid., 1923, p. 36; Ibid., 1925, p. 37; Ibid., p. 21; Ibid. 1928, p. 30.

---

565. The prevailing major diseases were malaria, eye diseases and of digestive organs, Administration Report 1913, p. 43; Idem 1914, p. 16; Idem 1923, p. 36

566. Administration Report 1923, p. 36; Idem 1925, p. 37. In nearby Basidu, on the island of Qeshm the British army had since 1823 a small military base, which included a small hospital. This hospital remained functional until the 1883 when the base was abandoned. The derelict hospital building was still there in 1925. There is no evidence that the services of this hospital were available to the population of Basidu. For a description of the military hospital of Basidu in 1856 see Shepherd 1857, pp. 71, 73, 75-76, 97. See also Administration Report 1882-83, p. 6; Wilson 1928, p. 212. For a photo, see IOR, Mss Eur F111/354, f 9.

In 1927, Ass. surgeon J.W. Woodsell, M.C. IMD was quarantine physician and in charge of dispensary. Woodsell remained till 23 February 1928 when he was replaced by ass. surgeon E.R. Hill IMD. At the end of August 1928 he was replaced by Dr. Mohammad Khan Faqihi, who was sent by Tehran, as a consequence of the transfer of the quarantine service to the Iranian government.[567] Because the British Consulate was discontinued on 28 May 1929, the charitable dispensary was also closed.[568] In 1934 it was reported that the town's health officer cared "little for the sick or poor but a great deal for money." He had few or no medicines, which most could not afford anyway, and, if really sick, people went to Bahrain or Muscat for treatment by the American missionary doctors.[569]

Malayer

In 1920, Dowlatabad or Malayer was a town of 8,000 people. The city was 70 km by caravan road and 100 km by car from Hamadan. US missionaries started working there in 1914, originally with an educational program, but 15 years later its work was mostly evangelical in nature. Because the wife of the evangelist (Rev. George Zoeckler) was a physician (Dr. Mary Zoeckler, née Dr. Allen),[570] she opened a small dispensary in the fall of 1914 in the basement of a rented house, where she lived with her husband, who preached the Gospel and ran a school. The dispensary was open every other day, but there were no regular hours, as patients were treated when they came. At first, Dr. Zoeckler had a large number of patients, because people expected miracles from the *khanom ferangi*. However, after a while they realized that she was no miracle worker and that like traditional Persian physicians she gave them pills and powders and, moreover, asked for money. As a result, the number of patients fell. Therefore,

---

567. Administration Report 1927, p. 18; Administraton Report 1928, p. 30.
568. Administration Report 1929, p. 34.
569. Administraton Report 1934, p. 31.
570. She had arrived in Hamadan in 1913, where she worked in the dispensary and hospital there (see above).

between 1 October 1914 and 30 June 1915, a total of 765 patients were seen, of whom about 200 were new ones. Dr. Zoeckler also made 120 house calls and had one in-patient. Because the basement room was flooded the dispensary had to be moved upstairs. Because the owner never repaired the basement, the dispensary was later moved to yet another room. When a patient really needed an operation the dispensary became OR and hospital ward. Using two *korsi*s [wooden frames]⁵⁷¹ and the mission's travel mattresses a bed was made. Mr. Zoeckler had to act as anesthetist, while all the local women looked on. A clean night gown was used as an operating gown. Although this was a better treatment than the patient would have gotten at home, Dr. Zoeckler felt the need to have at least one separate room for such occasional patients. Although the fiscal year ended in the black at one time she feared to be in the red, because when medicines and supplies ordered in Great Britain did not arrive she had to buy them at very high cost in the Hamadan bazaar. However, an unexpected fee case meant that the year closed with a surplus. Although the Persians liked to bargain, from the very beginning Dr. Zoeckler established fixed prices and rules, which, however, had a lowering effect on the number of patients. Rather than choosing for a free dispensary she had opted for the fee-for service system, which allowed her to become self-supporting and have her work grow slowly and not loose time and energy with bargaining. She only treated free patients, if these really could not afford to pay. Dr. Zoeckler was not the only foreign-trained physician in Dowlatabad, but the other one did not really practice. Apart from a few cases, all her patients were women and children. Despite the fact that patients paid, there still was a widespread prejudice against modern medicine, but she expected this sentiment to diminish over time, once people got accustomed to these foreign methods. Because of the make-shift condition and location of her dispensary, Dr. Zoeckler asked for permission to build a small dispensary on the Mission's premises with the balance of the money she had earned that year.⁵⁷²

---

571. On the *korsi*, see Willem Floor, 'Korsi," iranicaonline. org.
572. RG 280-1-10, Report of Medical Work for Women, Daulatabad,

Despite the unrest in the province in 1915-16, Dr. Zoeckler's medical work saw some progress in the following year. Also, for three winters, Dowlatabad was closed off from the outside world, not even having contact with its neighboring villages. Because inside the city conditions were also very disturbed, those who could, sent their family to some village, while those who remained behind hardly dared to go out into the streets. This also meant that visits to the dispensary fell compared with the previous year. For three months there was practically no activity at all in the dispensary, apart from treating scratches and bruises of boys playing at war or giving medicine for headaches for those families staying in the Mission compound. Attendance remained negligible during the fall and only picked up once the Russians had taken the province, although patients were still relatively few in number, it was more than the average of the last two years. The dispensary also treated a German lieutenant and some Austrian prisoners, who had fled from Russia as well as some Bakhtiyaris, who were allied with the Germans. Later Dr. Zoeckler also had wounded Russians among her patients, who in total numbered 539 cases of which about 130 new cases. She also made 125 house calls as well as visited a few villages on some Fridays, which were among her busiest days, treating an additional 383 patients. The year again ended with a surplus of 150 *tuman*s, which she put aside for the construction of a dispensary. Although she continued her fixed fee policy in the city, in the villages she only charged fixed fees for medicines. As many villagers also were among her city patients, she expected that the fixed fee policy would become less of a problem in the future and have no longer a downward pressure among the growth of her practice. However, the supply of drugs might become a problem, because only those that she had ordered from Baghdad prior to the opening of the dispensary in Dowlatabad were available to her. Some essential drugs had been finished and imports were impossible, while those available in the local bazaars were much adulterated, and thus practically useless, and exorbitantly expensive, if available at all.[573] In

---

1914-1915; Presbyterian Church 1916, p. 295.
573. RG 280-1-10, Report of Medical Work, Daulatabad, 1915-1916.

early 1916, there were even two American physicians, two American nurses and one British nurse from the Red Cross providing temporary medical and surgical care, because of nearby military operations.[574]

Despite the war,[575] medical work in Dowlatabad made progress; only the itinerations suffered in some small measure. 1,100 patients were seen at the dispensary and 515 house calls were made, while 816 patients in the villages were treated, or a total of 1,474. A few cases were surgical and some minor operations were performed, because the facilities (an OR, and assistants) were lacking. The year ended again in the black, partly because there was hardly any expenditure for drugs, which were unavailable. Another positive development was the successful treatment of an influential elegist or *rowzeh-khvan*, who had been given up by local Iranian physicians. Although Dr. Zoeckler had doubt about his recovery he did and even was able to perform the *rowzeh-khan*s during Moharram, where he confessed that he had always been against the work of the American missionaries and had spoken against their school, but he would never do so again. He later only spoke in very positive terms about them.[576] During these 4.5 months 520 patients were seen, of almost 100 were new cases, while 72 house calls were made and five operations were performed (two were harelips). Dr. Zoeckler regretted that she had to leave as her work

---

574. Presbyterian Church 1917, p. 298.

575. After the Russians returned to Dowlatabad for the second time in April 1917, they made George Zoeckler governor of the city, which function he occupied against his liking, for five days. "It isn't exactly an easy task managing a Persian city at such a time, especially when provisions for 2,000 soldiers and their horses have to be wrung from a more or less hostile people who have already been bled by another army to almost as great an extent as they can stand." For a description how the war between the Russians and Ottomans affected the people and region of Dowlatabad, see RG 280-1-8, Mary Allen Zoeckler to the Women's Guild, North Church, Buffalo, 16/05/1917.

576. RG 280-1-8, Report of Medical Work. Daulatabad 1916-1917. For a report what happened during the itineration, see RG 280-1-8, Report on 25 Days Itineration, Malayir. July-August 1916.

was going so well.[577] With the departure of Mr. and Dr. Mrs. Zoeckler in November 1918 to Hamadan medical work in Dowlatabad was discontinued.[578] In Hamadan, Dr. Zoeckler had to take charge of the hospital there until the return of Dr. Funk. She relished the hospital work that she found more satifying than dispensary work.[579] She remained in Hamadan until the return of Dr. Funk, who took over on 1 April 1921. On 15 June 1921, Dr. Zoeckler reopened her dispensary in Dowlatabad after an absence of 3.5 years.[580]

The workload was more regular than in the previous period with an average of 10 patients/day, but, with all her other tasks, Dr. Zoeckler was very busy. In July 1921 she received an operating table, a gift from the Junior Guild of the North Church, Buffalo, NY. The dispensary had to be reorganized to make place for it. Although minor operations were performed, Dr. Zoeckler could not do major ones, because of the lack of assistants. Two Lor gun shot patients stayed for six weeks on a mattress under a tree. In the case of a hairlip operation she was paid two gold ear rings, six lbs of butter, six lbs of cheese and a goat. Money was scarce in Iran at that time, the percentage of free patients was higher than before, while expenses were higher, so that the fiscal year ended with a deficit (230 *qran*s).[581]

In early 1923, Dr. Zoeckler had little competition, except from a traditional Iranian physician, who was still the man to go to for the majority of the population. This changed when a pupil of Dr. Funk, who had previously worked in Malayer, returned and opened a practice. Also, Iranian troops were stationed there and with them came a physician, who was also kept busy with private patients. Moreover, in May 1923, a free hospital was opened by a pupil of the Dar al-Fonun, which

---

577. RG 280-1-8, Report of Medical Work, Daulatabad, July 1--Nov. 12, 1917.
578. Presbyterian Church 1919, p. 263.
579. RG 280-1-8, Mary Allen Zoeckler to the Women's Guild, North Church, Buffalo, 15/02/1921.
580. RG 280-1-8, Report of Medical Work Hamadan 1920-21.
581. RG 280-1-10, Medical Report. Daulatabad 1921-22 (New cases: 351; old cases: 338; house calls: 486 ; total new cases 417; old cases 1124 or total: 1531 patients).

was financed by Seyf al-Dowleh, a Qajar prince and major landowner, who also laid out a beautiful park just outside the city, which was the pride of every one. In 1920, the prince had left one-fifth of his estate for charitable purposes, in particular for a hospital, a school and an orphanage. Even allowing for pilfering by the administrators, the endowment was expected to yield 6,000 *tumans*/year, of which 2,000 was set aside for the hospital. The latter was established in Seyf al-Dowleh's women's quarters (*andarun*). It did not have yet all instruments, but it opened with six beds, which were all filled. Dr. Zoekckler saw a significant increase of obstetrical work. In one case, Dr. Zoeckler was called to resolve a confinement in a village where the traditional midwife had given up. "When I arrived I found the woman lying in ashes and the color of charcoal to the waist with freshly killed opened up and tied over her abdomen." It took one hour to clean the woman and then five minutes to complete the delivery. In mid-winter the city governor asked Dr. Zoeckler to take his wife into her house and look after her. She had been ill with puerperal fever, which had been misdiagnosed by the gendarmerie doctor. Despite his vigorous, but wrong treatment, the patient's condition had grown worse. When she came, it was with five family members and many servants and stayed for two weeks, when she died. The governor was grateful and did not hold Dr. Zoeckler responsible for the death, although in the city there were voices who said differently. Because many dispensary patients came from the surrounding villages, Dr. Zoeckler wanted to go one day per week to some of the nearby villages, but unfortunately other duties often intervened. The fiscal year ended with a surplus, including after having paid off last year's deficit.[582]

In the early 1920s, the dispensary's equipment was simple:

---

582. RG 280-1-10, Report of Medical Work, Daulatabad 1922-23 (Dispensary- new cases: 429; old cases: 718; total : 1147. Seen in villages: 159 new cases. In-patients: two. City calls: old 86, new 121, total 207. Total new: 656; old: 859; total: 1515; 13 operations); Zahereddini 1966, p. 38; Gilmour 1924, pp. 29-30; Momeni 1976, pp. 46, 49.

An operating table, a small sterlizer, not pressure, a microscope with oil immersion lens, a fair supply of instruments including a blood pressure apparatus, and a fairly adequate supply of drugs. Brief records are kept of all patients, and only simple operations are performed; there are no in-patient facilities. Most patients come from within a radius of 16 km. Some time is spent on itineration (Nehavand, Soltanabad, villages), more so during the last two years, as home responsibilites are less and school work has closed. The dispensary has no outside financing at all, and in most years it had a small surplus.[583]

A positive development was the friendly cooperation with the physician in charge of the hospital in the Park. She sent patients to him, who could not go to the hospital in Hamadan, while he sent her cases that required difficult operations. Although the hospital was not ideal it really provided a service to the community. Dr. Zoeckler's plan to visit nearby villages on Fridays again suffered from other calls on her time, but in July 1924 she made a 10-day trip to Nehavand seeing 275 patients.[584] The next year was the busiest so far. A total of 1,606 patients were seen, and only 1917-18 was more with 2,511, due to the 896 patients seen during an itineration, whereas in 1924-25 she saw only 144 patients during a 10-day trip. City work was very busy with many night calls and increased obstetrical work. Although she had no hospital it sometimes felt that way with some patients. One of the missionaries gave child birth, which

> Was one maternity case in Daulatabad where no one pawned the patient's chuddar at the nearest grocery shop for a few dates, or hung on the latch of the door to make the baby's coming easier; where the patient was allowed all the water she wanted and not made to drink a quart or so of grease so that she would get well quicker; and where no precautions at all were taken to keep the 'Aul' away. The Persians here have a great fear at such times that the aul, which belongs to the race of jinns, will come and

---

583. RG 280-1-10, Report of Medical Work, Daulatabad 1924-25 (Last year: 573 patients, house calls 165, total outpatients 1053, Operations: 7 major, 10 minor. Most patients are women).

584. RG 280-1-10, Report of Medical Work, Daulatabad 1924-25.

snatch out the heart and liver of the patient and then disappear in which case the patient will surely die. Sometimes instead of killing the mother the aul will substitute a jinn child for the real one. In order to keep the aul away the never for a minute leave the patient or child alone. They put an onion on an iron spit and tap the walls of the room all around, one asking "for the sake of whom" and another replying "For the sake of Mary and her son Jesus." The the spit with the onion and some other sharp object, a sword or a pair of scissors, is put at the patient's head to frighten the Aul away. The 7th night is the most dangerous time. On that night they put a black rope all around the patient's bed and invite many guests who help to keep the patient awake till after midnight when the danger is supposed to be past.[585]

Cooperation with the Hamadan hospital, whose reputation increased in Malayer, grew. Patients needed operations that could not be done in the city were sent to Hamadan. Dr. Funk also made a short visit to Dowlatabad and saw many patients. Together with Dr. Zoeckler he made an itineration to Nehavand. At that time, Dr. Funk was more popular than her and many women were quarreling to have him see them. In spring there was an outbreak of measles in the villages and city, with high mortality due to broncho-pneumonia complications.

In 1925, it looked as is the Park hospital would be closed. The funds set aside were used to pay taxes or were otherwise misappropriated. The physician in charge became discouraged, resigned and took an army position. One of Dr. Funk's pupils in town, who had a private practice intended to go into the more remunerating carpet business in Soltanabad, which meant that there was a need for Iranian physicians in Dowlatabad. The fiscal year ended with a surplus of 61 *tuman*s, after having bought next year's supplies.[586] The year 1925-26 (of 40 weeks presence here) was a calm one and no surprises, medical or otherwise. Dr. Zoeckler made 343 house calls, which were time- and energy-consuming. Pressure was high, because other duties, such as home-schooling her daughter, took much time. Therefore, Dr. Zoeckler

---

585. On the *Al*, see Eilers 1979.
586. RG 280-1-10, Report of Medical Work, Daulatabad 1924-25.

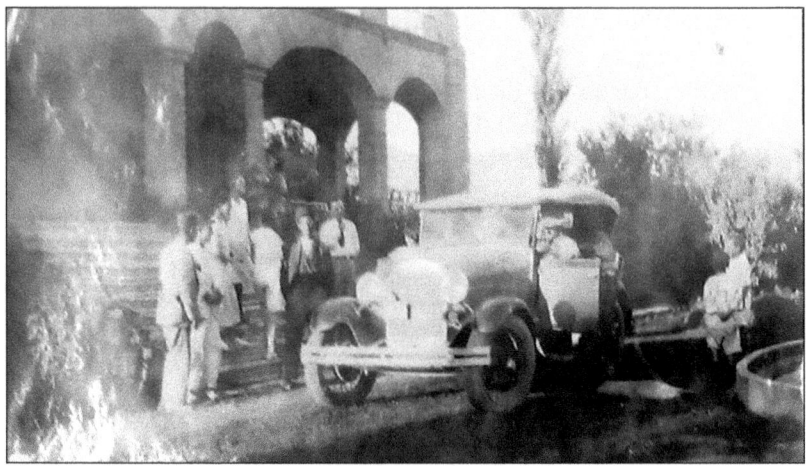

Above and opposite: American missionaries meeting at mission residence in Malayer, 1925.

expected that when she returned from furlough, she would have to reduce her medical work. The fiscal year again ended with a positive balance.[587] During Juy-November 1926, Dr. Zoeckler saw 121 patients in the disensary and 160 old cases, while 58 house calls were made of which 28 were new patients. This period also was concluded in the black and with her departure on furlough.[588]

Although Dr. Zoeckler returned on 18 May, she only opened the dispensary on 28 May 1928. She totally re-arranged her dispensary schedule, due to her home-schooling duties. She wrote a letter and sent it to the notables in town, who, in the past, had made use of her services. She also posted a copy of the letter at the door of the missionary compound. The letter explained the reasons for the change and announced that the dispensary would be open five days/week from 11 a.m. to 12 a.m. and also listed a slightly changed fee schedule. Although the opening time was an inconvenient one for people it was well respected, better than when the dispensary had been open all morning, leaving the morning entirely free for home-schooling.

---

587. RG 280-1-10, Report of Medical Work, Daulatabad 1925-26.
588. RG 280-1-10, Report of Medical Work, Daulatabad. July 1-Nov. 1, 1926.

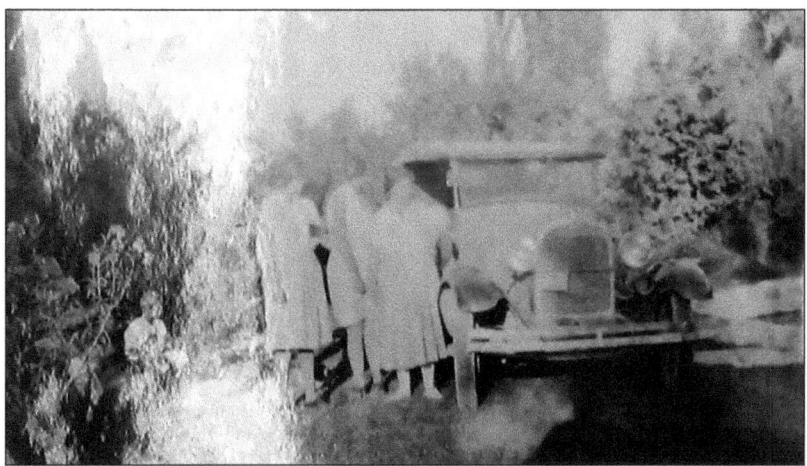

During the period of 28 May-June 20, Dr. Zoeckler saw 47 new and 36 old patients, she made 37 house calls of which 20 old ones.[589]

In 1928-29, the dispensary was open the entire year and the number of patients was controlled by the limited dispensary hours and slightly higher fees. She was pleased with the result, but the patients less so, who often came 2-3 hours before the opening hour. Despite this, there not that many fewer patients, while about 50% were either non-paying or paid less than the fixed fee. Many house calls (often obstetrical) were made, usually in the afternoons, or when the children she was home schooling were doing sums or writing compositions, or by getting up early, seeing the patients before breakfast. One interesting case was the daughter of the leading *mojtahed*, who had been very hostile. Against their better knowledge some relatives brought the daughter to Dr. Zoeckler as last resort, who said she needed to use forceps to deliver the child. This required to permission of the Aqa, so she hurried to his house. He first wanted to cut the Qur'an, but one of the leading merchants convinced him to leave fate in the doctor's hands. After grudgingly having given permission, Dr. Zoeckler hurried back and wanted to start the procedure. However, somebody sneezed and thus, she had to wait until somebody else sneezed, and this happened

---

589. RG 280-1-10, Report of Medical Work, Daulatabad May 28-June 20, 1928.

three times. Finally, she could start and delivered a dead baby at 10 p.m. although the child's head had already been visible since 3 p.m. In that year, the Park Hospital had a new physician, who was little inclined to cooperate with Dr. Zoeckler.[590]

During 1929-30, the dispensary was closed during five months, and during the rest of the year was frequently interrupted by other demands (itinerations, Hamadan trip) on her time. The number of patients seen was about the same as in the previous year, but that was because she saw many more in a day. Although she had no hospital, in the fall she had three in-patients. In compliance with government regulations a special cupboard for poison was built in the dispensary.[591]

In 1930-31, as many as 6,060 patients were seen, which was five times more than the previous year, and three times more than the previous highest number. This was because half of the patients were seen on four itinerations and with the children away at school Dr. Zoeckler could spent more time at the dispensary, which was open five days a week from morning till noon. In the late summer, the dispensary was swamped with patients after some free patients had told that the government had commissioned the missionary dispensary to give free treatment and drugs. Among the poor also many who could pay were found. When asked to pay they replied: "If we were able to pay, do you think we would have come to you? We would go to a real doctor." To prevent that the dispensary would go bankrupt Dr. Zoeckler introduced a ticket system, with tickets of five, three *qran*s and free. The five *qran*s was the usual fee, the three *qran*s was a discount. Immediately the number of patients decreased. The year ended in the black.[592]

In 1931–32, half as many patients were seen than the previous year, because of fewer itinerations and the impact of the ticket system. The two other physicians in town with a diploma left, but Dr. Zoeckler's practice did not grow. However, a large number of house calls (>500)

---

590. RG 280-1-10, Report of Medical Work, Daulatabad 1928-1929.
591. RG 280-1-10, Report of Medical Work, Daulatabad 1929-1930.
592. RG 280-1-10, Report of Daulatabad Medical Work 1930-1931.

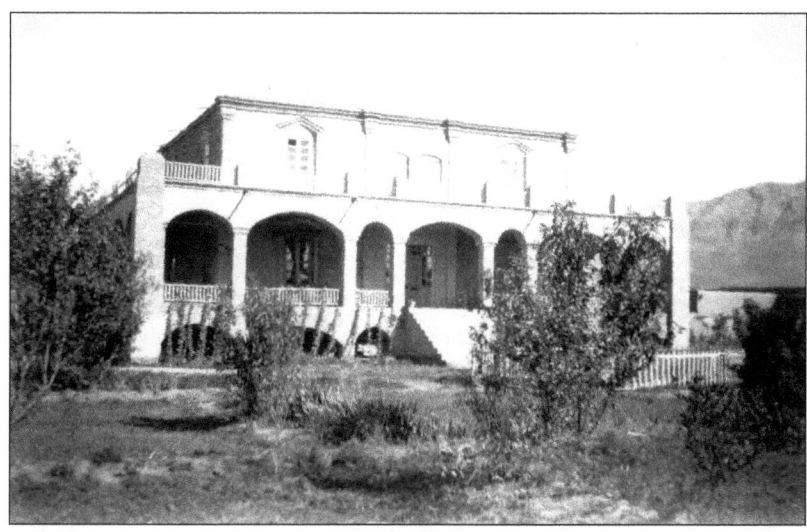
Mission residence in Malayer

might also account for this as they were time consuming. There were three psychatric cases that Dr. Zoeckler treated. Relatives advised marriage for one, disregarding the fate of the bride, even suggesting that he marry his equally mad cousin. They also urged the process of *tas neshastan* or "sitting around the bowl," which they had tried already on his praecox demention cousin without success. This was a method to oust the evil spirit by hypnotism. A sayyed was the leading actor. "He and the patient and a young girl are seated around a bowl of water, the girl wrapped in a sheet." The sayyed said some prayers, wrote some on a piece of paper that he threw into the water. He then asked the girl what she saw. Dr. Zoeckler was not allowed to attend the seance, but she learned some of the questions by listening. They were leading questions strongly urging the girl to see what the sayyed wanted her to see. In this case, she saw that a *pari* or fairy had fallen in love with the patient and he could not get well until she was separated from him. After the seance, the sayyed wrote prayers to protect the patient from the wiles of the *pari*, but the result was that only the nature of his delusion was changed. He repeatedly asked: Why have you taken away my companion?" In another case, it apparently worked; the person had inadvertently killed the child of a djinn, who tormented him in revenge. After having appropriated the djinn he recovered. Because of this experience Dr. Zoeckler submitted that there was a need for a psychiatric hospital in Iran. Financially 1931-32, was a good year.[593]

In 1932-33, there were two epidemics, in March influenza and in winter the whooping cough. Fortunately, both were mild in nature so few deaths occurred. Also, tuberculosis seemed to be on the rise. Despite all this and the fact that there were fewer physicians in the city, Dr. Zoeckler's work did not increase much. She ascribed this to the fact that people believed that there was no medicine and cure for the flue and the cough, which she did not disagree with.[594]

For the first time since 1929, the number of patients dropped below 2,000, because Dr. Zoeckler only worked 40 doctor weeks, and did less itinerations, while there were more patents seen in the city than in 1932-33. The city and region had barely recovered from the whooping cough epidemic, when it was struck by malaria, which caused many deaths in the villages. In the winter of 1933-34, puerperal fever and erysipelas became so widespread that it was almost an epidemic, causing much maternal deaths. That year Dr. Zoeckler was also consulted more than usual about medico-legal issues. Normally, she was consulted in case of suspected rape, but this year the local prosecutor was a graduate of the Boys School in Hamadan and in case of suspicious death or violence (suicide or murder) he often asked for her professional advice. She found it difficult cases, because she lacked the proper training and autopsies were not allowed, except in one case, where she was able to show that death was due to a third party. This result brought her greater repute than all her previous medical work. A sign that Iranian society was changing was the increased number of wives, who lodged a complaint when beaten by their husbands, something that was allowed by law. Apart from an itineration to Nehavand, the old plan to visit villages on Fridays was, as before, interfered with by other duties. In mid-1934, a new director

---

593. RG 280-1-10, Report of Daulatabad Medical Work 1931-1932; Presbyterian Church 1936, p. 151.

594. RG 280-1-10, Report of Daulatabad Medical Work 1932-1933.

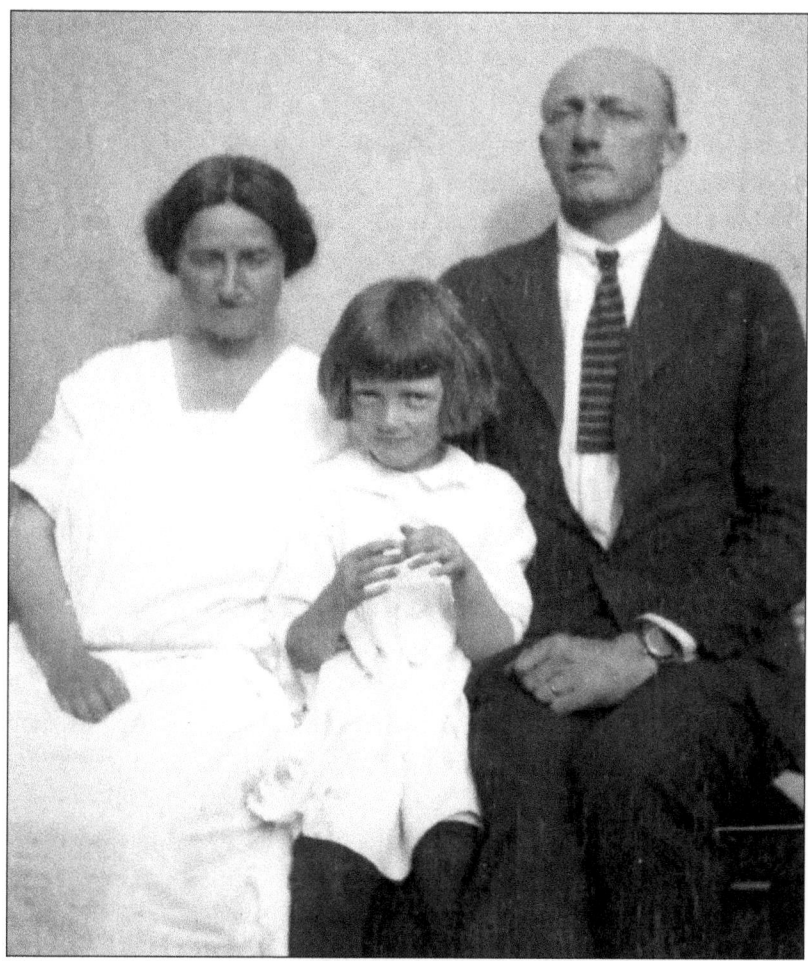

The Zoeckler family

of the Health Department arrived, who also doubled as director of the Park Hospital. He was an Iranian of British parentage and German education, and she hoped for more cooperation with him than had existed with his predecessors.[595] In 1934-35, Dr. Zoeckler made two itinerations, one to Lilahan and Kandeh, Armenian villages, and the other to Borujerd. The latter was not without problems, because new government rules stipulated where foreign physicians was allowed

---

595. RG 280-1-10, Report of Daulatabad Medical Work 1933-1934.

to work, which, in case of a hostile health director, might hamper medical work.[596]

In 1935, Dr. Zoeckler went on furlough and closed her dispensary. On her return, after having been closed for 3.5 years, the Dowlatabad dispensary was reopened (after some repairs) in early January 1938. During Dr. Zoeckler's absence there had been many changes. The Park Hospital was in charge of a young physician, who had trained under Dr. Carr of the CMS. He was far better than any other Iranian doctor who previously held the position. The 12-bed hospital had become a clean and efficient place, and he was known as a good surgeon (hernias, hemorrhoids, bone infections, but not abdominal). His beds were usually full and in 1937 he had treated 11,000 patients. He was very cooperative, called Dr. Zoeckler for consultation and offered the use of his hospital for her patients. In addition, with the gift of a wealthy woman, another hospital was under construction; earlier she had constructed the first girl's school in town. This hospital was closer to the city and being designed as a hospital, therefore, was better fitted for that purpose. It was being discussed to combine the two endowments such that the new hospital would be used as such and as out-patient clinic, while the Park Hospital be used as a home for incurables. If this would be realized, keeping the CMS trained physician, then Malayer would be in a better position than any other city in Iran. Moreover, an Iranian midwife, trained in Beirut, had arrived. When Dr. Zoeckler arrived in January 1938 the midwife situation was very bad. The one who treated upper class women had died the year before, and her successors (three old women, and some who had no experience at all) were worse. The arrival of a trained midwife, therefore, was a boon, be it that on the negative side, such trained women tended also to present themselves as a gynecologist, which they were not. Despite these changes, Dr. Zoeckler had plenty of work. One complaint of women was sterility, even though they already had eight children. But their reply was: "I have none left, or sometimes only one daughter, and my husband may divorce me." This situation stood in contrast with that of Hamadan and Kermanshah

---

596. RG 280-1-10, Report of Daulatabad Medical Work 1934-1935.

where missionary doctors were often called to rescue more sophisticated women from the ill-effects of self-induced abortions, or to provide contraceptive information. Favus also demanded more of her attention; the thallium acetate treatment for favus was very popular. Dr. Zoeckler had not wanted to use the treatment, because she lacked the proper scales to weigh the patients. However, because the cap or *charqad* could not cover the bald spot any longer and children with favus were sent away from school the treatment was in great demand. Also, the public baths were closed until showers had been installed, so that the almost universal favus scourge might finally belong to the past. After her return, Dr. Zoeckler found that collecting her fee was never so easy, perhaps because her work was better appreciated after her long absence.[597]

In 1939-40, two months were spent in Hamadan for backstopping and another month for meetings, so that only nine months medical work was done in town. Nevertheless, the patient-doctor weeks ratio was higher than in any year before, mostly due to itinerations. Financially, despite high cost for drugs, it was also a good year. There was excellent cooperation with the Park hospital, which resulted in operations that otherwise would have had to be sent to Hamadan, or would have remained untreated as the patients had no money to pay for the travel cost. The midwife was a disappointment; she did good work, but was dissatisfied with her income and left in April 1940. Favus and sterility remained the main cases, while measles, whooping cough and mumps were treated at home. It remained a problem to convince patients to rid themselves of favus infected caps. Also, a challenge was to train a young diabetic how to inject himself with insulin and calculate his carbohydrate and other calories. She had to use US diet tables and convert these to Iranian foods, especially to the various stews and soups that were very popular, "but contain a bewildering variety of articles all cooked up together."[598]

The year 1940-41 was a busy year with 5,154 patients, of which 861 favus cases. Many of the latter came from outlying districts,

---

597. RG 280-1-10, Report of Daulatabad Medical Work 1938 [-1939].
598. RG 280-1-10, Report of Daulatabad Medical Work 1939-1940.

because in the city it had almost been eradicated. There was a serious outbreak of whooping cough and measles, the latter caused quite a few deaths. Both typhoid (like in the previous year) and typhus were rife that year and the supply of dirty ice (due to a mild winter) might have had something to do with that. Income had never been as high; nevertheless, she decided to start using the ticket system again, although it was bothersome. However, too many people who were able to pay wanted to avoid paying anything. One itineration was made to the Armenian villages in the Burburud and Kamareh districts. The former were a hotbed of trachoma, and Dr. Zoeckler convinced one woman to continue the eye drop treatment for the children after her departure, which had a noticeable effect.[599] In 1940, the Malayer dispensary must have been temporarily closed, because Dr. Mary Zoeckler replaced Dr. Packard in Hamadan.[600] The year 1941-42 was a busy one, although less patients were treated. This was due to one month absence (meetings; backstopping in Kermanshah) and because many people left to their villages or hesitated to leave their houses, during the beginning of the British occupation. Dr. Zoeckler also made a number of itinerations. Dr. Rastan was the doctor of the Park hospital. More than 600 favus cases were treated, which seemed to present an inexhaustible supply. British Army doctors made a malaria survey in the district and found that <5% of the children under ten had an enlarged spleen, which was very good news. Financially it was was a banner year.[601] In 1942, the Malayer dispensary was only open part of the year, because in September 1942, the Packard family moved to the US. This meant that of that moment the Malayer dispensary was closed down, because Dr. Zoeckler replaced Dr. Packard in the Hamadan hospital.[602] The

---

599. RG 280-1-10, Report of Daulatabad Medical Work 1940-1941.
600. RG 91-19-27, Healing in Hamadan 1939-1940.
601. RG 280-1-10, Report of Daulatabad Medical Work 1941-1942.
602. RG 91-19-27, Report of Medical Work Hamadan 1942-1943. Dr. Zoeckler went on furlough in September and Ms Enderson took over on 1 July 1945. RG 91-19-27, Hamadan Hospital Report 1945-1946; Presbyterian Church 1943, p. 84.

Malayer dispensary was not reopened thereafter. However, the Park hospital with ten beds was still in use in the 1960s.[603]

At the Malayer dispensary brief records were kept of all patients, but only simple operations were performed. Although there were no in-patient facilities, at times Dr. Zoeckler had in-patients in the dispensary or in her house. Most patients were women, who came from within a radius of 16 km of Dowlatabad. Being a missionary, Dr. Zoeckler also went on itineration (Nehavand, Soltanabad, Borujerd, villages). Initially, when the children in the missionary compound were small, whom she home-schooled, she went less than later, when home responsibilites were less and there was no home-schooling any longer. Throughout the entire period that the dispensary was functioning, it received no outside financing at all. It was entirely self-financed and in most years it had a small surplus. The Presbyterian Board approvingly remarked that the Dowlatabad station "never asks for an appropriation and each year turns a profit."

Mashhad

As a major pilgrimage city, part of the population of Mashhad was fluctuating, sometimes doubling in size from its 50,000 size. Before the 1920s, there was no real hospital, although there was a *dar al-shafa* at the shrine of Imam Reza at Mashhad, which was the old Safavid one.[604] However, its *motavalli*s showed little interested in its proper operation.[605] When in 1860 Sayyed Mirza Ja`far Khan Moshir al-Dowleh was appointed *motavalli* of the Shrine, the old hospice building had not been changed since Safavid times, apart from the addition of the phlebotomy rooms in 1702. Although repaired several times it was very small. It was situated situated adjacent to the Friday or Gowharshad Mosque, and had fallen into complete disuse. Since Moshir al-Dowleh

---

603. Zahereddini 1966, p. 38; Momeni 1976, pp. 46, 49.
604. E`temad al-Saltaneh1294-97, vol. 1, p. 552; Ibid., 1301-03, vol. 2, p. 235; Asaf al-Dowleh 1377, vol. 1, pp. 20 (*marizkhaneh*), 39 (*dar al-shafa*); Rosta'i 1382, vol. 2, p. 512.
605. Sureshjani 1395, p. 207 (only Mirza Musa Khan Farahani made some efforts, Idem, pp. 199-202); Khakestar 1395, p. 54.

had been educated in Europe and knew about modern medicine he tried to make the *dar al-shafa* a better institution. Therefore, he moved the hospice to a new location and building, which he financed with his own funds. The new building was built in Bala Khiyaban, in a nice quiet garden. It had a separate male and female ward, while the rooms for people with contagious diseases were separated from the other wards. Unfortunately, Moshir al-Dowleh died after two years having been in function, so that the new hospice building was completed by his son. The new hospice had a separate female section, which in the old building shared the same space with the male section.[606] In 1862, Eastwick visited Mashhad and reported that he had visited "the new hospital, built by the Mashir [sic: Moshir al-Dowleh] for eighty sick persons. It is in a fine large garden, and the Mashir told me he intended to endow it with funds."[607] Because the hospital was not completed during Moshir al-Dowleh's tenure his son, Mohammad Sadeq Khan completed the building with funds his father had endowed for that purpose.[608] The new building replaced the old *dar al-shafa*, because it was reported that it was the only medical facility in the city.[609] The old building later became known as the *Sara-ye Naseri*.

---

606. E`temad al-Saltaneh1301-03, vol. 2, pp. 237, 268; Mo'taman 1348, p. 403; Sureshjani 1395, pp. 203-06, 220 (with a capacity of 15-20 patients. The entire building, including the court yard and offices, was 300 m long); Khakestar 1395, pp. 55-56.

607. Eastwick 1976, vol. 2, 213.

608. Elgood 1951, pp. 511-512; Nafisi 1325, pp. 56-57; E`temad al-Saltaneh 1301-03, vol. 2, pp. 237, 268; Utaredi 1371, pp. 498-501; Tajbakhsh 1379, pp. 247-248. According to Mohammad Hasan Khan, Malek al-Hokama, who was the public health officer (*hafez al-sehheh*) of Mashhad at that time, Naser al-Din Shah took this decision after he had submitted a paper to the Shah outlining 32 defects of the *dar al-shafa*. Prior to that decision he had already modernized its surgery and pharmacy. For details see Rosta'i 1382, vol. 2, pp. 512-513.

609. Hakim al-Mamalek 1356, p. 259; Nafisi 1329-31, p. 20. In 1881 it was reported that some mad people were brought to the *dar al-shafa* for treatment. *Ruznameh-ye Iran* 1375, p. 1868 (9 Shavval 1298/4 September 1881); E`temad al-Saltaneh1301-03, vol. 2, pp. 237, 268; Mo'taman 1348, p. 403.

Table 22: Staff of the *Dar al-Shafa* of Mashhad and their wages (ca. 1870).

Name and function	Remuneration (in *tumans*)
Hajj Molla Hoseyn *Nazer* (overseer) of the hospital	15
Hajj Molla Hoseyn *Nazer* of food and medicines	5
Mirza Mohammad *Tabib* (physician)	17.5
Mirza Baqer *Moshref* (inspector)	7
Aqa Mohammad Esma`il	10
Mirza Abū'l-Qasem	5
Molla `Abd al-Rahman	5
Orderlies: male 6; female: 2	14 (males: 8 + 5 *qerans*; females: 5 + 5 *qerans*)
Molla Karim, the druggist	9

Source: Utaredi 1371, pp. 501-502. The following functions are also mentioned among the orderlies: *parastari, rakht-shu'i* and *kohneh-shu'i*. Jashemi 1389, p. 13.

As is clear from Table 22, the *dar al-shafa* of the Shrine was under a general manager, who also doubled as the overseer of food and medicines. The hospital only employed one physician, whose prescriptions for drugs were supplied by the druggist. The latter did not receive much money, thus suggesting that there was no great demand for his services. It is of no surprise to find that the hospital employed both male and female orderlies as there was both a male and female ward. The other persons listed presumably had administrative and/or religious functions. What is also noteworthy is that the official number of hospice staff seems much less than in Safavid times. However, when Naser al-Din Shah visited Mashhad in 1868, the *dar al-shafa* employed 24 persons such two physicians (*tabib*), a surgeon (*jarrah*), a herbalist (`attar*), a barber, two doorkeepers, sick attendants (*bimardaran* - both for men and women) and administrative staff.[610] Thereafter, the staff increased in size.

---

610. Sureshjani 1395, pp. 214-16. Other functions mentioned are

Not much is known about the quality of medical service offered by the Razavi Hospital. From one description it is clear that officially much of the *dar al-shafa*'s work was devoted to "the preparation of food and medicines, so that the sufferers, the sick and ill from among the strangers, travelers, and pilgrims of the holy land with the help of the staff of that institution: the physician, the overseer, the eye-doctor, the surgeon, the orderly, the nurse, Koran reciter, and assistant may find healing for their illnesses and diseases in that place and after having taken the food and medicine may become healthy."[611] Although the new building made a good impression it is unlikely that the hospice functioned as required by its endowment and as suggested above. In 1882, Hajj Sayyah bemoaned the fact that the Shrine's allocated revenues were not spent for the purposes they were meant to and that "the hospital was dilapidated and absolutely no healing was done there."[612] In 1884, Afzal al-Molk Kerman was somewhat more positive in his opinion about the hospice that employed 30 people and even opium addicts treated in the hospice were given their daily opium dosage the same like other patients received their food and medicine.[613] In 1900, Yate wrote that men, who had been punished to be subjected to mutilations by a court of law, "with the maimed feet and hands duly turned up for treatment at the British Consulate dispensary. I have never heard of any one going to the Persian hospital in the shrine under such circumstances, though that was the place that ought to have been open to all."[614] Around 1905 the

---

parastari, rakht-shu'i and *kohneh-shu'i*. Jashemi 1389, p. 13. E'temad al-Saltaneh described the *dar al-shafa* as "narrow and unfit."

611. Utaredi 1371, p. 498.

612. Hajj Sayyah 1346, p. 134; Sureshjani 1395, p. 218. According to Nafisi 1325, p. 57, in 1881 Mirza Ali Akbar Khan Nazem al-Atebba went to Mashhad for one year, where he founded a new *bimarestan-e Razavi* on European principles, which, given what Hajj Sayyah reported, cannot be true. According to Rahnama 1332, p. 56, he merely put it into good order, but even that was not the case, according to Hajj Sayyah.

613. Sureshjani 1395, p. 221; Khakestar 1395, pp. 57-58.

614. Yate 1900, p. 336.

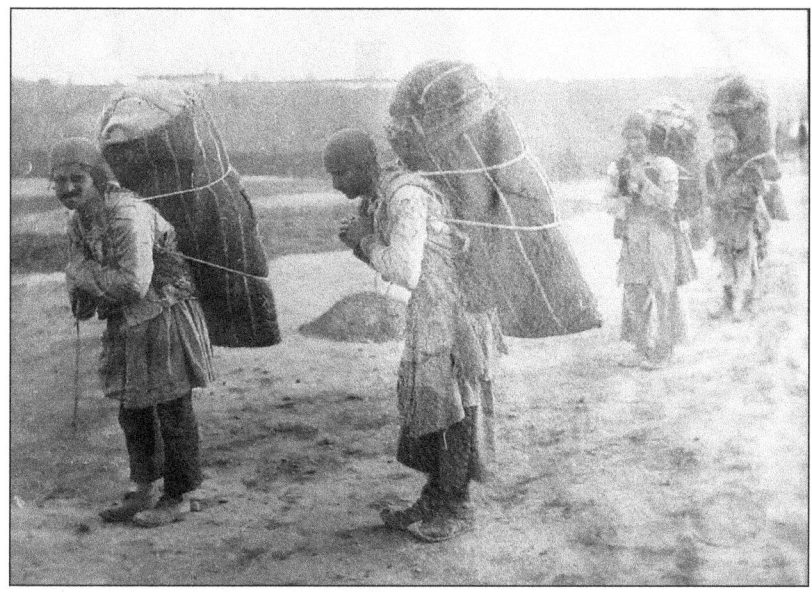

Transporting manure

Shrine hospital had "a staff of about five or six native physicians. The hospital is nearly always full, and some kinds of surgical operations are undertaken, but not often with satisfactory results. This hospital is used mostly by pilgrims."[615] Dr. Hoffman noticed that conditions had much deteriorated at the Shrine hospital. He stated that before 1915, "it was a place where men went only to die; hardly a pane of glass in the whole place, wooden bedsteads without sheets or pillow cases, a dirt floor, and no stove."[616]

---

615. Adamec 1981, vol. 2, p. 486. Although there are many documents showing how much was spent on wages, food and medicines this does not necessarily mean that these expenditures really happened. The fact that in 1901 a member of an investigation commission was impressed with the quality of the clothes and shoes of the patients suggests that these patients had been dressed up for the occasion. The more, because the same person one year later wrote that the Shrine's hospice had become 'a worse place than a Jewish cemetery and a Zoroastrian tower of silence." Sureshjani 1395, pp. 229-31; see also, Khakestar 1395, pp. 61-62 and Eyn al-Saltaneh 1376, vol. 1, p. 1748.

616. Morton 1940, p. 253.

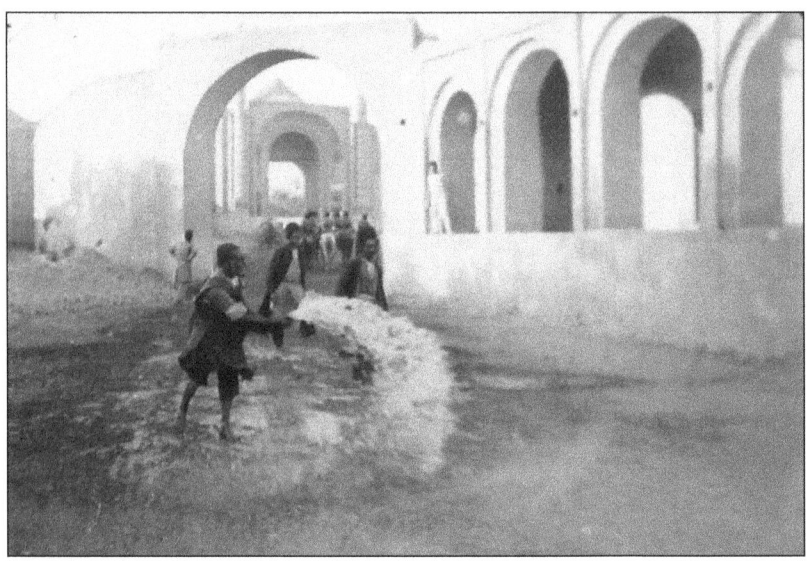

Above and opposite: Watering the streets using goat-skin water bags before there was paving.

In December 1909, a Note was submitted to the government outlining the management and financial problems as well as the corruption at the Shrine. Concerning the *dar al-shafa* the Note submitted that its expenditures had dropped from 18,000 to 2,000 *tuman*s, because most of its funds were used for the private use of the Shrine officials. But the government for a variety of reasons was unable to take action and the situation remained bad, so that hardly food and medicines were distributed in the hospice, where conditions were unhygienic. In fact, it was reported that if a patient asked for water he/she had to pay first.[617] Finally, the *Majles* took action and passed a law concerning the management of the Shrine on 19 November 1911. Art. 12 stated that the *dar al-shafa* needed to be run on sound medical principles and its physicians needed to be experienced and knowledgeable and approved by the Ministry of Endowments. Further, that its income

---

617. Khakestar 1395, pp. 61-62; Sureshjani 1395, pp. 235-43, 256 (in particular, Sheikh al-Ra'is and his brother Hashem Mirza were held responsible for the embezzlement of Shrine funds over the last 50 years!).

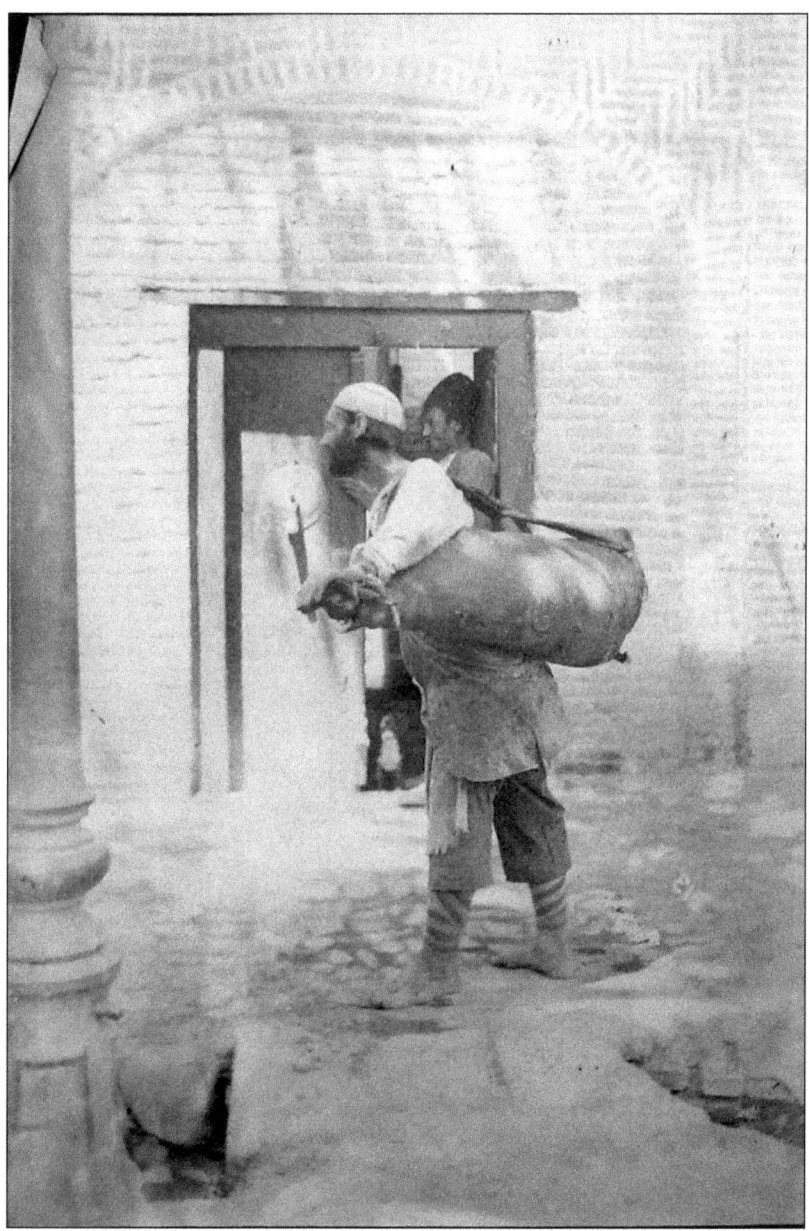

and expenditures should be in balance.⁶¹⁸ The fact that one month later the *Majles* was dissolved, the country was beset by financial

---

618. Sureshjani 1395, pp. 350-51.

and political problems (incursion by the ex-Shah and the rebellion by Salar al-Dowleh) impeded any swift action. In November 1914, the Ministry made a list of all *dar al-shafa*'s endowments and by telegram tried to initiate some reforms. It also announced that it would send Dr. Amir Khan A`lam al-Mamalek to implement the reforms, who on 14 December 1914 arrived in Mashhad. However, this had not the desired result, because Sayyed Javad Zahir al-Eslam, the new *motavalli* was a very cautious man, and so nothing happened and it seems that the hospice stopped functioning altogether.[619] Although the *dar al-shafa* of Mashhad hardly functioned any longer, it continued to receive endowments, such as in 1915-16 and 1919-20. Thus lack of funds cannot have been the reason for its negligence and the discontinuation of its operations.[620]

It was only in 1917, prodded by the success of the Christian hospital, that the Shrine authorities decided to improve their hospital.[621] "The old, crude sick-house owned by the Sacred Shrine and called the 'Place of Healing' was first rebuilt in 1917, then removed to another location.[622] In 1918, the Ministry of Endowments and Education sent Dr. Amir Khan A`lam al-Mamalek as its representative to Mashhad. The purpose of his visit was to assist the Shrine authorities in improving the work of the *dar al-shafa* as well as to continue the competition of who offered the best medical services in Mashhad, a competition that they had begun in slow motion in 1917 by repairing the old *dar al-shafa*.[623] Dr. Amir A`lam and the new *motavalli* had instructions to build a new *dar al-shafa-ye Razavi* and to improve its medical services.

---

619. Sureshjani 1395, pp. 351-54. Although the *dar al-shafa* of Mashhad had ceased to operate the hospital continued to receive new endowments, such as in 1915-16 and 1919-20, therefore, lack of funds cannot have been the reason for its negligence and the discontinuation of its operations. Setudeh 1366, vol. 7, pp. 561-562; vol. 8, pp. 257-258.
620. Setudeh 1366, vol. 7, pp. 561-562; vol. 8, pp. 257-258.
621. Khalifeh and Najafzadeh 1390, p. 14. In 1916, it also received a new pharmacy. Khakestar 1395, p. 79.
622. RG 91-20-2, Mashad Medical Report 1934-1935.
623. Khalifeh and Najafzadeh 1390, p. 14.

Dr. Amir A'lam (*ra'is-e edareh-ye hafez al-sehheh*) had the old *dar al-shafa* destroyed and began the construction of a new 2-storey and more spacious building on the same site. On 1 August 1918, the first part of the new building was opened, which, like the entire completed building, was built with funding by many individuals from all over Iran. Apart from a separate male and female section, there also was a section for VD diseases, surgery, and a lab. In Safavid times the hospice's capacity had been 20 beds and by 1918 it was 15-20 beds; thereafter its capacity was further increased. There also was place for new-borns and for the mad outside the city.[624]

These changes were clearly aimed to undercut the success and influence of the American hospital. Dr. Hoffman commented on this development as follows:

> Our work was disturbing the Shrine authorities, whose 'Dara-Shafa' (Place of Healing) was merely a crude refuge for dying pilgrims. Dr. Mir Aalam, head of the Tehran medical school came and got a new building erected, with an operating room, white sheets for the beds and white gowns for the helpers. A young surgeon was brought from Tehran, and a few operations were attempted, but of the three whose legs were amputated, all died. Then the surgeon himself got typhus fever, and after weeks of illness, died. Then Dr. Hejazi, again head of the hospital, asked me to do some surgery in their new operating room. On two days I did several small operations, taking the needed instruments with me. Then no more invitations, a Christian could not be tolerated in the Sacred Shrine hospital.[625]

---

624. Sureshjani 1395, pp. 259-66, 285, 299-90; Khakestar 1395, pp. 62-68. I think that when Gilmour 1924, pp. 29-30 reported that in 1919, the president of the Sanitary Council made a pilgrimage to Mashhad and at the time took steps to re-open the two run-down and neglected Iranian hospitals as well as to organize a public health service for the province of Khorasan, he referred to Dr. Amir A'lam's visit in 1918-19.

625. RG 231-1-6, Pioneering in Meshed, pp. 48-49 (Dr. Hoffman was near collapse; he had started too soon working after his 1918 typhus and was sent for a medical check-up in Tehran. He closed the hospital and because the examination was not available in Tehran, via iterations he went to

Dr. Amir A'lam drew up new regulations for budget, for the internal revenues and the overall management of the *dar al-shafa*. As of 22 March 1918, the treasury of the hospice was separated from Shrine; the renters of endowment lands had to give a written commitment to pay their rent on time and to publish this statement in the newspapers, while the manager of the endowments had to see to it that revenues would increase. A respected wealthy merchant would be appointed as the hospice's financial agent (*tahvildar*), who also would sell its in kind revenues, except what was needed for the auto-consumption of the *dar al-shafa*, the amount to be determined by the provincial Sanitary Council. The *tahvildar* had to give an accounting at the end of the year and many more rules, too many to mention them all. The overall thrust of the new regulations was to increase efficiency, transparency, and accountability.[626]

Dr. Amir A'lam stayed for one year in Mashhad, but then returned to Tehran and appointed in his stead Dr. Mozayyan al-Soltan as director of the *dar al-shafa*. During his tenure of office problems arose, because the budget was insufficient for the rising number of patients. The *motavalli* Sayyed Javad Zahir al-Eslam wrote him only to accept patients for which there was a bed available; the others had to be sent into the street. Dr. Mozayyan al-Soltan died after one year, after which the management of the hospital and its endowments reverted to its age old practice of neglect and misuse of funds.[627] When in May 1920, the city of Mashhad became a municipality, the *motavalli* Sayyed Javad Zahir al-Eslam wrote to this new body that in the past the *dar al-shafa* had taken charge of those afflicted with mental disease and foundlings, but that the municipality should shoulder this

---

Istanbul; where they said that he was able to travel to the US).
626. Sureshjani 1395, pp. 267-81 (here all articles of the three sets of regulations are given), 282-85; Khakestar 1395, pp. 64-65. For a list and documents of drugs stocked, diseases, names of doctors, *nazeran, darbanan, jarrahan, kahallan, bimardaran, `attar* and others at the *dar al-shafa*, including their wages as well as examples of prescriptions, see Sureshjani 1395, pp. 321-67.
627. Sureshjani 1395, pp. 295-307.

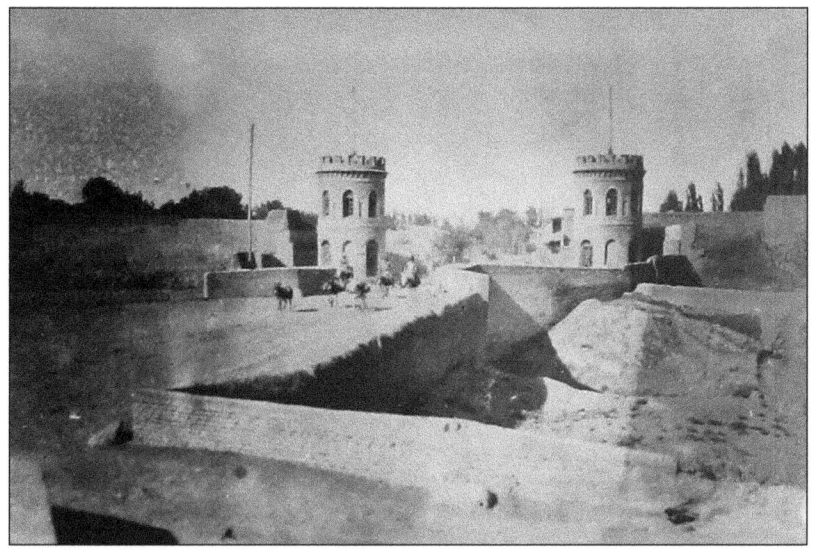

The Ark Gate of Mashhad (demolished in 1930)

burden and that as of 11 June 1920 the *dar al-shafa* would no longer be involved in this matter.[628] From Tehran, Dr. Amir A`lam tried to influence the management of the *dar al-shafa* and improve the scope of its activities. He promised that Mashhad would become a center of learning in medicine and that if reforms were introduced it would soon have a medical school, where even students from neighboring countries would come and study. To that end he wanted to establish a Dar al-Fonun in Mashhad, while he founded a philantropical *Sun and Lion Society* and in 1923 ensured that it would be of service to the poor, who could not afford a doctor and drugs.[629] In the mid-1920s, Mohammad Vali Khan Asadi, the deputy Shrine manager considered the *dar al-shafa* unfit for medical care and he proposed to move it to a new location where a larger number of patients could be treated. This did not happen, but he was able to hire physicians who had been trained in Europe. The move to a new building probably did not happen, because in 1926 order had been given to begin with the design for a

---

628. Sureshjani 1395, pp. 316-17.
629. Khalifeh and Najafzadeh 1390, pp. 14, 17-18; Sureshjani 1395, pp. 305-09.

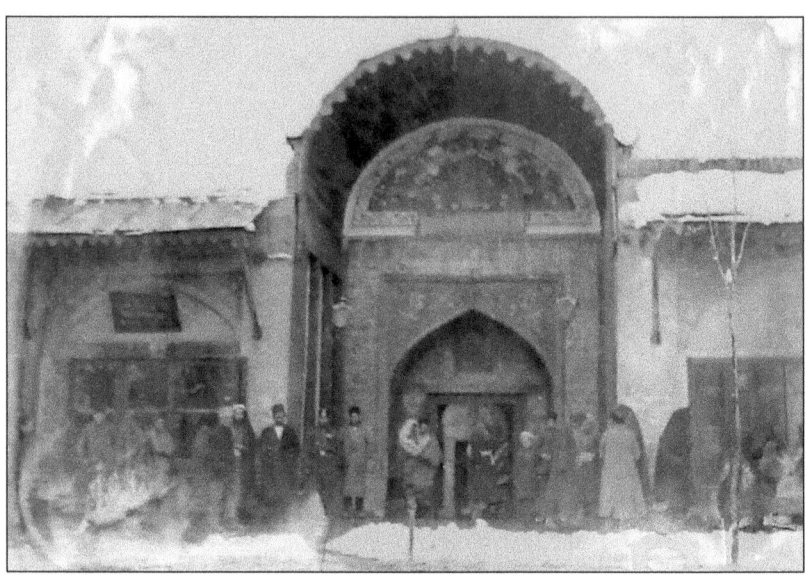

Entrance to the Shrine hospital; in 1922 functioned as a dispensary only.

totally new hospital. Meanwhile, in 1928, the house of Taj Khanom was rented and used as a women's ward, while in 1929, a permanent duty doctor was appointed.[630] In 1927-28, the *dar al-shafa* had 1,001 in-patients, of whom 146 died or 14.5% of the total. In 1929, the *dar al-shafa* had 65 beds, seven physicians, five interns, eight orderlies, and one pharmacist. In that year the dispensary saw 56,977 patients of whom 14,151 were treated free of charge. The hospital also had a laboratory and did 306 simple tests. Its surgery department had 282 patients of who 19 or 6% died. The surgeries performed consisted of simple cases such as tumors, circumcision, burns, bladder stone, broken bones, and the like.[631]

Although change had been slow in coming, but in the early 1930s, Mashhad was changing significantly. The British Consul-General reported that: "Half of Mashhad has now piped water. The streets are cleaned and continually sprinkled with water."[632] This picture of

---

630. Khakestar 1395, pp. 70-71, 103.
631. Khakestar 1395, pp. 71-76.
632. Secret. Diary for February 1935. HBM ConsGen Khorasan and

progress was enhanced by a large new Shrine hospital that was being built as of 1930 to replace the old moribund *dar al-shafa* building. For the competition begun by the Shrine authorities in 1917 had continued during the following two decades, although there also was collaboration concerning the leprosarium and as of 1934 with the exhange of medical services (see below). Dr. Hoffman of the American missionary hospital reported about the course of this competition as follows:

> But in 1917 there was a reform; it [the Shrine hospital] was rebuilt; a new doctor was secured, and the workers put on white gowns; a new operating suite was built, and surgery was begun on a small scale. Again, when we secured a larger and better hospital building in 1919, the Shrine hospital was moved into a larger and better house and more doctors were added to its staff. And when, again, in 1924, the Mission hospital advanced a decided step forward, through securing its own land and erecting a good building, along with many other reforms, the Sacred Shrine authorities soon began planning a really modern hospital building, which was begun three years later, a very elaborate series of buildings, costing around one million dollars![633]

The number of beds of the new Shah Reza hospital was to be increased from 50 to 150, and ultimately it would have 300 beds. However, in 1945, it still only had 150 beds and departments for pathology, dermatology, gynecology, and bacteriology as well as a dispensary.[634] The hospital's construction was not without financial

---

Sistan, IOR/L/PS/12/3406, Coll 28/10 'Persia. Diaries; Meshed Consular Jany 1931 – May 1940. Khorassan Political 1934 – May 1940. Khorassan Fortnightly Reports', f. 451.

633. Morton 1940, p. 254. Dr. Hoffman considered this competition a good thing as it was his policy to slowly give up one sphere of activity after another to Iranian hospitals, because finally the Mission hospital "seeks to eliminate itself."

634. Government of Great Britain 1945, p. 410. The hospital was designed by Taher Karimzadeh Behzad, a Tabrizi native, who had received his education in Istanbul and Berlin. He returned to Iran in

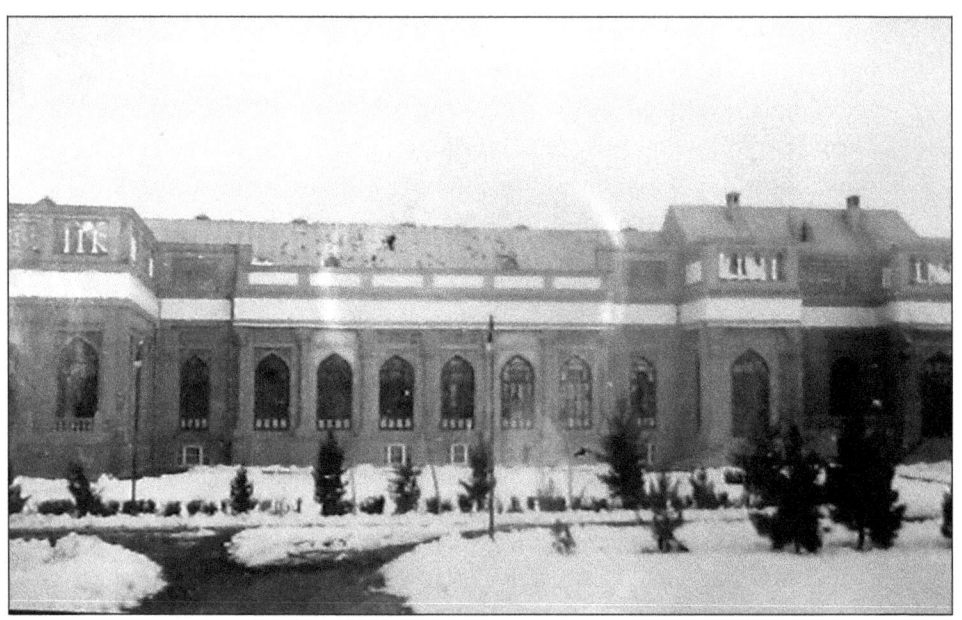

Parts of the main building of the Shah Reza Hospital, 1938.

problems, however. According to Dr. Hoffman: "The carrying out of grandiose schemes for immence [sic; immense] hospitals and new roads, as well as presents to those in high places, render it impossible for the Shrine to find money for the purposes for which the Waqfs they administer were originally created."[635] However, Reza Shah was the driving force behind this project and thus, failure or delay was not an option. As a result, work on the 300-bed Shah Reza hospital continued day and night so that Reza Shah might open it in 1934. At that time, 6.5 million Rls had been spent in construction and another 1.5 million was needed to complete it.[636] To resolve the shortfall of

---

1926 and was employed by the Municipality. He was chosen to design the Shah Reza hospital and in 1928 he began with its construction. Khakestar 1395, pp. 103-04.

635. IOR/L/PS/12/3607, Meshed Consular Diary no. 24 for the period ending 31at December 1931, Coll 29/45 'General reorganization of consular posts', p. 2.

636. IOR/L/PS/12/3415, Annual Commercial Report for the Province of Khurasan and Zabulistan for the Persian Year 1312 (21st March 1933 to

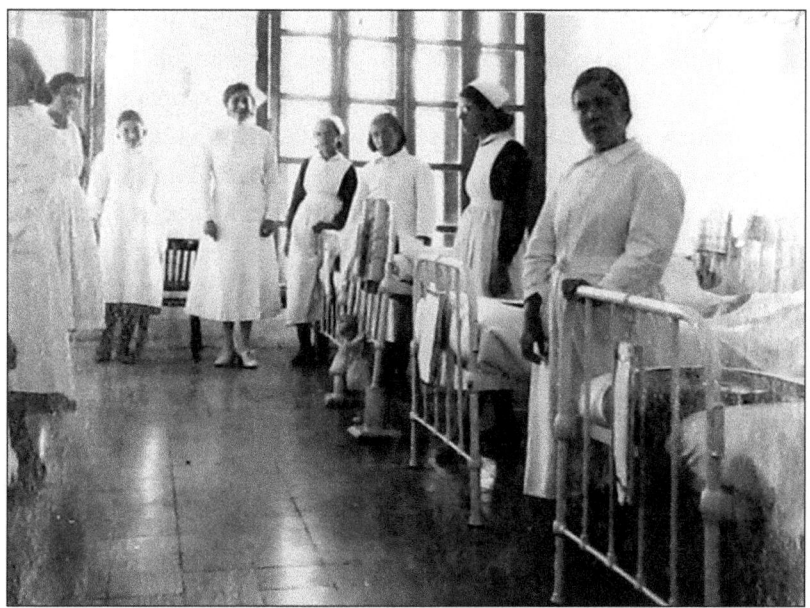

Emma Degner and nurses at an eight-bed ward of the Shah Reza Hospital. The nurses with caps are seniors.

financing of the hospital and other modernization projects, the village of Alamdasht, the property of Mahdavi, a former deputy for Khorasan, was declared to be the property of the Shrine by the Court. "It is to be sold and the proceeds to be used for purchase of pipes for piped water supply to Mashhad. The tax for water supplied will be devoted to the maintenance of the Shah Reza Hospital. The difficult problem of financing the water supply and the hospital has thus been happily solved at the cost of the unfortunate Mahdavi."[637]

The Shah Reza Hospital was built on Shrine land outside the city. It consisted of a number of buildings, of which the principal one was 650 feet long. In addition, there were half a dozen departmental buildings, widely spaced around about- for kitchen, X-ray, surgery, obstetrics, laboratory, etc. Over 100 gardeners worked at setting out shrubs and trees in the huge garden. Dr. Hoffman commented that it

---

20th March 1934), p. 6.
637. IOR/L/PS/12/3406, Secret. Diary for February 1935, f. 451.

was a standing joke to that you needed "to use roller skates or bikes to get around the widely scattered buildings." The hospital's size also meant higher maintenance cost than for a more compact building. Before the Shah officially opened the hospital in 1934, the American hospital was asked to lend "bed linen, wash basins and towels, to equip a few beds for show. Much of the constructions had been so shoddy that pipes leaked, floors caved in and roofs leaked. But a start has been made, and over the years came improvements."[638]

Dr. Hoffman enthusiastically wrote: "for the first time a specialist in Meshed is better equipped than us."[639] Three German 'professors', Jewish doctors eager to get out of Nazi Germany, were imported, also several German nurses, a lab technician and a German roentgenologist. Equipment bought in Germany included five X-ray machines (a 200 kilo-volt X-ray machine), plus diathermy, ultra-violet lights and other equipment but very few films, and more fancy surgical instruments than practical. One of the German doctors, Dr. Hammerschlag, a gynecologist was the hospital's superintendent, who arrived in the fall of 1934. A German nurse managed the obstetrical department and a German technician helped with the X-ray work. One of the nurses of the American hospital left to become its OR nurse. Although, the Shah Reza hospital was now officially up-and-running, "the local organization is inadequate to handle such a big place and as yet fewer than half the proposed 300 beds are in use." In 1936 Hoffman wrote: "There are about 250 beds, of which 60 are occupied by the army medical corps, around 30 by the sick from the prison, another section by the Municipality's contagious cases, and the rest are divided among the surgical, medical, eye and obstetrical-gynecological departments." It did mean less work for the American hospital, because the Shah Reza treated the poor, which was an indication of the vast need for medical care.[640] Already in 1936, the Shah Reza hospital lost two of

---

638. RG 231-1-6, Hoffman, Pioneering in Meshed, pp. 100-01.
639. RG 91-20-2, Mashad Medical Report 1935-1936.
640. RG 231-1-6, Hoffman, Pioneering in Meshed, pp. 100-01; RG 91-20-2, Mashad Medical Report 1935-1936; Khakestar 1395, pp. 105-08.

its three German doctors, but was able to hire an Iranian lab specialist trained in France and an Iranian pediatrician.[641]

After the invasion of Iran in August 1941, the whole staff of the Shah Reza hospital left on 28 August, the day the Russians bombed the Mashhad airport and barracks. The only ones who remained were "the Czech surgeon Baruch and his wife and the old German director Hammerschlag. [...] For a period of 28 hours there was nobody but these three foreigners to tend the patients, including eighteen Persian soldiers who had been wounded in the bombing of the aerodrome and the barracks."[642] The hospital's soliditude did not last long for the Russians commandeered a large part of it. In 1943, moreover, they took away the German roentgenologist. As a result, the Shah Reza Hospital's elaborate X-ray machines had only a locally trained technician and outside physicians, such as the Americans, had to do their own interpretation of films.[643] However, it was well supplied with equipment and medicines.[644] In the remaining years of WW II the situation did not improve. Dr. Hoffman commented that: "Medical practice in the other hospitals in the city has deteriorated. The large Shah Reza Hospital has only one European doctor, a surgeon, instead of three it had a few years back. A large section of its main building is still occupied by the Russians as a military hospital. Its elaborate X-ray installations have only a locally trained technician to operate them, and films are scarce and expensive. Since it is the only X-ray in the whole province, we are compelled to carry on as best as we can without much help from X-ray."[645]

---

641. RG 91-20-2, Mashhad Medical Report 1936-1937. For the names and the specialities of the physicians employed in the hospital, see Khakestar 1395, pp. 109-20.

642. Skrine 1962, p. 106. After the German staff left in 1941, Dr. Baruch was in charge of surgery at the Shah Reza hospital; later he was succeeded by the French Prof. Botaru, who was assisted by French nurses. Jashemi 1389, p. 15.

643. RG 231-1-6, Hoffman, Pioneering in Meshed, p. 142.

644. RG 91-20-2, Mashad Medical Report 1942-43

645. RG 91-20-2, Mashhad Medical Report 1944-45.

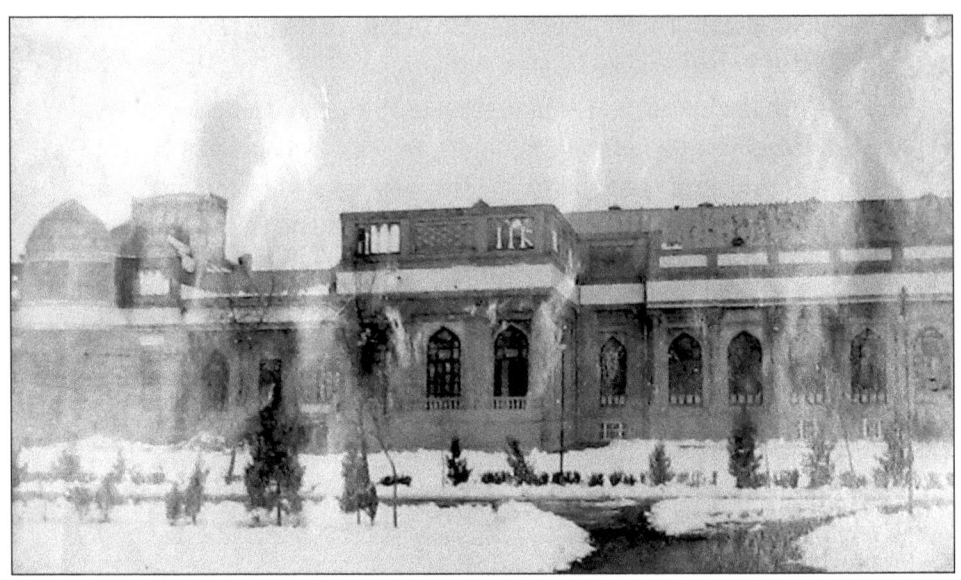

Shah Reza Hospital in winter, 1935.

When the Russians left in 1946, this did not mean an improvement for the Shah Reza hospital. According to the American physicians, its last European doctor left, so that its surgical facilities were even weaker than in the previous year. Its doctors often sent patients to the American hospital for surgery. The Shah Reza hospital had only one local technician to 'take pictures' with its several X-ray machines. Because all five machines were of German make, they were increasingly difficult to maintain. Moreover, sometimes there were no films, often they were disappointing and there was a big delay and large expense. The hospital's maternity service accepted 50-60 women/month. Dr. Hoffman concluded from the hospital situation in Mashhad in 1946 that he needed a second doctor, an X-ray machine, a better laboratory, an improved school of nursing, and better buildings.[646]

OTHER IRANIAN MEDICAL INSTITUTIONS

In 1885, in addition to the Razavi hospice there was a clean and well-provisioned dispensary, established by Mirza Molla Hoseyn

---

646. RG 91-20-2, Mashhad Medical Report 1945-46.

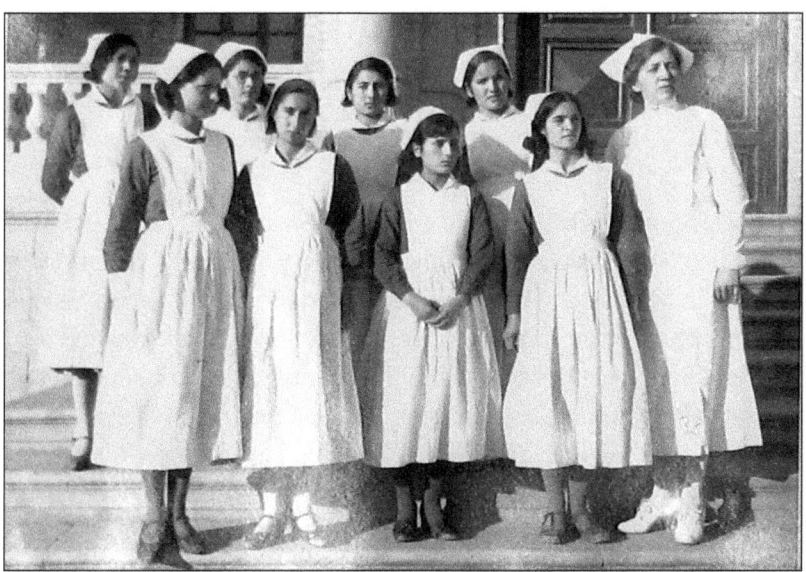

Shah Reza Hospital nurses with Ms Degner

Hakim-Bashi-ye Nezam-e Khorasan, which reportedly took good care of the troops in Mashhad.[647] Whether this dispensary continued to operate is not known, but seems unlikely.

There was also another Iranian hospital in Mashhad. During his life, Hajj Mohammad Hasan Mirza Montaser al-Molk had deeded a number of villages to his fourth wife, Ehteram al-Saltaneh, on condition that she used those properties to build a hospital in Mashhad. In 1918, she used the funds from the sale of part of that property to buy a piece of land of 3,500 sq. cubits situated on the Khiyaban-e Darvazeh-ye Jinnat and constructed there the Montasariyeh Hospital. She endowed the hospital with the remainder of the property. She remained the endowment manager until she died, when the management was transferred to the Shrine.[648] The hospital was not explicitly mentioned by Gilmour when he made his inventory of medical institutions in Iran. Therefore, it is likely that it was included in his observation that the

---

647. Asaf al-Dowleh 1377, vol. 1, p. 176.
648. Mo'taman 1348, p. 414 (with a picture of the hospital); `Atardi 1371, pp. 509-510; Sureshjani 1395, p. 288

two endowed and private hospitals of Mashhad (that of the Shrine and this one; the one with 70 and the other with 20 beds), which had suffered great neglect had been closed, because their funds had run out.[649] The 25-bed hospital was still open for business at the end of the 1940s.[650]

In 1935, the little semi-private hospital designed by Dr. Cook was still in use. There also was a gendarmerie hospital as well as a military hospital in Mashhad, where recruits were operated for hernia instead of being excused from the service. Furthermore, there was the Red Lion and Sun Society (later the health department), whose four doctors conducted free clinics for the poor and vaccinated children against smallpox with vaccine made in Iran, which relieved the pressure to see all who came to the American hospital.[651] Other hospitals mentioned include the 90-bed hospital for contagious diseases (*bimarestan-e vagirdarha*) founded before 1940, the 40-bed municipal hospital founded in 1941, the 150-bed maternity hospital founded in 1947, the city's prison 19-bed hospital founded in 1932, and as of 1953 a mental asylum (*timarestan*).[652]

In 1939, the British Consul General reported that "a charitable hospital containing 150 beds has been opened in Mashhad land also a dispensary at Turghabeh, the principal summer resort some 14 miles from the city,"[653] about which I have not found any further information. The Red Lion and Sun Society with $5,000 received

---

649. Gilmour 1924, p. 29.
650. For details see Khakestar 1395, p. 97.
651. RG 231-1-2 Rolla Hoffman Correspondence 1910-1919, Hoffman to McClanahan, 03/07/1932; RG 231-1-6, Pioneering in Meshed, p. 119; RG 91-20-2, Mashhad Medical Report 1934-1935; Khakestar 1395, pp. 189-95, 201-03, who also mentions two clinics, the *darmangah-e Saleh* (as of 1943) and the *darmangah-e Razi* (as of 1948).
652. Khakestari 1395, pp. 197-99.
653. IOR/L/PS/12/3406, Khorasan Political Diary for November 1939, p. 2 [Persia. Diaries; Meshed Consular Jany 1931 – May 1940. Khorassan Political 1934 – May 1940. Khorassan Fortnightly Reports']

from the American Red Cross built a large poor-house for 1,000 crippled, blind and helpless people, who during winter time were fed and housed there.[654] In 1935, Dr. Hoffman reported that there was "a well-organized orphanage with >300 poor children with regular school and medical supervision and are well fed; are often taken to cinema if they behaved well. Beggars are taken off the streets and kept in a very clean poor house where they have a visiting doctor, who often sends us cases for operation.[655]

In addition to these hospitals there was a leprosarium, which had been established one km outside Mashhad in 1884 or 1885 in the old castle of Mehrab Khan. Prior to that time lepers had lived among the people and congregated near the shrine to beg. Given the contagious nature of the disease it was therefore decided to concentrate them outside the city.[656]

FOREIGN HOSPITALS

As indicated above, the impact of the Razavi Hospital clearly was negligible for there was a growing demand, also from pilgrims, for the other hospital services available at Mashhad. The foreign medical establishments were the only source of modern medical service, for in 1914, because "there were only a few half-trained Persian doctors in the entire province of Khurasan" and no other hospital.[657] Although the number of foreign medical institutions would soon thereafter fall in numbers, but, in 1915 there were still three foreign hospital/dispensaries

---

654. RG 91-20-2, Mashad Medical Report 1929-1930, p. 9. The asylum for invalids (*navan-khaneh* or *dar al-`ajazeh*) had room for 3,000 persons and a 65-bed hospital; it was founded in 1923. Khakestar 1395, p. 196.

655. Mashad Medical Report, 1935-36 [img1850-65]; see further Khakestar 1395, pp. 98-101, who mentions that there were two. One was the *parvareshgah-e atfal* established in 1926 and the other, *parvareshgah-e aytam-e dar al-tarbiyeh*, established in 1928.

656. See Floor 2020, pp. 284–312.

657. Donaldson 1972, p. 108. Although there were many Russian troops in Mashhad apparently there was no Russian military hospital, or its medical service was considered to be inadequate, as Russian soldiers came for treatment to the American hospital. Idem, p. 112.

operating in Mashhad: (i) the British Consulate-General dispensary/hospital; (ii) the Russian Consulate-General dispensary; (iii) the Russian Bank dispensary; and, a recent newcomer, (iv) the American missionary hospital/dispensary. The two Mashhad Iranian hospitals (the Shrine's *dar al-shafa* with 70 beds and the Montasariyeh with 20 beds) had been totally neglected and had almost ceased to operate, allegedly due to lack of funds, after 1920. As to the foreign hospitals:

British hospital

As of 1889 there was a British Consulate-General in Mashhad, which had a small British Consulate hospital with 12 beds, 6 for men and 6 for women.[658] It had one British doctor and one Indian hospital assistant, who treated about 6,000 patients per year around 1900. In the doctor's absence the hospital assistant ran the dispensary.[659] Until the arrival of the American missionaries,

> The British Consulate-General hospital is the only one in the city which is equipped for the reception and scientific treatment of in-patients, and for the undertaking of serious surgical work. It has recently been largely repaired, renovated and altered; also a good deal of modern equipment has been added, an operating room fitted out and an ophthalmoscopic 'dark room'. The average daily attendance of out-patients throughout the year is 112. During the year 1904-05, before the renovations and re-equipment were completed, 41 major operations and a large number of minor operations were performed. Eye operations have hitherto formed the large proportion of the major operations. About 36,000 patients are seen annually.[660]

All patients received treatment and drugs free-of-charge, while the poor were fed at the British hospital's expense. Wealthy, presumably

---

658. Gilmour 1924, pp. 29-30; Grothe 1911, p. 131; Khakestar 1395, pp. 153, 159-63.
659. Yate 1900, p. 336; Wright 2001, p. 126. I have not been unable to find out when it began operating, but most likely when the British Consulate was opened in Mashhad in 1889.
660. Adamec 1981, vol. 2, p. 487.

paying, patients received house-calls. The hospital's services, therefore, were becoming popular by 1905; it even received patients from as far as Herat. Therefore, the government of India, in February 1905 allocated a sum of 5,000 Rupees for the re-equipment of the hospital, and later additional funds were made available to completely repair and renovate the hospital buildings.[661]

Table 23: Number of patients treated in the British hospital at Mashad in 1904-05.

	Male	Female	Children	Total	Remarks
Out-patients (new and old)	21,814	11,387	2,561	35,762	
Out-patients (new only)	7,926	3,082	1,195	12,203	
In-patients (new and old)	33	12	7	52	From April 1 to November 11,1904, surgical in-patients only were registered. From November 12, 1904 to March 31,1905 both medical and surgical are included
Major operations	27	10	4	41	Cataract, 28; bone, 2; liver abscess, 2; amputation, 2; litholapaxy, 1; lithotom, 3; suprapubic lithomy,1; other operations, 2
Total (excluding operations)	29,773	14,481	3,763	48,017	

Source: Sykes 1905, p. 22. The average daily attendance of out-patients (new and old) was 114.25. The average daily attendance of new out-patients was 39.00.

The British free dispensary did not close in summer, except to give the doctor a month vacation. Before WW I there was a fully qualified British doctor of the IMS with the rank of assistant Consul. Therefore, a large amount of his work was political, but he gave 2-3

---

661. Sykes 1905, p. 22.

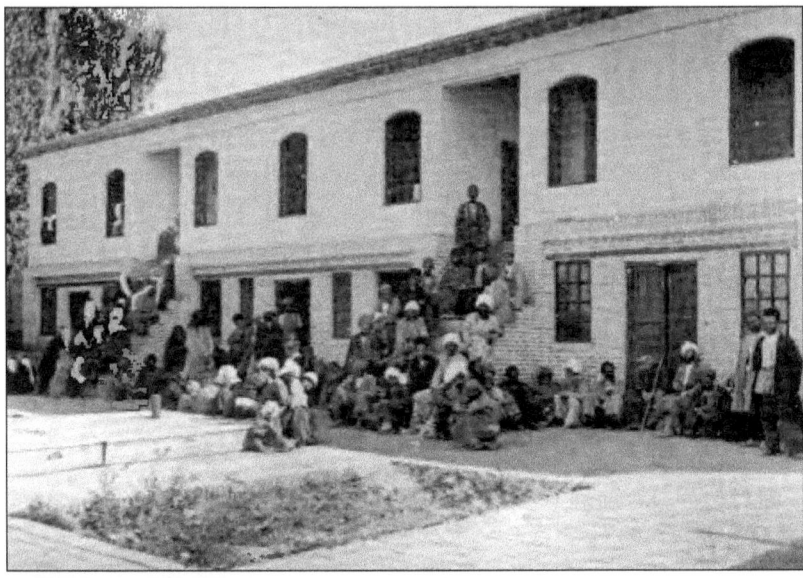
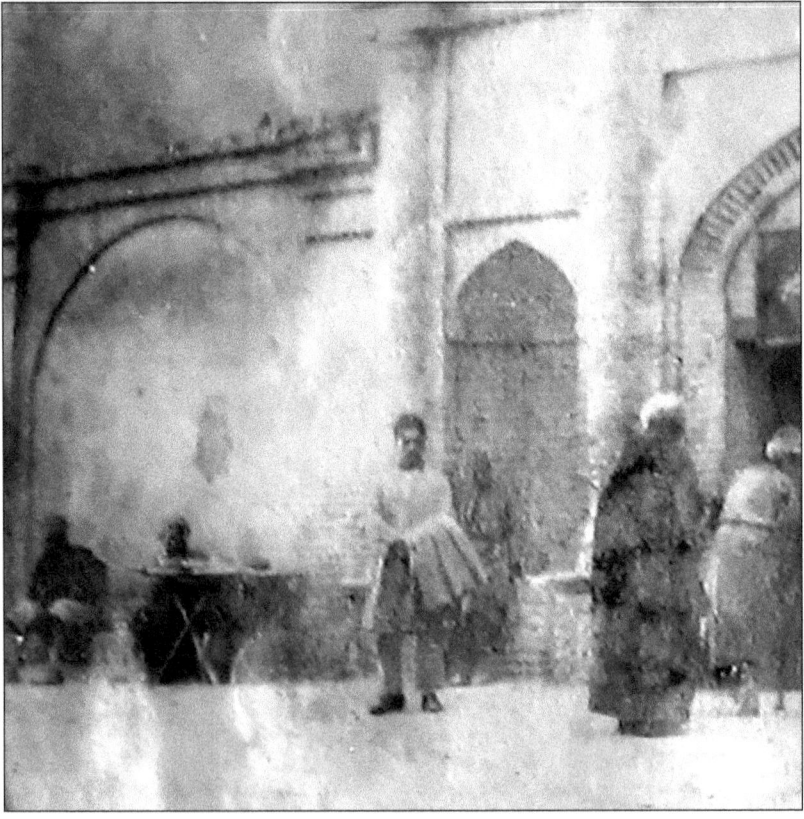

Top: Charitable British dispensary, Mashhad.
Above: British Consulate's free dispensary.

hours/day to the dispensary; he had an Indian assistant and saw about 22,000 patients per year.⁶⁶² When in early May 1917, British-Indian troops came, Capt. J.A. Sinton, V.C. I.M.S. set up a hospital in rented houses.⁶⁶³ In 1919 it was described as follows: "The British Consulate had a free dispensary with an Indian doctor who saw 150 to 200 patients mornings, and did a few operations afternoons, the patient's friends doing the nursing. One Persian and one Russian drugstore had a few medicines. The Shrine had a small hospital, a crude place where suffering pilgrims could at least get out of the rain."⁶⁶⁴ The British Consulate hospital was closed when the British troops left in April 1921. However, its dispensary was continued. In 1928, the British Consulate closed its free dispensary.⁶⁶⁵

The closure of the British consular dispensary was a loss in terms of local capacity of medical care for the poor, because over the years it had treated many needy patients. An indication of its importance is given by the data for the year 1919.

Table 24: British Mashhad Consulate Hospital Patients for 1919

	Male	Female	Children	Total	Average daily attendance for No of days hospital was opened.	Daily average No of In-patients in hospital for the year.	Average No of days in hospital for each patient.	Deaths
Out patients new only	10782	9005	4980	24767	107.21	-	-	-
Out patients new and old	22950	18586	10402	51938	224.84	-	-	-
Indoor patients	113	8	6	127	-	-	12.00	4
Major operations	71	30	15	116	-	0.66	9.44	2

Source: FO 248/1291, unfoliated.

Note- Hospital was closed altogether for 134 days in the year including Fridays, Sundays and other holidays. The 116 surgical operations were distributed as follows: Cataract 24, other eye operations 31, Tubercular glands 7, Benign Tumours 12, Malignant Tumours 4, Ovarian cyst 1, Caies and Necrosia of bones 9, Stone in Bladder 2, Hernia 15, Contractions tendons hand after burn 5, Haemourrhoids 2, Imperforated anus 1, all other causes 3. There were 6 deaths amongst the indoor patients as follows: (I) Very debilitated patient died of heart failure 2 days after operation (II) A case of very advanced Sercoma of the thigh died after amputation

662. RG 23 I-1-6; enclosure in letter Hoffman to Sykes, 4 October 1918.
663. RG 23 I-1-6; Hoffman, Pioneering in Meshed, p. 44.
664. RG 23 I-1-6; Hoffman, Pioneering in Meshed, p. 34; The British Consulate hospital has a new Indian doctor, RG 23 L-1-2, Hoffman to Donaldson, Mashhad, October 10, Saitnè 2680.
665. RG 23 I-1-6; Hoffman, Pioneering in Meshed, p. 68.

(III) Of four cases of Khurasan Levy Corps who died in Hospital two had died of acute dysentery and two of Broncho Pneumonia. Meshed, Sd. Mumtaz Ali Khan, K.S., Subedar, IMD. Acting Agency Surgeon.

Russian Hospital

The British medical service was not enough to satisfy demand, for there was a small hospital or charitable dispensary led by the Russian consular physician. It had "a daily attendance of about 40 to 50 out-patients in the summer; in the winter it is less."[666] When the Russian consular physician had finished his duties at the Russian dispensary "he proceeds to the [Russian] Bank dispensary, where he sees all the male patients. The female patients are seen by a Russian lady doctor, the wife of one of the bank employees. The average attendance here in the summer is about 70, and less in winter. The dispensary was established as a 'draw' for the Russian Banque d'Escompte de Perse."[667] In 1904-05, the dispensary treated 36,000 patients and performed 41 operations.[668]

As of 1912, Russia had a large military presence in Mashhad and its province of Khorasan, which in fact it had occupied. However, the medical services it was able to offer its soldiers were totally inadequate. In fact, ironically, wounded Russian soldiers came to the free hospital attached to the British Consulate-General.[669] To do away with this slight to its local importance, the Russian government wanted to build a hospital in Mashhad right across from the British

---

666. Adamec 1981, vol. 2, p. 486; Grothe 1911, p. 131. In 1911, the British Consul General in Mashhad reported that "the Russian colony is in a state of panic. They sleep in their clothes with their jewelry sewn up in the lining. They have transferred their funds and also their dispensary to their garden outside the city, where the clerks keep sentry day and night. They are especially afraid of their guard of Persian Cossacks, and until my colleague sent them ten Russian Cossacks, their state was one of wild alarm." IOR/L/PS/10/209, Meshed Consular Diary No. 50 for the week ending 11th December 1911, p. 1.

667. Adamec 1981, vol. 2, p. 486.

668. Khakestar 1395, p. 130

669. IOR/L/PS/10/209, Diary of the Military Attache, Meshed, no. 30, for the week ending August 3rd, 1912, p. 2.

Consulate-General. This was unacceptable to Great Britain and, therefore, the British Minister protested. To assuage British hurt feelings, Tehran agreed that the Russians might build the hospital in the Ark garden, but that the entrance should not be made opposite to the main gate of the British Consulate-General.[670] Fortunately for British amour-propre the hospital was not built. In fact, by late 1917, the two Russian dispensaries stopped functioning.[671]

In 1944, the Anjoman-e Ravabet-e Farhang-e Iran va Shuravi was established in Mashhad. Under the auspices of the health commission of this association, as of 28 November 1944 a free clinic was operated managed by a Russian doctor. During 1944-45, the clinic treated 5,008 patients.[672]

It was only in 1943 that the Russians again opened a hospital in Mashhad. Their hospital had three doctors, who spoke neither Persian nor English and did practically no free work. When the Red Army left in April 1946 they stripped the building they had rented of locks, hinges, even doors and windows. After the departure of the Russian army, the Russian government opened a 30-bed hospital in Mashhad on 30 June 1946, their fourth in Iran (Tehran, Tabriz and Rasht). The hospital had an X-ray machine, "almost a duplicate of the old German machine we had in Tehran, also several diathermy, quartz lamp and physiotherapy gadgets." Although the Russian hospital had three doctors (a radiologist, a surgeon and an internist) they did not begin working immediately, possibly because none of them spoke Persian or English. Although additional hospital capacity was always welcome given the total inadequacy of hospital facilities and the need in the province, the Russian hospital accepted few poor people.[673]

---

670. IOR/L/PS/10/209, Meshed Consular Diary no. 6, for the week ending 8th February 1913, p.1

671. The Soviet government did not claim the Russian Bank dispensary's pharmacy, when in November 1925 it did not consider it part of the Bank's assets. Khakestar 1395, p. 129.

672. Khakestar 1395, pp. 133-34.

673. RG 231-1-6, Hoffman, Pioneering in Meshed, p. 147; see also Khakestar 1395, pp. 134-49 (Russian hospital, anti-typhus actvities, Russian phycisians).

The American Christian Hospital

The Rev. Lewis F. Esselstyn began missionary work in Tehran in 1887.[674] He made his first visit to Mashhad in 1894. His missionary work there caused a riot and he had to flee for his life. In 1911, he returned and this time his evangelic work caused no outrage. In 1915, he was joined by the American missionary physician Dr. Joseph W. Cook, who started medical work in Mashhad.[675] To that end, just before X-mass 1915, Esselstyn had rented a poorly built, small house of 11 rooms in the Russian (south) part of the city and opened a 10-12 bed hospital. "It consists of 3 rooms upstairs, a surgery, a men's ward, a women's ward. A curtain in the waiting room divided it in a men's and women's part." Dr. Cook was in charge of the hospital, while he also did the dispensary. The largest number of patients treated in a single day was 265, in one week 2,266 with 36 operations, in one month 5,061 patients with 122 operations, all done by Dr. Cook with one Iranian assistant. Dr. Cook remained in Mashhad until the end of June 1916, when he had treated more than 17,000 patients, clearly the vast majority being out-patients. The patients came from all over Khorasan and even Afghanistan and Turkistan. Receipts of 12,163 *qran*s from patients were enough to furnish the hospital for immediate use and pay all running cost.[676] Dr. Cook returned to Tehran in July 1916. The number of dispensary patients fell off when Dr. Rolla Hoffman, with little knowledge of Persian, took over. Hoffman and Esselstyn opened the clinic in September, 1916. "A few sufferers came in much fear, to the 'infidel' foreign, unclean Christian doctor." Hoffman's work schedule was dispensary during six mornings/week and house

---

674. Presbyterian Church 1888, p. 77.
675. Donaldson 1972, pp. 108, 113; Elgood 1951, pp. 511-512, 534; Funk 1920, p. 153. According to Miller 1989, p. 50, Dr. and Mrs. Cook spent only a few months in Mashhad to see whether there was potential for medical mission work and Dr. Hoffman only came in 1916.
676. Presbyterian Church 1917, pp. 301-02; Anonymous 1918, p. 303; RG 231-1-6, Hoffman, Pioneering in Meshed, pp. 13 (Dr. Cook from Mashhad writes that people are flocking to his dispensary; he needs supplies, our stocks are low, little is imported due to war), 57; Donaldson 1920, p. 534; Donaldson 1972, pp. 108, 113; Elgood 1951, pp. 511-512, 534; Funk 1920, p. 153; Miller 1989, p. 50.

calls whenever time could be found. The afternoons he reserved for operations, of which he did some, but under local anesthesia to avoid deaths, which would have been disastrous.[677]

> I began work, with nine month knowledge of Persia, a roll of instruments. There was no nurse, nor other trained helpers, no sanitary water supply, no electric current, no health department, very little money. There was only a small, rented house, with a few crude beds, tables and chairs, wood-burning stoves, primus kerosene stoves for boiling instruments ... no surgical supplies or stock of medicines. Dr. Esselstyn managed the kitchen and laundry, scoured the bazaar for materials for gowns, sheets, towels, surgical sponges, for pitchers and basins, samovars for sterile water, quilts and blankets, even some medicines. He had a coppersmith make a live-steam sterilizer on the model of the British dispensary's sterilizer. I taught Mrs. Bess Donaldson how to make surgical sponges, towels and gowns, and had a carpenter make a wooden operating table.[678]

Hoffman's mission was supported by the First Presbyterian Church in New Castle, Pennsylvania. In return, he had to write something for their church news bulletin. They even sent him a car, but as there were neither garages nor gas or car mechanics in Mashhad, Hoffman sold the car to the British army who were very glad to have it and he used the money to buy hospital equipment.[679] He also received help from some members of the local medical community.

> The 'Chief Doctor,' - Sadr-ol-Atteba, sent a young man who had been his apprentice to be my assistant. Mirza Hajji Agha, about eighteen, had about a ninth grade education, knew some Russian, but no English. ... Then Dr. Moosa (Moses) Khan sent his nephew, Mirza Morteza, to be my second assistant. Those

---

677. RG 231-1-6, Hoffman, Pioneering in Meshed, pp. 23, 37; Presbyterian Church 1918, p. 287. Dr. Hoffman arrived in Tehran at the end of 1915 and worked a few months in the Tehran hospital before moving to Mashhad.
678. RG 231-1-6, Hoffman, Pioneering in Meshed, pp. 36-37.
679. RG 231-1-6, Hoffman, Pioneering in Meshed, pp. 3-4.

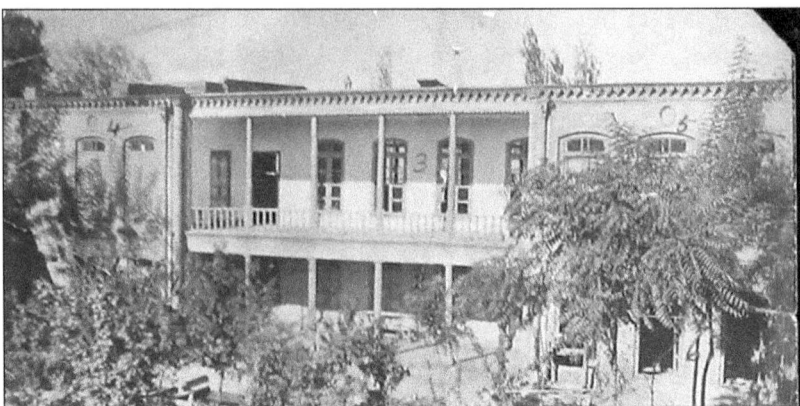

The first American hospital in Mashhad (1915-18) in a rented building in the Russian-Armenian quarter. Dispensary downstairs, in-patients upstairs (12 beds).

> two worked for a nominal wage, on the apprentice basis. I taught them to take temperatures, give injections, administer chloroform anesthesia, scrub up and assist at operations.[680]

Although Dr. Hoffman lacked a professional assistant, the Rev. Esselstyn was "always willing to put his beard under his gown, scrub and help, and give chloroform, until my mirzas had learnt enough to be trusted." Several local doctors came to watch operations and wondered at the magic of anesthesia. Soon it was said: "No one dies at the American hospital." A few major operations were done (senile cataract, stones in the bladder, inguinal hernia), but the most useful and impressive was the operation for entropion, inturned eyelashes from trachoma. "They were quickly done under local anesthesia and the black silk sutures, left long and affixed to the forehead with adhesive plaster, were a walking advertisement." The patients loudly praising the doctor who had 'cured' them. Some mullahs preached against the American doctor, but this was good advertisement, because nobody believed it. Also, Malek al-Atteba and his son Masih al-Saltaneh were

---

680. RG 231-1-6, Hoffman, Pioneering in Meshed, p. 36.

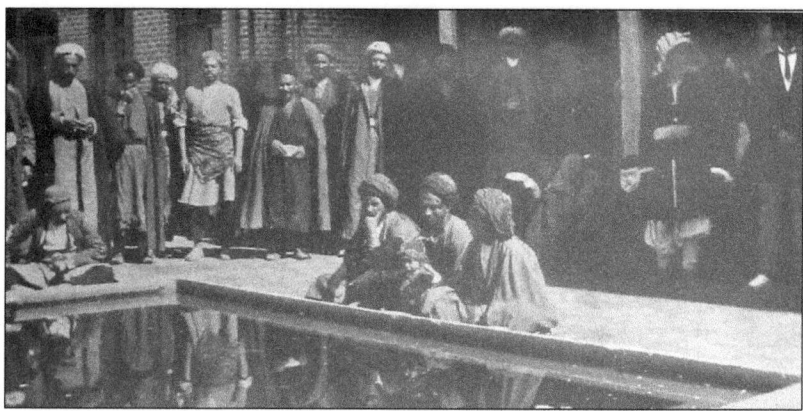

Waiting room at the American hospital with patients, Mashhad, 1916.

very friendly. Dr. Hoffman cooperated with the son in promoting smallpox vaccination, even importing vaccine from India.[681]

From April 1916 until early 1918 practically no rain had fallen in Khorasan. In the summer of 1917 several villages were abandoned, because of the drought and its inhabitants fled to Mazandaran. During August-October a mild cholera epidemic visited the province; nevertheless in the rural areas hundreds of people died. By December 1917 the price of bread had risen to 5.5 *qran*s or 5.5 times more than normal. At the end of December 1917, the Rev. Esselstyn started a relief fund with money received from the European community and a few rich Iranians, which enabled him to feed several hundred people. The American Relief Fund also donated a considerable amount of money to this fund.[682] During that period Hoffman was asked to become director of public health, so the hospital was closed. The hospital and dispensary were changed into a soup kitchen to provide relief to thousands of hungry poor and sufferers of a cholera epidemic.[683]

> In 1917 came a mild epidemic of cholera. The governor called some dozen physicians to form a sanitary commission to advise

---

681. RG 231-1-6, Hoffman, Pioneering in Meshed, p. 38.
682. RG 231-1-6, Report of Famine Relief Work; see also, RG 231-1-2, Hoffman to Parents, 16/04/1918.
683. RG 231-1-6, Hoffman, Pioneering in Meshed, p. 46-47. Presbyterian Church 1919, p. 269.

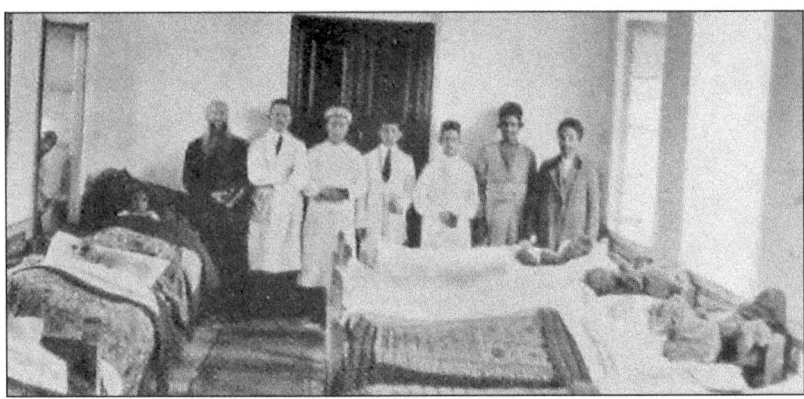

American hospital Mashhad 1918 with Rev. Esselstyn and next to him Dr. Hoffman

him regarding its control. Placards were posted in the bazaar, advising people to eat only cooked foods, boil drinking water and wash the hands after handling a sick person. Of course, a report got out that cholera sufferers were being killed to stop the epidemic. After the epidemic, the sanitary commission continued to advise the governor on health measures. It urged that contagious diseases be reported, that burying inside the city be stopped, that the water in public baths be changed once a month. But none of these measures were carried out. The thinking of the people was not yet ready for reforms. Disease had a free rein, often aided by the treatment used.[684]

In May 1918, both Esselstyn and Hoffman fell ill, victims of a very severe typhoid epidemic that raged in the city, with a lot of typhus and relapsing fever on top of it; Esselstyn died on 30 May, but Hoffman survived, be it in a weak condition. Capt. Sinton, the physician of the British Consulate-general, discharged the few patients in the missionary hospital and closed it. On the last of August the typhus epidemic was followed by the worldwide influenza epidemic.[685] The Rev. Murray wrote:

---

684. RG 231-1-6, Hoffman, Pioneering in Meshed, p. 39 img2835
685. RG 231-1-6, Hoffman, Pioneering in Meshed, p. 45; IOR/L/PS/10/211, Meshed Diary no. 22 for the week ending the 1st June 1918, p. 1. Hoffman wrote to friends in March 1918: "We are planning to open the dispensary on Monday and today I heard that Mr. Murray from Rasht will join me. ... Grippe epidemic started." RG 231-1-2,

One epidemic after another has afflicted this whole region
--- typhoid, typhus, relapsing fever, and recently a most severe wave of influenza, which seems to have attacked nearly 100% of the population, causing a considerable number of deaths; and it is being followed by a very severe malignant malaria. It is said that many nearby villages have been completely depopulated, and others reduced to one fourth of their former population by recent epidemics. In places, it is said, the harvest is still rotting in the fields, because there are no villagers to reap the grain. Apparently there has been no cholera in Meshed itself, but it has appeared as a mild epidemic in many nearby places.[686]

On 9 September 1918, although still weak, Dr. Hoffman re-opened the hospital and dispensary, which had been closed all summer. On the first day he saw 45 patients, among whom several women from Herat. He also accepted six in-patients. Attendance at dispensary grew; the record was 109 in one day. A large number were surgical cases. Patients came from allover the province and country; most of them were on pilgrimage. The dispensary was closed on Fridays and Sundays, because he decided to take it slowly, as the number of patients grew, the pace became too fast for him, drugs were scarce and very expensive. Also, one of his two assistants had left to Tehran to study in the 'Medical School' there[687] and the other was not in good health. He tried two replacements, but that did not work out, so that they were let go after two weeks. Hoffman decided to close all medical work in December and January, as he was still very fatigued. At that time, Dr. Hoffman asked Presbyterian Headquarters in New York for a second doctor, because the need of patients was great and they ran the risk to find the door closed, because he had been able to keep his doors open only for two-thirds of the time. In December 1918, his Turkish landlord served formal notice that he had to vacate the building used

---

Donaldson? to friends, Mashhad 20/07/1918; Idem, NN to friends, Mashhad 30/08/1918. On the impact of the influenza pandemic on Mashhad in particular, and Iran in general, see Floor 2018 a, p. 100.

686. RG 231-1-2, Murray to Speer, Mashad 12/10/1918. Idem, Hoffman to parents, Mashad 02/10/1918 ("There is a lot of malaria now.")

687. On the medical school in Tehran, see Floor 2020, pp. 1–73.

as hospital/dispensary in January 1919. Because the building was rundown, Hoffman started to look for another house and he found a better and cheaper place. It was one of the best built houses in town. Its designer, Mirza Ali Akbar, had wanted to live there but died. It was situated a mere 6 minutes walk from the public square in the center of the city. Also, its water supply came from the city's only pump station and was pure spring water brought by iron pipes without contamination - the best water in town. The dispensary was open for business five days per week, although it was still problematic to obtain medical supplies. The hospital also began to draw many patients from across the border.[688] The hospital, which had only a few beds, as well as its lone American physician, was locally known as *Yengi Donya*, i.e., the 'New World.' "The villagers would sometimes say that they had gone to America when they had visited the hospital!"[689]

In February 1919, medical work was resumed in the 'Telephone House', so-called, because the telephone exchange had been there. Hoffman adopted the schedule of Tehran hospital, where he had worked the first 9 months after his arrival in Iran. Dispensary openings were cut to three weekly, but this meant longer hours. The other three days were for surgery, house calls, and sometimes tennis at the British and Russian Consulates-general. In April 1919, he saw 126 to 278 patients per day during three days/week and did 157 operations with only locally trained helpers. He was exhausted, because he had done too much work after his typhus. Therefore, the Tehran mission told Hoffman to come and have himself checked out. However, the Tehran hospital was unable to do the required tests and after in vain having tried hospitals in Baku and Tiflis, Hoffman went to Istanbul, where tests showed that he was healthy. Hoffman then returned to Mashhad via Tehran, where he met a nurse, Ms Easton, whom he married.[690] Getting medicines became a problem. In 1919, Hoffman

---

688. RG 231-1-6, Hoffman, Pioneering in Meshed, pp. 46-47; Presbyterian Church 1919, p. 269; RG 231-1-2, Murray to Speer, Meshed 12/10/1918.

689. Donaldson 1972, pp. 108, 113; Donaldson 1920, p. 534; Elgood 1951, pp. 511-512, 534; Funk 1920, p. 153.

690. RG 231-1-6, Hoffman, Pioneering in Meshed, p. 48-50; RG 231-1-2,

could not rely on local pharmacies any longer; they substituted so much in filling prescriptions that he was forced to give patients his own hospital's medicines. This required much time to scour the city to find the ingredients. He ordered from India, which, because of transport, cost four times more than in India for bulky drugs such as boric acid and more than 10-50% higher for expensive and concentrated drugs. This enabled him to help his patients, but this was only possible by using part of the famine relief funds for the supply of medicines for the poor. Patients were from all over the province and Herat as well as from Tun and Tabas and Qa'en as well as pilgrims from the rest of Iran. What was encouraging was that people were more willing to accept surgical treatment for certain conditions.[691]

Medical work was closed the last eight months of 1919 due to his absence from Mashhad, but, as of 1920, Hoffman was not alone any longer, because Dr. Hartman Lichtwardt had joined him as well as Khanom Sharifeh, a graduate nurse. Hoffman took charge of the male patients, while Lichtwardt took care of the women and children. During first six months of 1920, they resumed medical work with an increased staff. A new consulting room was prepared and, in March 1920, Lichtwardt began to see some out-patients, with Khanom Sharifeh as interpreter. In June 1920, fortunately the ordered equipment came. So far they worked with the few instruments that "I packed into the corner of my trunk when I came in 1915, supplemented by a few which the Tehran hospital was able to spare us and a few more that I was able to pick up in the local pharmacies." Now they had enough for general operating and eye work to run two operating rooms at the same time. Both Hoffman and Lichtwardt had married a nurse, who also worked in the hospital, while they also had one Iranian trained nurse, Khanom Sharifeh. Hilda Lichtwardt supervised the operating room and dispensary nursing, with Khanom Sharifeh as interpreter. Helen Hoffman had the kitchen, laundry and ward nursing; she knew Turkish from her childhood in Urmiyeh and needed no interpreter, as

---

Hoffman to parents. Tehran, 10/10/1919 (announces his marriage to Ms Easton).

691. Presbyterian Church 1920, pp. 320-21.

almost the entire staff knew Turkish. Khanom Sharifeh also helped in the operating room and dispensary. The three nurses told the doctors "that we had been keeping a pretty dirty hospital." Cleaner and better cloths for the patient, white aprons and uniforms on the helpers and general cleanliness of the places showed that a "hospital without a nurse is no hospital."[692]

Because there were now two physicians, for the first time hospital was open the whole year, and was not closed during summer. The dispensary was open 3 days/week. Although the hospital building was a comfortable one with thick walls, high ceilings and wide porches, it was too small for a 2-doctor team. Therefore, an adjoining yard and 3-room house was added, from which the door was opened into the yard of the hospital.[693]

When the British army left in early 1921,[694] Hoffman bought almost all their hospital furniture, drugs, canned food at reduced prices. Then followed the threat of a Bolshevik invasion and local uprisings. Therefore, in March 1921 all Europeans left Mashhad, except the Donaldsons. The American doctors closed the hospital and sold the furniture at an auction. They went to Zabol, 1,000 km to the south, where the Mashhad team established a medical station (see Zabol section below). In July 1921 they returned to Mashhad and were able to buy back what they had sold; they repaired the hospital building and with the Lichtwardts back in September 1921 Hoffman opened the hospital.[695] Dr Lichtwardt did the women's dispensary with Khanom Sharifeh and Dr. Hoffman the men's part. For the first

---

692. Presbyterian Church 1921, p. 338; RG 231-1-6, Hoffman, Pioneering in Meshed, pp. 51-52.

693. Presbyterian Church 1922, p. 371.

694. The Sistan Force had taken control over the border with Afghanistan as of April 1915 to prevent German and Ottoman agents from entering that country and foment trouble for the British, see e.g., James, Frank 1934, *Faraway Campaign. Experiences of an Indian Army Cavalry Officer in Persia and Russia*. London: Grayson & Grayson; Dickson, W. E. R. 1924, *East Persia. A Backwater of the Great War*. London: Edward Arnold & Co.

695. RG 231-1-6, Hoffman, Pioneering in Meshed, pp. 52, 54-55.

time the hospital was not closed throughout summer and the building was comfortable during the hot weather, although too small for a two doctor hospital. Its capacity was enlarged by securing an adjoining yard and a 3-room house.[696]

The Iowa Synodical Society had adopted the Mashhad hospital and contributed $50,000 for property, and also sent it White Cross dry goods. Cleveland doctors gave it $600 in instruments, and the New Castle church medicines. They all made suggestions for the new hospital and this led to the plan for a $30,000 building plus residence for the Hoffmans. In December 1924, they moved into the new permanent hospital. Hoffman noted that he had changed hospitals three times (1916, 1919, 1924) and that each time, when he moved, the hospital had doubled in capacity. The new and third hospital building had 44 rooms, was much larger and better. It was hoped to soon to have 50 beds, a second nurse, and more. Also, its "red painted roof" was like a great red finger toward the sky, and was situated in the northern part of the city, near the Shrine. "Without piped water, laundry machinery, central heating, electric lighting, X-ray or a real laboratory, it still represented a forward step, for there was no other as good within many hundreds.[697]

When Dr. Lichtwardt returned from furlough he brought an electric generator with a storage battery of 110 volts and a small X-ray machine. The Rev. Charles Murray, one of the evangelists of the Mashhad mission, erected a tower for the windmill that ran the generator. In this way, the hospital had electric lights during evening only; after 9 p.m. kerosene lamps and Dietz lanterns were used. Then they found a kerosene engine to run the generator. Later they bought power from a commercial local company and had light until midnight. The use of

---

696. Presbyterian Church 1922, p. 371 (Hoffman had a contract with the IBP to treat its employees).

697. Presbyterian Church 1926, pp. 206, 217; RG 231-1-6, Hoffman, Pioneering in Meshed, pp. 57-59. Hoffman made already a plea for funds to build a bigger hospital in 1919, suggesting to the readers of his newsletter to 'buy' $10 shares in his hospital, so that the necessary amount might be collected.

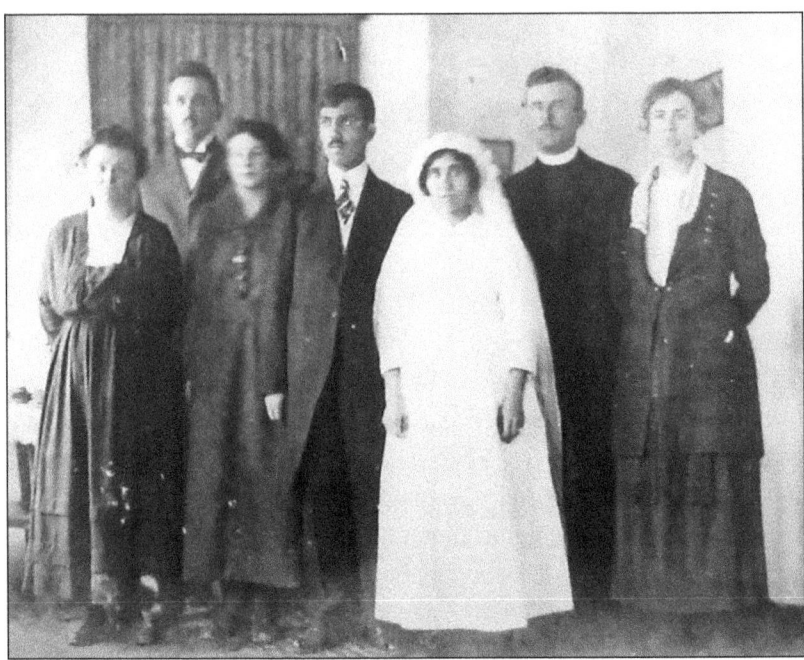

Wedding party of Khanom Sharifeh and Mirza Abdol-Hoseyn Khan, (1921). Helen Hoffman is on the right. Khanom was the first Moslem woman to become a graduate nurse at the American Tehran hospital, class of 1919.

the X-ray was limited to the evenings.[698] In 1928, the British consulate closed its free dispensary. The American hospital purchased its medicines and equipment and the British and Russian Consulates made a contract with it to look after their sick; this was good for income, but demanded time. It also meant that there always had to be one doctor, and made it difficult to do vaccinations during furlough.[699]

Dr. Hoffman visited Isfahan and saw the CMS system of 'family wards' that allowed the entire family to live with the patients, feeding and nursing all patients.[700] In Mashhad they did not go that far, but

---

698. RG 231-1-6, Hoffman, Pioneering in Meshed, p. 63.
699. RG 231-1-6, Hoffman, Pioneering in Meshed, p. 68.
700. RG 231-1-6, Hoffman, Pioneering in Meshed, p. 68.

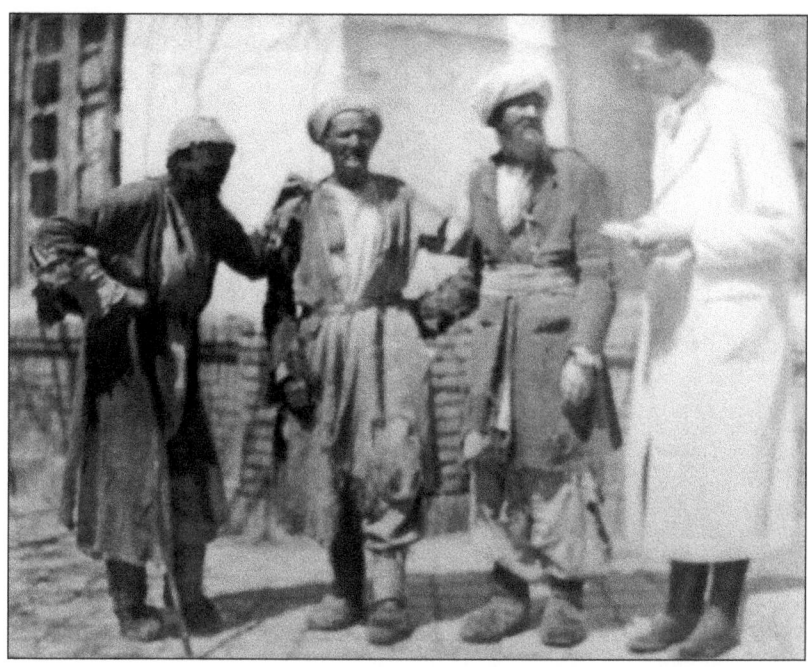

Dr. Lichtwardt with Afghan (Barbari) patients at the
Mashhad American Hospital

they were not strict about visiting hours, which were all afternoons daily, nor about noise, although there were limits.[701]

The X-ray machine was a great asset, especially for bone work, but it was too small for abdominal work, except in case of very thin people. The hospital did not as yet have an upright fluoroscope or Bucky diaphragm. The hospital's small electric generator supplied the X-ray and part of the year the building. But it was too small to get satisfactory lighting for the hospital and the residencies and supply adequate current to the X-ray machine and therefore, they needed a larger generator. Unfortunately, not one of the 7-8 electric lighting companies of the city was near the hospital. Moreover, these plants were small, unreliable and expensive, and only supplied from sunset to about 11 p.m. To be able to do that as well as to maintain work and enable us to employ better helpers the hospital needed an

---

701. RG 91-20-2, Mashhad Medical Report, Year 1932-1933.

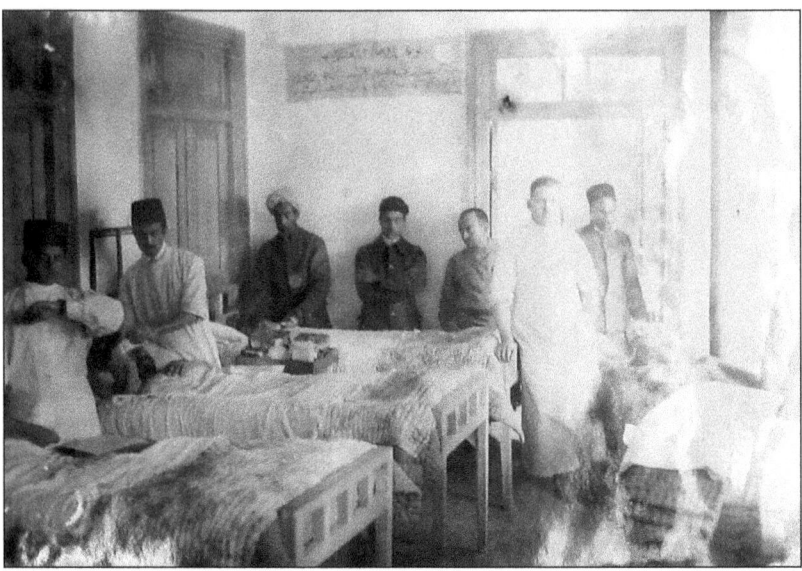

Men's ward with Dr. Hoffman in American hospital, a rented building, 1921.

extra $5,000/year. What Hoffman also wanted was a second Indian physician assistant and a trained lab technician.[702] He referred to Dr. Piyara Singh Ranjit, a graduate of the Lahore Medical College, who as of January worked in the dispensary.[703] In 1931-32, the electric-light plant was overhauled, while their own amateurish wiring was taken out and the building was rewired. Also, new storage batteries were installed and, as a result, the X-ray and lights were working better. Better, but not what was needed, because its capacity was much too small. Therefore, Hoffman repeated that the hospital needed a bigger dynamo, and new supplies such as a diathermy outfit and a Bucky diaphragm for the X-ray machine.[704]

Because medical work continued to grow, the major problem was how to control or limit the ever-increasing numbers. The more

---

702. RG 91-20-2, Mashhad Medical Report 1929-1930. For the electricity situation in Mashhad, see Hamed and Habibi 1376.
703. RG 91-20-2, Mashhad Medical Report 1929-1930; RG 91-20-2, Mashhad Medical Report, 1935-1936.
704. RG 91-20-2, Mashhad Medical Report 1931-1932.

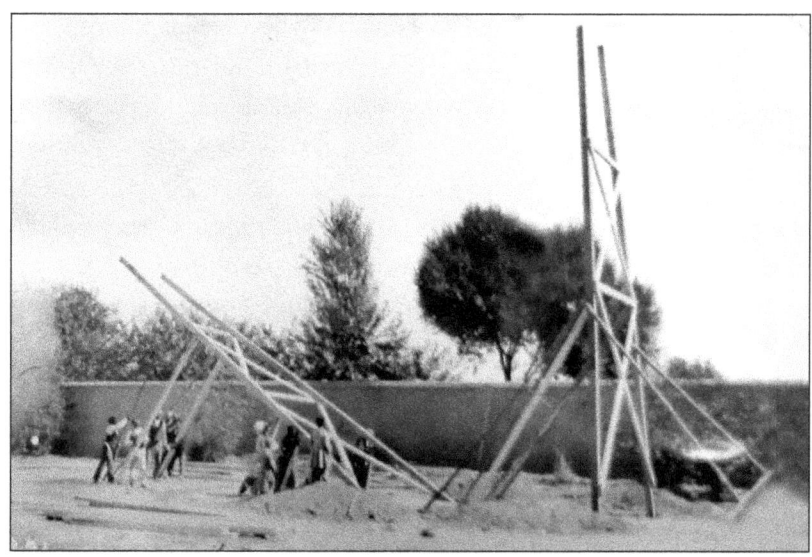

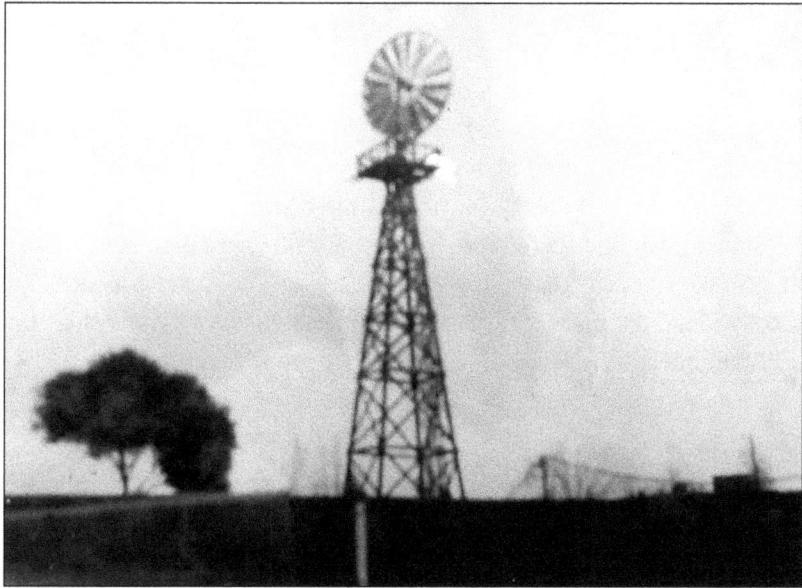

Erecting a windmill to supply electricity to the American hospital, Mashhad, 1926

so, since Hoffman complained that he had to spent time overseeing construction and other tasks that could be done by helpers. Fortunately, with the arrival of Dr. Adelaide Kibbe in 1931 the hospital had three physicians, which enabled the hospital to satisfy the long felt need for better medical work for women.[705] In April 1933, Dr. No-ee (No'i?) was hired. He was a young Iranian with limited training, but with a permit to practice, but the hospital budget could not afford to hire a first-class assistant.[706]

There was a fall in number of patients and thus in the percentage of bed capacity used, but there was an increase of over 500 in total number of in-patients. This attempt to reduce hospital stay helped reducing congestion in the wards and allowed them to help more patients. Hoffman argued that the rating capacity of 60 beds in summer and 54 beds in winter, when the porches were not available, was too high and was only achieved due to crowding. Even with the drop in bed occupancy there were at times moments of unavoidable congestion, especially in winter, unless needy patients were turned away, who had nowhere else to go.

Their big problem was the isolation of contagious patients for which there was no such a place, unless one of the private rooms happened to be empty, which reduced hospital income. A separate contagious ward would be a great help and lessen danger of spread to the hospital, and therefore, was on the doctors' wish list.[707] In the Mashhad hospital "seldom are beds empty for more than a few hours at a time. On occasion we have to use various cots and couches and sofas around the place, or to have a dismissed patient sit in a chair for a few hours till his relatives come, while we fill the bed with a new and a more urgent case."[708]

Medical work continued to be carried on with many staff handicaps, many vacancies, occasioned by retirement and resignations.[709] In 1940, Dr. Walter Norem had come to Mashhad and his wife, a highly trained

---

705. Presbyterian Church 1932, p. 181; RG 231-1-2, Hoffman to Friends 10/03/1930.

706. RG 91-20-2, Mashhad Medical Report 1932-1933.

707. RG 91-20-2, Mashhad Medical Report 1939-1940 .

708. Presbyterian Church 1945, p. 71; RG 91-20-2, Mashhad Medical Report 1942-1943.

709. Presbyterian Church 1943, p. 84.

lab technician, who improved the lab and trained Tooba Rezail to be a technician. However, in 1942, Dr. Norem resigned and returned to the US Army, leaving Dr. Cochran alone. Fortunately, Dr. Hoffman returned to Mashhad on 20 October 1942 with Ms Shamsi Borumand, an operating room nurse, and two student nurses.[710] Because of an epidemic in 1942-43, two wards were filled with typhus and typhoid patients. Thanks to the American-Iranian Relief Commission (AIRC) the US physicians were able to help the very poor; many remained in the hospital for a week and when they left they were given coupons for rice or charcoal or bread or shoes paid by AIRC.[711] This was not appreciated by the pro-Russian local newspaper *Atash-ye Sharq* (Fire of the East), which in February 1943 wrote that in the American hospital they draw people's blood to make them spies, while it staff propagates Christianity so as turn patients into Christians. Moreover, their care was expensive and it was a dirty and unhygienic place.[712] The hospital was closed from 15 July to 15 August 1944 for vacations and again 18 days in April 1945, because of the doctor's illness. Because no US doctors were found for the Christian hospital in Mashhad, the Board had given funds to get Iranian doctors. In the summer of 1944, a young doctor was tried out, but he was let go. Finally, an Assyrian doctor from Beirut was hired, but after one month he got typhus and died. The choice of hiring physicians was limited, because the hospital could not employ non-Christian doctors, because it would be "better [to] have no hospital than one with a doctor hostile to our Cause."[713] In July 1945, the hospital was closed. Since October 1945 the hospital employed a graduate Iranian doctor Dr. Nurollah Hakim-A`lam from Tehran, in full-time service. The other goods news was that the hospital finally a good fridge for the first time in 31 years,

---

710. RG 231-1-6, Pioneering in Meshed, p.138.
711. RG 91-20-2, Mashhad Medical Report 1942-1943.
712. Khakestar 1395, p. 181. Although Khakestar writes that this happened during WW II, his reference gives the date of 12/02/1331 or 21 February 1953. It is likely that 1331 is a printer's error for 1321, which gives the date of 21 February 1943.
713. RG 91-20-2, Mashhad Medical Report 1944-45.

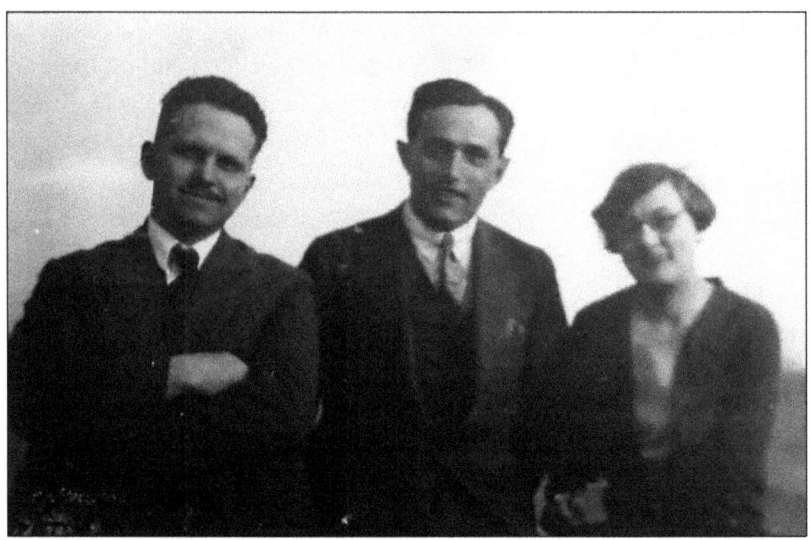

Drs. Hoffman, Lichtwardt, and Kibbe, 1932

which allowed it to store medicines like penicillin, sulfonamides and arsenicals, which were then available and at lower cost. The hospital also received a large quantity of US Army surplus medicines and some medical equipment.[714] In January 1945, Dr. Cochran went to the US, so that there were only two doctors to take care of 55 in-patients, plus the clinic of 150-200 patients, three days/week, which allowed very little free time.[715] Early in 1947 Dr. Cochran helped by Dr. Thomas Murray, new from the US, and Dr. Hakim took over the hospital.[716] Dr. Hoffman had gone to Rasht to take over from Dr. Kibbe. In 1960, the Christian hospital of Mashhad was closed due to lack of funds and staff and it was transferred to the Ministry of Health.[717]

---

714. RG 91-20-2, Mashhad Medical Report 1945-1946.

715. RG 231-1-6, Hoffman, Pioneering in Meshed, p. 141.

716. RG 231-1-6, Pioneering in Meshed, p. 148. Other American physicians working in the hospital after 1950 include Dr. Mary Ziegler, Dr. Rice and Dr. Daks [?]. Khakestar 1395, p. 185.

717. Khakestar 1395, p. 182.

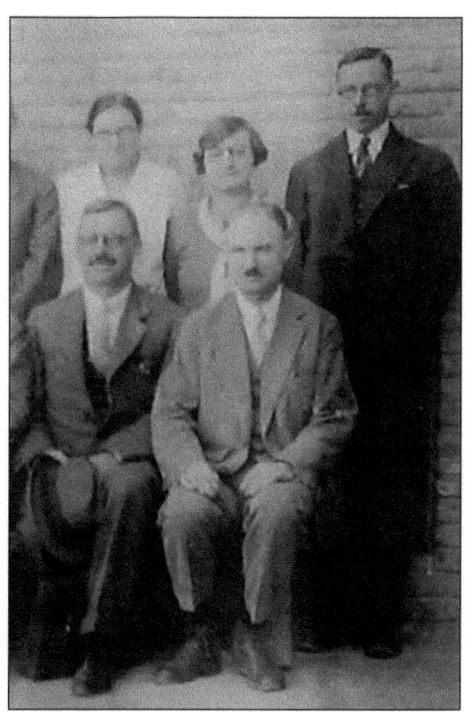

Top, from left: Nurse Taillie, Dr. Kibbe, Dr. McDowell; *Seated:* Drs. Frame and Blair

RENOVATION OF THE HOSPITAL

In the hospital built in 1924, there were about 20 beds for women patients, divided over three wards, which were all light and cheerful with the morning sun. Those patients, who were able to were put on the porch for sun treatment. Many had to be refused admittance.[718] In the summer of 1932, the doctors prepared a tennis court; friends came to play including an Iranian doctor. All what was needed were shoes, for they supplied balls and rackets. A shower bath was also installed. In winter, there was a ping-pong table with bats and balls, and the proposed new addition offered the nurses a rest room, for resting, reading or games in time-off.[719]

---

718. RG 91-20-2, Mashhad Medical Report 1930-1931.

719. RG 91-20-2, Mashhad Medical Report 1932-1933; Idem, Mashhad Medical Report 1937-1938.

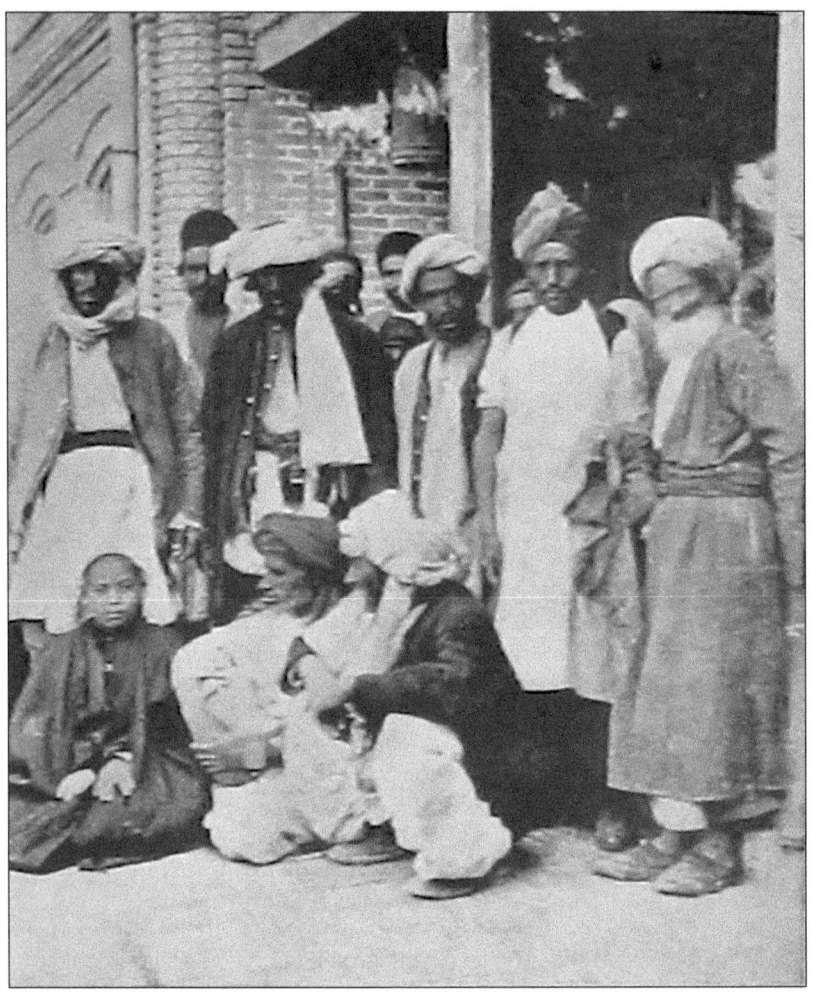

Mashhad dispensary with Barbari patients

In 1929, Mrs. Hoffman took charge of the cleaning of the hospital, tinting of the rooms and other repairs,[720] because the hospital began showing signs of its heavy use. In 1930, the mud roof fell in. It was replaced with a tin roof, costing $1,000. In 1924 there was not enough money for metal to cover the roof and, therefore, part was covered with mud. Hoffman submitted that the hospital really needed an

---

720. RG 91-20-2, Mashhad Medical Report 1928-1929.

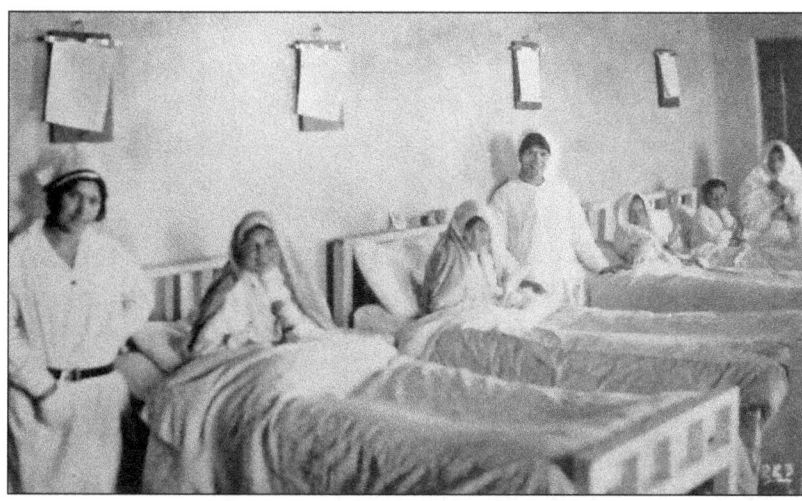

Children in the American hospital, Mashhad, 1928. The two nurses in the background are Christian girls trained in the hospital. The nurse on the left is a graduate of the Tabriz Nursing School.

overhaul.[721] In 1932, the hospital's name was changed to The American Christian Hospital, which did not arouse any adverse criticism.[722] In 1930-31, the New Castle church raised $15,000 for a new wing to the Mashhad hospital, but due to the Great Depression half of this fund was 'frozen' in the bank and the church, needing the money itself, diverted the other half to local use. When the money was 'unfrozen', the hospital received $500 and in driblets $1,000, which enabled the wing to be built.[723] However, there was another wait, "because first the Municipality of Mashhad had to lay out the proposed new avenue cutting off a small corner of our yard, before we erect the proposed Women's wing". The whole building cost less than $30,000 and mainly was made of mud bricks and poplar timbers and was paid for by the New Castle Church. In 10 years it had served some 320,000 dispensary patients and housed 103,000 or 230 years of in-patients

---

721. RG 91-20-2, Mashhad Medical Report 1934-1935.
722. RG 91-20-2, Mashhad Medical Report 1929-1930; Presbyterian Church 1932, p. 181.
723. RG 231-1-6, Hoffman, Pioneering in Meshed, p. 4; RG 231-1-2, Hoffman to the New Castle church (31/07/1934).

and 15,000 surgeries were done. In 1934, Japanese white tiles, water pumps, the first septic tank in Mashhad, wiring for electric lighting, cement floor tiles and paint on all woodwork made it fit for better work.[724] The renovation was not only done, because it was needed for technical and capacity reasons, but also because the Christian Hospital had to look good on the outside, for people would compare it with the recently completed new Shah Reza hospital.[725] In 1942, Hoffman wrote in this connection: "No one visiting Meshed can fail to be impressed by the contrast between the beautiful flower gardens encircling the magnificent buildings of the Shrine Hospital, operated by the government in one part of the city, and the crowd of suffering human beings who mill around the modest Mission Hospital, located in a neat but unpretentious yard."[726]

The hospital employed two mechanics, who maintained and operated the new small electric plants it had received as well as the electric pump to pump water from a well to irrigate the hospital grounds.[727] In 1936-37, a number of improvements were made in the hospital. The workers' dining room floor was cemented, a store room made over the dining room for the women nurses; a drying room was fixed up for the laundry; a nice obstetrical delivery room was prepared, also with a cement brick floor, and the former X-ray room was moved downstairs to what used to be the nurses' bedroom. The other room of the former nurses' suite was used as the business office for Ali Soheyli; the former gate-keeper's room was transformed into a morgue. All these changes and improvements increased the hospital's working space with five rooms and had been made possible by a gift of $500 from the New Castle church. The cost of the changes was higher than expected due to the absence of skilled plumbers in the city and the high cost of cement.[728] Thanks to a $300 gift, Mrs. Hoffman,

---

724. RG 91-20-2, Mashhad Medical Report 1932-1933; RG 231-1-6, Hoffman, Pioneering in Meshed, p. 122.
725. RG 91-20-2, Mashhad Medical Report 1934-1935.
726. Presbyterian Church 1943, p. 84.
727. RG 231-1-6, Hoffman, Pioneering in Meshed, p. 121.
728. RG 91-20-2, Mashhad Medical Report 1936-1937.

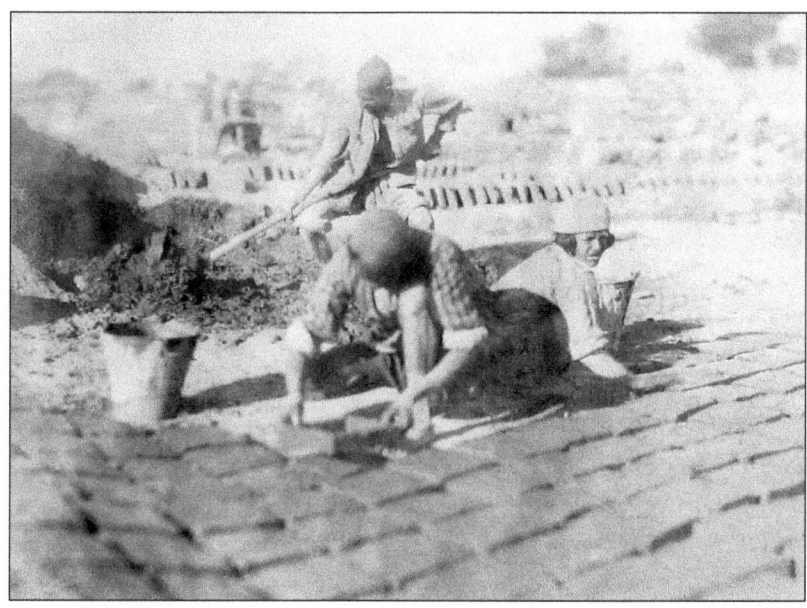

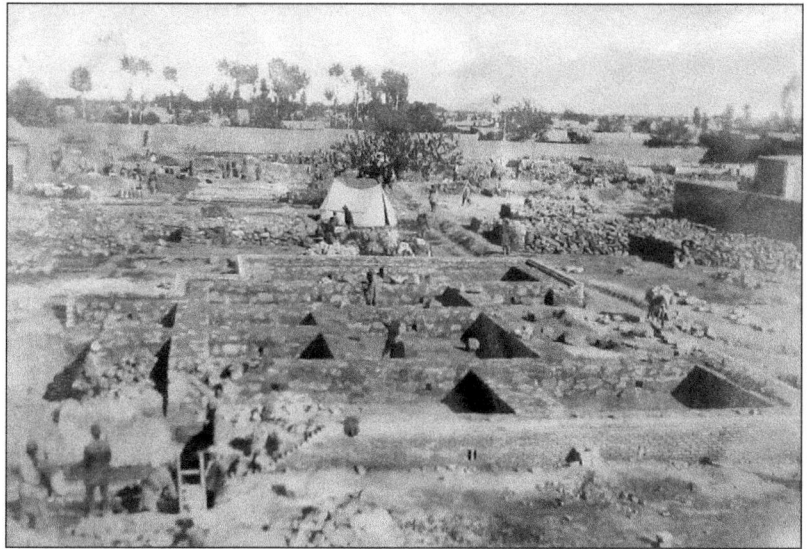

Building the American hospital and houses of the physicians, Mashhad, 1924. *Top:* Making mud bricks. *Below:* Building the foundations.

who was matron throughout the 1920-30s and much of the 1940s, replenished the stock of linens, OR gowns, stored the chinaware and glassware and in such a way that it could easily and efficiently be

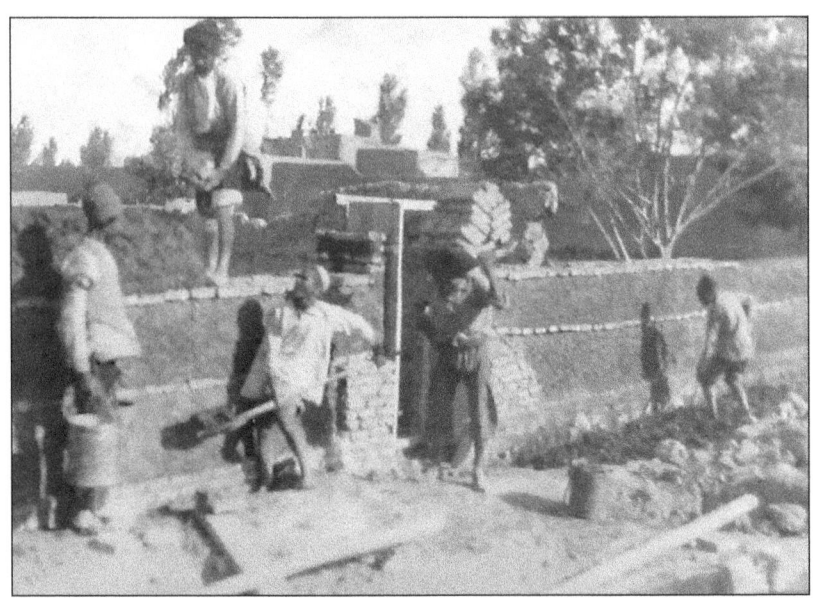

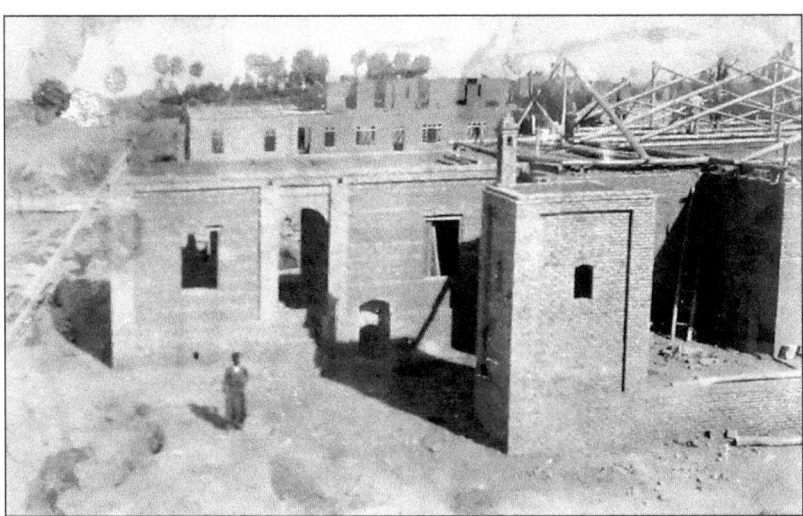

Construction of the American hospital and houses of the physicians, Mashhad, 1924.

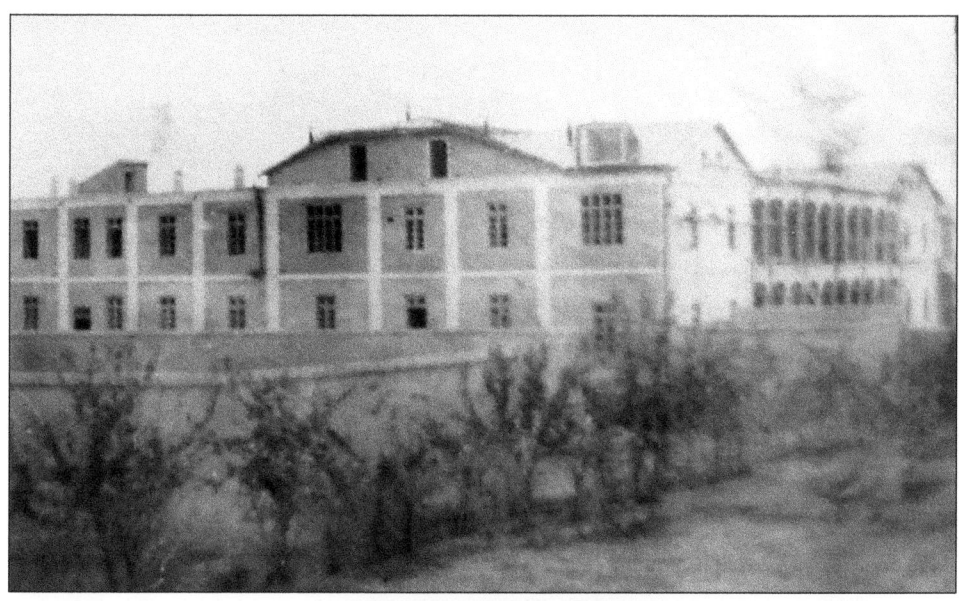

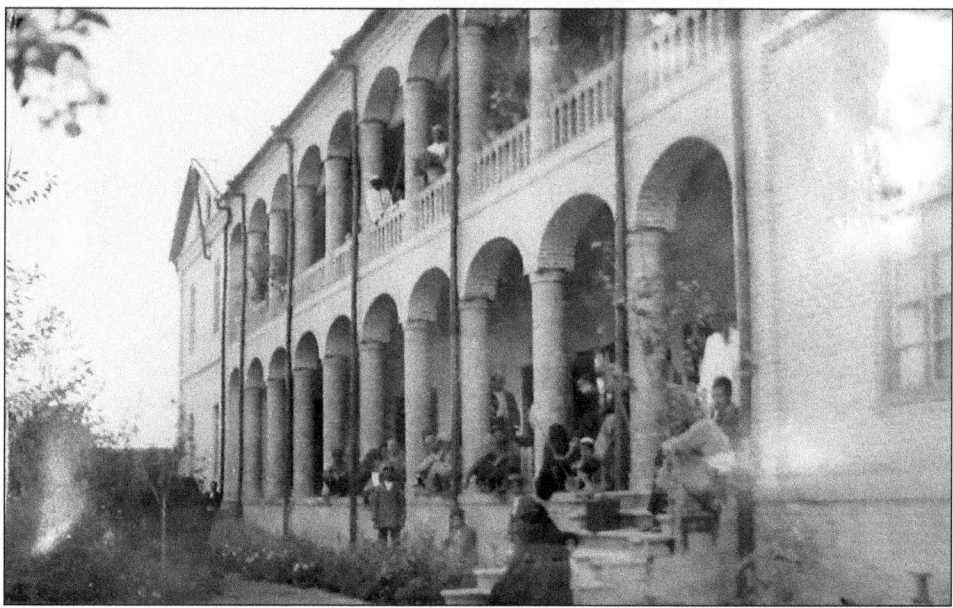

Top: Finished American hospital and houses of the physicians, Mashhad.
Above: The front of the American hospital, Mashhad. Downstairs behind the veranda is the out-patient department, with its 3 waiting rooms, 7 office and treatment rooms, and pharmacy at the far end of the veranda. Upstairs in this wing are the men's wards and at the far end the operating suite.

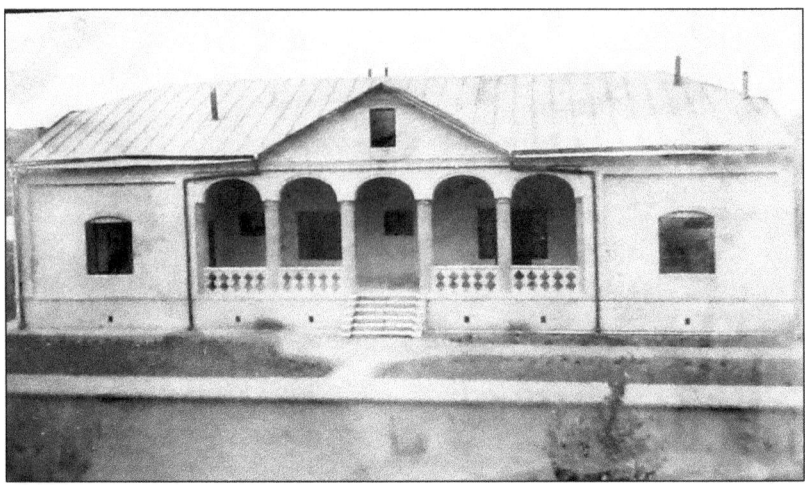

Dr. Hoffman's house in Mashhad.

found. Also, a simple piped water system was installed and the women's porch was screened against flies.[729] In 1938, again with New Castle church funds, the hospital bought a sterilizer; the old one was kept in reserve. The New Castle money also made possible an addition to the women's wing, a nurses' sitting room, a sun balcony, and a bath room and store closet to meet the needs of women. Underneath it was a large room used for storing wood, which, once finished, could be used for other uses.

> Formerly much of our water had to be carried in pails
> from the underground water cisterns; now we are grateful
> for our simple but quite adequate system which carries
> pumped water to some thirteen most necessary points
> in the building. A bath room and toilet for the men has
> also been installed with funds from the same source;
> and improvements have been made in the laundry.[730]

---

729. RG 91-20-2, Mashhad Medical Report 1937-1938.

730. RG 91-20-2, The American Christian Hospital, M. Report for year 1938-39.

In 1939-40, the lawns and planted hedges among the walks were re-grassed, although, despite the wires strung, it was difficult to prevent the hordes waiting before the clinic from destroying the planting. The loose old brick railing on the upstairs front porch was replaced by a strong steel pipe, which made it a safe place for patients. The back porch was re-roofed. The obstetrical and women's ward were repainted.[731] Although by the end of WW II, the building was in good repair, thanks to the supervision by Mrs. Hoffman, but after 21 years of use its wear and tear was obvious. The halls needed cementing, for which often funds had been requested. The hospital's crying need was a Nurses Home; most nurses lived at home, and a dozen employees lived scattered in various residences, which were not needed by the reduced missionary force.[732] Dr. Hoffman continued to ask for funds for repairs to the hospital, a new X-ray machine for the hospital even before he left for Rasht.[733]

DISPENSARY

From December 1915 to 28 February 1919, the American missionary hospital and dispensary were open for 27 months and 53,545 patients were treated, or an average of about 2,000/month.[734] These figures show the success and, at the same time, the problem of the hospital. On the one hand the medical care provided really satisfied a need, but, given that often only one physician was available, per force, this care was provided in a hasty manner. It was, of course, also good policy to have those numbers, because back home those supporting the hospital were encouraged by this. Therefore, in 1926, the Presbyterian Board proudly published the report that the Mashhad dispensary held the record with 375 patients seen in one day, but, at the same time observing that in the American missionary hospital of Tabriz more patients had

---

731. RG 91-20-2, Mashhad Medical Report 1939-1940.
732. RG 91-20-2, Mashhad Medical Report 1944-1945.
733. RG 91-20-2, Hoffman to Allen 03/12/1947 asking for money for various repairs to the hospital img1742; RG 91-20-2, Allen to Hoffman 25/06/1946 money for X-ray.
734. Donaldson 1920, p. 534.

been seen, despite the fact that it had less staff than Mashhad.[735] In 1933, Hoffman and Lichtwardt proudly reported that since 1924, when the new hospital was occupied, nearly 300,000 treatments had been carried out in the dispensary.[736]

These high and even increasing numbers of dispensary patients were not only driven by need, although people were awakening to the need of medical care faster than the medical profession was able to rise to that need. Modernization of society also was a driving force, because in the 1920s there were better cars with gasoline (which was obtainable in five gallon tins in the larger cities) and better roads. Better roads and more cars brought the hospital more patients.[737] In 1915, when Dr. Cook came from Tehran it took 22 days to reach Mashhad, in 1935 it was done in two days by bus.[738] But showing up at the dispensary did not automatically that you were seen by a doctor. Many were turned away and many others were discouraged by the long wait and didn't return. Therefore, Hoffman commented, "it is good that we foreigners don't draw away clients from the growing native professionals and who are working as hard as we are; for doctors are at a premium here." He saw the role of the medical missionaries as bringers of the latest knowledge to the field of medical care. "Except in very few and narrow fields our hospitals still keep the lead in quality of work done in this land and are stimulating ever higher standards for local profession. Iranian doctors sent us referrals, esp. for the Kline test.[739]

The methods and routine of giving medical care to an ever larger growing group of patients developed and changed over time, not only concerning the opening hours, but also organization became more professional and formalized as more trained staff became available. From the beginning, the dispensary had been open for business five days per week, with men and women separated by a curtain in the

---

735. Presbyterian Church 1927, p. 121.
736. RG 91-20-2, Mashhad Medical Report 1932-1933.
737. RG 231-1-6, Hoffman, Pioneering in Meshed, pp. 63-64, 71.
738. RG 91-20-2, Mashhad Medical Report 1934-1935.
739. RG 91-20-2, Mashhad Medical Report 1936-1937.

waiting room.[740] However, after the gruelling experience during 1917-18 (famine relief, epidemics, long and exhausting working hours), in the fall of 1918, the dispensary was closed on Fridays and Sundays, because Hoffman decided to take it slowly, because the number of patients was growing, the pace became too fast for him; drugs were scarce and very expensive.[741] In 1919, Dr. Hoffman decided to cut dispensary days to three per week, although this meant longer hours.[742] When in 1920, Hoffman was joined by Dr. Lichtwardt he did not change this schedule, but he himself took charge of the male patients, while Lichtwardt took care of the women and children. The latter's wife, Hilda Lichtwardt, assisted in the dispensary with Khanom Sharifeh, an Iranian nurse, as interpreter[743] The three days per week dispensary schedule did not change and neither did the separation of men and women. In the new hospital dispensary (built in 1924), the patients followed a planned route from waiting room to the doctor's office, dressing room, injection room and finally the drug room. Fees were collected in advance by a man who sold tickets. Helpers did dressings, injections, bargained about fees for those needed operations and in-patient care, and explained about diets, bathing, etc. It was not safe to give medicines for more than three days as illiterate patients might swallow them in one go, or take a liniment by mouth, "for to take it at all if someone should sneeze. Some would even boil the prescription paper and drink the water." Bottles were few, so patients had to take their own containers, which ranged from dirty broken bottles to leaves and rinds. The mirzas were very good in giving injections and "patients complained if they did not get the needle."[744]

---

740. RG 231-1-6, Hoffman, Pioneering in Meshed, p. 46-47; RG 231-1-2, Murray to Speer, Meshed 12/10/1918.
741. RG 231-1-6, Hoffman, Pioneering in Meshed, p. 46-47.
742. RG 231-1-6, Hoffman, Pioneering in Meshed, p. 48-50.
743. Presbyterian Church 1921, p. 338; RG 231-1-6, Hoffman, Pioneering in Meshed, pp. 51-52.
744. Hoffman, Pioneering in Meshed, p. 60; Presbyterian Church 1922, p. 371.

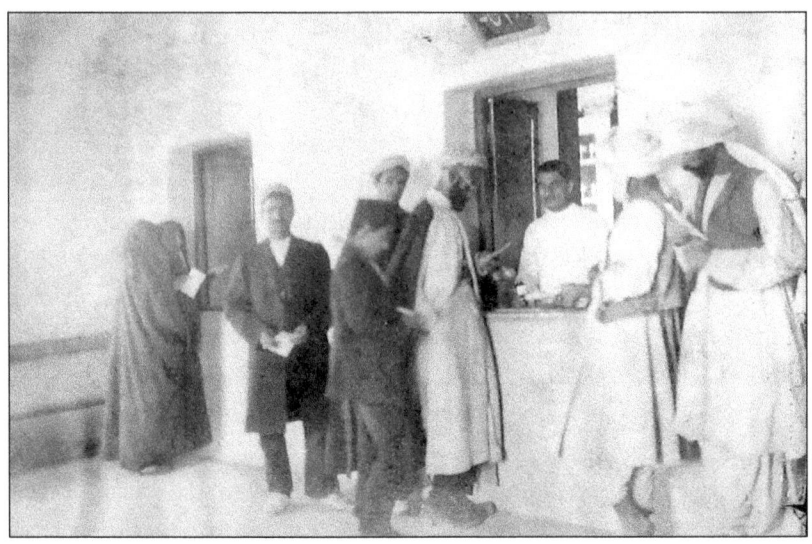

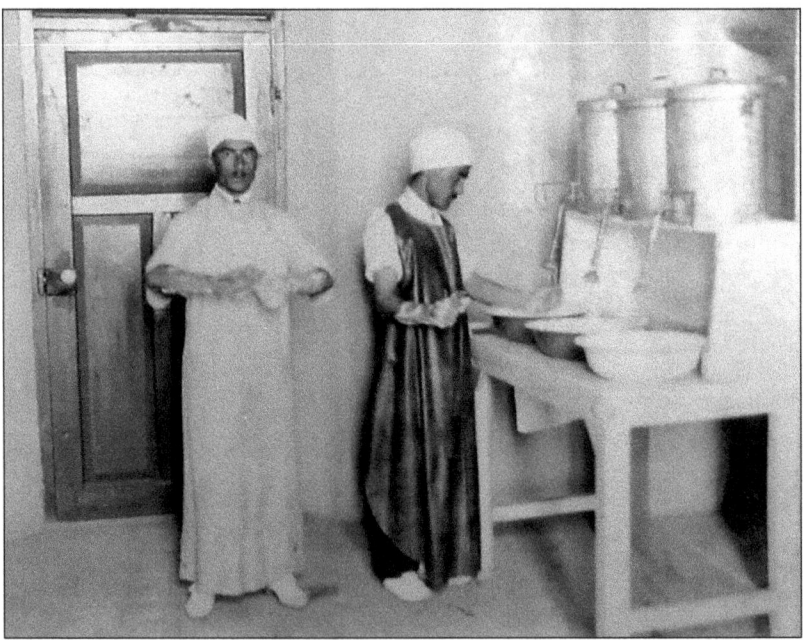

Top: Pharmacy window with Sayyed Abu'l-Qasem. *Above:* Scrub-up room with Naser Khan and Loqman (Malek al-Fatehi).

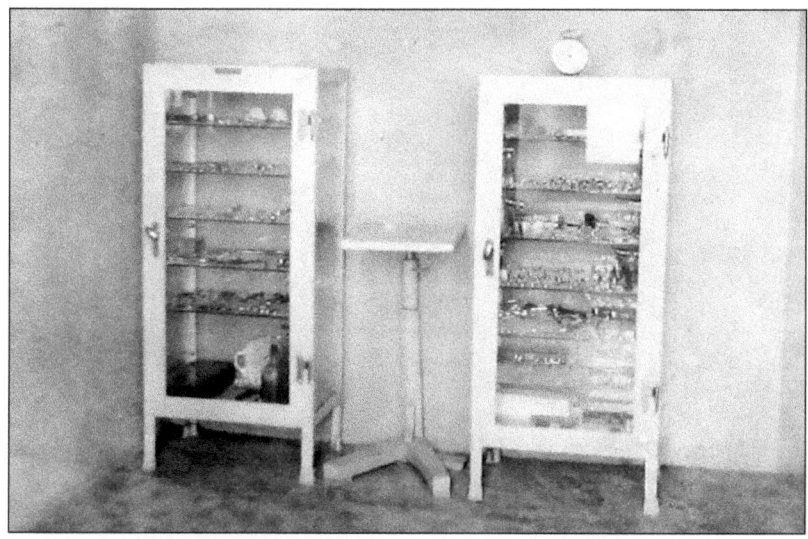

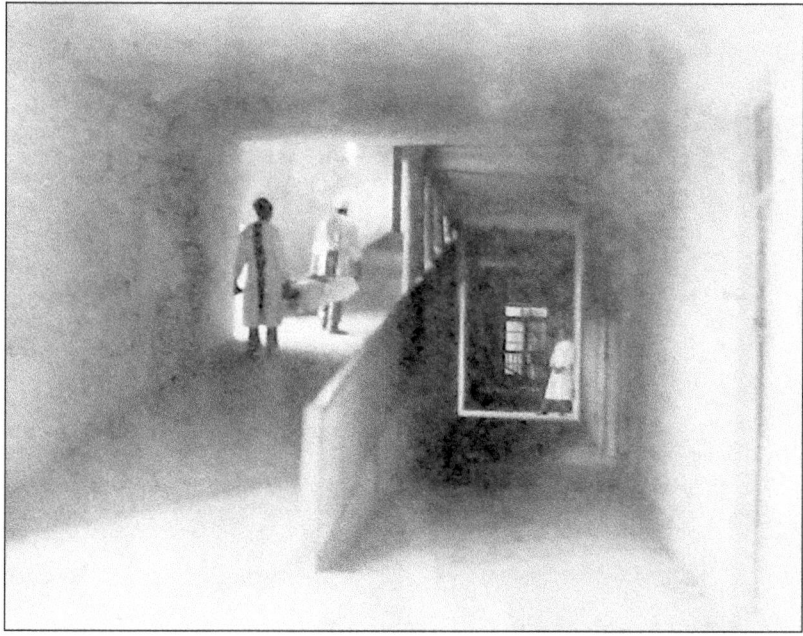

Top: Surgical instrument cases bought from the British army. *Above:* lacking an elevator, the hospital was designed with inclined ramps to facilitate transport of patients and heavy goods.

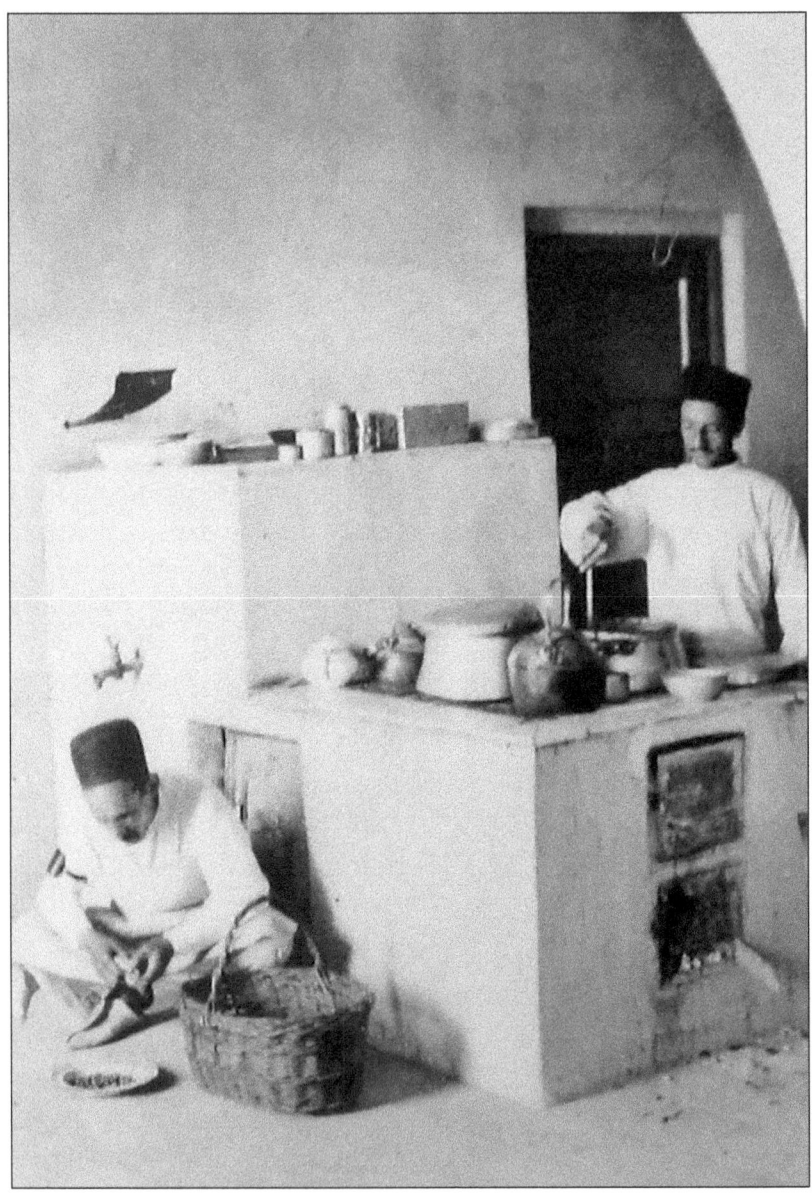

Hospital kitchen with Russian stove and Mohammad and cook Ebrahim.

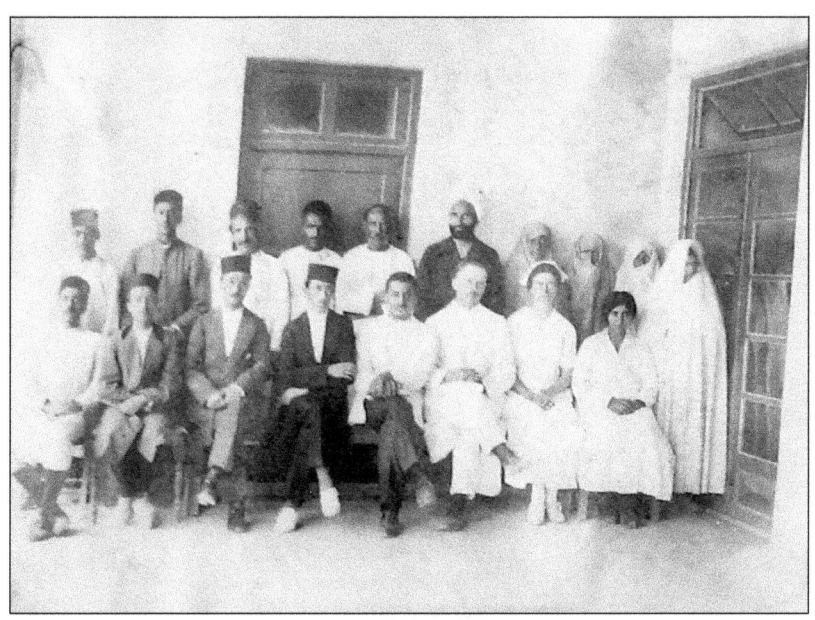

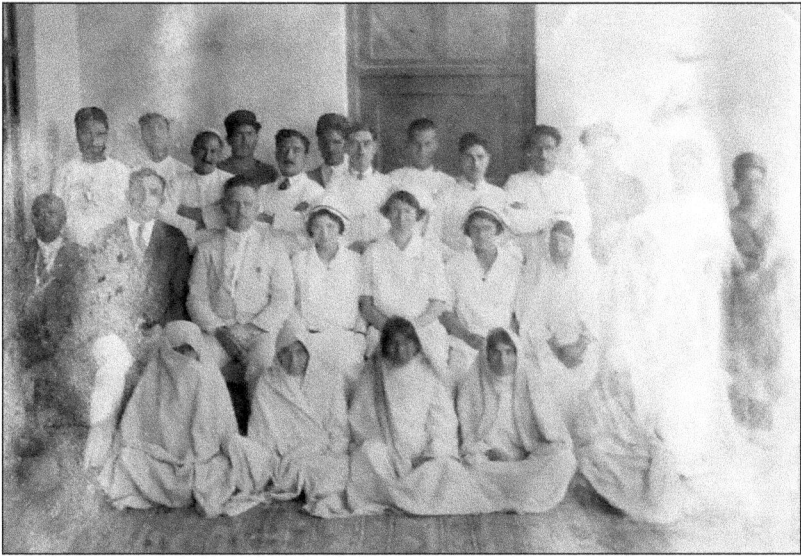

Mashhad American hospital staff in 1925 *(top)* and 1929 *(above)*

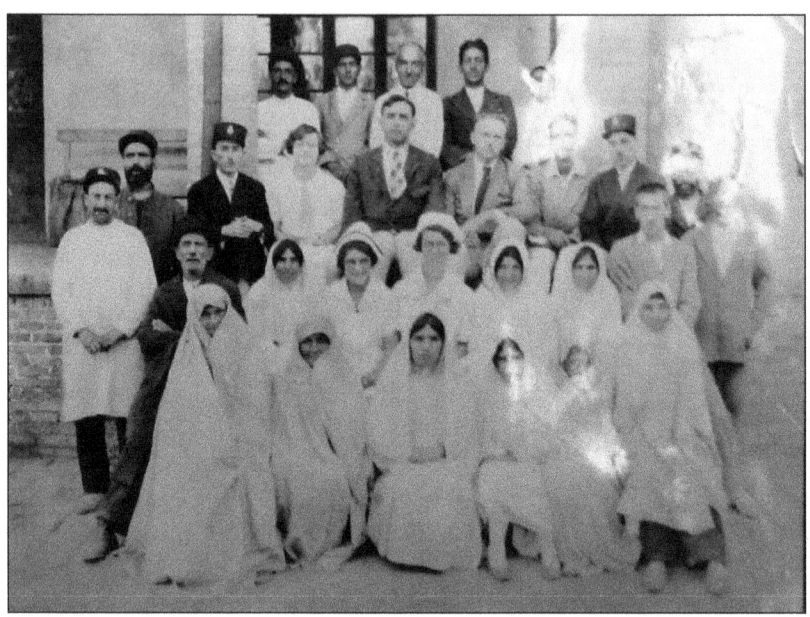

Mashhad American hospital staff in 1930

Even with two physicians the work load was heavy, and always there were more out-patients than they were able to see, but what to do, who to turn away? To reduce the number of return patients, "Old chronic cases are given sufficient medicine for a week and told to return no sooner: hypochondriacs and those with incurable diseases are gently refused treatment," but even then there were too many.[745] An additional problem was the availability of support staff. In 1930, because of the Depression, the hospital suffered from a lack of funds, higher exchange rate, customs rates, etc. Therefore, it had to cut down the number of its local staff by one-third. This meant that the doctors had to reduce the number of patients, also because they would be unable to give each of them the attention they deserved. "For each patient sees an American doctor first, then is sent to the dressing rooms where the Persian assistants care for him." The only solution they saw was that everyone had to buy a ticket, according to his/her ability, from 2 *qran*s to 10 *qran*s (10 c to 50 c), because, so the doctors argued, everybody who can had to pay at least a little.

---

745. RG 91-20-2, Mashhad Medical Report 1928-1929.

On arrival, patients had to buy a ticket from the record clerk, which covered being seen by the doctor, treatment, medicines, injections, dressings etc. Many believed in injections as a miracle cure and want it; many were given, "because of the frequency of default in taking oral medication." Anyone arriving after the tickets for new cases had been given out was turned away. It was sad but the doctors had no choice to do quality work. Despite this undesired decision, the doctors were amazed how many in the end were able to buy a ticket and continue to buy them on return visits. In 1933, Hoffman reported that people liked the one-fee-per-visit system; receipts were also better, because they received 200 to 500Rls/day each of the three dispensary days. At the end of the morning there remained a small handful of patients that were seen free. As a result, by 1933 only 15-20% of dispensary patients were given totally free care, while a few years ago that had been 50%, when the doctors saw 250-300 cases/day. This policy reduced the number of dispensary patients somewhat, while it increased the quality of care and gave the doctors more time for record keeping of each patient. It also brought in more money.[746]

In March 1933, Hoffman returned from furlough to Mashhad. He made it his first task was to set up new record system, because theirs was very poor. It was an experimental project granted to the Mashhad hospital by the last annual Iran Mission meeting. Therefore, he brought Ms Hioanoosh Muradian, a teacher to manage it. As a result of the introduction of the record system dispensary work much improved. The system was based on that of the mission hospital in Tripoli (Syria), viz. a loose card file with name index in a book. Each patient was given a number and all his or her information was filed under that number. Also, by means of a names index a patient's record could be found even after many years. Inpatient records were clipped to the cards, so that there was a single file for out- and inpatients, and each person's complete record was instantly available on return visits. The records were kept in English, although many items were recorded in Persian and even in French. A section of the waiting room was walled off,

---

746. RG 91-20-2, Mashhad Medical Report 1930-1931; Idem, Mashhad Medical Report 1932-1933.

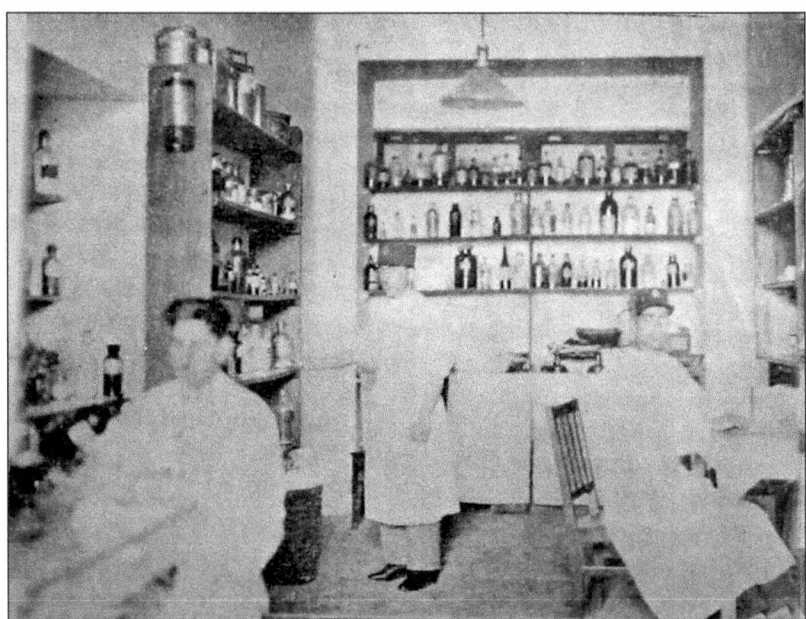

Above: A corner of the pharmacy room, where the druggist and his assistants prepare the medicines for use in the hospital. *Opposite:* Drugstore room of the American hospital, Mashhad.

cabinets were made, each drawer to hold 1,000 case records with a smaller cabinet for the name index cards. Two name index cards were used for each patient, one for the first name, the other for the family name (*sejil*) because many had not yet taken family names; some even forgot what they were! It was run by Poulos Sagda, an Assyrian from Urmiyeh, who was a teacher of the closed mission school.

> Some people caused trouble. They would change their names after a serious illness, to thwart the evil eye. Some gave false names, fearing that information might reach the government authorities and lead to trouble. Some borrowed identification cards from well-meaning friends, since the number of new cases was limited, usually to forty a day. Once three sisters were found using the same case number and name. The doctor might find that No. 1, 211, who had no teeth at his first visit, now had a good set, and his age had change from 60 to 16! An amusing case was that of Seeb-gul (apple blossom). A visitor in

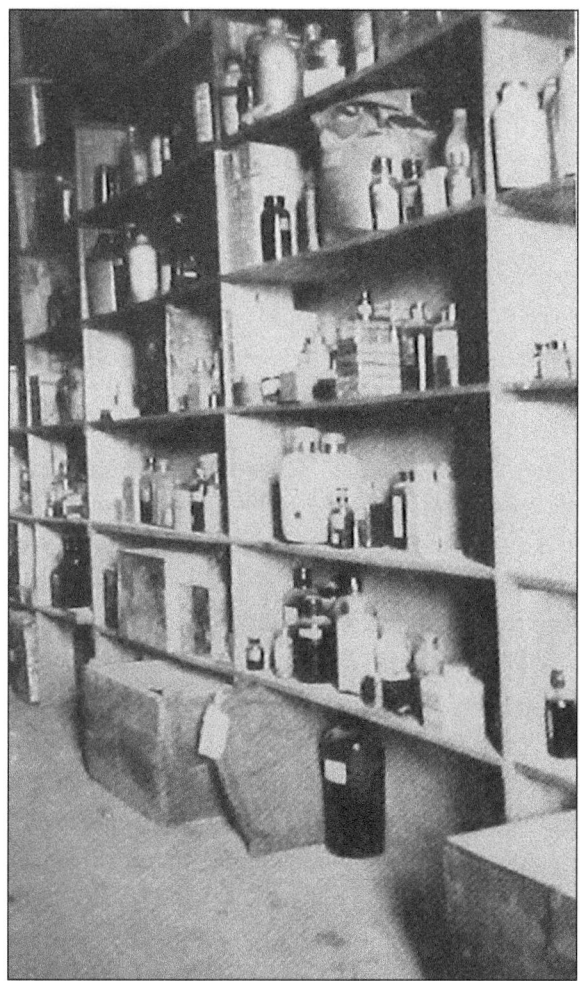

the ward saw her and exclaimed, "Why Seeb-gul! The people in our village think you are dead; someone came here and asked for you and a nurse told him that there was no one by that name here." She had borrowed a friend's card, bearing the name of Gulabtoon.

Poulos would sometimes find that he already had a name card with some new patient's name and data; he would point the finger at that man and say –"Why didn't you tell me you were here last year?" The man would tremble and mutter – "This man can read my thoughts!" Newborn babies may not be given a name until they have been taken to the public bath, or may be given a temporary name until their circumcision at four or five years of age. Jewish folks usually had two names, one Moslem, one Jewish. This was because a couple of hundred years ago, they had been persecuted and forced to profess Islam, hence they were called Jadeeds (new ones). Some women changed their first names as well as their family names when they married. Some took the husband's name, some kept their father's, others even took entirely new names. But most patients treasured their identification cards, so that as the years passed, the records increased in value, the hospital's statistics became accurate and even a new doctor or nurse could know the patient's history. Iranian doctors would send notes, asking about their patients who had been in the hospital, saying we had the only reliable records in Meshed.[747]

The American doctors were trying to limit the number of new outpatients to 20 or 40/day, depending on the number of doctors 'sitting.' In addition, there were 70-100 return visits, making a total of 90-150 with three doctors working. Dr. No-ee [Nu'i?] did the return visits that were referred to him.[748] Often Hoffman was working till sunset, seeing sometimes up to 200 cases. Some 50 of these received return treatment, while a few were admitted to the hospital, usually for an operation and then they had to bargain how much they were able to pay. Many patients were half-starved from poverty or by following the wrong diet, "abstaining from certainly supposedly 'wind-producing' foods, from 'hot' or 'cold' foods, instead if making a logical attempt to get enough of the right kind of food, and ignoring vitamins."[749]

One of the objectives of the record and the ticket system was to better manage, i.e. to reduce the number of patients. This worked to a certain extent, but sometimes the three dispensary days were a nightmare for the lone doctor, for even when there were two they had to refuse patients. In fact, in July 1945, Hoffman closed the dispensary for one month to take a breather, for even with the 'obstacle race' to the dispensary there were always more patients than he could see. Patients started coming in the early morning. After chapel, Hoffman did rounds of his >50 in-patients, gave nurses instructions to that day's treatments and dismissals, and then there were already some 500

---

747. RG 231-1-6, Hoffman, Pioneering in Meshed, pp. 117-18.
748. RG 91-20-2, Mashhad Medical Report 1932-1933.
749. RG 91-20-2, Mashhad Medical Report 1944-45. "The waiting crowds are enormous and some people have to wait till the afternoon; we have made this less confusing with the system of tickets. The ticket seller has to be astute, can the patient pay 1 or more Rls." RG 91-20-2, Mashhad Medical Report 1939-1940.

people waiting, of whom 110 were patients. It was quite normal that each patient was accompanied by 3-5 relatives and/or friends. They filled the waiting rooms and the large porch and flowed over into the yard. In the driveway, cars and vehicles were waiting. Tickets were sold to collect fees in advance, records were issued, while several hospital employees tried to keep some order. The card had to be shown to verify that fees had been paid, which were raised to 240 rials ($7.50) in 1942; several more paid 100 rials after having waited for several days. Many come from faraway places. The poor had to wait till the end- 7 to 8 hours; many had brought lunch and ate on the grass. While the first patient was sitting in the doctor's office, the next half-dozen were already in the hall between his office and the waiting room, whose doors were locked. Even here the routine was regimented.

> When we ring the bell for another patient, the servant in the hall opens the door and sends one in. In his hand is his history-record, dated, the prescription blank also dated, and the 'ticket' for the fee he has paid. On the record are also written a few salient facts as to the patient's age, sex, marital status, and address. Polus also keeps the record of the hospital in-patients, and has the months' and years' statistics in order at all times.[750]

Once the patients had seen the doctor, s/he was handed over to the assistants and nurses in the dispensary, who took care of giving injections, dressing wounds, weighing patients, and preparing them for special exams. The lab tech did the general run of exams, and the druggist carefully and promptly filled the prescriptions, using as far as possible stock formulas to save his and the doctor's time. In total there were some 15 workers in the dispensary from 7 a.m. till 4-5 p.m.[751]

---

750. RG 91-20-2, Mashhad Medical Report 1942-1943. Hoffman wrote about his record clerk Polus, who spoke Russian, Turkish, Assyrian, Persian and English, so that the record system would be less without him.

751. RG 91-20-2, Mashhad Medical Report 1942-1943 (Ali Soheyl the business manager bargained and collected the fees.)

Hoffman's hospital staff was essential to enable him to do his work and they relieved him of many activities and thus, saved him time. In 1944-45, an average of about 180 patients per day was seen. Of these, 50-75 were seen by the locally trained dresser Ajari. These were patients on the mend or merely needed their ulcers of post-op wounds dressed, or were old patients with chronic conditions, who received an injection or other remedies that Ajari could order. Besides these, during office hours, he took care of people for extraction of infected tooth roots, tapping of ascites, putting on splints or removal of plaster casts, taking of blood pressure, and incision of abscesses. On OR days, Ajari did the operations for in-turned eyelashes-entropion and various other minor operations, besides giving general anesthesia -chloroform or ether- or sometime the intravenous pentothal sodium; in the afternoons he went to the leper village to supervise work there. Another 405 out-patients were seen by Dr. Hakim-A`la, who brought Hoffman half a dozen patients for consultation. The rest were seen by Hoffman, while the graduate nurses were helping with weighing patients, taking temps, preparing women for special exams, dressing wounds and giving injections. The lab tech examined blood for malaria and relapsing fever, of which there was an epidemic in 1945-46; counting blood cells and taking specimens for serological tests to be done next day. Another male dresser was busy giving the 100 or 200 or more injections, which the doctors had ordered, and carried out special treatments assigned to him. The pharmacist and his helper were busy dispensing medicines ordered and gave instruction how to use and apply them. The record clerk registered everybody, got their old histories, saw to it that they had paid their fees as he collected the tickets sold to them by the *farrash*. The steward bargained with those who needed operations and in-patient care, collected their fees, took the kitchen accounts, answered telephone calls and attended the business affairs of the hospital.[752]

In short, the record keeping was a stimulus for more careful work and helped the doctors preparing the monthly report for the Health Department. Also, the record system systematized the work

---

752. RG 91-20-2, Mashhad Medical Report 1945-1946.

of dispensary and hospital. Those with puzzling symptoms were kept for observation in the hospital of which a record was kept, which were of permanent cumulative value. More and more patients valued these records and cooperated in keeping them.[753] Not only patients appreciated the records, but so did local Iranian doctors, who would send Hoffman notes asking about their patients, who had been to the hospital, saying the Christian hospital had the only reliable records in Mashhad.[754]

Operations

The emphasis on preventive care did not mean a reduction in curative care. On the contrary, the number of patients only increased, in particular of surgical cases. This was only an expected development, because 'The Mission's American Hospital was the only place where surgery was done; there were no Persian surgeons.'"[755] In fact, even as late as 1936, there was only one other surgeon in the whole of Khorasan.[756] The increase in the number of operations was due to a change in patients' attitude towards operations. At first, it was difficult to persuade them to have an operation, although Dr. Hoffman from the very beginning of his sojourn in Mashhad did quite a few of them. In December 1915 he wrote that: "Dr. Cook left on 11 November 1915; I came of 4 October and since his departure I did 29 cataract operations, in total 60 operations, about 30 major ones, not counting trachoma, abscesses, etc.[757] In July 1920 he reported that the men's ward was full and that he was doing 10-12 operations/week.[758]

There were two problems that needed to be resolved before surgical work would increase and be more successful. The first one was the fact that there was insufficient and competent medical staff in Khorasan, or for that matter in the entire country. There were old

---

753. RG 91-20-2, Mashhad Medical Report 1935-1936.
754. RG 231-1-6, Hoffman, Pioneering in Meshed, p. 118
755. RG 231-1-6, Hoffman, Pioneering in Meshed, p. 31
756. RG 91-20-2, Mashhad Medical Report 1935-1936; Idem, Mashhad Medical Report 1944-45.
757. RG 231-1-2, Hoffman to Friends, Tehran, 26/12/1915.
758. RG 231-1-2, Hoffman to parents, 25/07/1920.

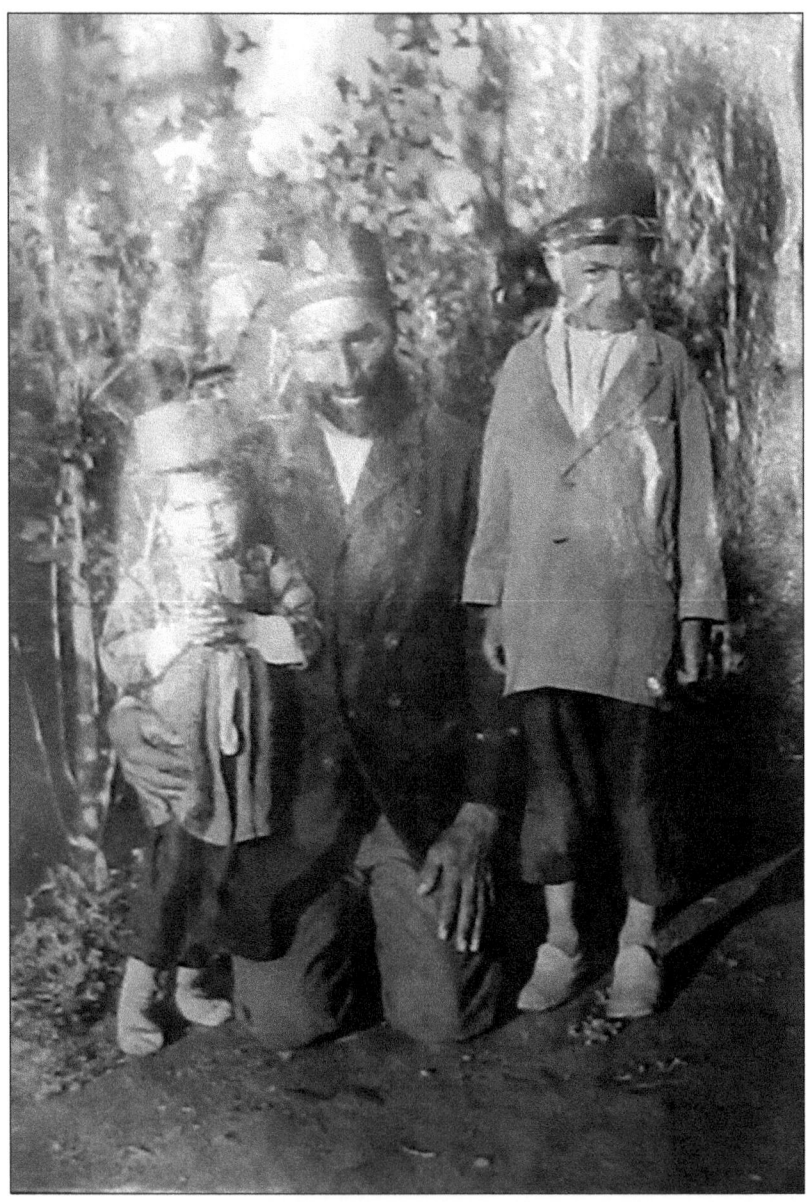

Above: Kerbela'i Hoseyn, hospital servant for 14 years with his 2 boys. *Opposite, top:* Ajari, lab technician. *Opposite bottom:* Employees of the American Hospital, Mashhad, 1934.

Hospitals in Qajar & Pahlavi Iran • 1794–1950

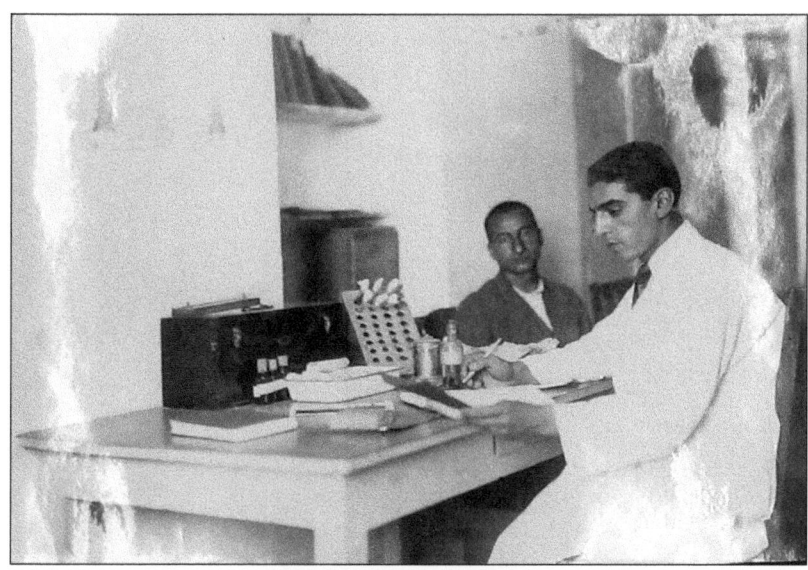

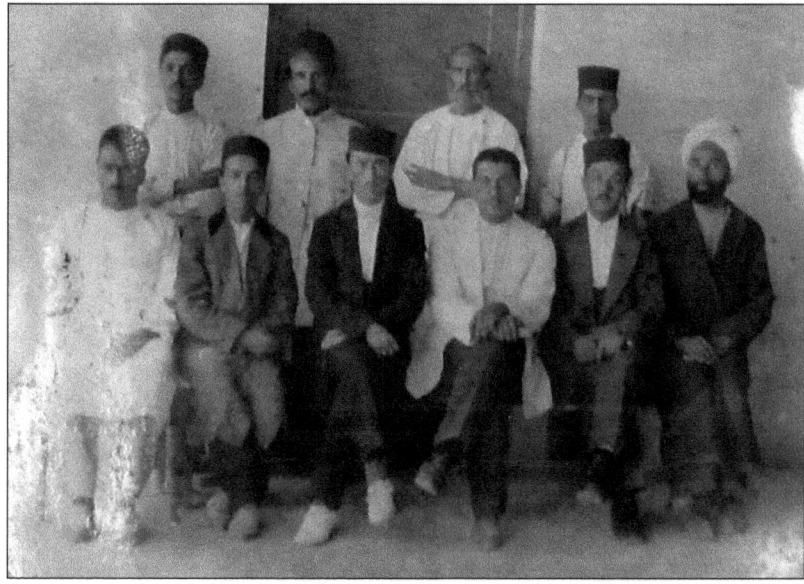

hakims or herb doctors and a "dozen with a smattering of modern

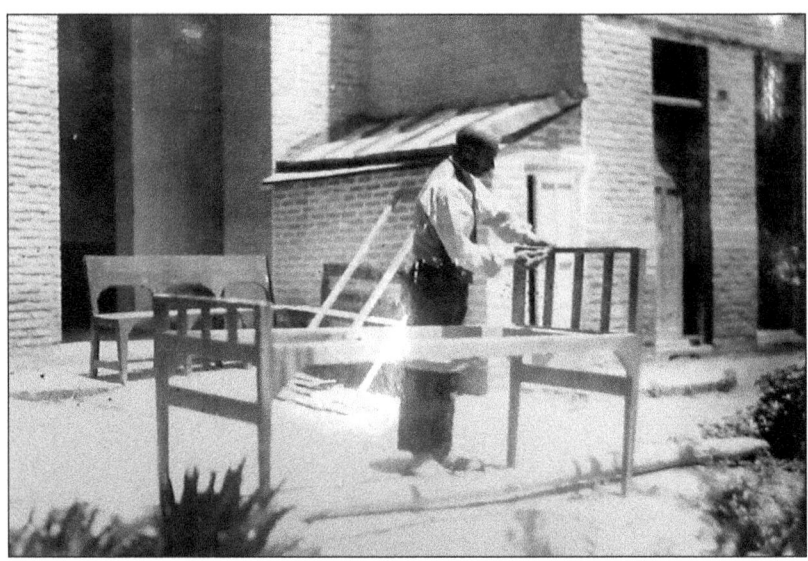

Above: Ali the carpenter makes wooden bed-steads, 1930s.
Opposite American hospital Mashhad laundry at work.

medicine."[759] In October 1920, Dr. Hoffman reported that, "Yesterday at the Shrine Hospital the new Persian doctor amputated a man's leg, who died shortly afterward. This was the new doctor's first operation in Mashhad and the third amputation done there, each by a different doctor, and all the patients died; a mortality of 100%! It is good for us, but to-day I had 161 patients more than we can properly can handle with current staff."[760] The lack of trained Iranian surgeons was a major problem, even in Tehran. In the summer of 1936, three students of the University of Tehran worked with the Christian Hospital in Mashhad for credit in surgery, for there was a shortage of surgery in Tehran.[761] This remained a persistent problem, for in 1945-46, Dr. Hakim-A`la worked for nine months in Mashhad and assisted in the OR, because surgical training in Tehran university was sketchy. He took over most tonsillectomies, pneumo-thorax refills, tuberculous

---

759. RG 231-1-6, Hoffman, Pioneering in Meshed, p. 37.
760. RG 231-1-2, incomplete letter Hoffman to Speer, October 1918.
761. RG 231-1-6, Hoffman, Pioneering in Meshed, p. 123.

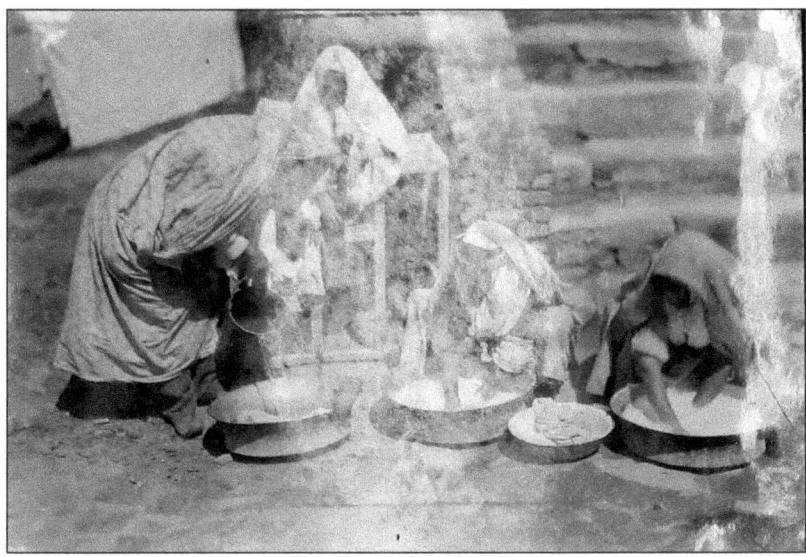

glands, removal of small tumors and other minor operations.[762] The second main problem was that, because of their reluctance to have an operation, people came late, "partly due to fatalism, partly due to lack of confidence in doctors in general, mainly due to their ignorance of the urgency of the symptoms."[763] Moreover, the patients' problems often were made worse by the quacks they went to see first, before going to the dispensary.[764]

By 1929 the number of operations was increasing. Since 1924 over 2,600 major operations and 11,000 minor operations were done.[765] In 1936, Dr. Hoffman was kept very busy. He wrote to his mother: "I usually have 2 to 5 major operations each operating day, in addition to several minors- some of which are not so small at that."[766] Also, due to an increase of equipment, the US doctors were able to do more. Having seen other patients being relieved by surgery, more patients also demanded that intervention. The use of local and spinal

---

762. RG 91-20-2, Mashhad Medical Report 1945-1946.
763. Presbyterian Church 1921, pp. 337-38.
764. RG 91-20-2, Mashhad Medical Report 1930-1931.
765. RG 91-20-2, Mashhad Medical Report 1932-1933.
766. RG 231-1-2, Hoffman to Mother, 14/06/1936

anesthesia made that operations were more popular than when done under general anesthesia.[767] Conditions in the OR also improved. "The sepsis in the OR is reliable, post op care can be relied upon, dressings are done without cross-infection, and over-worked doctors are relieved of much worry."[768]

Most operations were of a minor nature such as trachoma and its complications, mainly entropies, in-turned eyelashes scratching the cornea. Further, allegedly infertile women, whose husband threatened to divorce them; unmarriageable girls "because of 'tender' eyes or sores of faces or scalp, showing their blemishes with many blushes." Many were urged to come to the hospital in Mashhad for operations (hernia, stones, tumors, harelip). These minor operations were a major thing for the sufferer, who, if s/he became blind had to beg. There also were traditional alternative eye operations. "Women with small forceps pull out the offending hairs for temporary relief. One local doctor operates by pulling up a fold of skin of the upper eyelid and tying it between two stick so that the sins sloughs off and the scar pulls the lid away from the cornea. He watched us operate, and we sold him a few instruments, which we trust will help his technique. Mirza Loghman did 260 of the 415 lids operated on this trip."[769] Doctors also had to be inventive to get the tools they needed. For example, a set of Thomas splints was made by a local iron maker, so that broken arms and legs could be splinted without delay.[770]

Conditions in the OR were somewhat unusual. The steaming samovar was its hot water source. Initially, patient's relatives were allowed in the OR. However, by 1930, Hoffman and Lichtwardt tried to persuade them that it was better to stay out. They were unable to do away with it entirely, because "when something is taken out from the

---

767. RG 91-20-2, Mashhad Medical Report 1928-1929.
768. RG 91-20-2, Mashhad Medical Report 1945-1946.
769. RG 231-1-6, Hoffman, Pioneering in Meshed, pp. 78-79.
770. RG 231-1-6, Hoffman, Pioneering in Meshed, p. 71.

patients his relatives want to see and even keep it from teeth, bladder stones to TB glands and tonsils."[771]

MASJED-E SOLEYMAN

In 1914, the APOC established one of the most modern hospitals in the Middle East, in the Fields (near Meydan-e Naft), as it had been known for a long time, which later developed into the town of Masjed-e Soleyman. This was part of a comprehensive hospital construction and health development program led by Dr. Young. The Fields hospital had a capacity of 88 beds (administrative staff 27; workmen 57 plus two beds for European ladies and another ward for two beds for clerks' wives), a dispensary, two operating rooms (one for septic, the other for aseptic cases), a laboratory, and a radiology unit. The number of patients treated in the Fields numbered more than 128,000 in 1926.

Table 25: Number of patients treated and of activities undertaken in the Fields APOC hospital (1926).

Activity	Number
Hospital in-patients	1,666
Out-patients (a) new cases	38,270
(b) attendances	88,913
Major operations	290
Minor operations	1,378
Pathological examinations	6,039
Dental cases	607
X-ray photographs	483

Source: Williamson 1927, pp. 127-128

In the Fields, the APOC employed a senior medical officer, two resident medical officers, a visiting medical officer, a consulting surgeon, a pathologist, and an ophthalmologist. These were assisted by 26 local nurses under a European matron with by eight European

---

[771]. RG 91-20-2, Mashhad Medical Report 1930-1931 (A cataract operation for a wealthy Persian cost 50 *tuma*ns).

nurses.[772] In 1942, the AIOC hospital was air cooled with 70 beds, which could be extended to 100. It had X-ray equipment and a pathology lab.[773]

Mohammerah

Mohammarah had an estimated population of 25,000 after the Great War[774] and no medical institutions until the establishment of a charitable dispensary by the British government. It is unclear when this took place, but most likely it must have been around 1908. It was run by the Quarantine medical officer for the government of India. The annual cost was 150 rupees plus the cost of free medicines. In 1909 it was open to the public throughout the year.[775] In 1911, 242 patients were treated monthly. There was a severe outbreak of cholera in July, while malaria was epidemic, representing 11% of the cases seen in the dispensary. Eye diseases were also prevalant, such as corneal opacitus, etropion, cataract, etc. Many children suffered from ophthalmia and 14% of patients were eye cases. Venereal diseases were 7%, but it was estimated that 50% was a fair estimate for its incidence among the urban population. Skin diseases 6%; respiratory diseases (sub-acute and chronic bronchitis) 5%; rheumatic affections 3%, TB 15%.[776] The dispensary clearly satisfied a felt need as the growing number of visits indicates (See Table 26).

Table 26: Number of out-patients treated at the Mohammarah British dispensary

---

772. Isolation hospitals for quarantine purposes were also maintained by APOC. Williamson 1927, pp. 123-128; Shahri 1374, pp. 320-321; Gilmour 1924, p. 39.
773. IOR/L/MIL/17/15/24, 'Military Report on Oilfield Area', p. 49.
774. Administration Report 1919, p. 10.
775. Administration Report 1909, p. 38.
776. The annual dispensary cost were 150 Rupees plus free medicines, Administration Report 1909, p. 38; Administration Report 1911, p. 67. For a discussion of the most common diseases and their frequency as well as of the lack of hygiene in the town, see Administration Report 1912, p. 65; Idem 1913, p. 86.

(1911-1925).

Year	Outdoor patients
1911	2,209
1912	3,395
1913	4,275
1921	>5,500
1924	>4,000
1925	3,800

Source: Administration Report 1913, p. 86; Idem., 1921, p. 38; Idem., 1924, p. 49; Idem., 1925, p. 60.

For the years between 1913 and 1924 the British reports only mention that the dispensary was "well attended."[777]

Table 27: The common diseases treated in the Mohammarah British dispensary (1911-1913).

Disease/year	1911	1912	1913
All diseases	2,909	3,395	4,275
Malarial fever	213	312	415
Eye Diseases	430	491	618
Skin Diseases	182	265	280
Digestive system	272	487	683
Venereal	212	220	307
Total named diseases	1,309 (45%)	1,775 (52%)	2,303 (54%)

Source: Administration Report 1913, p. 86; see also Ibid., 1912, p. 65 ("Eye diseases are exceedingly common. 66 minor operations were performed.").

Given the rising demand for medical services, the establishment of a hospital was proposed. This plan was put in jeopardy when in 1913 the medical officer left. The British consul commented, this "has been very unfortunate since not the least of the methods which we should employ to mark our predominance and to extend our

---

777. Administration 1914, p. 36; Idem, 1916, p. 53; Idem, 1918, p. 42; Idem, 1919, p. 43; Idem, 1920, p. 40; Idem, 1923, p. 62.

influence is by the erection of a Hospital. It is to be trusted that His Majesty's Government will realize the importance of this point." He further noted that despite this set-back, the plans for a hospital were being submitted.[778] The enthusiasm for the hospital was tempered by the outbreak of WWI, for "Owing to the disturbed state of the country no progress was made with the proposal to build a hospital. The dispensary maintained by the Government continued to do good work staffed by Quarantine Medical officer."[779] In 1916, it is reported that the "Charitable Dispensary in the town continued to be well attended." This may have been partly due to an outbreak of cholera and plague during that year.[780] There also were British and Indian Convalescent Depots at Mohammarah since 1916. The Imperial Bank of Persia offered its accountant's house as a hospital, which the medical authorities accepted. As a result, this building began to be used as hospital on 1 July 1917 under the charge of Assistant Surgeon K.S. Dick, who was replaced by Civil Surgeon Captain T.H. Bishop, IMS on 11 September.[781] In 1918, the charitable dispensary continued to be well attended. There was an outbreak of the plague as well of the Spanish influenza from the beginning of October until the end of November, which resulted in a considerable loss of life among the population.[782] The dispensary continued to be well attended in 1919; in June-August some cases of the plague occurred.[783]

---

778. Administration Report 1913, p. 86.
779. Administration Report 1914, p. 36.
780. Ass. Surgeon C.H. Lincoln was the quarantine officer, Administration Report 1916, p. 53.
781. Administration Report 1917, pp. 36; Administration Report 1916, p. 52. The British convalescent depot was closed as per 1 December 1918, but the Indian one was continued. Administration Report 1918, p. 41. It was closed and moved to Basra in April 1919, Administration Report 1919, p. 43.
782. Administration Report 1918, p. 42. Captain Kirk, RAMC relieved Captain Bishop, IMS as civil surgeon Arabistan, until November Major Napier, IMS was appointed. Both also acted as assistant political officers. Idem, p. 39.
783. Administration Report 1919, p. 43; Administration Report 1920, p. 40; Administration Report 1922, p. 40.

In 1921, Hajj Ra'is al-Tojjar, C.I.E., a leading merchant, had started to build a 20-bed hospital in Mohammerah for the use of the local population, with adequate accomodation for the European and clerical staff of local firms in case of an emergency. The APOC donated the entire equipment of the hospital. Sheikh Khaz`al "generously agreed to endow this Hospital in perpetuity on a scale adequate for its needs." The hospital, which was named in his honor *Aqdasiyeh*, was formally opened by Sardar-e Aqdas (Sheikh Khaz`al) on 8 January 1923. The hospital board consisted of the British vice-consul (president and secretary), the general manager of APOC, the manager of the IBP and Hajji Ra'is al-Tojjar. The hospital was managed by Dr. A. Dias.[784] In 1924, the Charitable Dispensary treated over 4,000 out-patients, amongst which 40 cases of plague and 26 cases of cholera.[785] In 1925, it treated about 3,800 out-patients.[786] There is no further information available on this dispensary, but its function seems to have been taken over by the dispensary established by the APOC in Mohammarah.[787]

In 1942, there was an Iranian hospital near the city with 50 beds. The building was new and reportedly clean and sanitary. In association with the hospital of Masjed-e Soleyman, it maintained dispensaries at: Tembi, Meydan-e Naftun, Chasm-e Ali and Haft Kel.[788]

QAZVIN

In 1898, American missionaries were the first to offer modern medical treatment to the population of Qazvin, a town of some 40,000 inhabitants. The fact that this medical work was done by two women, Ms Dale and Ms Bartlett, be it under the supervision of Dr. Bedrosian, one of the graduates of the Urmiyeh medical school, was quite remarkable for Iran in those days.[789] In 1902, Dr. Jessie Wilson from

---

784. Administration Report 1923, p. 60-61, 62; Gilmour 1924, p. 30.
785. Administration Report 1924, p. 49.
786. Administration Report 1925, p. 60.
787. Williamson 1927, p. 129.
788. IOR/L/MIL/17/15/24, 'Military Report on Oilfield Area', p. 49.
789. Presbyterian Church 1899 pp. 188, 191.

Hamadan went permanently to Qazvin. In 1904, she married Dr. E. T. Lawrence, then in Rasht, and both were assigned to Qazvin.[790] After their marriage, Dr. and Mrs. Dr. E.T. Lawrence continued the dispensary in Qazvin. It was situated in the center of the town, near the post-house and hotel.[791] The dispensary was open daily, except Sundays, where the Lawrences treated many women and men. They reported that a large number of out-patients visited their dispensary. In addition to medical treatment, the Lawrences also tried to convert Moslems to Christianity, but this did not prevent that "even mullahs call us to their homes."[792] Apart from preaching and treating people in his dispensary, Dr. Lawrence also spent much of 1906 itinerating in the city's environing villages.[793] In 1907, to make their work place more appealing to visitors, the Lawrences cleaned the old dispensary building and made it more sanitary. Many of the local Armenians frequented the dispensary and they also asked Dr. Lawrence to make house calls. He was also asked to go to Bakandeh, where there was a large Russian colony that was engaged in road making.[794] In 1909 the Lawrences returned to the US on furlough, but in 1912 they returned and immediately opened a dispensary in Qazvin.[795] As before their furlough, the dispensary was open every day of the week, except Sunday. Because this time Dr. Lawrence was better equipped than before 1908 medical work was done more efficiently. This also meant that his income from medical fees, although small, was higher than before.[796] However, Dr. Lawrence ran his dispensary to get a crowd and to be able to preach, because he preferred preaching to medical

---

790. Presbyterian Church 1903, p. 249. Dr. Lawrence had arrived in Iran the previous year. Idem, p. 246.
791. Wishard 1908, p. 80; Grothe 1911, p. 131; Funk 1920, p. 142; Richter 1910, p. 322; Presbyterian Church 1919, p. 260; Idem 1920, p. 314; Speer - Russell 1922, p. 348.
792. Presbyterian Church 1905, p. 276.
793. Presbyterian Church 1906, p. 293.
794. Presbyterian Church 1907, pp. 306-07.
795. Presbyterian Church 1912, p. 356.
796. Presbyterian Church 1913, p. 318.

work.[797] In 1917, the Lawrences had dispensary work six days a week, during which time the Gospel was preached to the waiting patients. Dr. Lawrence often made itinerations and after his evangelic work in the villages he held an open dispensary during which he wrote 3,500 prescriptions; receipts were less than 1 *qran* per piece, so his receipts amounted to about 300 *tumans*.[798] However, as of April 1918, the dispensary was 'temporarily' closed due to lack of staff, but it was still closed in 1922,[799] and the Presbyterian annual reports don't mention any missionary activity, medical or otherwise, in Qazvin after the 1918 closure of the dispensary.

The Russian Road Company established the first modern, though small, hospital in Qazvin, which took care of the medical problems of its staff. In 1923, when its assets were transferred to the government of Iran, the Tehran municipality wanted to transfer all its equipment to Tehran, against which the population of Qazvin protested. Nevertheless, despite assurances to the contrary the transfer took place.[800] The Russian government had established an additional Zemsky Zayust hospital in Qazvin at the beginning of World War I, when the Russian army transformed the Sepahdar mansion in Qazvin into a hospital. The Russian Orthodox Sisters of Compassion managed it till 1918, when the Russians left they handed it over to the British.[801] It would

---

797. Hoffman 1916, p. 589.
798. Presbyterian Church 1918, p. 281.
799. Wishard 1908, p. 80; Grothe 1911, p. 131; Funk 1920, p. 142; Richter 1910, p. 322; Presbyterian Church 1919, p. 260; Idem 1920, p. 314; Speer - Russell 1922, p. 348.
800. Varjavand 1377, vol. 2, p. 1822.
801. Teymuri 1363, pp. 269-271; Elgood 1951, p. 512; Varjavand 1377, vol. 3, pp. 1818, 1822; Presbyterian Church 1918, p. 281. On 12 February 1916 American Red Cross medical staff left to Qazvin where a Red-Cross hospital had been established. Here they treated a woman who had just been married and had tried to commit suicide with large doses of opium and strychnine. Her husband had whipped her, which she resented. He said that "he beat all his wives once per month whether they needed it or not just to show them their place." History of American Red Cross Nursing. American National Red Cross. Nursing Service– 1922, pp. 159-60.

appear that the British had established a military hospital in Qazvin as well, which, by early 1919, was empty.⁸⁰²

In 1917, at the initiative of Hajj Mohammad ʿAli Amini, the Amini Hospital (*mariz-khaneh-ye Amini*) was built in Qazvin. It had 25-30 beds and a dispensary. For the operational cost Hajj Mohammad Ali Amini had endowed some villages to the hospital. Although the hospital was practically moribund after 1919, due to mismanagement by the founder's sons, it continued to function till 1927. By that time, due to insuffcient endowment funds to keep it operational and needed repairs it was take over by the State.⁸⁰³

Qom

As one would expect, there was a *dar al-shafa* attached to the shrine of Fatimah in Qom, a town of about 30,000 inhabitants, which was visited by Mozaffar al-Din Shah in 1903.⁸⁰⁴ This may have been the same as the one built, or perhaps renovated, by Fath ʿAli Shah (r. 1797-1834), north of the Feyziyeh madraseh, for the use of travelers and pilgrims of the shrine. Fath ʿAli Shah had assigned the income of a village for the annual wages of a physician and surgeon, who had to treat ailing pilgrims and travelers. It is not known when, but later the hospital was transformed into a madraseh and dormitory for theological students, which, of course, was called *madraseh-ye dar al-shafa*.⁸⁰⁵ At least in 1849, an infirmary still existed at the shrine at Qom, when Abbott visited the shrine city and reported that: "A small annual allowance was formerly made from the revenues of the country for the maintenance of this establishment." Abbott continues, "but at

---

802. Griscom 1921, p. 239.
803. Varjavand 1377, vol. 3, p. 1820; Ebrahimnejad 2014, p. 159; Rezai 2012, pp. 123-24 (partial text of the endowment deed).
804. *Ruznameh-ye soltani va Iran* 1380, p. 156 (11 Ramadan 1321/1 December 1901)
805. Ṭabaṭabaʾi 2535, vol. 1, pp. 28-30; vol. 2, p. 140; Hedayat 1338-39, vol. 10, p. 106. Whether in the same building or in a new one, but there still seems to have been a *dar al-shafa* in Qom at a later date. Rostaʾi 1382, vol. 2, p. 199,

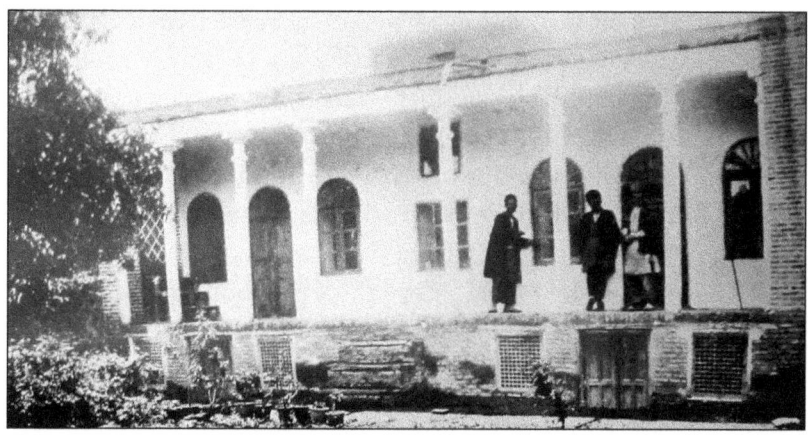

American dispensary at Qazvin, 1912.

present, beyond the accommodation afforded by the bare apartments, there is no provision for distress and sickness."[806] There also existed a charitable hopital (*bimarestan-e sehamiyeh*) in Qom, probably as of the early 1920s. It had been built by Ayatollah Hajj Sheikh Abdol-Karim Ha'eri from the charitable funds sent to him; initially it only had 12 beds.[807]

Rafsanjan

In 1945, a new hospital was opened in Rafsanjan for the poor. The governor of Kerman "made many attempts to raise the funds for their treatment."[808]

Rasht

In the fall of 1903, Dr. and Mrs. Schuler began educational and evangelistic work in Rasht, then a town of some 40,000 inhabitants. At the same time, Dr. N. T. Lawrence was also assigned to Rasht for medical

---

806. Abbott 1855, p. 9. Louise de la Marnierre, who visited the *Dar al-Shafa* in 1836, does not mention the presence of any patients or medical care in the building. Calmard 2019, p. 240.
807. *Ruznameh-ye Ettela'at* 1329, p. 57; Tajbakhsh 1379, pp. 245-246.
808. Administration Report 1945, p. 8.

work, but, after his marriage in 1904, he was transferred to Qazvin.[809] Lawrence was not the only physician in the city, because in addition to a few other foreign physicians, there were traditional Iranian medical practitioners, and in 1903, there also was a non-traditional Iranian physician in Rasht, who was married to a Swedish woman. He had worked for the Swedish mission in Turkistan and had received his training in an Iranian hospital and the Shah's college (presumably the Dar al-Fonun) in Tehran. Nevertheless, the inexperienced and youthful governor of Rasht Prince Abu'l-Fazl Mirza Azod al-Soltan, the governor of Rasht (1903-06), asked Schuler to send him an American physician.[810] Like the rest of the country, Rasht was also ravaged by the cholera epidemic of 1904. The Schulers could not do much but provide help to those afflicted, although Mrs. Schuler had some experience in hospital work and had a small supply of drugs and helped cholera sufferers. She also handed out the booklet written in Persian by Dr. Wishard of the American mission hospital in Tehran about what to do to prevent cholera and how to treat cholera patients. In Rasht this booklet seems to have had some impact. Because afterwards, Mrs. Schuler saw a change in the attitude of the local people towards the missionaries, "for as we walked through the bazaars we could but note the changed attitude of many; and again when later the little children in the streets, who had formerly not hesitated to call out behind us 'Christian dogs' now stopped in their play to salaam profoundly as we passed."[811] In 1905, the *anjoman-e kheyriyeh* (charitable association) established a hospital in a stand-alone house that belonged to Aqa Sayyed `Ali Aqa Fumeni and his sister, and, therefore, the hospital

---

809. RG 91-19-19, "History of the Resht Station (1934), p. 1; `Eyn al-Saltaneh 1376, vol. 1, pp. 377, 865; UNESCO 1343, vol. 2, pp. 1449-1451; Elgood 1951, pp. 511-512, 534; Wishard 1908, p. 76; Waterfield 1973, p. 139; Richter 1910, p. 322. Dr. Lawrence arrived in Iran in 1902. Presbyterian Church 1903, p. 246.

810. Presbyterian Church 1904, p. 239. He was the fourth son of Mozaffar al-Din Shah. As to his lack of administrative skills and bad government, see Sepehr 1368, pt. 2, pp. 50, 164, 310, 319.

811. Presbyterian Church 1905, p. 276; RG 91-19-9, "History of Resht Station," p. 1.

was named after him. It was a two-story house; the upper level had two big rooms with each six beds. The beds were donated by wealthy notables and on each bed hung a sign with their name. The lower level served as dispensary. The hospital services (for males only) were gratis and patients, who wanted to pay, gave the money as a donation. The hospital, known as *bimarestan-e melli* or national hospital, continued to function in this way for almost three years. Because demand for hospital services grew a hospital with a larger capacity was needed. Therefore, the *anjoman-e kheyriyeh* decided to establish a second and larger hospital (see below).[812]

In that same year, at the initiative of Azod al-Soltan, the governor of Rasht, a hospital was built by subscriptions to which the governor himself donated £1,800 from his own private funds. According to an article in a British journal, "The hospital is situated in a well-chosen and healthy locality. It contains seven wards, each to accommodate ten to fifteen patients. It has [a] consulting-room, [an] operating-room, and all appliances of a modern hospital. The furniture for the place was brought from Russia."[813] Azod al-Soltan invited the American missionaries to send a physician to manage the hospital. In the fall of 1905, Dr. John D. Frame arrived and began negotiations about the terms of the management of the hospital.[814] However, the long

---

812. Ta'eb 1384, pp. 23-24; Ebrahimnezhad 2014, p.152.
813. Anonymous 1905, p. 458. Given the laudatory nature of the article it has all the trappings of an article commissioned by and ghost-written for the prince. Sepehr 1368, pt. 2, p.104. The prince may have been induced to this initiative by his chief executive (*pishkar*) and physician Dr. Mo'addab al-Dowleh Nafisi. Fakhra'i 1353, p. 32.
814. Presbyterian Church 1906 p. 293. In 1905, the *anjoman-e kheyriyeh* also had established a hospital in a two-storey house, called *Bimarestan-e Aqa Sayyed `Ali Aqa*, after the owner of the house. The beds were given by local notables, whose names were written on a note affixed to each bed. There were only male patients and the hospital had four male orderlies. At the lower level was a dispensary (*darmangah*) for patients not in need of hospital care. Local doctors in turn made their services available for a few house each day. Apparently, this hospital functioned for three years. Thereafter, the *anjoman-e kheyriyeh* moved it to a larger place, about which no further information is available. Ta'eb 1384, pp. 23-24. This hospital in not mentioned by Dr.

negotiations with local officers concerning the Government Hospital, of which the Mission had been invited to take charge, did not turn out satisfactorily. Initially, negotiations went fairly well; 1,000 *tuman*s for start-up expenditures were paid, and there was reason to believe that a 5-year contract would be soon signed, but the Russians opposed the planned arrangement and the contract could not be signed. Nevertheless, Dr. Frame opened the hospital the last of December 1906 and worked there until mid-April 1907, "the Sardar [Mansur] agreeing to furnish the expenses monthly in advance until the regular contract could be sealed." The number of patients agreed upon was 12; during these three months Dr. Frame saw 78 patients and did minor surgeries. But in April the contract was still not signed. Dr. Frame gave notice and the Sardar dismissed the patients and closed the hospital. Some days later he gave the keys to the Italian Dr. Sterlini, who had been in Rasht for some years, but had left in 1903. He was not in the country when the prince-governor began the negotiations with the American missionaries. Sterlini had returned from Europe as physician for the Russian consulate shortly prior to Dr. Frame's arrival and he had been consulted by Iranian officials and given estimates for running the hospital. After the failed negotiations, Dr. Frame continued with his own dispensary, which was right in the center of the city.[815] As far as Frame knew, at that time, the only other European physician between Rasht and Astarabad was a Greek, who resided in Mashhad-e Sar.[816] In 1908, Dr. Frame was a good part of the year in Tehran, but, when working in his dispensary in Rasht, he, at first, had to turn away some patients due to limited room, which was something that Persians didn't understand. "They think it is a confession of incompetence,"

Frame.

815. Presbyterian Church 1907, pp. 304-06; `Eyn al-Saltaneh 1376, vol. 1, pp. 377, 865; UNESCO 1343, vol. 2, pp. 1449-1451; Elgood 1951, pp. 511-512, 534; Wishard 1908, p. 76; Waterfield 1973, p. 139; Richter 1910, p. 322; RG 91-19-9, "History of Resht Station," p. 2; RG 91-19-9, "Resht Medical Work." Sardar Mansur had endowed the hospital with 4,000 *tuman*s per year. Sepehr 1368, pt. 2, pp. 50, 164, 310, 319.

816. Presbyterian Church 1908, p. 344; RG 91-19-19, "History of the Resht Station (1934), p. 2.

and so those whom we asked to return later did not. In August 1908, Dr. Frame had 47 new cases, in September 98 and over 180 return visits, or over 278 consultations. This was because Iranians thought that "fall is the most favorable time to take treatment." Dr. Frame also noted that, "It is now the exception rather than the rule for a woman to object to a proper examination of her features."[817]

American Missionary Dispensary

In 1909, the dispensary, where most work was done, had four rooms. There were separate waiting-rooms for men and women, a consultation room and a tiny drug room. During the summer, patients arrived at 6.30 a.m. and each arrival was handed a numbered card by a servant. At 7.30 a.m. Dr. Frame began his daily work with prayer in the men's room; then he saw the patients one by one. Although he had reserved three days in the week for the poor there was no sharp division between rich and poor in the waiting room. Each one had to take his or her turn and to pay what he was able for his drugs and treatment. Dr. Frame was called to assist in caring for the wounded when revolutionary forces captured the city in February 1909.[818] In the summer of 1910, Enzeli and environs again suffered an outbreak of cholera, but in Rasht it did not amount to much. The authorities asked the foreign physicians for advice but, as usual Frame comments, did nothing. The increase in the number of patients was less than Frame expected, probably because the local assembly had opened a dispensary for the poor, which was under the care of an Iranian physician for a few months. Also, there was an influx of Iranian doctors, who all advertised that they treated the poor for free. According to Frame, some of them were

---

817. Presbyterian Church 1909, pp. 347-48 (In July he was itinerating).
818. Presbyterian Church 1910, pp. 329-31 (New cases 1,008; return visits 2,570 Total during 8.5 months: 3,587 seen on trips to neighboring bazaars: 294; seen on itineration 369. Total for the year 4,250. Of those in Resht were: house calls 331; in-patients 0; minor operations 0. In fees and gifts *qran*s 6,165; for drugs: 2,375 or Total 8,540 = $780, which makes my work self-supporting. In May-June I will go itinerating.). On the capture of Rasht, see Pezhman Dailami, "Gilan viiia. In the Constitutional Revolution of 1905-11," iranicaonline.org.

fairly capable, while others were unmitigated quacks. On the whole, the quality of the local doctors was improving and Iranians were doing more for their poor than before. In the late summer and early fall of 1910 many foreign physicians were absent, which meant more dispensary and private work for Frame. In December, however, all was back to normal. Dispensary and private work continued; i.e. a free clinic three days/week and drugs at cost, and as much private work as he was able to handle. In April 1911, Frame

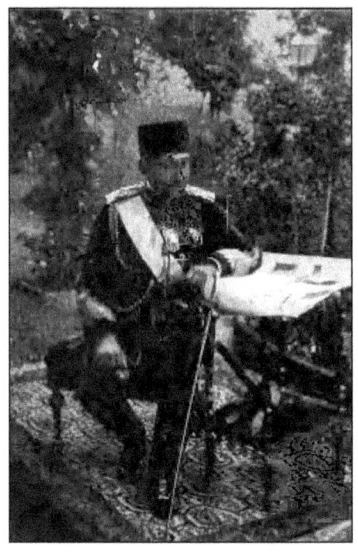

went itinerating and the US trained Dr. Tashjiantz agreed to take charge of his dispensary.[819] For the next few years Frame had a routine of dispensary, house calls and private consultations, until the fall of 1914 when he left for the USA.[820] In September 1915, Dr. Frame returned from furlough and acquired two assistants. In Baku, he had bought a piano, which was unloaded with much difficulty, while in October 1915 he married Ms Grace Murray.[821] In 1916, Frame observed that the number of doctors in the city was increasing, some of whom were of fair ability, in his opinion. Because he was a missionary and not a medical competitor, Frame didn't want just to practice like the others, but to provide services that others could not. Therefore, he offered: testing of the eyes for glasses and better ophthalmic work generally as well as better lab methods for diagnosis.[822] In 1917, Frame only treated about 300 patients, which was partly due to a serious lack of drugs.

---

819. RG 91-1-12, Report of Resht Station 1910-1911 (New cases: 2.432; return visits to see the doctor: 3,498; treatments and dressings by the assistants: 3,703 or a total of: 9.638. Of these 404 were house calls. The total for last year when we were 10 months in the city was 3,587.)

820. Presbyterian Church 1911 p. 320; RG 91-1-12, Report of Resht Station, 1910-1911; Presbyterian Church 1914, p. 332.

821. Hoffman 1916, p. 586.

822. Presbyterian Church 1917, p. 300.

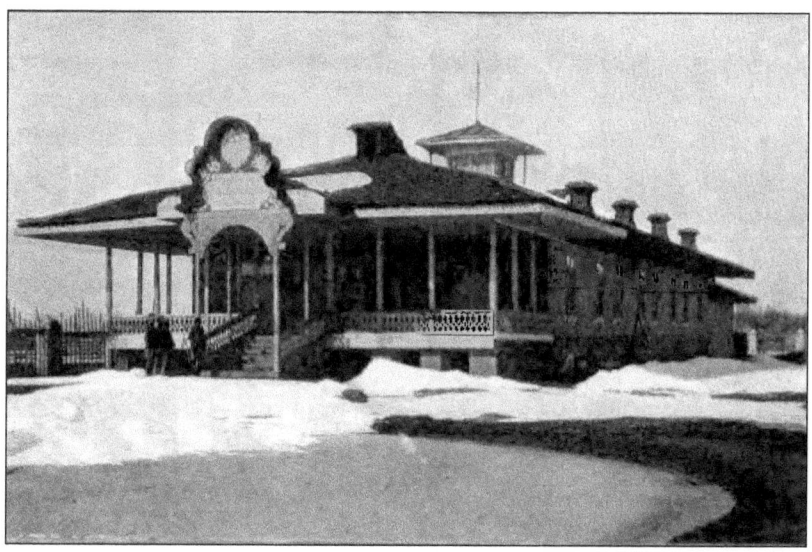

The hospital in Rasht, and its princely founder (*opposite*)

He was often demanded as a consultant and surgeon, which brought in money. He also organized a vaccine campaign for the government, which resulted in 5,000 vaccinations in two months. He also was the unofficial physician and surgeon for the Police Department.[823]

The period after the end of WW I was a hectic and troublesome one for the province of Gilan and its inhabitants. The revolutionary Jangali movement took control over much of the province, including Rasht.[824] At the same time, trade with Russia, which was the main importer of Gilan's products, was reduced to a low single digit number, due to the Bolshevik takeover. As a result, people in Gilan were poor, because there were no buyers for their goods and services, while the continued insecurity further reduced economic activity. In 1919, Frame was mainly occupied providing relief aid (see hospital section). Although fiercely nationalist, the Jangalis were friendly towards the American missionaries and even partnered with them in carrying out

---

823. Presbyterian Church 1918, p. 285; RG 91-19-9, Resht Medical Report, 10/07/1919.

824. On the Jangalis, see Pezhman Dailami, "Jangali Movement," iranicaonline.org.

relief work. The effect of the political and economic turmoil was also evident in the widely fluctuating number of patients coming to Frame's dispensary. He wrote: "In the old days when the Russian dispensary was open we had a rather select class of the more respectable poor, who wished to pay for their medicines at least." However, the Russian dispensary was gone and with the increased poverty this class was almost gone. In fact, most patients were very poor. Therefore, in larger numbers than before, he had to treat patients gratis. What was new in 1919 was the large number of Turkic speakers, who came down from the mountains, necessitating interpreters more than ever before. The dispensary was closed most of the summer of 1918. In the fall and winter, under Dr. Tashjiantz, it had an average of 35 patients/day in winter, but in the spring about 100/day. In the summer the number of patients typically rose and was a busy time, but in the summer of 1919 the Rasht dispensary was closed due to lack of funds. [825]

The number of out-patients grew, even though Frame only irregularly attended the dispensary in summer, but it grew under his assistant, Baron Hagop's supervision. In the fall, instead of decreasing, as was normal, it increased and continued to do so in winter. Usually Frame saw from 100 up to 200 patients per day. In 1919-20, Frame saw a total of 8,217 new patients and 15,195 old ones. The fall malaria epidemic continued in winter. Leprosy was also seen, and more common than usual, but no provision was made for them. Because of the availability of nurses more effective treatments were given to women. VD was "one of the most frequent the doctor has to face." During the war the newer methods were too costly, even when found, and too complicated for Frame's limited staff. But in 1919-20, neosalvaran was available (left in large quantity in the Caucasus by the Germans) and its substitutes were smuggled to Rasht at a reasonable price. Therefore, he had a syphilis treatment clinic twice week, usually treating 10-30 patients/day. A total of 935 superfascial injections of neosalvaran were given from November 1918 until June 1919, and the results seemed to justify

---

825. RG 91-19-9, "History of Resht Station," p. 2; Idem, Resht Medical Report, 10/07/1919. For an overview of the medical staff helping the Jangalis, see Ta'eb 1384, pp. 34-38.

the expense. Because Frame had to spend most of his time providing relief to refugees, he reduced his private practice as well as his medical care of the military. These were important decisions, because so far Frame had run his dispensary supported solely by his private practice of better class paying patients. Also, the Sanitary Council in Tehran wanted to resume public vaccinations after the defeat of the Jangalis. Frame had been chairman of the Gilan section for two years. The province was still too disturbed, but he had established two stations in Rasht and Lahejan and intended go into some mountain districts in the summer. The governor asked Frame to establish a permanent hospital for the police force, but he had to refuse given his imminent departure from Iran to go on furlough.[826] In fact, the entire American mission (consisting of Dr. and Mrs. Frame and Ms Amerman, who ran the school) left Rasht in 1920 on furlough. The Frames returned in the late summer of 1921.[827] During 1921-22, Frame saw an average of 100 patients per day during three days/week in the winter and 50/60 patients/day in the spring. He came to the conclusion that you could not adequately treat 100 patients in an afternoon, "But it is easy as a rule to recognize tuberculosis and impossible to offer an effective program for treatment of a man who supports a family on 25 c a day." [828]

In the out-patient department the problem was that patients came once or twice, but Dr. Frame was unable to follow up whether they had been cured or not. There was also the problem that patients were unaccustomed to modern medicines. One woman refused internal treatment; she wanted an injection as before; after the first injection her problem had disappeared and therefore, she wanted the injections like the previous time. She felt she had to come back as it had worked so easy. Therefore, Frame realized that he had to educate not only his medical assistants, but also his patients. "Given so much ignorance, poor social conditions and insufficient medical care education aimed

---

826. RG 91-19-9, Report Medical Work 1919-20; Idem, "History of Resht Station," p. 2.
827. RG 91-19-9, Resht Medical Report 1923-24.
828. RG 91-19-9, Medical Report Resht 1921-22; Idem, Report Medical Work 1919-20.

at setting standards training helpers and leading the people themselves to understand the possibilities of better care for themselves." Because there were less out-patients, Frame had more time for those who came and record keeping. "We find the number of cases, carefully recorded varies inversely to the total attendance. The records showed 2,176 new cases and 7,624 total visits."[829]

In August 1923, Dr. Frame gave up the rented building in which he held his free dispensary, because he had no place until the new hospital was ready in March 1924.[830] Although Frame was of the opinion that the hospital-dispensary should be closed in summer and the staff be given a vacation during July-August, the dispensary was kept open throughout the summer in 1926-27 and there was a fair amount of work. On 22 October 1926, Dr. Brinkman arrived and Frame left on 12 April 1927 on furlough. During that overlap time they divided the work. Dr. Frame did the daily morning clinics; Brinkman took the dispensary during the three afternoons of free clinics. That year Brinkman was kept busy 30 hours/week in the clinics and operating the rest of the time.[831] A Turkish speaking boy helped the doctor in the male dispensary. One of the Armenian nurses helped with the women; a Persian speaking boy worked in the reception room, running errands, washing bottles, i.e. he was a general handyman.[832] In 1928-29, there was a slight increase in the number of out-patients, despite the free treatment at the National Hospital (the American physicians tried to charge for drugs) and because Frame was too busy to always regularly attend dispensary. In the dispensary a set of electrically lighted instruments for eye, ear and throat was daily helpful. Formerly, Frame was the only one specializing in these specialties, but a few years earlier a Russian doctor had set up a practice as a specialist. For a time, he held the field, but patients were returning to Frame and local doctors referred them to him.[833] During 1928-29, Frame and Brinkman were

---

829. RG 91-19-9, Resht Medical Report 1924-25.
830. RG 91-19-9, Resht Medical Report 1923-24.
831. RG 91-1-12, Report Resht Medical Work 1926-1927.
832. RG 91-19-9, Medical Report Resht Station 1927-1928.
833. RG 91-19-9, Resht Medical Report 1928-1929.

busier than usual, working from 1 September to 31 May and closed shop during the summer. The two doctors had seen an average of 470 patients per month, an increase of 30%, despite an increase of other hospital facilities in the city.[834] There was another change in 1930. In 1920, the American missionary dispensary was the only free one in Rasht and was flooded with 100-250 cases a day. Now there were two Iranian free dispensaries to share the burden, so that Frame could devote more time to what he called the better class poor, who could pay for drugs.[835]

Because in 1933 Dr. Brinkman, who went to Tehran relieving Dr. Blair, was absent, Dr. Frame asked Dr. Ali Khan Shafa, one of the better Iranian local doctors, to take care of the men's dispensary during his absence. He came three afternoons per week without payment. He remained in close touch with the American hospital thereafter. Frame wished he would be able to establish more such relationships with local doctors.[836] Frame went on furlough to the US in April 1935. Because Dr. Brinkman would be alone and because there was too much work for one doctor, before Frame left, they asked Dr. Shafa to take charge of the men's clinic for three days/week, but he suddenly died of typhus. He had frequently helped out in the free clinics without payment, when one of the American doctors was gone. He also did much charity work in his private practice and therefore, his Iranian colleagues had criticized him.[837]

In the spring of 1934, there a most noticeable increase in out-patients. Never before since the relief days of 1919-20 had attendance been so large at the free clinic, although most had to pay for the drugs. Tuesday, Thursday and Saturday afternoons were reserved for free consultation, and, if need be, patients returned in the morning for special treatments. During that year it was normal that the doctors saw 100 patients in one afternoon, the record was 200. Dr. Brinkman

---

834. RG 91-19-9, Resht Medical Report 1928-1929.
835. RG 91-19-9, Resht Medical Report 1929-1930.
836. RG 91-19-9, Resht Medical Report 1932-1933.
837. RG 91-19-9, Report Resht Medical Work 1934-1935.

remained in charge of the men's side and also gave special attention to chest and urinary conditions among women. Frame looked after women and children and eye, ear, and throat diseases among men. In mid-1934, Brinkman was still studying the language. At the women's side of the dispensary Miryam Khanom was the doorkeeper and interpreter; a nurse stood ready in the dressing room on one side of the office and her brother Bahram was in the lab on the other side to make urgent tests and looked after favus cases. The free clinic was

> Nothing but a clearing and sorting station. This woman
> complains about dimness of vision, watering of the mouth,
> discomfort in the stomach, and perhaps thinks she has latent
> fever. Do not stop! She is convinced that she has worms
> and will accept nothing but worm medicine. Argument
> will prove useless. Miriam Khamum gives the directions
> while the doctor meekly writes the prescription.
>   The next marshalls in three children with head disease. They
> are referred to Behram who will examine the urine, enter their
> names in his special list if the examination is favorable, weigh
> them carefully, measure out give instructions for cleaning and
> urge faithfulness in after care which is the price of success.
> The next holds out her hands as she approached. Itch!
> Scrub your hands thoroughly at night with soap and
> water and wrap them up with this ointment! Next.
> Next however is a woman who had been coughing
> six months. She must go into the next room where the
> nurse helps her remove her voluminous clothing for
> careful chest examination. She is to bring a specimen of
> sputum the next morning or is the case is urgent will be
> detained until dusk for an X-ray examination."[838]

Because Dr. Shafa had died, Dr. Vartan Oganessian, another of the better physicians in Rasht, was willing to come on Thursdays,

---

838. RG 91-19-9, Resht Medical Report 1933-1934. The report continues to describe in some detail the routine of the daily workload. The woman with the cough had to wait for the X-ray, because electricity was only available as of nightfall.

the busiest day. The other days Brinkman started earlier and saw patients as they came. In- and out-patients showed a slight decrease, because the clinic had practically no TB patients, who stayed long.[839] Sometimes the constant complaints at the free clinic overwhelmed Dr. Brinkman. Fortunately, Dr. Vartan Oganessian continued to come every Thursday afternoon, usually the heaviest day, and saw male patients. As a result, Brinkman did not feel so rushed on that day. They realized that out-patients suffered quality wise, of course.[840] In 1936-37, the doctors trained a young woman for women's dispensary work. She had entered nurses training, but left to be married. However, after the birth of her baby the spouses separated, but, as a married woman, she was not eligible for nurses training.[841] By 1938, the workload at the free dispensary (three afternoons) had grown out-of-all bounds. Under these conditions, Frame and Brinkman were unable to maintain the quality of work as desired. They did not choose to set limits to the number of patients, because then more urgent cases might be turned away. To increase efficiency they introduced individual record cards, but they had not yet found a man to take charge of the system and perhaps exercise a selection of cases.[842]

After morning rounds in the hospital, followed the dispensary.[843] During 1938-39, the doctors did a complete reorganization of the out-patients department. The change had already begun in 1937-38, with the introduction of the record system with the individual names of patients to limit inflow, because the quantity of patients hurt the quality of care. The major problem, of course, remained the selection of cases. With the limitation of the numbers, patients came earlier at 7 or 8 a.m. although the dispensary did not open till 2 p.m. They made so much noise and looked so pitiful that the doctors decided to care for them as early as possible. For financial reasons they could refuse non-paying patients, who also stood in need of their services.

---

839. RG 91-19-9, Report Resht Medical Work 1934-1935.
840. RG 91-19-9, Medical Report Resht 1935-1936.
841. RG 91-20-8. Resht Medical Report 1936-1937.
842. RG 91-19-7, Resht Hospital Report, 1937-1938.
843. RG 231-1-5, Hoffman/Rasht to Friends, 12/09/1948.

Drs. Kibbe and Frame tried to see 25-30 poor patients on the fixed three dispensary days of the week, in addition to what paying patients might come, although this still meant that poor patients had to wait till afternoon. Because the individual record system required a qualified person they employed a pharmacist, so that their first assistant could do the records, admission of patients, correspondence, etc. Also, the government demanded more data, according to its system as well as statistical reports, so this was a full-time job. Nevertheless, this assistant still remained the chief anesthetist and often helped with operations.[844]

During 1940-41, three mornings per week, the out-patient department was formally open for patients, i.e. for those who were able to pay. "On most days it is necessary to limit both paying and free patients, the covered tickets being handed out as nearly as possible in the order of arrival or pressing physical need of the patients." Almost all patients were accompanied by friends or relatives, so a group of 4-5 represented 1-2 patients. Even on free mornings paying patients came to see that doctor that day. On top of that there were also emergencies. Over 100 prescriptions were free each month. These were presented at the pharmacy of the mission hospital's former pharmacist and charged to the hospital at the end of the month, representing 3,000 rials in 1940. The rising cost of everything and the increasing poverty was expected to increase this post. Toward the west of the building, the lab and man's dressing room, there were large numbers of patients above the number of ticket holders waiting for a change of gauze, irrigation, medicine or treatment for favus. During the spring and fall women, babies and small children waited for vaccinations or confirmation of the 'take' of the vaccination. In 1939-40, 537 vaccinations were done. To the east of the dispensary was a small waiting room where women and children, also not numbered among the ticket holders, waited for hypos, douches, etc. A nurse was in charge there, but as it adjoined the doctor's office, a professional eye was kept on all cases. The lab also did outside work as it had time and equipment. Urine and feces of all hospitalized patients were routinely examined. Sputum, blood and other special tests were only done at the doctor's orders. Frame

---

844. RG 91-19-7, Resht Hospital Report 1938-1939.

was firmly convinced that without a lab they could not work. During 1940-41, a total of 2,438 lab exams were done, besides 2,200 men's dressings and 1,581 favus treatments.[845]

HOSPITAL

In mid-1909, Dr. Frame rented a small building for hospital purposes and took possession of it in July. It was 100 m from his house door. It "was a small one-story building with a whitened room for operations and two unfinished rooms and a verandah for patients." One of these unfinished rooms was for the servants and the third room accommodated 2-3 patients. On the wide verandah was place for 3-4 patients, at night once even five patients were accommodated there. He had bedding for only two patients and no kitchen, but many patients brought their own bedding and supplied their own food; for others he sent for food from the nearby bazaar.[846] In 1910, Frame's main interest was surgery and in the hospital his two beds were generally occupied, and often 2-3 patients were sleeping on the floor. During winter admissions were lower. In May 1910, he closed hospital for itinerating, because he soon had come to the realization that: "Only the poorest and most needy would go to such an institution [hospital]." Later he made efforts to make the premises more attractive and suitable, but income was insufficient to continue the hospital, without outside appropriations. In short, "The hospital was too humble to attract well-to-do patients, and we did not have the means to treat many poor unless they could furnish their own food."[847] After the departure of the Schulers in 1910, Dr. Frame, with his assistant and his wife (Deghan Yaghut) as housekeeper, moved into the Schulers' residence and transformed the former school and residence building into a hospital. Evangelical meetings were held in the parlor. Medical work demanded most of his time, which was all routine work. In the 'new' hospital he had

---

845. RG 91-19-7, Resht Hospital Report 1940-1941 (in 1939-40, a total of 3,017 cases were seen).
846. Presbyterian Church 1910, pp. 329-31 (in May-June itinerating.).
847. Presbyterian Church 1911, p. 320; RG 91-19-9, "Resht Medical Work."

seven beds in the winter. Frame gave a few patients free treatment and food, but most paid for their food or had it brought from outside; a few also paid for their room and Frame's services. Therefore, the hospital beds were never fully occupied and sometimes he had no in-patients at all. But Frame considered it a good start and a basis to continue. Even if he had the money he argued that it would not be effective to only offer free service in the hospital, although he would run a free ward. In 1911, a local Iranian hospital was opened, which was supported by a subscription of Iranians and foreigners. In the spring it burnt down and it was doubtful whether it would be rebuilt. Therefore, the need for a hospital was greater than ever. Frame hoped to rent a new building that would be more suitably located than the current one; otherwise he intended to continue as before.[848] This hope was not shared by the Presbyterian Board, because it noted that 1912 was for Dr. Frame the most disappointing year. The Board opined that it would be better "If Dr. Frame devote himself to the dispensary and itinerating work and the opening of branch drug rooms, such as the Lahijan dispensary, rather than continue to confine himself (to any locality) by establishing a hospital, the center for such work to be determined later."[849]

During WWI no effort was made to continue the hospital, although a suitable house for a hospital had been found in 1917. However, there was no money to open a hospital in the true sense of the word. With other doctors, Frame asked 100 notables what to do, but only a few replied. Therefore, he took a few private patients, who could supply their own food or pay for it, while he occasionally helped poor patients. Without nurses he could not even think about doing operations. The arrival of the Dunsterforce in mid-June 1918 resulted

---

848. RG 91-1-12 Station Reports East Persia 1910-12, Report of Resht Station 1910-1911; Presbyterian Church 1912, p. 356. This is perhaps the hospital to which Zell al-Soltan contributed in 1909. On arrival in Rasht he was arrested and only released after promising to pay 300,000 *tuman*s, of which only one-third was paid. Later he gave 12,000 *tuman*s, his monthly salary, for education (*ma'aref*) and the hospital of Rasht. Fakhra'i 1353, p. 144.

849. Presbyterian Church 1913, p. 319.

in three-days of fighting between British troops and the Jangalis in the streets. There were Jangali and civilian wounded in the hospital and there was a major threat of an Armenian massacre. The British threatened to burn the town if the Armenians were injured and the situation improved, although that was only realized afterwards. On 24 July 1918, British airplanes flew over the city and scared the Jangalis out of the city. Frame did not stop caring for the Jangalis. Later they made peace with the British and thereafter took control of the province. Throughout the winter they sent Frame their wounded, which their doctors could not treat.[850]

Meanwhile, there was no food to be had in the city, neither rice nor flour. After the fighting was over, the British offered the American missionaries transport to a less exciting place. Frame's Armenian assistant left with his family and so did his colleagues. Many other people also made preparations for flight out of fear for the expected arrival of the Turks, who were advancing on Baku. After several false alarms, Frame wanted to leave as well and started packing, while many Christians finally fled on 1 August 1918. Then the news got better and Frame opened the dispensary and tried to obtain food for the poor patients that he saw, who needed food more than medicines. Mrs. Frame fell ill and with a borrowed British motor ambulance Dr. Frame took her to Enzeli, where he could look better after her and the weather was better. He then learnt that the British had evacuated Baku in October 1918, so the Frames returned to Rasht. On his return to Rasht, Frame found a trained nurse from Van, who had fled from there, whom he hired as nurse and matron. However, she got consumption and died on her way home. Meanwhile, about 2,000 Armenians from Baku had come to Rasht. The local Armenian committee asked Frame to care for them by offering 25 beds, for which they would pay. With nurses found among the refugees he set up shop. In November 1918, Dr. Wilbur N. Post of Chicago arrived, who worked for the American-Persian Relief Committee (APRC). Famine also struck Resht

---

850. For the medical staff of the Jangalis and their activities, see Ta'eb 1384, pp. 34-38. On the Dunsterforce in Rasht, see Dunsterville 1920, pp. 165-66.

at year's end of 1918, which went hand in hand with a combined epidemic of typhus, typhoid, and relapsing fever that swept over the city and took many lives. Men and women died in the streets without anyone to bury them; 25 were counted per day. The APRC buried 500 in one month, Frame was told. Finally cholera appeared which did not prove to be severe.

The APRC asked Dr. Frame to take charge of their relief work in the Caspian district, but he told them the British organized the work in Enzeli and local Armenians did a good job in Rasht. They offered him enough money for operating a hospital (Armenians and locals) for 60 beds and to look after the Gilani highlanders, who were poor and hungry. Frame agreed to do the relief work, provided the APRC offered a substitute for the hospital, which they did. Dr. Tashjiantz [Tashchiyan], who was trained in the US, took charge of the hospital and the dispensary work. Then the British consul asked Frame to take care of additional Armenian refugees for whom there was no room in Enzeli. Would he be able to provide for 6,000 refugees in Rasht? Frame was all alone, for the British consul had left. The first group arrived 48 hours later. Most of them were villagers, who had fled from the Turks to Baku and from Baku to Enzeli. There was no place for them; they had been shipped up to the lagoon of Enzeli and from there by the small railroad to Rasht.[851] They had to walk the last 3 kms to the relief camps. Of this first lot of 1,500 some 300 were in immediate need of hospital care. Unfortunately, the doctor hired was totally incompetent and indifferent to his responsibilities and for a few days, while Frame was arranging the relief work, they received no medical care at all. Frame was able to secure a nurse from the earlier refugee wave, who was "enthusiastic, faithful, and tireless." Some 8-10 rooms had been attached to the camp and three large barracks that accommodated 35 patients. Each received pajamas, a comfort and pillow. Heat, shelter and food were most needed. Shortly thereafter, Capt. Warren was appointed political officer and took care of the administration. They never got the doctors well organized and

---

851. On this railroad, see Shireen Mahdavi, *For God, Mammon, and Country*. Boulder: Westview, 1999, pp. 126-31.

Frame lacked the language skills, but he found some young doctor who did fairly well. The matron gradually gathered a staff, but then cholera was reported. Drs. Tashchiyan and Frame went to the camp, where 6-7 patients were crowded in a small room. As the nurse did not panic Frame took heart. Fortunately it was false alarm. The refugees began to return and soon the local Armenian committee took care of those that remained. By mid-December 1918 the number of patients was so small that they were moved to the hospital in the city and the relief camp was closed.

Capt. Warren and Dr. Frame then turned to improving the camp for poor Iranians. These were mostly mountaineers who had fled the 1918 famine. Among them were very few able-bodied men. Most were women and children, who were too emaciated to work, even if they had to organize work, which they did not. Warren and Frame rented two adjacent caravanserais, covered the walls with reeds and established a simple men's and women's hospital and organized food distribution. At one time, they had 2,500 refugees. Once they were sheltered and fed the high death rate dropped. In the spring of 1919 dysentery appeared, but it was a mild one. In May the refugees were given a suit of clothes and many left home before the final payment was given them. The Jangalis, who controlled the province, became his partners in the relief work for Iranians.

Once the Armenians were returning and relief for the Iranians was organized, Frame turned to his own hospital and dispensary. Dr. Tashchian and the nurse (until she fell ill in December 1918) had been working faithfully. Frame visited the hospital to see the few Iranian patients, but all was in Tashchiyan's good hands. He was in charge till the end of March 1919, when he was charged with the task of sending the Iranian refugees home. Frame then realized that he needed a bigger place for the hospital, which he found. Here he accommodated as many as 90 patients by putting them on the floor. The space was fit for 60 beds and the APRC offered Frame 2,000 *tumans*/month through May 1919 as a starter. But there was hardly a demand for 60 beds and it was more effective to bring the dispensary into the hospital, so that he could be near the work all the time. This reduced the number of beds to 45.

Frame used Russian-Armenian nurses who did not know Persian. These were gradually replaced by local Armenian girls with whom Frame was able to talk. Although untrained, they picked up the nursing fundamentals quickly. Frame's assistant had returned from Hamadan and helped as well. After the refugees had left and Frame had returned to his hospital his troubles were not over. A severe epidemic of paratyphoid broke out among the nurses; six of them became ill and then three more. In the city were also many cases, who came to the hospital. By carefully changing clothes no cases developed among the patients, while none of the nurses died. During the winter of 1918-19, he had 332 refugee patients in the hospital and 300 from the city with a total of 9,040 days of treatment.

In January 1919, Frame finally started the main regular hospital work, i.e. surgery, as the APRC had decided to support it though the winter for the relief of locals and refugees. In the city Frame had found a pressure sterilizer, but it took till February 1919 to train the nurses in its use and preparation for surgery. There were some emergency operations (amputation in case of gangrene), but whenever possible Frame postponed surgery until the rush of relief work was over. As OR nurse Frame had a graduate from the missionary Girls' School, who knew English and had been working in a drugstore. The number of operations was not large, because people had become used to refusal and did not realize that the situation had improved. Frame did 50 major operations, including ovarian cyst, hernias, but limited fearing infection, liver abscesses, bladder stones, cataract, neocrosed bones with sequestra, and removal of bullets. The well-to-do preferred to go to better-equipped surgeons in Baku. Although, the APRC had started the hospital, Frame and his staff were continuing with it when it discontinued its operations.[852]

---

852. The above is based on Presbyterian Church 1919, pp. 264-65; RG 91-19-9, "History of Resht Station," p. 2; Presbyterian Church 1920, pp. 315-16; RG 91-19-9, Resht Medical Work 10/07/1919; Idem, Resht Medical Work 1919-1920.

Dr. Frame had intended to close the hospital for the summer, but in the spring of 1920 the Iranian government sent troops to put down the Jangalis. Thinking having achieved their objective they closed the military hospital. However, fighting broke out anew and Frame was asked to admit the government wounded and all through summer and fall wounded came. Sometimes 25 beds were occupied; in all 65 military were admitted, of whom 55 were wounded. In September 1919, he wondered how he would be able to maintain the size of the hospital. The rooms were so arranged that he could accommodate either 15 or 35, but not an intermediate number. If he only kept 15 beds then the soldiers might occupy all beds and leave no room for civilians. If he kept 35 beds there was no money to do so, unless government paid for this larger number. As it was more economical to run a large hospital he decided to keep 35 beds and close it in early spring when funds would dry up. After the departure of the soldiers the hospital again became a relief institution. The number of paying patients was very low. Because business activity was low and because Frame was unable to spend much time on private practice as before, prospects for a substantial income for hospital was low. A shipment of sugar and condensed milk from APRC as well as a donation of cash and medical supplies, helped greatly and friends in the city donated 280 pounds of rice. This enabled Frame to keep the hospital open until 1 March 1920, a few weeks prior to his furlough.

Help from the staff was great as was the arrival of Ms Taillie RN in the fall of 1920, who left after a few months to help in Hamadan. One graduate of the missionary school was matron nurse as before (see above). She was in charge especially of the OR and the preparation of sterile dressing. She was so good that Frame could do an operation at one hour's notice. Housekeeping was done by a girl of 17, the assistant matron. At the beginning of the year they went over the food available and dishes Iranians generally used, and worked out a diet for the patients together. "Persians have few invalid dishes and do not care much for our sick room concoctions. Fortunately, however most of them enjoyed the sweetened condensed milk," which simplified care of the more seriously ill. The other nurses did well and showed that theirs was not a job, but a service to the poor. Baron Hagop, the medical assistant, worked in the out-patients department and Yezneek took charge of the dressings and the lab work. Frame tried to train him in lab work, but lack of essential material hampered that; he was good at certain exams. Sometimes Frame thought he had to close the hospital, due to lack of supplies. When he was out of cedar oil, he read in old books that methyl alcohol was a good substitute. In Frame's view the hospital offered the advantage of better "diagnosis and the study of diseases of the community."

The military episode was medically interesting for Frame, because he saw tetanus, gas gangrene and he was able to try the celebrated Dakin's solution and Bipp. There was no epidemic as in previous years. In February 1920, influenza threatened to become serious; some nurses were affected, but few patients. Fortunately there was heavy snowfall (1.2-1.5 m), which prevented many patients from coming. Nevertheless, Dr. Frame commented that: "We still have to overcome some prejudice against going to a hospital or having an operation." This was more marked among city people. Non-residents came quicker. As modern medicine was gaining the confidence of the people and if carefully approached and explained patients accepted to be operated. But old school Iranian doctors still doubted the success of hernia operations. Nevertheless, hernia and stone operations were the most frequent ones. Cataract operations were few as it was very uncommon in Gilan, although quite a few among the refugees and the mountaineer day-laborers were afflicted with it.

Before his departure on furlough in May 1920, Dr. Frame made an assessment of his past experience, raised the question whether the Iran Mission should continue in Rasht with medical or non-medical missionary work, and what possible steps needed to be taken in the future. Rasht was a commercial center, one of the densely populated areas in Iran. It had 60-70,000 inhabitants, with those in its environs in a of 60 kms radius, there were some 300,000 people. S.W. of the Rasht district was the Turkic speaking mountain area with no doctor; the mountaineers migrated seasonally. Given the dispersed single farm-house habitation in the province itinerating was unlike in the rest of Iran, while in the city he had a captive market. His was the only hospital in the province. Frame submitted that the hospital that he had established in 1919 with funds from the APRC had shown that there was a demand for it. In six months he treated 300 cases and did 50 major operations. For the past years the dispensary had been supported solely by Frame's private practice. More recently, he generally had a few beds available for in-patients, who could pay or could provide for their own nursing.

Because the Presbyterian HQ in New York had decided to continue with a missionary-physician in Rasht, Frame submitted that in that case a 15-20 bed hospital would suffice. However, given the limited earning capacity of one physician, 2,000 *tuman*s needed to be appropriated. Even with the presence of a second doctor, which would mean more income, that amount still would be required. Because it was not possible to make the hospital a financially self-supporting institution, because of the poverty of the people and, consequently, low fees the hospital could charge, while operating cost were high. Income possibilities were also low, because foreign doctors charged lower fees than in Tehran or Mashhad. "To collect 20,000 Krans in 5 and 10 Kran fees [1Kr=10c] takes time." The above-mentioned 50 operations paid less 4,150 *qran*s and the 300 patients paid about 9,500 *qran*s for board. He averaged less than $8 and $3 /patient for board, while expenses were 200 *qran*s per patient. Also, Baku was very accessible and those who had money preferred to go there to better known and better equipped hospitals. Therefore, Frame was stuck with those who were unable to pay fees, although he expected that to change over time. In short, according to Frame, running a 40-bed hospital cost 10,000 *tuman*s per year. Assuming that patients would pay about 500 *tuman*s per month, the out-patient department would show a surplus of 1,000 leaving 4,000 and 2,000 *tuman*s to be supplied from outside ($4,000 and 2,000 at normal rates, which was two times higher in 1921). Also, the cost of nursing was higher than in other missionary hospitals. A second doctor would increase earning. As to the OR, there was a fist class although well-used sterilizer and a failing complete list of instruments. There was a wooden operating table with a hinged end; before the war it was enameled, but enamel paint was unavailable. The instrument tables were rough painted pine, while the instrument closet was a many times repaired old wooden set of drawers and shelves, but hopeless to use any longer. Frame also stressed the need for a proper lab, because they needed to do more careful exams in digestive cases. There was much stomach trouble, which was hard to treat, because Iranians had a vague terminology for their symptoms. Having an X-ray machine, especially in case of patients with bullet wounds, would make things simpler and even save lives, of which he cited various examples.[853]

During Frame's furlough, the Russians invaded Gilan (June 1920 until September 1921).[854] They had no doctor and, therefore, they seized the missionary hospital and its equipment, using it as a hospital as long as they were in the city and finally took all medical equipment with them to Russia. Frame returned to Rasht in the late summer of 1921, a few days before government troops re-occupied the city on 23 September. One of the last acts of the head of the city government, a Kurd, was to release all Frame's supplies from the local tax office. The new government gave him permission to establish a hospital and duty-free import of supplies. Visiting his former hospital, Frame found that all hospital equipment had been taken to Russia, except the microscope and the surgical instruments, which faithful servants had saved. Frame rented the former building, acquired a small amount of equipment, and, the hospital was open for business. Lack of supplies in the city made it difficult to fully re-equip the hospital, but he and his team made the best of it and got through the winter. In the spring of 1922 a large shipment of supplies came. What Frame really needed was a good sterilizer. Fortunately, a local iron worker produced one in six months, but Frame could not find a burner to heat it. Therefore, he used the kitchen steamer, despite this make-shift apparatus there were no post-operative infections. The hospital had an X-ray machine offered by the Sunday School, but unfortunately the wrong tubes were sent. This was a setback, the more so, because an adjacent cinema

---

853. RG 91-19-7, Resht Medical Report, 10.7.1919; Idem, Report Medical Work 1919-1920; Presbyterian Church 1921, pp. 332-34.

854. On this episode in the history of Gilan, see Chaqueri 1995 and Persits 1996.

had offered free electricity. Fortunately, the Tehran mission hospital needed this type of machine, so Frame gave it to them, hoping that a friend would bring a new one.

For a few weeks Frame still received some funds from the APRC, but when this source dried up he had to close the hospital, due to lack of funds. Because trade with Russia stagnated people had no money. Also, the cost of drugs and dressing were much higher. E.g., formerly he could get 10 c. for drugs costing 8-9 c. from out-patients, now they cost 25-30 c., but patients had no money. Surgical gauze cost 4 c/yard, now cost 35c. It was so scarce that, instead of gauze, Frame used a cheap voile costing 35c. The hospital also had to reduce salaries. The very young Armenian matron-nurse tried to keep cost down. During the formal hospital's closure she stayed on at a lower salary. She also suggested hiring less efficient help even though this meant more work for her. Furthermore, she suggested that when patients would get food from outside she would care for them, even staying at night. In this way, the hospital had 5-6 patients, even though it was 'closed.' Fortunately, times were getting better and the number of private patients was increasing, but these were still fewer than before. This gave Frame more time for record keeping and more careful examinations. He noted that his hospital was getting a reputation in four areas: general surgery, skin, eye, and women's diseases. In surgery there was still much fear and patients tried to go to Baku, but this was changing. Also, there was an increasing freedom with which women came to see a male physician. A daughter of a chief mullah came to see Frame that year, while 10 years ago her sister chose death rather than allow him to treat her after confinement.

Because the Mission owned no land in Rasht it could not build. Therefore, in 1922 money was made available and a piece of land was bought with "a Persian bungalow which had been remodelled for the use of unmarried ladies. There was also another Persian building, which was incorporated in the physician's residence." The Frames started remodeling the house and with the remaining funds they intended to build small hospital next to it, one with 10 beds and two private rooms.

The complete plans for a 40-bed hospital required $10,000.[855] On the whole there was less work in 1921-22, due to hard times, which kept paying patients away as well as Dr. Frame's inability to treat poor patients with the same liberality as before, in particular concerning free drugs and hospitalization. Therefore, income was about 150 *tuman*s per month lower than expenditure. The 1,000 *tuman*s appropriation only lasted six months; although he kept the dispensary open all year. Because spring time was slack time in Gilan, Frame closed the hospital in March 1922 and intended to reopen it in November, when he expected the new hospital building to be ready. However, even when closed he usually had 3-4 emergency patients, who came from afar. Because boat service had resumed on the Caspian Sea, his hospital also received more patients from Ardabil, Tonakebun and Mazandaran than before, and even more from Zanjan.[856]

On 1 June 1923 ground was broken for the new hospital in the Cheragh-e Barq lane.[857] Frame had intended to do so in January and to begin using the new building in early spring 1923, but the uncertain political outlook made him postpone it. The building was completed on 15 November. In August there was a flood, several feet of the hospital's foundation of the hospital had been under water, but there was no damage. The real cause of delay was the rain, which made that the walls were not dry enough to bear the roof or to be able to finish the inside. Also, he only had funds for the bare building without any special equipment. Frame had estimated the total cost at $25,000, but after buying the land he only had $10,000 left of the $16,000 appropriated by the 1920 Sunday School Christmas Offering. To complete the modest main building, measuring only 15 x 24 yards, would cost $13,000 without outbuildings. Therefore, he decided to leave one end of the building unfinished. By mid-November 1923 ready were: the men's ward, the women's ward, two private rooms, with beds

---

855. RG 91-19-7, Medical Report Resht 1921-1922; Idem, Report Medical Work 1919-1920; Idem, "History of Resht Station," p. 3.
856. RG 91-19-7, Medical Report Resht 1921-22.
857. `Eyn al-Saltaneh 1376, vol. 1, pp. 377, 865; UNESCO 1343, vol. 2, pp. 1449-1451; Elgood 1951, pp. 511-512, 534; Waterfield 1973, p. 139.

for 12 to 15 patients, the operating and sterilizing rooms, the rooms for nurses, the X-ray machine and the bath. On the first floor, there were two waiting rooms, two dressing rooms, and the consultation and drug rooms. The waiting rooms had been designed in such a way that when thrown together these were able to seat >100 people with women secluded from men, to hold Sunday preaching services. Although the hospital was still small for his needs it was more and better than what he had before. Frame was also pleased with his two nurses and the likelihood that he might get a third one.[858] In 1925, some electric lights and a water system (bath, stationary wash stands, drainage etc.) were added, partly paid from special gifts and partly from receipts. That the additions could be paid from receipts indicated that great changes had taken place in the local attitude to surgery and hospital care since the war. Well-to-do Iranians came to realize the advantage of hospital care and surgical treatment. The establishment of a local Iranian hospital for the poor relieved the pressure on the missionary hospital and enabled it to give better service to all patients. In 1931, a small wing was added to the hospital to be able to admit more female patients and provide more adequate arrangements for the nurses. Despite all this, there was no accommodation for the nurses to live in the hospital. In 1932, a beginning was made for an outside shelter for TB patients, which was enlarged in 1934. Much of these additions were paid from receipts.[859]

Less work was done in 1923-24, due to lack of funds and the transition from the old to the new building. The high points of that year were the completion of the hospital and the arrival of Ms Ellen D. Nicholson, the first American RN for Rasht. Because of the combination of the lack of funds, Nowruz (21 March) and Ramazan (starting on 17 April 1923) Frame decide to close the hospital in March, earlier than in the previous year. The same held true for 1924 with Ramadan

---

858. RG 91-19-7, Resht Medical Report 1923-1924; Idem, Resht Medical Report 1922-1923; Idem, Medical Report Resht 1921-1922.

859. RG 91-19-7, "History of Resht Station," p. 3; Idem, Resht Medical Report 1924-1925; Idem, Resht Medical Report 1931-1932.

starting on 6 April 1923. Nevertheless, the hospital continued to receive in-patients, in case of emergencies (e.g. extra-uterine pregnancy).[860]

In 1924-25, funds were sufficient to keep the hospital open all year, although not at full capacity. The hospital opened in August 1924. Because of uncertainty of funds, Frame planned to care for 10 patients on average and in December 1924 he reached this goal. In January-February 1925 heavy storms kept villagers away. In April, despite Ramadan, he exceeded his target of 300 patient days. In May he had even more, so that the staff had to put patients on the floor, while they also put together four old wooden beds in the downstairs corridor. The highest daily number was 18 patients and two new-borns. In May 1925, the hospital had 478 patient-days and total receipts of 675 *tuman*s. Frame's greatest problem was keeping his patients accommodated in accordance with their gender and social standing. If there was over-demand for private rooms he used the nurses' relaxation room and the X-ray room as well. He realized that this was an additional burden for the nurses, because when the work load was heaviest they needed a room to rest. Frame was surprised that well-to-do women were willing to come to the private rooms. In fact, demand exceeded his expectations.

> One doctor sent his wife, another his sister, and third a relative, and a fourth paid full price for his Russian housekeeper in a private room. One lady of means came into the hospital for a small operation. The day she went home she felt somewhat faint and giddy and returned next morning asking to be readmitted. Her reluctance to leave became embarrassing as we needed the room for more urgent cases. A wealthy landlord from Lahijan suffering from neglected carbuncle literally turned pale when I suggest he come to the hospital offering any sum if would name if I would treat him in his friend's house. After a few days in the hospital he refused to leave saying he was more comfortable in the hospital than could be elsewhere. He stayed twenty days and reluctant to leave before his wound had entirely healed.

---

860. RG 91-19-7, Resht Medical Report 1923-1924.

Despite trade depression in the bazaar many patients were able to pay and hospital income was higher than Frame had hoped for. It was not sufficient, however, to keep the hospital open for poor patients. But during the winter he received a gift from a friend in the US for this very purpose. Also, Frame received a case of dressing and linen supplies from the Brookline Church with a gift in cash for freight and customs. He also received some gifts from local people. The Northumberland Presbytery promised to send more dressing. Although the new hospital was more popular than Frame expected, still more needed to be done to gain people's confidence and teach them the advantage of hospital care. On the back of his prescriptions he had printed a statement about the advantages of hospital treatment, mentioning especially surgery, obstetrics, diagnosis and better care for certain medical ailments.

The hospital's strong point and comparative advantage was surgery, because there was hardly any one else in Gilan who did so. Nevertheless, people were still reluctant to come to the hospital for surgery. Frame submitted that he needed to avoid risky desperate cases, so as not to scare away less desperate ones. He had developed a technique for local anesthesia, because people feared total anesthesia. Frame did 80 major and 176 minor operations in 1924-25. Although, he realized that it would take a long time before Iranian women would come to the hospital for confinement, but sometimes there were a few who realized the advantage. Frame was encouraged that he had some positive responses to his suggestion to remain in the hospital for a few days for the diagnosis. Not only the poor, but also the rich were beginning to realize the advantages of hospital as a nursing institution. Frame also tried to induce diabetes patients to come. He had insulin from Lilly of Indianapolis. However, the first case refused: "saying he'd rather die than being the first case in the city on whom we experimented the drug; he died."[861]

In 1926-27, the hospital was kept open throughout the summer and there was a fair amount of work. Nevertheless, Dr. Frame was

---

861. RG 91-19-7, Resht Medical Report 1924-1925.

of the opinion that the hospital should be closed in summer and the staff be given a vacation during July-August. Because Frame left on furlough April 1927, Dr. Bussdicker from Kermanshah arrived on 22 October 1926 to substitute for him until his return on 1 April 1928. During the overlapping time they divided the work load. With this division labor they could do more and see more patients. Also, they were able to do more accurate diagnosis, because before the doctor was kept busy 30 hours/week in the clinics and operating the rest of the time. However, when Frame left people thought that Dr. Bussdicker was not able to do surgery and there was a drop in surgical cases, although this notion was gradually changing.[862]

With the funds available the hospital tried to treat as many free patients as possible, many of whom were surgical cases and had to remain for a long time in the hospital. People in private rooms had difficulty sleeping alone as they were not accustomed to that and they complained that the room was too small. Also, they wanted a light on during the night. Nevertheless, the number of paying patients for private or semi-private rooms and special treatment was growing, but in general there were fewer patients. Because Frame was gone people thought that the 'real' work of the hospital had stopped. But Dr. Bussdicker soon was sought after when they learned that he would go to the US, when Frame returned. But when he did, a lot of 'saved' up cases came and April 1928 showed more patients and cash receipts than any previous month in the hospital's history. Because Frame had to go to conferences the hospital was closed from 15 June to 15 August. However there were some dispensary patients throughout July, and one every day in August. "These last three years we have gradually accumulated sufficient linens, ward and surgery and patients' supplies so that now the nurses have a comfortable feeling instead of one of panic when we have a week of rain and an influx of new patients," thanks to the ladies of Northumberland Presbytery. Also, the hospital had more rooms with clean plaster, newly painted woodwork than ever before and the bed-side tables were clean, painted and ready for

---

862. RG 91-1-12, Report Resht Medical Work 1926-1927.

years of service. This really was a luxury compared with their previous condition, thanks to savings and to a village painter under supervision.[863]

In 1928-29, more patients came for non-operative conditions. The fear for the hospital was diminishing. There were fewer hernias (in the past 50%) and thus, there was a greater variety of surgical procedures. A most noteworthy addition to its physical equipment was the 'electrification' of the hospital. A gift allowed the wiring of the entire hospital. Better service in the city line improved lighting, which was a great help. Nevertheless, electric service was only for a limited period at night, which constrained hospital activities. There was a promise of day light service in the near future, in which case Frame intended to add more equipment. The hospital also had some light cradles made for use in the wards, which was a boon to many patients. Frame also bought a cystoscope, but only four cases were willing to submit to it since its arrival in November 1928.[864]

In 1929-30, the volume of work was like in the previous year, which was unexpected, because the National and the City Women's Hospitals by then had larger and better quarters than before and were well filled. Frame also noted that people's attitude to hospital care had changed from "that a hospital is a place for a poor man to die" to one that was appreciated for its care.[865] In 1929-30, Frame thought that he had reached the limit of his expansion, but free from mission responsibilities he was able to keep the hospital open all year, a 20% increase over last year. In fact, the year 1929-30 was the best year since the relief years and with the highest income, which belied the notion held by some that the hospital has reached the limit of its possible expansion with the present capacity, equipment and staff. The population demanded more hospital care instead of just medical care. Therefore, Frame had to turn away more female patients, because the hospital lacked adequate facilities for them. Income increased by 58%

---

863. RG 91-19-7, Medical Report Resht 1927-1928.
864. RG 91-19-7, Resht Medical Report 1928-1929. Cystoscopy is a procedure that lets a physician view the inside of the bladder and urethra in detail.
865. RG 91-19-7, Resht Medical Report 1929-1930.

and statistics showed a 40% increase in patients, except in operations. The hospital had more women patients than before; the women's ward was so crowded that an extra bed was kept in a space for four adults, and, sometimes, there were six adults and 1-2 children in that space. Obstetrics cases increased by 48% and 45% of major operations were gynecological or obstetrical. With infectious cases, abscesses, pneumonia, and influenza it was increasingly difficult to provide proper safeguards for obstetrical and clean operative cases. Therefore, Frame was very happy with a donation of $1,000 from Mrs. Meytag to add a small wing for women's patients and nurses' rooms. He intended to add seven beds, be it in small units. One was a small room for new born babies, which until then were kept in the operating room, when not used or were parked somewhere in the hospital if it was. The same held for new mothers, who should not be in the general ward with cases of influenza, pneumonia, septic condition etc. Therefore, he also wanted to add a small ward for clean cases, separate from the general ward as well as a sun parlor for three beds. There were many patients who needed a sun parlor treatment. On the first floor of the addition two necessary needed administrative improvements were going to be built. One, a light airy storeroom for the linen supplies, which until then were scattered in closets. The other, a room was for day time sleeping for the night nurses. The hospital's nurses lived at home and, therefore, they seldom had the opportunity of a proper quiet day for sleeping. Various other gifts allowed the replacement of the old army and wooden beds.[866]

In August 1931, Frame had eight obstetrics cases in nine days, which filled the female ward and private rooms to capacity. At that time, the addition was almost finished only lacking the final plaster coat, the woodwork was unpainted, etc., but the rooms were habitable, so the 10th patient was moved in after 10 minutes. The addition accommodated five beds and the sun parlor 3-4 patients. The sun parlor was immediately put to use for some children with hip joint disease and a TB patient on which he did a phrenectomy. The addition also freed

---

866. RG 91-19-7, Resht Medical Report 1930-1931; RG 91-20-8, Frame/R to Speer/NY 17/02/1931.

space in the main building for obstetrics and the care for babies. This was essential given the increase of obstetric cases from 33 in 1930-31 to 53 in 1931-32, and the babies to be cared for from 25 to 35. The desperate nature of these cases was indicated by 40 major operations on 53 cases. "Nevertheless such is the resistance of the women to the mishandling of Persian midwives before admission that only four died, one of them moribund on admission." Sometimes, the women traveled many kms on horse or by car after many days of labor in the villages. In October 1931, Dr. Harry Brinkman arrived. Their first thought was not how to increase the quantity of work, but, through consultation, do more detailed examinations and better lab work, and keep more careful records, to improve quality. However, the National Hospital had to reduce its generous policy of free drugs with the result that many patients came to the missionary dispensary, on the principle that if they had to pay they preferred to come there. Dr. Brinkman's presence allowed them to divide the men's and women's dispensary and by its efficiency attracted 70% more patients. Dr. Brinkman had training in TB work and genito-urinary diseases. Therefore, his experience with the cystoscope opened the field of urology in the hospital, so that they were able to operate on long standing cases of kidney stones and other cases. Also, his familiarity with the newer chest surgery encouraged them to operate a number of tubercular cases and led to the creation of the TB shelter.[867]

Despite the absence of the various American members of the medical staff (each for several weeks) and poor economic conditions, in 1933-34 the hospital's income was the second largest it its history and only 10% below that of the previous year. This was due to better and specialized service the hospital offered. Due to the increase in patients the hospital was sometimes overcrowded, although it was not always full in all departments. Therefore, in cases of overflow, a bed was added in a ward, or a convalescent patient was sent to the outside ward, or a patient was put in the corridor. Demand for semi-private rooms was such that it was decided to wall off one end of the larger

---

867. RG 91-19-7, Resht Medical Report 1931-1932; Idem, Resht Medical Work 1933-1934.

men's ward. The new room thus formed became a relaxation room for the nurses, while their relaxation room was transformed into a two-bed ward.[868]

Frame went on furlough to the US in April 1935, which meant too much work for the one remaining doctor. There was indeed an increase in surgery, which showed an increase in the confidence in operations.[869] During the spring of 1936 painting and renovating was done. Before the walls were plain white plastered, now they were covered with a good oil paint, which permitted washing when dirty. The same was done in the large waiting room downstairs, the OR, the obstetrical and service rooms, two hallways, the women's 4-bed ward and all but one private room. The private rooms were painted in various pleasant colors to lend variety. Also, new linoleum was laid in the OR and service room and in one of the hallways, which added much to appearance and cleanliness of the hospital.

It not infrequently happened that bodies of medico-legal cases that died in the hospital had to be kept, sometimes too long, until permission came from the department of justice. As the hospital had no morgue, there was no choice but to keep the body in one of the private rooms or in one of the waiting rooms. Therefore, in 1936 a morgue was constructed, a small brick room with a cement floor built against one of the walls of the hospital near a large gate and from where the bodies could be stored and taken without attracting too much public attention. This brought much peace of mind and less anxiety.[870]

In 1937, the doctors were surprised by the large number of 'acute abdomens' they saw. They explained that as an indication of people becoming more conscious of the value of hospital treatment. Also on the increase were accidents due to cars, heavy construction works, factories, etc. Foreign companies especially sent their fracture cases to the missionary hospital, because of the new laws as to workmen's compensation. Some of these cases came from 300 km distance. These cases were problematic, because without a portable X-ray machine

---

868. RG 91-19-7, Resht Medical Report 1933-1934.
869. RG 91-19-7, Report Resht Medical Work 1934-1935.
870. RG 91-19-7, Medical Report Resht 1935-1936.

it was not possible to examine patients in bed. The hospital's homemade Balkan frames were often not adequate to a particular case. Sometimes adhesive did not arrive on time from abroad. Therefore, it took much ingenuity by doctors and nurses to keep these patients in good condition. To create more space for female patients, the sleeping quarter of the night nurse was relocated to a separate building. At the same time, more space around beds rather than more beds became the norm, while it also created a semi-isolated alcove for special cases.[871]

Dr. Adelaide Kibbe arrived in October 1937. It was a new experience for the city to have a female doctor, who was an obstetrician and a surgeon. She did a Caesarean without the help of other doctors, which amazed a British doctor working in the National hospital. During Hoffman's illness, one male patient left the doctor's office saying he wanted a doctor not a midwife, but a former patient said he would take his chance with the female physician.[872] In 1940, Dr. Dodds visited and agreed that the hospital needed better facilities for its 30 beds. It was also hoped to get funding for this as well as for the Nurses' Home on the plot east to the hospital.[873] As Dr. Frame's wife had died in September 1939, he married Dr. Kibbe on 11 January 1941. In early December 1941, she gave birth to a daughter. Dr. Kibbe-Frame carried work on part-time thereafter. In 1941-42, the hospital was closed for 13 weeks; four weeks in the summer for vacation and nine weeks in December-February due to Dr. Frame's illness. Despite closure etc. much work was done, including house calls. After the hospital's closure many patients showed up when it reopened. In August-September 1941, the town was bombarded, which was the inception of many diseases. People fled to the villages and even months later they came with a fractured wrist, due to a fall from a horse during the flight; or malaria and dysentery developed while living in the village, etc. There also were a few bomb casualties, mostly infected wounds and fractures. The doctors were very pleased that the hospital had a Kirschner Traction Pin outfit, which was often in use. Dr. Frame started

---

871. RG 91-20-8, Resht Medical Report 1936-1937.
872. RG 91-19-7, Resht Hospital Report, 1937-1938.
873. RG 91-20-8, Resht Medical Report 1944-1945.

working again from mid-February until mid-May 1942; he died on 11 June. Dr. Kibbe-Frame worked part-time thereafter.[874]

In August 1942, the hospital was re-opened. In November, Dr. Mohammad Kar, a German-French schooled Christian physician, came on a 1-year contract to work part-time, especially in the mornings in the out-patient clinic. He did three mornings in the free clinic and three mornings for those who could pay. Dr Kibbe-Frame's clinic was divided about equally between them. He did not do surgery, being basically a lab rat. This was somewhat of a disappointment, because Dr. Kibbe-Frame had hoped for a physician who did surgery and took night calls. The surgeon of the National Hospital resigned and left to Tehran and so that hospital was converted into a place to receive typhoid-typhus cases.[875] In June 1944, Dr. Kibbe-Frame wrote that the Rasht Christian hospital, which was

> an integrated, efficient, busy institution, is about to collapse. The sterilizer is completely worn out, the large primus for heating it is gone, several instruments like the cystoscope, needed for exams, have broken due to constant use. The running water system after 15-20 year of use has collapsed; the flooring is breaking through in places from dampness, the linoleum is worn out and looks untidy; the X-ray machine and tubes are on their last legs and the whole instrument is outmoded and too small. Stoves and heating arrangements will have to be renovated and changed, and even the doctor, needs a bit of mental, spiritual, perhaps even physical repair work.

In short, the hospital was in a crisis and limping along. Not only equipment and material was collapsing, "but the very heart is in a

---

874. RG 91-19-7, Medical Report Resht Hospital 1941-1942. Kirschner wires or pins are sterilized, sharpened, smooth stainless steel pins. Introduced in 1909 by Martin Kirschner, the wires are now widely used in medical surgery. In Rasht the interesting operation this year was extraction of a four-prong dental plate from a woman's esophagus." Presbyterian Church 1943, p. 84.

875. RG 91-19-7, Resht Hospital Report 1942-1943.

weakened state." Dr Kibbe-Frame was supposed to work only half-days and the other time devote to her daughter and home. But patients were demanding and most of that free time was spent in the hospital. Then Ms Benz went on furlough, which meant that Ms Nicholson R.N. had to do the work of several people, viz. (i) superintendent of nursing and of the nursing school, in which she did much of the teaching, and (ii) being matron of the hospital involving the difficulty of getting supplies, and (iii) after the hospital treasurer left she became the keeper of the books. This was too much for one person, and she stayed only so that the dispensary and X-ray unit could be kept going. Dr. Kar worked the morning clinic, which relieved some of the congestion. He also was in the baby clinic one afternoon for consultation and two afternoons per week in the TB clinic. Even when two nurses fell ill with dysentery the hospital staff persevered and did a lot of work.

Rising prices and thus, of living wages, made the hospital's financial situation weak. Dr. Kibbe-Frame was forced to increase the prices of the dispensary tickets, the private rooms, operations, etc. and although income rose an amazing amount had to be paid in wages, supplies, food, firewood, and the like. The support from the Board was used for a bonus to the Iranian staff and for expensive medicines and drugs. The Red Cross helped out with bandages, some drugs, blankets and surgical supplies, which kept the surgery department going. Gauze and cotton were sold in the bazaar at exorbitant prices.[876] In the fall of 1944, Dr. Kibbe-Frame went on furlough, so the lonely US nurse, Ms Gertrude Benz, was in charge of the hospital. Together with the other staff she kept the hospital open in a 'reduced and quiet way." People were grateful; they knew that there was no US doctor, "but feeling that whatever our hospital offers will be first-class." Fortunately, Dr. Kar continued to work part-time as did the hospital's druggist, Ali Aqa Nizkad. Most of the time, there were four nurses to help in a reorganized nursery. For better protection, the gardener and orderly were moved onto the hospital compound, because there was a lot of thievery in town. Meanwhile, everybody was waiting for the

---

876. RG 91-19-7, Resht Hospital Report 1943-1944.

return of Dr. A.E. Kibbe-Frame and her stepson, Dr. John D. Frame Jr. after he finished with his army service.[877]

After Dr. Kibbe-Frame's return in 1945, she still was the only doctor of the 30-bed hospital. She resumed her normal routine, of going to the dispensary after morning rounds in the hospital. Operating days were Tuesdays, Thursdays and Saturdays, although it was often at night, in case of emergencies. Because the city's electricity supply and quality were unreliable the hospital had an emergency battery box always ready. Iranian doctors continued to send some surgical patients to the Christian hospital. Dr. Kibbe wrote that, "There is a fairly nice Iranian hospital, but no one there is doing surgery. The Russian hospital does no charity work." Because malaria was prevalent, the Near East Foundation sprayed all the hospital buildings with DDT. Dr. Kibbe-Frame was assisted by one US nurse, Ms Eunice Baber, who kept the nursing school running in spite of uncertainty and finally the closing of the hospital, when Dr. Adelaide Kibbe-Frame resigned in June 1948, and closed the hospital. Her replacement, Dr. Rolla Hoffman, who came from Mashhad, arrived in Rasht in July 1948 and opened the hospital in August.[878] The Iranian assistant, Dr. Kar, had just resigned as well, induced by better pay at the AIOC. Hoffman wanted an Iranian physician to help him. He wrote: "The US doctor needs at least to have one qualified national doctor, else he is like a car driver who begins his trip without a spare tire." Fortunately, Hoffman's former assistant, Dr. Nurolllah Hakim-A`lam, a young Christian doctor, who had worked with him over three years in Mashhad, was willing to fill in for six months. He did much of the surgery, taught nurses, and for three months was alone in charge of the hospital. He then moved to Detroit, where he worked at the women's hospital, where Dr. Lichtwardt, a former colleague was medical director. To replace him Hoffman hired Dr. A. Muradian, another young Christian doctor. Ali Nikzad continued as the hospital steward and pharmacist, also as

---

877. RG 91-20-8, Resht Hospital Social Service Center 1944-1945.
878. Mrs. Helen Hoffman died in early 1949; in 1950 Dr. Adelaide Kibbe returned to Rasht and married Dr. Hoffman. They had to leave Iran in 1957, because of the compulsory retirement age of 70. RG 231-1-7, Pioneering in Meshed, p. 148.

record clerk, until a new one was hired. The "Frame" hospital as it was commonly called, because of the nearly forty years of outstanding service of Dr. John D. Frame, enjoyed a high reputation, although the hospital rooms were too small and the building was in need of repairs.[879]

Dr. Hoffman wanted a new and above all, a better hospital. Therefore, he made a request of $50,000 for new building and $10,000 for a nurses' home and furnishings. Hoffman didn't want to compete with the new Pahlavi hospital, because "Iranian institutions tended to be grandiose with showy ill-equipped shells of buildings, lacking in convenience and especially in trained nurses. But its presence made the Christian hospital look gloomy and a modern hospital was needed." Apart from extensive repairs, a new X-ray machine was installed. Also, a better record system where patients were indexed by name was introduced. The repairs, the new sterilizers, the suction pump, the well pumps, various instruments and some electric fans were paid for by gifts from friends in the US. In May 1949, income was at an all high of 168,000 rials ($3,000).[880] Despite the high revenues, the hospital was 5,000 rials in the red, due to rising local cost. Dr. Hoffman tried to absorb that deficit by adjusting salaries and collecting more fees, but he feared that this might harm maintenance. Therefore, he asked for an extra monthly appropriation of 500 rials. He believed that an investment in space for 10 beds, private, for men and women would increase revenues. Lodging both American and Iranian hospital nurses was going to be a problem, because of the growth of the mission's staff and the development of the school for nurses. He also needed

---

879. RG 231-1-5, Hoffman/Rasht to Friends, 12/09/1948; RG 231-1-6, Personal Report 1949 and Hospital Report (with details on the extensive hospital repairs and its general condition), RG 231-1-5 Rolla Hoffman Correspondence 1930-1949. (Mrs. Hoffman fell ill in December 1948 and Dr. Hoffman had her transferred to the Hospital of the National Bank in Tehran, where the nurses were mostly from the US mission hospitals. Dr. Raji, an eminent Tehrani surgeon, trained in Europe, attended Mrs. Hoffman, who had cancer and died on 4 February 1949).

880. RG 231-1-6, Personal Report 1949 and Hospital Report R.E. Hoffman (It takes 6-9 months to get supplies from the US due to shipping delays and red tape).

a record clerk, because the government asked for records, reports, etc. Furthermore, special equipment was needed such as: a small portable X-ray for bedside work, an electric refrigerator, the rewiring of the hospital for safety and capacity, and a Persian typewriter for government correspondence.[881] The hospital continued to function until 1960, when it was closed.

IRANIAN HOSPITALS

The hospital established by the philantropical association (*anjoman-e kheyriyeh*), presumably around 1909, after the first one had become too small (see above), is not mentioned by Dr. Frame at all until 20 years later. Although this hospital, which was known as the *Melli* or National hospital, used the services of Dr. Tashchiyan, with whom Frame had a very close relationship. This hospital had 24 beds, of which 8 for surgical cases. In the surgical section, three beds had been set aside for maternity cases. There also was a room for the distribution of drugs. The hospital was supported by gifts to which end collection boxes hung in the bazaar. However, people were poor, so much money came from the notables. The hospital was managed by the *anjoman-e kheyriyeh*. The *Melli* used the services of Dr. Yadollah Khan, a famous surgeon. Dr. Tashchiyan and Ms Taku'i were in charge of the women's section. The *Melli* hospital's services were in great demand by the Jangalis and apart from Dr. Yadollah Khan, Dr. Abu'l-Qasem Khan Farbod, Dr. Aqa Khan Tub, Dr. `Ali Khan Shafa, and Dr. Sayyed Mohammad Khan provided their services to them both in the hospital and in the forest.[882] In May 1911 the hospital was destroyed by fire and the *anjoman-e kheyriyeh* tried to collect funds to rebuild the hospital. In this it was eventually successful, because the *Melli* hospital continued to operate until 6/3/1308 or 27 May 1929, when

---

881. RG 231-1-6, Memo Medical Needs Rasht Hospital undated, probably 1948.
882. Ta'eb 1384, pp. 25-27. For the funding of the first *Melli* hospital, see Ta'eb 1384, pp. 117-18.

it moved into a new larger building at the time when Frame returned from furlough.[883]

The new hospital was built on a lot of seven hectares, which was split into two. One part was for the general hospital, the other part for a girls' orphanage (*shirkhvargah*).[884] On the entrance of the terrain a sign said: *Bimarestan-e Melli-ye Rasht*. In 1939, following disagreement with the original founders and the public health authority the government took over the management of the hospital and the name was changed to *Bimarestan-e Pur Sina-ye Rasht*. The hospital was modern for its time with iron beds, a wooden commode and a moveable table so that patients could eat. All patients were separated by a moveable cloth screen encased in wood. Over time, due to the humidity, the buildings lost its pristine look and looked worn out, and, therefore, it was covered with cement and grouted (1951, 1968).

The building had high ceilings and windows, so that it was very bright inside even on cloudy days. At night candles and oil lamps were used, because electricity was only available for 2-4 hours at night. Heating of the rooms was with wood or coal in Russian stoves. The hospital had five departments: infectious diseases, internal diseases, surgery, administration and dispensary (*darmangah*), and kitchen, storage of drugs, and food. The infectious diseases department had one floor on the S.W. side and was practically isolated from the rest of the hospital. Its separate sections each had two rooms of 5 x 6 meters and one small room of 1.5 x 3 meters. In each room there were five beds; the small room was used to isolate patients that were near death. There was a male and a female part. Each section had its own dedicated nurse. The hospital had one 2-storey western wing, which houses the internal diseases department. Work on this part of the hospital had begun on 1927 and was completed in 1928, when it already took in patients, although it had not yet officially been opened. Both quadrangular floors were about 500 meters in area and were divided into five rooms (of 5 x 3 and 5 x 7 meters) with 4 meter high

---

883. Ebrahimnejad 2014, p. 214, n. 154; RG 91-19-7, Resht Medical Report 1928-1929.

884. On the functioning of this orphanage, see Ta`eb 1384, pp. 205-15.

ceilings and one glass lounge. There was a small room for patients who were in a bad condition and another room for patients who were recovering. Next there was a small room where nurses could relax and change, although it was sometimes used to put patients, while another room (5x5 meters) served as kitchen. From this room, three meals per day were served by the duty nurse, as instructed by the physician. At this level there also was a laboratory. On the second floor there were a bathroom and toilets. Here was one big glass lounge (13x20 meters with 24 beds) as well as a smaller one (8x13 meters) with 10 beds. The hospital's official capacity was 80 beds, but, for example, in both lounges more beds could be added, if needed. It also happened that sometimes patients had to be laid on the ground. Both floors had balconies. The lower floor was for men and the upper one for women.

The surgery was built with help from the *anjoman-e kheyriyeh*; work started in 1925 and was completed two years later. It had an area of about 350 square meters with many windows so as to benefit from natural light. It had one big room, which was the OR, and a number of small ones. One room, where the patients were prepared, another where the surgeons prepared for operation, while a third one was used to protect surgical dresses and materials against contamination. The OR had an autoclave to sterilize its instruments. There was a kitchen and a room for nurses to relax and change. The remaining rooms were occupied by patients (20 beds), apart from a small one room where patients in bad condition or dying were kept apart. Finally, there was a room for minor surgery and dressings. This department had two kinds of nurses; those who did the dressing of infectious wounds and those who did not. They were not allowed to take over from each other; the same strict separation was observed between OR nurses and ward nurses. The nurses of the surgery department had a Λ on their cap (one Λ for a nurse 3rd class; two Λ for a 2nd class, and three Λ for a 3rd class nurse). In the southern part of the building there was one big sunny room (8x13 meters) for post-op patients. In 1948, an entirely new surgical building was constructed, which was a gift from the Shah; it was opened in 1950. The old surgery building was used laboratorium and as ophthalmology and otolaryngy dispensary. In

1951, the administrative department had to share its previous space with the new radiology section.[885]

Frame observed that in 1931, although the National Hospital had increased the number of its beds, while financial considerations led many to go there, "there is still great prejudice in favor of our hospital, because of better service and nursing we offer."[886] And this came to the heart of the matter. Frame wanted the Christian hospital to be non-competitive, but better, in particular in those fields where it offered treatment that the others could not offer. This required continuous adjustment and learning to remain at the leading edge, and the missionary doctors did so with success. Given "the steady development of government health and general Persian medical services the permanence and need of Mission hospital work depends largely upon our ability to keep ahead of these programs and continue some contribution which the Persians are not yet making and thus continue pioneers in new lines of medical activity."[887]

There were other changes. In 1937, a competent military surgeon was transferred after several years. He also worked in the National Hospital and was a cooperative consultant in case of need.[888] After his departure Frame was asked by the National Hospital to be their surgeon, but being alone he had to decline. They then hired a young doctor from London. In 1938, Dr. Vartan and Dr. Badvagan of Enzeli, who sent Frame many surgical cases or for X-ray diagnosis, left for Tehran better opportunities.[889]

From 1941 to 1944 the Pur Sina hospital was in dire straits. Because the central government had no money, and its patients were mostly poor and were treated free-of-charge, it had no income. Things became so

---

885. Ta'eb 1384, pp. 103-16.
886. RG 91-19-7, Resht Medical Report 1932-1933.
887. RG 91-19-7, Rest Medical Report 1932-1933.
888. This was *Sarhang* Dr. Hoseyn Khan Moqaddam, see Ta'eb 1384, pp. 57, 131-32.
889. RG 91-19-7, Resht Hospital Report 1937-1938. It is interesting that these two surgeons are not mentioned in the list of surgeons found in Ta'eb 1384, pp. 132-36.

bad that the hospital did not even have paper to write a prescription. Henceforth, poor patients had to buy their own medicine and food and as result, despite cries for help, the hospital closed for some time.[890] Although the government hospital (that is what Frame called the Pur Sina) in Rasht reopened 1944, it did hardly any free work as their budget was too small. "When an operation is necessary, even one as small as the lancing of a boil, patients must first go to the bazaar and purchase gauze, bandages, iodine, cotton, alcohol and anesthetic if needed or desired."[891] This deplorable situation was not resolved very quickly. In September 1948, Dr. Hoffman wrote: "There is a fairly nice Iranian hospital, but no one there is doing surgery. They have an X-ray machine but no one who can operate it.[892] Fortunately, in that same year, once again with financial support from local notables, the Pur Sina Hospital was placed in a better and normal position to provide its services to the public, including, as mentioned above, a new surgical building.[893]

After the Allied invasion of Iran in August 1941, the Russians who occupied Gilan took over the military hospital that was located in the so-called Nobel barracks. However, officers and NCOs were taken to the Pur Sina hospital. Because it was a civil hospital for the general public, the Russians decided to establish a hospital in a building located in the *Bagh-e Ettehadiyeh*. Dr. Frame reported that in the fall of 1944, the Russians opened a 20-bed hospital "with much fanfare, bright carpets and upholstered furniture, but do not seem to provide competent doctors or nurses. They have a workable fluoroscopy and some therapeutic lamps for which the new-rich are glad to pay good prices. All their charges are very high."[894] The Russian hospital had X-ray equipment and Dr. Hoffman sent "some patients there for

---

890. Ta'eb 1384, p. 120 (he does not mention the temporary closure).
891. RG 91-20-8, Resht Hospital 1944-1945.
892. RG 231-1-5, Hoffman/Rasht to Friends, 12/09/1948.
893. Ta'eb 1384, pp. 120-21. For information about and photos of the medical staff as well as photos of the buildings, see Ta'eb 1384, pp. 119-205.
894. RG 91-20-8, Resht Hospital 1944-1945.

examination, with indifferent results; it does no charity work."[895] The hospital had a surgical and an internal disease department. It was under Dr. Kavaltarov, who was assisted by a few Russian orderlies. If need be he used Iranian physicians and surgeons, with whom he had a good relationship. The hospital also had a dispensary that treated poor patients, but apparently not after 1945, in view of Dr. Hoffman's observation. However, after the war Russia did not want to return the hospital. It was only in 1948 that a mixed committee was able to settle this problem and the property was transferred to the Ministry of Finance.[896]

When the Russians invaded Rasht the local board of the 'Institute for the protection of mothers and infants' (*Bongah-e hemayat-e maderan va nowzadan*), an institute founded by Reza Shah in December 1940, decided to establish a maternity clinic outside of the Pur Sina hospital (see above). To that end it rented a building and opened the 10-bed clinic on 10 April 1940. In 1944, the number of beds was increased to fifteen. The operating cost of the clinic was financed by a range of fees on, e.g. cinema tickets, sales tax on food and restaurants, and by money from collection boxes.[897] Although the board also had men as members clearly it was generally thought to be managed by women. In 1945, Dr. Hofmann reported that "the ten-bed hospital sponsored by some leading women for obstetrical work continued to give help to many. A Russian midwife did much of the work, but recently one of the Christian hospital's nurses joined their staff. The missionary doctors hoped that 'this civic project, financed by special taxes in cinema, team etc. will continue in this needy field." People also hoped that the Russians would leave soon.[898] With funding from the Shah a new maternity clinic was built, which was opened in 1950. It had 30 general beds and five for special obstetric cases.[899]

---

895. RG 231-1-5, Hoffman/Rasht to Friends, 12/09/1948.
896. Ta'eb 1384, pp. 217-19, with a photo of the building on Idem, p. 221.
897. Ta'eb 1384, pp. 225-26.
898. RG 91-20-8, Resht Hospital 1944-1945. Ta'eb 1384, p. 217, reports the same sentiment towards the Russians.
899. Ta'eb 1384, p. 227. For names of the staff, statistics and photos, see

In 1942, a hospital was opened for the treatment of venereal diseases (*bimarestan-e zahravi*), which had a high incidence among Iranians. It was located in a rented building. On the first floor there was patients' ward, while the dispensary was at street level. Dr. Kazemi, the head of the internal diseases department of the Pur Sina, was in charge of this hospital. When he left for Tehran in 1943, Dr. Hasan Niku replaced him. When typhus broke in Rasht in that year the hospital was used to treat typhus patients. Unfortunately, Dr. Niku became infected with typhus and died in 1944. He was replaced by Dr. Sirus; typhus had run its course by that time and the hospital was again exclusively used for VD patients. In 1945 the hospital was closed due to lack of income and VD patients turned to Pur Sina for treatment. This situation lasted until 1958, when in Rasht a center for the fight against VD was established.[900]

In 1949, Dr. Hoffman mentioned that the local maternity hospital cared for many cases, while the city hospital Rasht was getting a fine new surgical building, a gift from Shah. Moreover, two new private hospitals had been opened, with over 20 beds each.[901] It is quite likely that he meant the Dr. Milani Hospital and the `Adl Hospital. Dr. Milani's hospital was divided into two parts. One part with cheap rooms was for patients that were treated free-of-charge, and the other part with expensive rooms was for wealthy patients. This hospital only existed for a few years. Dr. Niri, an army major, who worked as a surgeon in the military hospital in Rasht, founded the `Adl hospital, which had a surgery department. When Dr. Niri was transferred to Tehran the `Adl hospital was closed down.[902]

Idem, pp. 227-34.
900. Ta'eb 1384, pp. 235-27 (with photo).
901. RG 231-1-5, Personal Report 1949 and Hospital Report R.E. Hoffman.
902. Ta'eb 1384, pp. 285-87, with a photo of the `Adl hospital on p. 289..

SABZAVAR

In 1919 or thereabouts, at the initiative of Dr. Ghani, a small hospital was constructed in Sabzavar, a town of some 15,000 people, which was financed by the local community.[903] In 1928, Dr. Rolla Hoffman of the American Hospital in Mashhad made an itineration tour to Sabzavar. By that time it had a population of 30,000 and it had a 100-bed hospital. It had just been closed due to lack of funds as these were cut off due to a budget readjustment after the departure of Millspaugh, the American Treasurer-General of Iran. The hospital was very clean and it was said that it would soon be opened again. Dr. Hasan Khan Eftekhari, the doctor in charge of the *Heshmatiyeh* hospital was a Persian "with a scientific spirit and free from fanaticism." He lent the American medical missionaries operating tables and many other things. He also offered them the hospital building itself, "but we reluctantly refused, for we know the fanatics would cause trouble to him if he allowed 'unclean heretics' to use it. So we rented two adjacent houses for hospital and residence." Dr. Eftekhari helped his American colleague daily as he had little surgical experience in his four-year training in Germany, and saw this as a chance to improve his skills.[904] No further information is available what happened to this hospital or about other medical developments in this town.

SALMAS

In 1895, Dr. Yohanan Sayaed, trained by Dr. Cochran, and finished at Medical College NY, ran a dispensary in Salmas treating 450 patients and 200 outside. Receipts in 5 months were $150.[905] Although the US missionaries continued their missionary and educational activities in Salmas, there seems to have been no further US medical activity.

---

903. Ghani 1367, vol. 1, pp. 190-191.
904. RG 231-1-2, Report Itinerating 4 April -19 May 1928; RG 231-1-7, Pioneering in Meshed, p. 81.
905. Presbyterian Church 1895, pp. 160-61.

Sari

In January 1920, Hasan Zahir al-Dowleh, governor of Sari at that time, bought a caravanserai outside the city and endowed it as a public civil hospital, which he called the *mariz-khaneh-ye Mahdavi*. However, the legator did not assign any other funds for the hospital's upkeep. Therefore, if the hospital functioned at all, it must have been one with ups and downs, due to its uncertain financial basis. It was demolished in the early 1930s, when on its site of about 2 ha, the new Pahlavi hospital was built. Several endowments constituted the financial basis for this hospital, which after the 1979 revolution was renamed Khomeyni hospital.[906]

Semnan

In or around 1885, the governor of Semnan, Anushirvan Mirza established a hospital (*mariz-khaneh*) in that town, which had a population of some 20,000. It probably fell into disuse after the end of his governorship in early 1888, for in July 1901 the inhabitants of Semnan raised money and established a *dar al-shafa* with a pharmacy as well as engaged two physicians and one surgeon to provide gratis treatment and medicines for the poor and pilgrims. The total cost amounted to 700 *tuman*s.[907] It is not known how long this institution lasted; it is not mentioned in local histories.

Shiraz

From 1900 until 1909, there had been a CMS dispensary in Shiraz, then a city of some 30,000 people, when it was closed due to lack of staff.[908] It would appear that Dr. Carr, a missionary physician from

---

906. Reza'i 2012, pp.125-27.
907. E'temad al-Saltaneh 1306, p. 79; *Ruznameh-ye Iran* 1374-78, p. 4020 (nr. 998, 12 Rabi` II 1319/29 July 1901).
908. Grothe 1911, p. 131; Cash 1930, p. 54. Although Grothe called it a hospital, this was not the case, because Richter 1910, p. 330 explicitly states that it was intended to build a hospital, but it had not yet been completed, when he wrote his book. In 1906, for some time, there was only one CMS staff in Shiraz, viz. Ms Malcolm M.B. 1905. *Mercy and*

Isfahan, was in charge of the dispensary. He was still reported to be in Shiraz in 1912, but later that year his address was in Liverpool.[909] During his absence, in 1910 Hajj `Ezz al-Molk endowed 5.5 `*oshr* of the revenues of two villages to buy a house and turn it into hospital. In 1912, he bought a garden just outside the Bagh-e Shah gate, in which the hopital was established. For the upkeep of the hospital `Ezz al-Molk deeded half of his property.[910] These annual cost were detailed as follows in the endowment document:

Table 28: Annual budgetted expenses of the `Ezz al-Molk hospital in Shiraz (1912)

Administration and supervision	Bookkeeper and hospital steward	1 `*oshr*
Repairs	Repairs, cleaning	0.5 `*oshr*
	Salary physician	
	Staff wages	
Hospital expenditures	Medicines, food, equipment, instruments	4 `*oshr*
Total		1,980 *tumans*

Source: Reza'i 2012, p. 123.

There is no information available about the actual functioning of this hospital and for how long. It is not mentioned in any of the sources consulted.

Medical CMS work started again in 1922 when Dr. Carr opened a dispensary in Shiraz with the help of Dr. Emmeline Stuart and Ms Alice Verinder, a British nurse, and a few local Christian nurses. They worked under difficult circumstances (cramped and crowded quarters, drugs in short supply), sometimes seeing 250 patients per morning.

Truth vol. 10 (1906), p. 378.

909. *Year Book* 1922, p. x, xiii. There also was Dr. Woollatt's dispensary at that time, about which I have found no further information. He was employed by the IETD. IOR/L/PS/20/224, Biographies of the notables of Fars and certain Persian officials who have served at Shiraz. Delhi: Government of India, 1925, p. 50 (see, 174. Mirza Muhammad Hasan Dast-Ghaib).

910. Reza 2012, pp. 121-23.

Initially, a building in a garden had been rented, but in 1924, with a donation of land by Hajj Mohammad Hoseyn Namazi, a maternity hospital was built. It was subsequently converted into a large general hospital with financial assistance of the IETD. The hospital, known as *Bimarestan-e Morsalin*, had a male and female ward, a midwifery department plus an out-patient department.[911] This hospital was the last one established by the CMS in Iran.

By 1932, Dr. J. Vaughn was in charge of the CMS Shiraz hospital, who received help from Dr. Sharp, the wife of Reverend Norman Sharp. The hospital had 20 beds in one large ward and a small operating room in a house nearby, where simple surgery was done under rather primitive conditions. According to Cash, describing the situation in 1928, "the hospital itself is a private house converted for the purpose. Every available corner of space has been utilized, but the congestion is terrible. However, a beginning has been made and the staff are bravely tackling the problems of extension."[912] In 1931, it was planned to replace the CMS hospital with a larger building that was under construction. At that time there was no other civil hospital in Shiraz,[913] although there was a military hospital. In 1931, the roof of the CMS hospital under construction was destroyed by fire, but construction continued and the building was almost finished at the end of 1932.[914] In 1935, the CMS opened its new 50-bed hospital on land donated by the former governor, Abdol-Hoseyn Farmanfarma. A female physician, Dr. E. T. Messe was in charge, who replaced Dr. Vaughn. Molly Williams was the nursing supervisor. The hospital also had a much improved maternity and obstetric service. After Dr. Messe, Dr. J. Coleman was in charge of the hospital for 16 years. At

---

911. Elgood 1951, pp. 534-535; Waterfield 1973, p. 166; Anonymous 1924, p. 182; Williams 1994, pp. 60-61; Azizi, Bahador, and Ghanbar 2014, p. 240. The move in 1922 had been facilitated by the fact that the IETD had asked the CMS to take over the medical care of its employees, on generous terms, when its own physician retired. Waterfield 1973, pp. 165-166.
912. Cash 1930, p. 54.
913. Administration Report 1931, p. 20.
914. Administration Report 1932, p. 17.

the end of 1935, Dr. Martin arrived to work in the CMS hospital.[915] In 1937, the CMS hospital was working at full capacity. Dr. Martin was transfered to Kerman, leaving a very energetic British female physician, Dr. E. T. Messe in charge with three nurses.[916] In 1945, Dr. S. Henriques seems to have been in charge of the CMS Shiraz hospital.[917] Like the other CMS hospitals in Iran it is likely that in 1954 the one in Shiraz also ceased operations.

Other Hospitals

The CMS hospital did not remain the only modern hospital in Shiraz for long. In 1931, "the military having acquired the two buildings given by the Persians in the past for use as hospitals."[918] The military hospital was under General Dr. Karim Hedayat, a graduate of the Paris Faculty of Medicine. He had only one assistant, a graduate from the Tehran medical school. Dr. Hedayat also had a private practice.[919] In 1924 Mohammad Hoseyn Namazi not only gave the CMS land to build a maternity, but he himself also built a small hospital, which was known as *Behbudestan-e Namazi*. Dr. Karim Hedayat was in charge, while Namazi paid all operating cost. After his death, the health department and the municipality fought over the control of this hospital and the allocation of funds and staff. As a result, in 1932 the hospital was closed down. Later in that same year, the municipality asked Dr. Zabih Ghorban to take charge of the *Behbudestan* and to have 30 beds available for the poor. There was no medical staff and Dr. Ghorban received no salary. Therefore, he only came to the hospital in the mornings, when from 8-10 a.m. he ran a dispensary, providing

---

915. Administraton Report 1935, p. 27; Administration Report 1936, p. 23 (The CMS hospital had some problem with the municipal health officer, was was settled through intervention of the governor-general).
916. Administraton Report 1937, p. 25; Ghorban 1989, p. 3.
917. IOR/L/PS/12/3713, Intelligence Summary no. 22 for the month December 1945.
918. Administration Report 1931, p. 20. In that year also Dr. Bahrami as new director of Public Health was appointed.
919. Ghorban 1989, p. 3.

patients with free drugs from the hospital's pharmacy. After 10 a.m. he performed minor surgeries and made rounds of the patients in the ward. In the afternoons he had his own private medical practice. However, like other Iranian physicians he lamented the fact that the number of drugs were few and most were of poor quality and effectiveness. "For the treatment of syphilis, we had only arsphenamine bismuth and mercury products, often risky for the patients. For treatment of gonorrhea, we used urethral irrigation with antispectics, such as a solution of permangate. For malaria we had only quinine, either tablets or injection, and we treated trachoma by scrubbing the conjunctiva and uding frops of silver nitrate or copper sulfate solutions." There were no modern pharmacies in Shiraz at that time and the five operating in the city were run by people who had no training in pharmacology and could not read Latin letters, so that physicians had to write their prescriptions in Persian.

When Dr. Ghorban's sister Keyhan graduated in nursing and midwifery from the American University in Beirut, he asked her to come and take charge of nursing, and train a few female staff members, whom he had convinced to volunteer for this task. All nurses went unveiled, which was before the abolition of the veil in 1936! This practice caused many people to come in large crowds to the hospital to see this phenomenon, while some newspapers protested against the working of unveiled women in the hospital. However, the governor-general, a progressive man, supported Dr. Ghorban's efforts and sent additional police to protect the nurses against any attack. In 1933, another family member, Ms Maimanat Dana, also trained in Beirut, reinforced the nursing staff. Also, Dr. G. Ovanessian came from Tehran to assist in the operating room. A local physician, Dr. T. `Oyun, who had been trained in Bombay in ophthalmology, began performing cataract and trachoma operations. In 1935 the Namazi hospital was transferred to the Department of Health as the municipality had no funds. However, this was no improvement, and, because working conditions had become impossible, Dr. Ghorban resigned and so did his entire female staff. The hospital was then downgraded to an outpatient dispensary for the poor. It was then known as Clinic no. 1 or *Darmangah-e Shomareh-ye Yek*.[920]

In 1936, at the initiative of `Ali Asghar Hekmat, then Minister of the Interior, and Dr. Zabih Ghorban, the government ordered the municipality to buy 20,000 sq. m. of land outside of Shiraz to build the Sa`di Hospital there (now renamed Shahid Faqihi hospital). However, when WW II broke out construction of the hospital was stopped. Because the government had no money, although disease was rampant and people were dying, Dr. Ghorban, who as of 1940 had become director-general of Health of Fars, appealed to the people of Shiraz to complete the hospital. The contributions were sufficient to buy beds and other furniture. With only limited staff and means only urgent cases could be treated. Fortunately, Dr. Ghorban was able to get his hands on some DDT so that the spread of lice causing recurrent fever and typhus could be brought under control to some extent. There was no treatment for typhus, but for recurrent fever one injection of neoarsphenamine (salvarsan) was found to be an adequate cure. The completion of the Sa`di Hospital only occurred at the end of 1945. Later it was expanded to a well-equipped 200-bed hospital, which also served as a teaching hospital for nurses and medical students.[921] In 1946, it had the following departments: internal medicine, surgery, ophthalmology, obstetrics and gynecology, and pediatrics.[922] In 1950, the construction of the new Namazi hospital, costing $2 million, and in 1962 of the Khalili hospital (1962) began. The 250-bed Namazi hospital was officially inaugurated in 1955, and since 1954 its income was ensured by the revenues of the waterworks, which also had been financed by Mr. Mohammad Namazi. However, those revenues proved to be insufficient and the government financed the shortfall, on condition that the hospital merged with the newly (1955) established University of Shiraz.[923] Also, there was not enough trained medical

---

920. Ghorban 1989, pp. 3-5; Azizi, Bahador, and Ghanbar 2014, p. 240.
921. Ghorban 1989, pp. 9-10; Administration Report 1936, pp. 18, 23.
922. Azizi, Bahador, and Ghanbar 2014, p. 240.
923. Ghorban 1989, p. 10; Azizi, Bahador, and Ghanbar 2014, pp. 241-42; Farahmandfar 1384, pp. 122-24.

staff to operate such a big hospital. Therefore, as an interim solution, with financial assistance of CARE, American doctors, nurses, dieticians and technicians were provided for the Namazi Hospital. To further resolve the staffing problem ICA provided special training programs in the United States for Iranian doctors, nurses and teachers for the Vocational School at the Namazi Hospital.[924]

Treatment of patients in a modern hospital requires having a trained nursing staff, which was in very short supply in Iran at that time. Therefore, in 1937, Ali Asghar Hekmat, the Minister of Education, organized the assistance of an American nurse, Ms A. Setzlar, to start a nursing school in Shiraz. A small building near the CMS hospital, where its students attended demonstrations, was rented as the teaching locale. To overcome the problem to find girls willing to become nurse Dr. Ghorban called on parents of girls, who had graduated from the ninth grade and persuaded some of them to allow their daughters to attend the training at the *Amuzeshgah-e Pezeshkyari*, or the School of Nursing Assistants. Finally six girls attended the two-year course, who were trained by Ms Metzlar, assisted by Ms Molly Williams, the CMS nurse, while Ms Soghra Namazi acted as interpreter. Dr. Ghorban taught some anatomy, physiology and medical terminology. When Ms Metzlar had to return to the USA because of WW II, the school was closed. Until then 20 nurse assistants (*pezeshkyar*s) had been trained, who worked in the Sa`di Hospital and the Health Department.[925] As a result of the agreement between the leaders of the 1945 tribal uprising and the government, a Village Doctors School (*Amuzeshgah-e `Ali-ye Behdari*) was established in Shiraz in October 1945.[926] With a new university that had a medical school as well as two modern Iranian hospitals and a nursing school Shiraz was well positioned to address the medical problems and challenges of Fars province. CARE provided

---

924. CARE 1961, p. 6 (CARE also developed a modern water system for Shiraz).
925. Ghorban 1989, pp. 11-12; Administraton Report 1938, p. 18.
926. Ghorban 1989, pp. 13-17; Farahmandfar 1384, pp. 118 (with the text of the agreement).

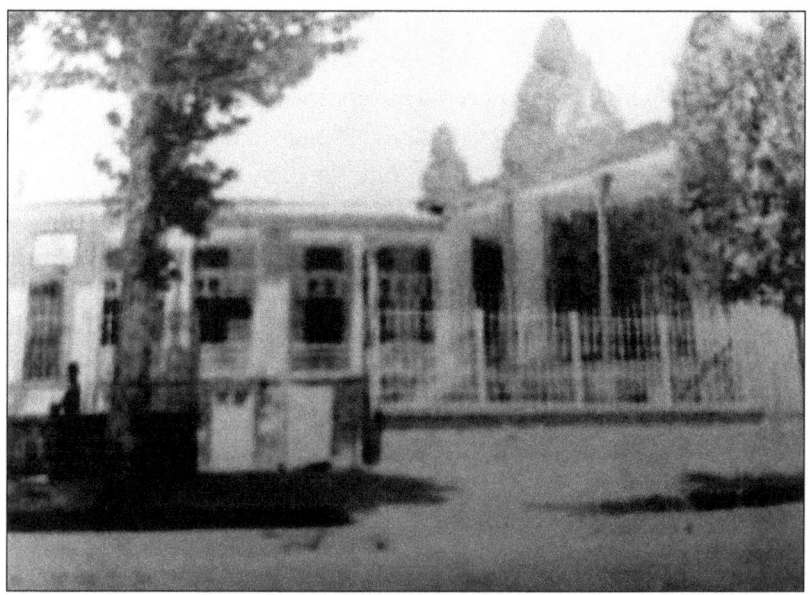

Behbudestan, Shiraz

the Namazi Foundation with a Director of the Nursing Services at the Namazi School of Nursing.[927]

SIRJAN

In 1945, the local health department of Kerman received 20,000 *tuman*s for the construction of a government hospital in Sirjan.[928]

TABRIZ

According to Eugene Aubin, about 1875, the American Presbyterian Missionary Society (APMS) established a 15-bed hospital with dispensary in Tabriz, which initially mainly served the Armenian population. However, APMS sources leave no doubt that missionary activity was started in 1873 (which Aubin misinterpreted to also mean missionary medical work), but it was only as of 1881 that Dr.

---

927. CARE 1961, p. 6.
928. Administration Report 1945, p. 6.

G. W. Holmes began his medical work in Tabriz,[929] and Dr. Mary Bradford, from 1888. Dr. Holmes was succeeded in 1892 by Dr. William Vanneman who served there for the next 40 years. By 1896, there were two dispensaries (although Waterfield mistakenly writes that it was a hospital as of 1893), one for men and one for women, with separate receiving rooms for them. It was only in 1898 that Dr. Mary Bradford established a hospital for women in Tabriz.[930]

Dr. Holmes had begun his work as a medical missionary in Urmiyeh, where he also had started training Iranian Moslem and Assyrian students as physicians. In 1878, he had been forced to discontinue his work there due to health reasons. Therefore, on his return to Iran in 1881, and this time to Tabriz, he employed one of his former students, Mirza Shimoil, who had completed his studies with Dr. Cochran in Urmiyeh, as his dispensary assistant. In his first report, Holmes stressed the great need for a hospital in Tabriz, a big city with 200,000 inhabitants.[931] Holmes' outcry in 1882 for the establishment of a hospital in Tabriz was heard, because in 1884 Mrs. W.H. Ferry donated $3,000 for the establishment of such a hospital, but the project was abandoned as it was too arduous a task for Dr. Holmes given his weak health.[932] However, the money was still available, and in 1890, the Tabriz Mission bought land for, among other things, a hospital,

---

929. No medical missionary is mentioned in Tabriz, see Presbyterian Church 1880, p. 42. In 1881, however, the return of Dr. Holmes was hailed by everybody desiring his service, which suggests that he had been there earlier. In fact, it is reported that: "Dr. Holmes has a medical class. One of his former students, Mirza Shimoil, who completed his studies with Cochran, is his dispensary assistant." Presbyterian Church 1882, p. 62.

930. Aubin 1908, p. 45; Wilson 1896, p. 259; UNESCO 1343, vol. 2, pp. 1449-1450; Waterfield 1973, p. 137. There was a physician of the Russian road company working in Tabriz. Grothe 1911, p. 131. Presbyterian Church 1899, pp. 208-09.

931. Presbyterian Church 1883, pp. 62-63 (One year later, Mirza Shimoil received a certificate that was equal to an MD degree. Another of Holmes' former students had become regimental surgeon in the Iranian army).

932. Presbyterian Church 1885, p. 76.

because in surgical cases patients could not be rightly treated at home. Also, there was not a single hospital in the Tabriz.[933]

Apparently, Dr. Bradford and Dr. Vanneman had prepared a hospital room in the female dispensary, for they reported that in 1893 that it was occupied during 131 days.[934] Although medical missionary work was free from persecution by the authorities in Tabriz, some people, who associated with the missionaries, suffered much by the behavior of their neighbors and families.[935] Nevertheless in 1893, induced by Armenians who resented conversions of their co-religionists, there was opposition by the government to the American Mission. The local authorities ordered the closure of the Mission school, which alarmed many Moslems, who did not dare to come for medical care to the Mission Compound. This may explain the empty hospital room in that year. Dr. Vanneman's extensive contacts among the highest echelons of government and of the Armenian community proved to be invaluable in conciliating the government and the hostile Armenians.[936] It is perhaps from that day onwards that the female dispensary occasionally had an in-patient. In fact, in 1894 Dr. Bradford's hospital room was in use for 202 days. In 1895, the hospital room was occupied 112 days by eight women,[937] for there was as yet no men's hospital room in Tabriz.

In 1897, on the property donated by Mr. and Mrs. Whipple, a hospital was built. This was made possible by special gifts by Mrs. Reid of Lake Forest, Ill. in memory of her daughter Mrs. Lillie Reid-Holt. Also, money was used that was given to the Memorial Funds by friends of the artist Theodore Child, who had died in Iran.[938] During

---

933. Presbyterian Church 1891, p. 176.
934. Presbyterian Church 1894, p. 191.
935. Presbyterian Church 1884, p. 66.
936. Presbyterian Church 1894, p. 191.
937. Presbyterian Church 1896, pp. 197-98.
938. Presbyterian Church 1898, p. 195 (Although the service of Dr. Bradford, a female physician was welcomed, the problem of possible defilement remained. Even when she finally was accepted into the house a Sayyed, "my every movement had been guarded with the utmost care that not a drop of water should fall on the carpet, nor even my finger come into contact with the faucet of the samovar.")

the winter and spring of 1897-98, the hospital was finished, assistants were trained, and eight patients were admitted.[939] Dr. Bradford was in charge of the Whipple Hospital, where since last September 18 patients had been admitted, 13 of whom were Moslems.[940] In 1900, Dr. Bradford had 20 in-patients in the women's hospital.[941] Although money was available for the construction of male hospital rooms, Dr. Vanneman believed that it was better not to open them, because his method of house calls was more effective. Dr. Bradford thought differently and in 1901 she had 20 in-patients[942] In 1902, the Whipple Hospital for women had 18 in-patients.[943]

In 1903, the Whipple Hospital for Women was closed during May-June and two weeks in August, because Dr. Bradford was itinerating, otherwise it was open all weekdays.[944] The three small dispensary wards and the operating room were finished in the late fall of 1904, too late for the patients of the cholera epidemic. The wards accommodated 12-14 beds. Of the $5,250 for the construction of the doctor's residence and the dispensary hospital, outbuildings and furnishing $2,300 were raised from the net of medical receipts. In 1906, Dr. Bradford returned to the US and did not return and thus, the Whipple Hospital for Women was closed, which up till that time had been well attended.[945] It was only in 1911 that a replacement for Dr. Bradford was found, viz. Dr. Orcutt, but she arrived in the fall and first had to learn Azeri. Therefore, the female dispensary and the Whipple Women's Hospital remained closed.[946] In 1912, when Dr. Vanneman returned from furlough work continued as before, but there was no trained assistant. As a result, the medical capacity of the American

---

939. Presbyterian Church 1899, pp. 208-09.
940. Presbyterian Church 1900, pp. 207-08.
941. Presbyterian Church 1901, pp. 255-56.
942. Presbyterian Church, 1902, pp. 236-37.
943. Presbyterian Church 1903, pp. 269-70.
944. Presbyterian Church 1904, p. 262.
945. Presbyterian Church 1905, p. 203; Idem 1906, p. 315 (attendance at dispensary higher than last year); Idem 1907, p. 329.
946. Presbyterian Church 1912, p. 368.

missionaries was insufficient to manage a hospital. However, the dispensary was open every weekday from 8.30 to 12. Many patients came from distant villages. Attendance was as in previous years, i.e. some 40 patients/day, most of which were Moslems. Dr. Vanneman considered house calls very important in his work. He did four per day in the afternoons. This made his dispensary self-supporting. He wrote: "A great part of these medical visits are consultations with the foreign trained native and other physicians, and therefore take considerable time."[947] In March 1913, Dr. Lamme arrived giving Dr. Vanneman time to oversee the construction of the new Mission compound. The Whipple-Kirkwood hospital dispensary was open; 12 obstetrical cases were attended to, all difficult cases and the ones in Moslem homes were "at the risk of the physician's reputation."[948]

In March 1914, a beginning was made with the construction of the Kirkwood Whipple Hospital for Women and the new hospital for men, both being under one roof. At that time Dr. Orcutt died, just when her influence among women was growing. In the fall of 1914, four rooms were made ready in the general dispensary building for Dr. Lamme's use to receive patients and use as a small hospital. These consisted of an operating room, a small drug room, and two small bedrooms. He then began having a daily surgical dispensary. Average attendance was about 10 cases per day. In March 1914, following the death of Dr. Orcutt, the large dispensary room was made into a sick room, giving Dr. Vanneman and Dr. Lamme room for five cases at a time. These beds were always full. Patients were there from one day to three months. Patients were required to bring their own food and caretakers, as the physicians could only provide medical care with their limited equipment. The hospital had only one trained nurse in October 1914, Ms Easton (later Mrs. Hoffman), who shouldered a large share of the work, especially as she knew Azeri, having grown up in Urmiyeh. When the new building was ready there was room for 36-40 patients, besides a house for the female physician and nurse and a dispensary for Dr. Lamme and the female doctor. Dr. Lamme did

---

947. Presbyterian Church 1913, p. 333.
948. Presbyterian Church 1914, p. 347.

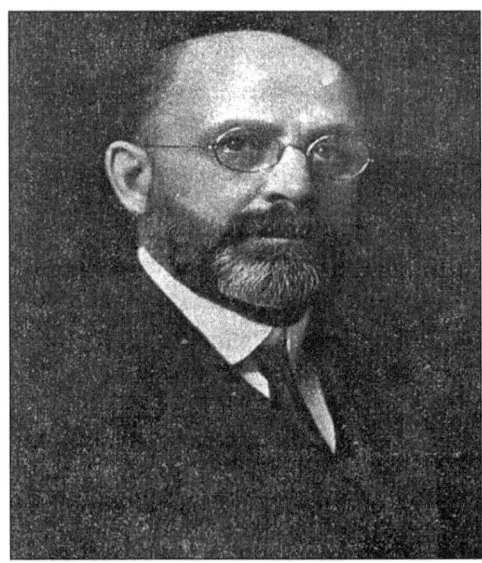
Dr. Vanneman

33 major operations and many minor ones; they had 35 in-patients; from all sources he received 820 *tuman*s, expenses were less.[949] Dr. Vanneman's dispensary work and house calls received more than $3,000 in 1915, enough to help support the Colton Memorial hospital and the Whipple Memorial for Women, both of which were then in a new building. Because there was no female doctor, work with women was less than possible.[950]

Dr. Vanneman had few cases in the hospital. Not only by preference, but also because the hospital was not yet fully equipped with beds. Most hospital cases were surgical in nature and were under the care of Dr. Lamme and Dr. Mary Fleming, the new female physician. The surplus of Dr. Vanneman's dispensary income again went to the hospital, which did well in 1916, despite the fact that it was able to deal only with 14 adult patients at the time. Moreover, many of its surgical instruments were very incomplete, old, and showing signs of wear. Another problem was that hospital supplies were expensive, some were difficult to get, while some were unobtainable at any price. Dr. Charles Lamme was in charge of the hospital, in addition to his

---

949. Presbyterian Church 1915, pp. 330-31.
950. Presbyterian Church 1916, pp. 302-03.

other medical work. From November to March 1916, Dr. Laura Müller (from Urmiyeh) kept the women's dispensary, receiving patients in the hospital, and assisting Dr. Lamme with operations. After Dr. Müller's return to Urmiyeh, Dr. Fleming had the women's dispensary two days per week, she received patients in the hospital and assisted Dr. Lamme with operations.[951] Part of 1917, the hospital was closed, in another part only urgent cases were received. However, after Dr. Lamme's return, the hospital was back on full schedule, and its beds were taxed to capacity.[952]

The work of the Tabriz medical mission was interrupted by the departure of the American staff for Hamadan on 30 May 1918, prior to the Turkish-Kurdish attack (14 June) and occupation of Tabriz, during which period the Turks and Tabrizis looted the American hospital. At that time, the staff of the Tabriz hospital consisted of Dr. Charles W. Lamme, who was the head of the so-called Colton Memorial hospital until May 1918, assisted by Dr. Edmund Dodd and Dr. Mary R. Fleming, who was in charge of the female section, known as the Whipple Memorial hospital. In reality, these two were wings of the same building. Other medical staff included Dr. W. S. Vanneman and Ms. E. Jean Wells, a nurse. At that time, they all had left Tabriz for Hamadan via Qazvin.[953]

In June 1918, the occupying Turks turned the American hospital into a Turkish one. It was then occupied by the regular Turkish army medical organization for five months and was used to its utmost capacity as indicated by the many wooden bedsteads and floor bunks in the basement. When in October 1919, the Turkish army withdrew these bedsteads were about the only moveable thing they did not take with them. Fortunately, Dr. Lamme's instruments had been taken to

---

951. Presbyterian Church 1917, p. 312.
952. Presbyterian Church 1918, p. 293.
953. New York Times 1918. The names of the hospitals are those of the families that made their construction financially possible. Prior their departure, Vanneman busy with dispensary, Lamme with hospital; he left Tabriz on 8 May 1918. Presbyterian Church 1919, pp. 271-80 (with details of what happened in Tabriz and Urmiyeh).

the Boys' School compound, while the hospital building was intact. In November 1919, Dr. E. M. Dodd of the Urmiyeh station reopened the Colton-Kirkwood-Whipple Memorial Hospital with 10 beds after having whitewashed, cleaned and repaired it. The available equipment was heterogeneous and limited. Beds and mattresses were lent by the Memorial School. Others were bought in the bazaar and a wooden operating table was constructed locally. The American physicians had very few drugs and mostly wrote prescriptions on the town's drugstores. The first three months they had few patients, unless they had been willing to take in typhus cases, in which case the hospital would have been full. In the spring of 1920 things went better, also because of the return of Dr. Fleming and Ms Wells in May. They received some instruments from the Persian-American Relief Commission, but needed bedsteads, general furnishings and supplies, including lab equipment. Ms Well's management improved patient care. In 1921, the hospital received some more equipment, while much maternity work was done among the Assyrian and Armenian refugees. At that time, the Colton-Kirkwood-Whipple hospital was the only modern hospital between Lake Urmiyeh and the Caspian, the Aras and Hamadan.[954]

The Colton-Kirkwood-Whipple hospital in Tabriz was closed for one month vacation. Ten days after the opening several hundred Moslem refugees from the Caucasus arrived. In November 1920 it was decided to depart from Tabriz, fearing an invasion of a Bolshevik army, and to close the hospital.[955] It was further decided to sell everything given the experience two years earlier, when the hospital was looted during the Turkish occupation. The hospital was sealed by the US consul and Iranian government guards were placed in the compound. Fortunately, the hospital remained undisturbed until the missionaries

---

954. Presbyterian Church 1920, p. 331-32; Idem 1921, p. 346; Speer 1920, p. 69.

955. On the Bolshevik threat and an account by one of the Caucasian refugees fleeing to Tabriz, see Hamideh Khanim, *Awake*. translated from Azeri by Hasan Javadi and Willem Floor with an Introduction and appendices. Washington D.C.: MAGE, 2016.

returned. In July 1921 the hospital was reopened; first work was begun in Dr. Vanneman's dispensary, where each weekday morning patients were seen. Meanwhile, repairs were done to the hospital; it was cleaned and equipment put back in place. Without the help of the Iranian army, which sold supplies to the hospital, it could not have been opened. As a result, a 30-bed hospital, with room for five babies, was functioning again. However, the lack of a female doctor was sorely felt, as Iranian women did not allow themselves to be examined by a male physician, even in their greatest need.[956]

In 1928, the bad news was that the hospital in Tabriz had to work with only half of the US doctors and nurses; the good news was that prejudice against the hospital had broken down. "Persian women are coming in greater numbers and the work among children has greatly increased. Follow-up work has had to be curtailed on account of the smallness of the hospital force."[957] The Tabriz hospital was becoming better known as one of the most efficiently conducted medical institutions in Iran. The number of patients from city and rural areas from all over the province coming for treatment was increasing.[958] This meant more work for the medical staff, which in 1929 had only one doctor during most of the year. This situation of a one-doctor hospital after Dr. Vanneman's death in 1933 did not change in the years thereafter.[959]

In the 1930 and 1940s, the Tabriz hospital was full of patients and busy with baby clinics, nurses' training classes, etc. Because of the depreciation of the rial after 1945, the high cost of living, and it being unreasonable to ask physicians to work without modern equipment, the Tabriz mission wrote to the Presbyterian Board that the appropriations had to be revised upwards. The current budget was based on the old rial value and the hospital budgets had long outgrown them. This had as consequence that, "We cater too much to the rich and turn away

---

956. Presbyterian Church 1922, pp. 377-78; Anonymous 1922 b, p. 146.
957. Presbyterian Church 1929, p. 103.
958. Presbyterian Church 1930, p. 194.
959. Presbyterian Church 1932, p. 175; Idem 1930, p. 165. Dr. Vanneman died in 1933.

many sufferers because they cannot pay, to secure from our practise the funds we must have."[960]

In April 1952, Dr. Lamme retired after 37 years of having served the people of Azerbaijan. His hospital work was continued by two young physicians, Dr. Ashton Stewart and Dr. Arnold Schneider. They observed that, "Of special interest is the increasing use of new drugs, new methods, new cooperation with local doctors and officials." In the spring of 1952, the hospital benefited from the expertise of four visiting American surgeons. In that same year, service to the lepers was re-established.[961]

Table 29: Patients seen, house calls made, receipts collected, hospital days, and operations performed in the American hospital in Tabriz (1884-1931)

Year	Vanneman's dispensary	Vanneman's house calls	Vannemans's receipts	Female dispensary	Female house calls	Hospital days	Male dispensary	hospital	Operations
1884	-	-	-	-	-		1200		
1886	-	-	-	-	-		3500		
1889	-	-	-	2669	-		-		
1891	1000	-	$125	3000	-		-		
1892	2000	-	-	-	-		-		
1893	4331	552	-	3025	582 hc		-		
1894	5348	742	$600	3013	625 hc	202	-		
1895	4320	-	$775	3095	-	112	-		
1896	5457	943	$1500	-	-		-		
1897	8579	1153	-	349	114		-		
1898	9300	833	-	2456	264	8 patients	-		
1899	-	-	-	3364	575	16 p	-	18	
1900	-	-	-	5068	672	20 p	0	0	

---

960. Presbyterian Church 1947, p. 55-56.
961. Presbyterian Church 1951, p. 67. There was a fire in the Tabriz hospital, see RG 161/3/51. For the history of treatment of lepers in Iran, see Floor 2020, pp. 271-318.

Year	Vanneman's dispensary	Vanneman's house calls	Vannemans's receipts	Female dispensary	Female house calls	Hospital days	Male dispensary	hospital	Operations
1901	8353	2080	1200	6155	885	20 p	-		
1902	1960	1320	1516 T	6856	999	18 p	-		
1903	7140	-	-	6893	699	10 p	-	-	34
1904	8152	1072	1800	-	-	-	-	-	
1905	8990	1406	2000 T	-	-	-	-	-	
1907	10905	1419	-	-	-	-	-	-	
1908	12737	1405	2800 T	-	-	-	-	-	
1909	13825	1200	2900 T	-	-	-	-	-	
1913	13250	1200	27340 qran	-	-	-	-	-	
1914	12118	1128	3000 T	-	-	-	-	-	
1915	11672	882	$3000	-	-	-	>2000		68
1916	13195	880	-	-	-	-	-	14	-
1917	12000								

Source: Presbyterian Church 1885, p. 76; Idem 1887, p. 81; Idem 1890, p. 175; Idem 1892, p. 212; Idem 1893, p. 182; Idem 1894, p. 190; Idem 1895, p. 159; Idem 1896, p. 197; Idem 1897, p. 167; Idem 1898, p. 195; Idem 1899, p. 209; Idem 1900, p. 207; Idem 1901, p. 255; Idem 1902, pp. 236-37: Idem 1903, p. 270: Idem 1904, pp. 262-63; Idem 1905, p. 302; Idem 1906, p. 315; Idem 1907, p. 330; Idem 1908, p. 367-68; Idem 1910, p. 342; Idem 1911, p. 332: Idem 1913, p. 333; Idem 1914, p. 347; Idem 1915, p. 331; Idem 1916, pp. 302-03; Idem 1917, p. 311; Idem 1918, p 293.

DISPENSARY

From the beginning of his stay in Tabriz in 1882, Dr. Holmes focused on his dispensary work where attendance was very large in his first year. He also did many consultations with many Iranian doctors at their request. He concluded that several of them "are really very well informed," but these had all been educated by European physicians.[962] Although money was available, Dr. Holmes decided not to build a

---

962. Presbyterian Church 1883, p. 63; Idem 1884, p. 67.

hospital given his state of health. The dispensary and house calls taxed his strength; in fact, in 1885, his medical work was interrupted due to his sickness.[963] Although Dr. Holmes worked the first six months of 1885, he again fell ill and then went to Urmiyeh to rest. On his return he re-opened the dispensary, but, due to reduced receipts, he had to let his valued assistant go, who had been with him for four years. The latter began his own lucrative practice.[964] In 1886, Dr. Holmes saw 3,500 patients. Receipts of the medical department made it almost self-supporting. His reputation led to his appointment as physician to the Crown prince Mozaffar al-Din Mirza, which was strongly opposed by the olama. Dr. Holmes, who first had declined the honor, finally accepted the post of Physician in Chief of the Crown prince for one year, which resulted in a successful practice at the palace.[965]

In the fall of 1888, Dr. Mary Bradford arrived, the first female physician in Iran. There was an enormous demand for a female physician and she would have been immediately overwhelmed with patients, if she did not have to study the language first. Nevertheless, she visited the palace twice per week, was training two medical students and also attended the dispensary.[966] After a few months she opened a female dispensary once/week as self-defense, because many patients came to her home at all hours. After a month she added a second day to her dispensary schedule; each day 3 hours. As of August 1889 she worked without interpreter.[967] In November 1890, Dr. and Mrs. W. (William) Vanneman arrived. In that year there was much sickness at Tabriz, including diphtheria, followed by almost universal measles and a wide prevalence of dengue fever. Scarlet fever also appeared. When Mr. Oldfather, an evangelist member of the mission, returned to the US, his house was made into a dispensary.[968] In 1891, Dr. Vanneman mainly studied the language, but he also wrote some

---

963. Presbyterian Church 1885, p. 76.
964. Presbyterian Church 1886, p. 86.
965. Presbyterian Church 1887, p. 81; Idem 1889, p. 85.
966. Presbyterian Church 1889, pp. 83, 85.
967. Presbyterian Church 1890, p. 175.
968. Presbyterian Church 1891, p. 176.

1,000 prescriptions and had a class of 4-5 Iranian students, which he also continued thereafter.[969] In 1893, "The removal of the women's dispensary to the church yard was an experiment, but is looked upon as a success." This move was made because Moslem women came to Dr. Bradford's house on Sundays either for Bible reading or medical treatment and thus, having the dispensary in the church yard facilitated evangelical work.[970] Among the cases seen eye diseases predominated, while respiratory diseases were second.[971]

It is perhaps from that day onwards that Dr. Vanneman had his male dispensary and Dr. Bradford her female dispensary. She also had started training a graduate of the Girls' School as a nurse.[972] In 1895 the hostile atmosphere in Tabriz had changed to a much friendlier one. The Crown prince called Dr. Vanneman several times to his palace, while there was a cordial relationship with local European and Iranian doctors. He also was called to the village of the chief *mojtahed* of Tabriz to treat him, where he stayed for two days and was looked after by the *mojtahed*'s family. Although Dr. Bradford's dispensary was full every morning, she also went to the leper village at 4 km distance from Tabriz. There were about 200 of them, who lived by begging.[973] In 1896, Vanneman had to close his dispensary for one month, when he had to attend to the new Shah, when he was moving to Tehran.[974] Dr. Bradford returned from furlough in July 1897 and resumed women's work.[975]

By that time both American physicians had settled in their daily routine. Because there was as yet no men's hospital in Tabriz, Dr. Vanneman only worked the dispensary and made house calls. The male dispensary was open every weekday morning for about 3.5 hours,

---

969. Presbyterian Church 1892, p. 212; Idem 1893, p. 181.
970. Presbyterian Church 1894, p. 191.
971. Presbyterian Church 1894, pp. 190-91.
972. Presbyterian Church 1895, p. 160.
973. Presbyterian Church 1896, pp. 197-98. On the occurrence and treatment of leprosy in Iran, see Floor 2020, pp. 271–318.
974. Presbyterian Church 1897, p. 167; Anonymous 1897, p. 431.
975. Presbyterian Church 1898, pp. 194-95.

where he noted that the poor were coming more than formerly. In the afternoon Dr. Vanneman made house calls. "It is our custom to charge every patient something. To the wealthy, the charge is about the same as the other European doctors charge; but to the poor the charge is merely nominal - only a cent or two- and this is taken with the idea to protect them from taking the medicine all at one dose, which they are inclined to do if it be given entirely free. Those poor whom we trust we don't charge anything." Dr. Bradford opened the new dispensary for women on 1 November 1898, although all construction work was not yet finished. The dispensary was open for seven months that year. She also visited the leper village twice.[976] In 1899, Dr. Vanneman went on furlough and so there was no medical work for men.[977] Dr. Bradford's outside visits were mostly to the poor, "who have no money, not even a rag." She further observed that: "Others with whom money was no question, have allowed a patient to suffer for hours and days before overcoming their prejudice, and calling in the doctor, who rendered everything unclean by her touch. ... Many women, too exclusive to think of coming to our houses, have thus been reached and often have become warm friends."[978]

Dr. Vanneman returned at the end of 1900 and settled in his old routine. In the morning (8.30-12) he was at the dispensary and oversaw the entire department. The Iranian Dr. Eshoo assisted him in the dispensary, preparing most of the medicine and seeing many patients, who were a mixture of the poor, the wealthy, and Europeans. "For the wealthy we have to have medicines that are palatable and that requires much time; most come from London." Patronage of the rich was important, because they paid and with their fees Dr. Vanneman was able to afford to treat the poor gratis. These were not only the urban poor, but also many villagers and pilgrims came; even some from as far as the Caucasus. In the afternoons, as was his practice, he made house calls.[979] Although the number of European and Iranian doctors

---

976. Presbyterian Church 1899, pp. 208-09.
977. Presbyterian Church 1900, pp. 207-08.
978. Presbyterian Church 1901, pp. 255-56.
979. Presbyterian Church 1908, pp. 368-69.

was growing in Tabriz, the number of patients in the American hospital dispensary was not affected; in fact, medical work was heavier than the previous year. Dr. Vanneman wrote: "in our dispensary everybody is treated the same way, a general has to wait his turn for a poor man, who does not pay."[980]

Dr. Vanneman believed that his method of house calls was more effective than hospital care. In Tabriz, a city with 200,000 people, there were 5-6 European trained physicians and a few trained in Iran itself (Moslems). In most of the 12 city districts there was an Iranian doctor, who had received some training in European medicine. In difficult cases they called Dr. Vanneman as an outside consultant. There was no trained surgeon in the city. True, the house calls, which were mostly consultations with Iranian and European doctors, took more time, but in this manner people could be better reached than in the dispensary, and, above all, no door was closed to the missionary doctor. Because these were all patients who were confined to bed, in fact, really hospital cases, and thus, Vanneman argued that he was actually doing hospital work in the homes. In this way he also was able to enter all homes, whether of the governor or the poor. He adhered to this rule, because his dispensary was in the center of a large city, and the sick were all around him, and, thus, it was impossible to answer every all. He only accepted distant cases as consultation to an Iranian doctor. In 1907, Dr. Vanneman made a total of 1,419 house calls. He went on horseback and stayed longer than in the US (0.5-1.5 hour). "We not only have to prescribe and give directions but also oversee the nursing, as there are no nurses in Persia." Because house calls took most of his time, he could only do four in the afternoon, but he was fully repaid for it.[981]

In 1903, Dr. Vanneman was able to construct a new building for medical work, and a physician's residence with a dispensary, which he financed from his medical receipts and gifts from US friends. Here, 7,140 male patients were seen. Dr. Bradford went itinerating in

---

980. Presbyterian Church 1902, pp. 236-37.
981. Presbyterian Church 1902, pp. 236-37; Idem 1903, p. 269 Idem 1908, pp. 368-69.

May-June and two weeks in August, otherwise the female dispensary was all weekdays open.[982] In 1904, Tabriz, like many other parts of Iran, was ravaged by an outbreak of cholera. The epidemic began in October and lasted more than two months. The American physicians thought that not less than 6,000 had died in Tabriz, while some others estimated the number of deaths at 10,000. During this time the dispensary was kept open every day and all day. Mrs. Vanneman and Mr. Jessup took care of medicines, while Dr. Vanneman made house calls. "Sometimes I was up all night. Nearly all foreign and native physicians had fled, while we were open."[983] In 1906, there was no women's work as Dr. Bradford was in the US. Dr. Vanneman continued to place emphasis on dispensary work (mornings) and house calls (afternoons). At that time, there were only 2-3 European trained doctors in Tabriz, and, therefore, people called the missionary doctors all the time to come to their homes.[984] An interesting development was that in 1909 Dr. Vanneman noticed that his weekday morning dispensary was increasingly well-attended by the wealthy, because of bad times they came there rather than have the doctor come to their homes.[985] In 1910, Dr. Vanneman went on furlough, while there still was no replacement for Dr. Bradford. Dr. Vanneman reported that 1909-10 had been the heaviest of the last 20 years. Attendance was much higher and house calls had been equal to the previous year. When he left in June 1910, the men's and women's department were closed.[986] In 1911, a replacement for Dr. Bradford was found, Dr. Orcutt, but she first had to learn Azeri. Therefore, the medical missionary dispensary and the Whipple Women's Hospital remained closed.[987] In 1912, Dr. Vanneman was back and work continued as before, but there he had no trained assistant. The American Tabriz medical staff was insufficient

---

982. Presbyterian Church 1904, p. 262.
983. Presbyterian Church 1905, p. 203; Idem 1906, p. 315 (attendance at dispensary higher than last year).
984. Presbyterian Church 1907, pp. 329-30.
985. Presbyterian Church 1910, pp. 341-42.
986. Presbyterian Church 1911, p. 332.
987. Presbyterian Church 1912, p. 368.

in strength for developing a hospital or touring the villages.[988] In 1913, the men's dispensary was open every weekday morning, in the afternoon house calls. The Whipple-Kirkwood hospital women's dispensary was open two mornings per week.[989]

In March 1913, Dr. Charles Lamme arrived and, after he had learnt Azeri, he and Dr. Vanneman divided the work between them. All medical work was in Dr. Vanneman's charge (mornings, dispensary with an average attendance of 40-45, afternoons, medical house calls). Mirza Ali and Israel Karam were Vanneman's assistants in the dispensary, the latter a third-year medical student of Dr. Packard in Urmiyeh. On 8 March 1913, Dr. Orcutt died of pneumonia just when her influence among women was growing. In the fall of 1914, four rooms were made ready in the general dispensary building for Dr. Vanneman's use to receive patients and as a small hospital.[990] Up to end June 1914, Dr. Vanneman had done 8,880 dressings on out-patients, apart from receiving 460 calls from other patients in the dispensary. He further made 184 house calls, many of which were consultations.[991] In 1915, Dr. Vanneman's receipts of >$3,000 were enough to help support the hospital. There was no female doctor, so work with women was not possible.[992] In 1916, Dr. Charles Lamm was in charge of the hospital and kept the hospital dispensary open for 6 days/week; he also did outside calls. In 1916, the stock of drugs was running out so that it became difficult to treat patients. Therefore, the American physicians themselves made substitutes for the chosen drugs.[993]

On 30 May 1918, almost the whole Tabriz missionary contingent left for Qazvin.[994] Only Dr. Vanneman and Mr. Jessup remained

---

988. Presbyterian Church 1913, p. 333.
989. Presbyterian Church 1914, p. 347.
990. Presbyterian Church 1914, pp. 347-48; Idem 1915, pp. 330-31.
991. Presbyterian Church 1915, pp. 330-31 (He received 820 *tuman*s, expenses were less).
992. Presbyterian Church 1916, p. 302-03.
993. Presbyterian Church 1917, p. 312; Dr. Mary R. Fleming started working in Urmiyeh in 1905. Presbyterian Church 1906, p. 301.
994. Presbyterian Church 1919, pp. 271-80.

behind, who were imprisoned by the Turks. However, such was their reputation among and appreciation by the Tabriz population that they were strongly defended by the two leading mullahs of the city. One, who was the head of one group of Shiites, preached in the mosque openly on their behalf. He said he had known them from their arrival in Tabriz, had only experienced good from them, and, if they were not released he would rouse the city on their behalf. The other one, who led another group of Shiites, even went in person to the Turkish pasha to defend them. A testimony by leading mullahs and merchants had been prepared in case the two men would have been court-martialed.[995]

In 1921, the dispensary was open five days per week.[996] In 1925, the hospitals and dispensaries in Urmiyeh and Tabriz treated more than 30,000 patients.[997] In Tabriz more patients were seen, despite fewer staff.[998] Each morning there was a dispensary at the hospital, whose reputation was widely known. Dr. Vanneman's dispensary in the center of the city was like "a Mecca for the sick of all races, so well known has it become that the street is named for it." Vanneman also continued his consulting practice with Iranian physicians.[999] In 1931, Dr. Vanneman saw more patients in his dispensary than ever before during his 40 years of work, i.e. >14,000. He also continued his consulting practice and was the Mission treasurer.[1000]

OTHER HOSPITALS

On 12 Ramazan 1326 (8 October 1908) the council of Tabriz decided to establish a municipal hospital a.k.a. *Melli*, which was opened in early January 1909.[1001] Nicholas reports on 29 December 1908 that the *anjoman* had established a hospital. The French Consulate had made

---

995. Presbyterian Church 1923, pp. 224-35.
996. Presbyterian Church 1922, pp. 377-378.
997. Presbyterian Church 1926, p. 222.
998. Presbyterian Church 1927, p. 212.
999. Presbyterian Church 1930, p. 194.
1000. Presbyterian Church 1932, p. 175.
1001. *Ruznameh-ye Anjoman*, vol. 1, p. 207, 321, 499, 500

an important contribution.[1002] The establishment of the hospital was the logical consquence of the law regulating the provincial *anjoman*s (art. 97), which assigned it the responsibility of establishing i.a. hospitals. A similar thrust had the Municipality Law (*qanun-e baladiyeh*).[1003] The actual construction was triggered by the fight between Constitutionalists and government troops.[1004] At first, the building was shared with the free care dispensary (*kheyriyeh*), but when the number of wounded rose, the building was exclusively used as a hospital and the *kheyriyeh* was moved elsewhere. Wounded enemy combatants were also treated. They were even given a bed with sheets. Sattar Khan, one of the leaders of the revolutionaries, visited the hospital and promised money and new clothes to one of the wounded enemy soldiers, after he had healed. The hospital depended on a monthly subsidy of 186 *tuman*s plus food and medicines from the *anjoman* as well as on private donations. Medicines were made available free of charge. Although initially under the *anjoman*'s supervision at the insistence of the foreign community the hospital was transferred to the Municipality. According to Kasravi, the hospital was located in a good building and had 25 beds distributed over seven rooms. It was in the Armenian quarter. The first director of the hospital was Mirza Mahmud Hakkak-bashi, while the medical director was Dr. Sarkis. According to the newspaper *Mosavat* the medical staff consisted in: 1 physician, 2 assistants, 4 day nurses, 4 night nurses, one cook, one cook helper, 1 clothes washer, and 2 servants. The hospital was operational until at least Moharram 1330 (starting 22 December 1911). After the Russian occupation of Tabriz on 27 December 1911, the hospital was transferred to the Russian physician Dr. Vahan, as a private hospital, and, as a consequence, no longer free treatment was given. Until November 1914, Dr. Vahan received a monthly subsidy/salary of 200 *tuman*s. Thereafter, the hospital was placed in the hands of Dr. A`lam al-Molk under the supervision of the Public

---

1002. Nasiri 2016, doc. 78, p. 345.
1003. Fardyar 1395, pp. 201-02.
1004. Nasiri 2016, doc. 77, 19 October 1908, p. 338. For the official opening, see *Ruznameh-ye Anjoman*, vol. 2, p. 910.

Health Office (*edareh-ye hefz al-sehheh*). However, Dr. A'lam did not consider the building suitable and moved to another one, where he opened the 32-bed Ahmadiyyeh hospital.[1005]

In 1924, the municipal hospital was reopened in Tabriz. It apparently was supposed to be a continuation of the old one, because it was said that it had been closed down at an unknown date. However, Gilmour, who reported this, was unable to obtain any information on its previous activities. It had 30 beds, but no other details are available about its activities.[1006]

In early 1925, the American Adventists opened a dispensary in Tabriz, which remained open till 1928. It was led by the Englishman Dr. H. E. Hargreaves.[1007] By 1930, a government hospital for both men and women was established.[1008]

Torbat-e Heydari

There were two small hospitals in Torbat-e Heydari, a town of 5,000 inhabitants. One, established by the British, was managed by the Consular physician, the other by the Russians, who likewise had opened a small hospital under the Russian Consular doctor. It is not known when these hospitals were established and how long these politically motivated establishments lasted.[1009] The Russian hospital was the first to be established. For the British consul reported in January 1904 that the British hospital was not yet in proper working order, but patients were already lining up for its services in great numbers. "A large proportion seem to be patients who have tried the Russian cure and are

---

1005. The above is based on Fardyar 1395 which has many photos of the building and staff.
1006. Gilmour 1924, p. 29.
1007. Sajjadi 1989, p. 261; Rühling 1934, p. 82.
1008. Presbyterian Church 1930, p. 165.
1009. The British Consulate had one medical officer, while the Russian Consulate had two doctors, one of whom was stationed at Kariz. The main work of the Russian physicians was the enforcement of quarantine regulations. Grothe 1911, p. 131; Adamec 1981, vol. 2, pp. 653-654; Bricteux 1908, p. 192.

now anxious to see if the English treatment is more successful. Special attention is paid to such cases, as, if they are treated successfully, it will at once raise the prestige of English methods."[1010] The Russian hospital may have remained open until 1917, because it constituted a link in the Russian sanitary barrier between Mashhad and Sistan.

URMIYEH

Following the establishment of a dispensary by Dr. Asahel Grant in 1835, American missionaries continued to provide medical assistance at Urmiyeh and its environs. After Grant's death in 1844, medical missionary work was continued by several physicians, including Dr. Austin Wright (1840-65), Dr. T. L. van Orden (1866-73), Ms K. Cochran (1871-75), and Dr. G. W. Holmes (1874-77). In those early days there was a hostile environment and little to work with. There was as yet no hospital, only a dispensary, followed by outreach work in the villages and thousands were treated. Not much is known about the early medical accomodations, but in 1876, Dr. Holmes reported that the dispensary moved to "commodious quarters and with its appointments merits the more comprehensive title of hospital. It is not designed to receive any in-patients, except for surgical treatment, as other duties have occupied the physician's time." Holmes not only engaged in curative and surgical medicine, but also developed prophylactic activities. Every year he

> held 'vaccination parties', when everyone was expected to present an arm. I have rubbed against the arm of a woman in a village holding a child terribly sick with smallpox. The people deliberately expose the children to measles, scarlet fever, and such diseases to get it over. Miss Holliday had smallpox but Dr. Holmes' treatment brought her through without one pockmark.[1011]

1010. Tchalenko 2006, p. 47, see also pp. 54-55.
1011. Johna 2003, pp. 47, 119.

In the fall of 1876, Dr. Holmes began a medical class. He further tried to make his medical department self-supporting.[1012] In 1877, medical activities at Urmiyeh were put on hold, because Dr. Holmes returned to the US for health reasons.[1013]

Dispensary

In 1878, Dr. Holmes was succeeded by Dr. Joseph Cochran, who wrote in April 1879 that "since arrival in December I've treated 5,000 patients in the dispensary and my house. Patients of all ethnic groups come listen to the religious service and receive treatment. Some came from 4 days distance on foot, some even father away. There is no skilled physician within 120 miles."[1014] Dr. Cochran's work program basically consisted in working in the dispensary and making house calls.[1015] He saw outpatients in: i. the hospital dispensary; ii. the city dispensary; iii. during visits to houses in the city; and iv. visits to villages. This same schedule was maintained throughout the existence of the Urmiyeh American mission. Most of Cochran's work and that of his assistants was in the dispensary, where twice/week (Tuesdays and Fridays) from 10 to 12, they saw 130 sick in the city dispensary, and the four remaining weekdays, in the forenoon, he prescribed for up to 70 patients at the hospital office. Of course, nearly every day there were five to 10 emergency cases outside regular dispensing hours. He also made 43 visits to villages and houses in the city. Also, his students and assistants saw several hundred patients alone in the city and villages. In 1898, in total almost 3,000 patients were seen at hospital dispensary; outside the dispensary twice as many. Although consultation was free, Dr. Cochran charged something for medicine and visits. In-patients also were charged, depending on their ability

---

1012. Presbyterian Church 1876, p. 42; Idem 1877, p. 42. Ms Cochran's "knowledge of medicine her thorough acquaintance with people, were humanly speaking all that saved Mr. S[tockig] from being buried by the side of his wife." Wells 1878, p. 26.
1013. Presbyterian Church 1878, p. 41.
1014. RG 91-20-7, Famous Urumia Hospital to be rebuilt.
1015. Presbyterian Church 1883, p. 60.

to pay and how much their treatment had cost.[1016] In the second half of 1888 and most of 1889, the two-day weekly city dispensary was under Hakim Oshanna Badal, the Iranian medical assistant, who saw about 100 out-patients per week.[1017]

In 1892, the arrival of Dr. Emma T. Müller was a most welcome addition to the medical team that now could extend its help to female patients. Dr. Cochran remained the head of the medical department, assisted by Dr. Emma Müller, who was the house physician of the women's department and supervised nursing there. She also shared the work in the dispensary with Dr. Cochran in the city dispensary, four days/week, where Dr. Isaac, the Nestorian assistant-physician also worked.[1018] In 1892, Iran was ravaged by yet another outbreak of cholera. Dr. Cochran in advance of cholera epidemic had published a pamphlet on the disease in Syriac and Persian on how to prevent and treat the disease. Both he and Dr. Müller were active treating patients during the cholera epidemic.[1019] In 1904, cholera again struck Iran. In Urmiyeh it came on 1 November 1904. In six weeks not less than 3,200 people died and in the villages the death rate was higher, because the villagers did not seek medical advice. In Urmiyeh, some 3,500 people were immunized with the prophylactic serum of Dr. Lustig, of Berne, of whom only five were attacked by cholera.[1020] After the

---

1016. Presbyterian Church 1884, p. 66; Idem 1885, p. 71; Idem 1886, p. 82; Idem 1892, p. 206; Idem 1899, p. 202; Idem 1918, p. 290. The need for medical treatment was great. People came in droves every day; "some on foot, others on horses, donkeys, oxen, or on the backs of their friends, or borne on litters." Presbyterian Church 1885, p. 72.

1017. Presbyterian Church 1889, pp. 82, 94 (Dr. Alexander of Hamadan was at Urmiyeh for some time); Presbyterian Church 1890, p. 168.

1018. Presbyterian Church 1892, p. 206; Idem 1894, p. 188; Idem 1895, p. 156; Idem 1900, p. 202.

1019. Presbyterian Church 1893, pp. 177-78. Although the text clearly states that the pamphlet was also written in Persian, I think that the editor must have made a mistake, for few people knew Persian in Azerbaijan. Therefore, it is more likely that the pamphlet was written in Syriac and Azeri.

1020. Presbyterian Church 1905, pp. 291-92 (doctors are stopped in

summer of 1905, cholera raged again at Urmiyeh for several weeks. Measures were taken to prevent its spread; 5,000 vaccinations were done, of the latter hardly any patient got cholera. The pamphlet made by Cochran in Persian and Syriac in 1894 was distributed.[1021]

Hospital

In 1878, Holmes was succeeded by Dr. Joseph Cochran. He immediately raised the need to erect a hospital in Urmiyeh, because surgical cases could not be treated successfully, unless they remained under his care and control.[1022] Moreover, as another missionary later emphasized, a hospital had "the advantage that it satisfied: i. the need of a merciful and Christ like provision for the sick; ii. the salutary influence upon the Mission work especially in disarming the prejudices of the Mussulmans and showing to all the spirit of Christ."[1023] This appeal received a positive reaction from the Presbyterian Westminster church in Buffalo, NY, which made funds available for the construction of the hospital that was begun in 1880. The building was erected 3 kms from Urmiyeh in a beautiful compound on the banks of a river of the same name.[1024] The so-called Westminster Hospital was completed in 1882. The hospital had to charge patients for its service, because a single bed for one year cost about $25. However, while some patients were able to pay board, others were not. Mrs. D.P. Cochran was the hospital matron, who made the rooms brighter and more attractive with help from ladies of the church in the USA.[1025] When the hospital was open for business the scope of surgical work increased.[1026] Nevertheless,

---

the road and asked for advice; house calls are important. We also take medical care of the German orphanage, the Russian mission and its school, often called at the British mission and the French schools).

1021. Presbyterian Church 1906, p. 308.
1022. RG 91-20-7, Famous Urumia Hospital; Presbyterian Church 1880, p. 40.
1023. RG 91-20-7, Famous Urumia Hospital.
1024. RG 91-20-7, Famous Urumia Hospital.
1025. Presbyterian Church 1883, p. 60; Idem 1884, p. 65; Idem 1885, p. 72.
1026. Presbyterian Church 1920, p. 326.

the beginning of the hospital was a difficult one, for there was no support structure whatsoever. There was no other doctor to consult about difficult cases, no anesthesiologist no pharmacy, and there were no nurses or orderlies. Basically, Dr. Cochran had to do many of these support tasks himself and to ease his task he had to train helpers. He compounded his own medicines, trained school boys and servants to give chloroform in the OR, he himself had to monitor the patient's pulse and breathing during the operation and had to organize his instruments in such a way that he could easily access them while operating. After the operation with the help of his 'assistants' he carried the patient to the hospital bed. For many years there was not even an autoclave in the surgery and lab work was quite sketchy. And yet Dr. Cochran's name and influence was great throughout the region.[1027]

In 1890, Mrs. George Howard of Buffalo, N.Y. gave $2,000 to erect another hospital building, while friends from Buffalo added $350 for furnishing the new wards. The new building was called the Howard Annex. "It is a square, three-story building, including the basement, faced with red brick. Aside from the rooms in the basement, which are used as wood or store rooms, there are four rooms for patients, besides a suite of rooms for the matron, Mrs. D.P. Cochran." It was located on one side of the main building, and on the other side the dispensary, with rooms for medical students and assistants. This building allowed the medical staff to separate men and women. The old building had been exclusively for men. In 1891, the Howard Annex for women had 121 in-patients.[1028] In 1900 and 1901, an important Iranian nobleman donated $40; a gift of the Lymans of Minneapolis funded the construction of a well-fitted and much-needed operating room, an addition, as a memorial to Mrs. Cochran.[1029] Later, the so-called Lyman Memorial, with a new operating room and an additional four-bed ward was added. Within the Compound there also were residencies for the physicians. Its main building was 75 x 30 feet, two stories high,

---

1027. RG 91-20-7, Last annual report of the Cochran Memorial Hospital, 1934.
1028. Presbyterian Church 1892, p. 206 (arrival of Dr. Emma T. Miller).
1029. Presbyterian Church 1901, p. 250; Idem1902, p. 232.

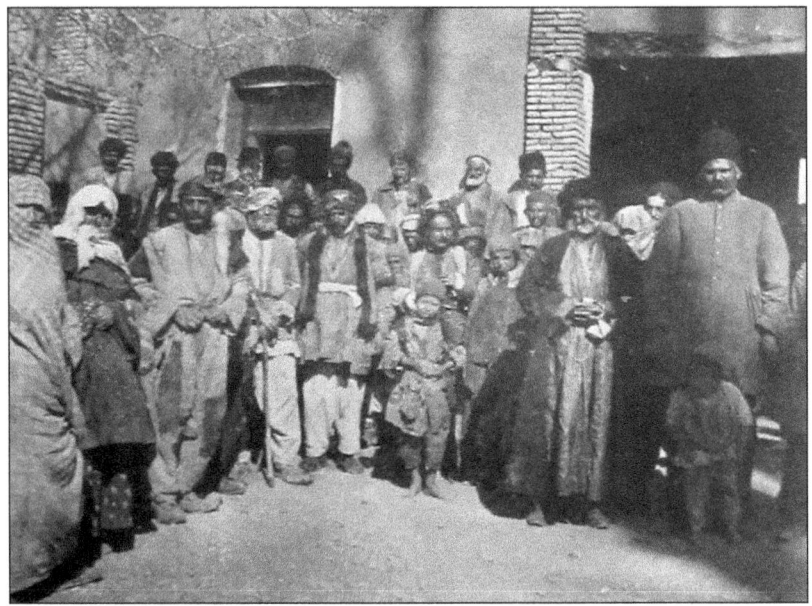

Above: Dispensary day at the Urmiyeh hospital. *Opposite:* Dr. Cochran with Kurdish chiefs at the hospital of Urmiyeh (ca. 1900)

and accommodated up to 30 patients.[1030] The so-called Westminster Hospital was built on a 15 hectares piece of land. When it reached its final dimension in 1906, it had become a 100-bed hospital. There was a morgue and a dissection room in the basement, while the upper floor had patient wards, two operating rooms, a pharmacy, and ten small isolation rooms. The new building connected the two older buildings, making an imposing front. As a result, the hospital had room for 75 in-patients, and better surgical equipment.[1031]

Due to demand on his time and limited funds, Dr. Cochran only was able to open the Westminster hospital part of the year; it usually closed during the summer months. In 1885, it was open for 9.5 months,

---

1030. Wilson 1896, pp. 74, 259; UNESCO 1343, vol. 2, p. 1449; Presbyterian Church 1920, p. 237. For some time the Anglican mission also had a medical missionary in Urmiyeh in the 1890s, but he returned after a while. Richter 1910, pp. 310, 313.

1031. Presbyterian Church 1909, p. 353.

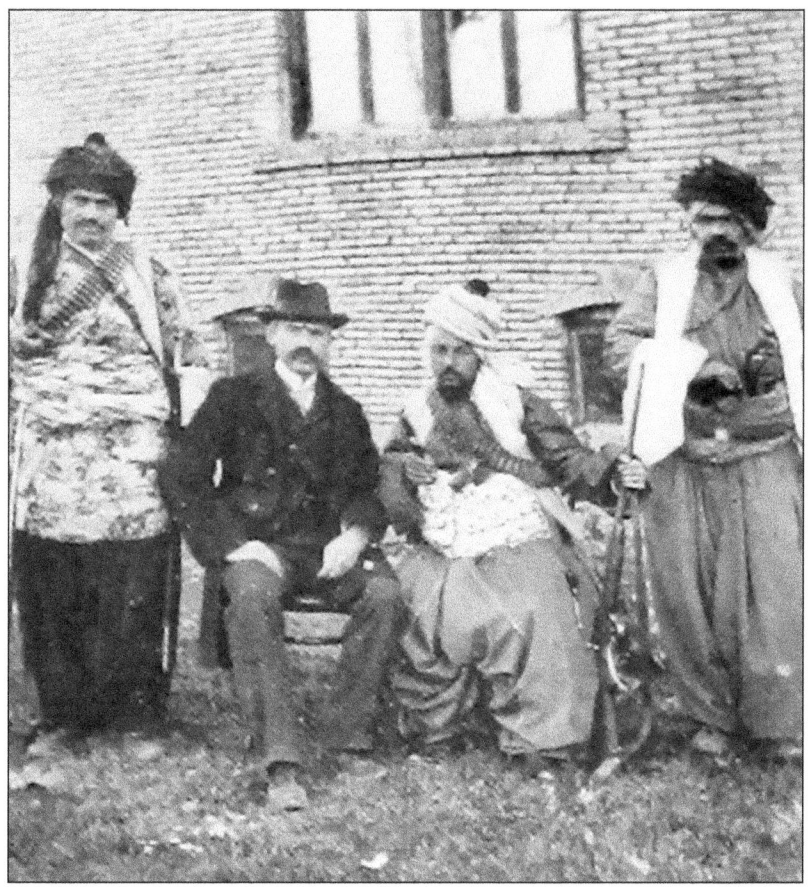

7-8 months in 1886, 8.5 months in 1890 and 9 months in 1894.[1032] Sometimes exceptions were made. In 1892, the staff had just closed the hospital when an important lady came, and thus, "we readied two rooms for her and her escort."[1033] In 1897, as usual, the hospital was closed during the 3 summer months; nevertheless a few patients, who came from afar, were admitted.[1034] In 1898, the hospital was open till

---

1032. Presbyterian Church 1886, p. 82; Idem 1887, p. 77; Idem 1891, p. 172; Idem 1895, pp. 155 -56 (because the fiscal year was from 1 July to 30 June, the hospital was actually open from 10/09/1893 to 20/06/1894).

1033. Presbyterian Church 1894, p. 188.

1034. Presbyterian Church 1898, p. 188.

the first June.[1035] Sometimes, the hospital was closed altogether such as in 1888, when, after 10 years of work, Dr. Cochran left on furlough in April.[1036] In 1889, the hospital reopened when Dr. Cochran returned early winter.[1037] But even in case of a complete closure exceptions were made, such as in 1899, when due to Dr. Cochran's absence the hospital was closed, 16 patients were admitted who could supply their own food.[1038]

In the beginning, the in-patients were mostly Assyrians; more men than women. More than half of them were surgical cases.[1039] Many patients remained for a long time, but lack of funds limited the number admitted.[1040] Some came from as far as the Caucasus and Nineveh. Very few were wealthy patients, who, after leaving, usually sent gifts. Most patients were so poor that they were unable to give anything and even had to be given clothes and a riding animal to return home. At that time, this was the only hospital outside Tehran. In 1893, the hospital had about 500 in-patients per year, a much larger number in dispensary and many noblemen were treated at home. In total, the hospital treated 4,000-8,000 patients per year.[1041] Although the majority of hospital patients still were Christians, but in 1901 more Moslems had been treated than before.[1042] With the new building and OR also came better surgical equipment.[1043] The latter was indeed a welcome addition; because the missionaries in Urmiyeh were so isolated that they always needed more surgical and medical appliances.[1044] They often had to deal with unnecessarily difficult cases. "In surgical practice we are always meeting with cases where the native surgeons

---

1035. Presbyterian Church 1899, p. 202.
1036. Presbyterian Church 1889, p. 82.
1037. Presbyterian Church 1890, p. 168.
1038. Presbyterian Church 1900, p. 202.
1039. Presbyterian Church 1886, p. 82.
1040. Presbyterian Church 1892, p. 206.
1041. Presbyterian Church 1894, p. 188.
1042. Presbyterian Church 1902, p. 232.
1043. Presbyterian Church 1909, p. 353.
1044. Presbyterian Church 1895, p. 155]-56.

have so maltreated the patient that either the case cannot be saved, or the result of long and difficult effort is only crowned by limited success."[1045] In 1904 the medical staff treated 12,754 patients of all creeds and ethnic groups.[1046]

In the 1890s, the hospital had an average of 300 in-patients, and performed a variety of operations, including those on the eye. In 1896 it had trained twelve Iranian physicians. The addition of a new operating room after 1906 made abdominal surgery possible, while 28 more beds were added to the hospital's capacity, which additions were called the Cochran Memorial, made possible by special gifts in honor and memory of the late Dr. Cochran.[1047] Dr. Joseph Plumb Cochran was born on January 14, 1855 and died on August 18, 1905 in Urmiyeh. His father, the Reverend Joseph J. Cochran, and his mother, Deborah Plumb, traveled to Iran in 1848 as first-generation American missionaries. His death was mourned by many; more than 10,000 attended in his funeral. He was buried on the other side of the steep Seer Mountain, in view of his wooden house, just opposite the boarding school of the Seer village, where his wife, Catherine, and her parents, were also buried. Through his work and that of his collaborators the fame of the name of the Urmiyeh hospital spread throughout Iran, eastern Turkey and even Southern Russia. For 27 years Dr. Cochran had served the community. "He was the first to send out physicians, natives of Persia, trained in western science." Because of this Dr. Cochran and Dr. Holmes both received the order of the lion and sun second-class and the Iranian doctors received titles.[1048]

In 1909, Dr. Packard, who came to Urmiyeh in 1906 and succeeded Dr. Cochran, wrote that in the new Memorial Hospital several operations

---

1045. Presbyterian Church 1905.

1046. Speer 1911, pp. 166, 270, 328-329.

1047. Speer 1911, chapter 16; Wilson 1896, pp. 267, 275; Presbyterian Church 1920, p. 237; Idem 1894, p. 188; Idem 1920, p. 326. http://www.ams.ac.ir/AIM/0252/0252127.htm.

1048. RG 91-20-7, Famous Urumia Hospital to be rebuilt; Yourdshaian et al. 2014, pp. 280-81. For the training of Iranian physicians by the American missionaries, see Floor 2020, pp. 75–82

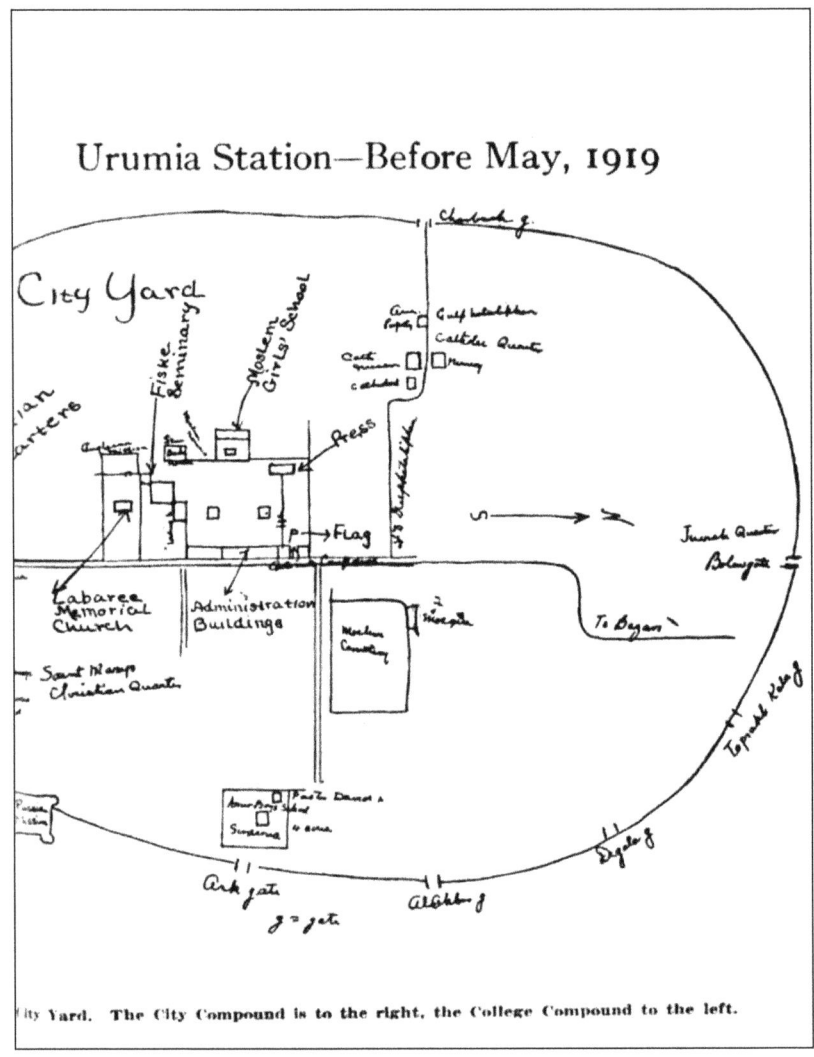

Above: Map of Urmiyeh indicating the location of the American Mission before 1919. *Opposite:* Map of Urmiyeh with the location of Galla (*below to the left*) and the location of the new missionary compound with hospital and schools. 1930.

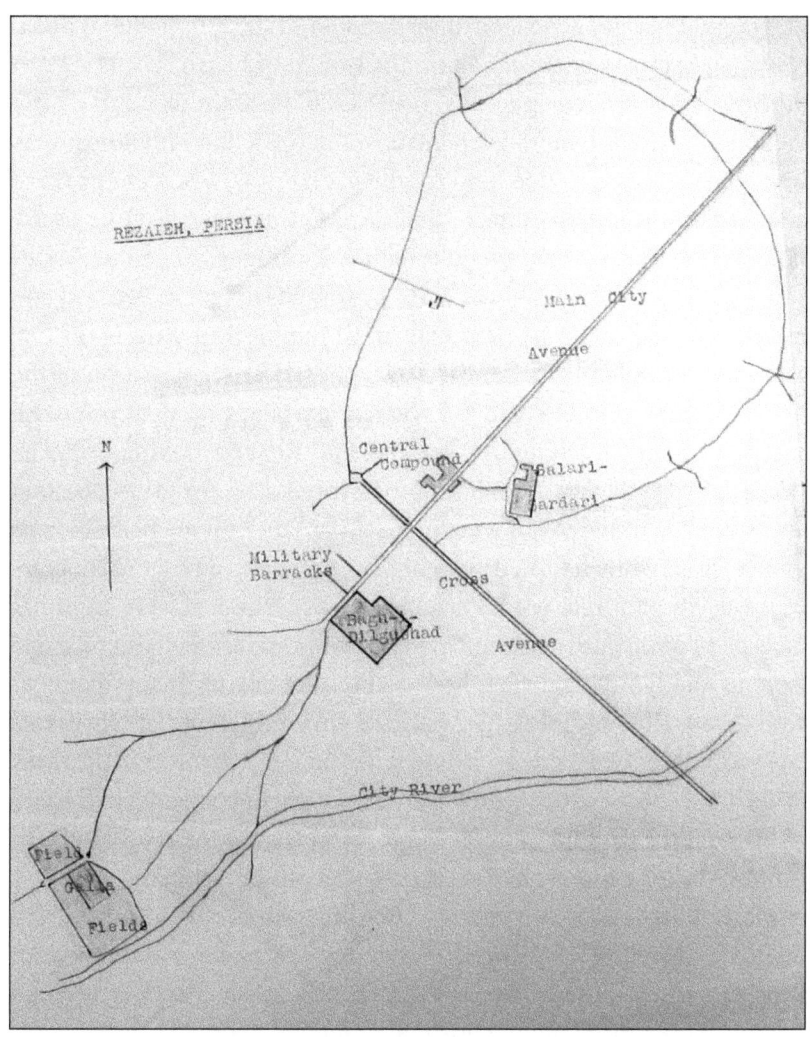

could be done, such as hernia, which they had been unable to do before.[1049] In 1911, the hospital was closed during the summer. After it opened on 1 October, the hospital was full of patients, "closets full of clean bedding, necessary servants. In the middle of previous winter we had as little as 10 patients; this year we never had less than 5-6 wards full."[1050] When in 1912, Dr. Packard returned from Hamadan

---

1049. Presbyterian Church 1910, p. 337.
1050. Presbyterian Church 1912, p. 363.

the hospital was reopened, but after two months he fell ill with typhoid fever, and so it was closed again for two months. In January 1913 the hospital was open again.[1051] In 1914, Dr. Packard was still ill, but the mission staff voted to keep the hospital open, but only to patients who were able to provide food for themselves.[1052] When Dr. Packard had recovered from his illness, the hospital was never so full; after 1 January 1915, it was submerged with war refugees. The number of sick was so great that medical work was impossible. Dr. Packard and his Iranian assistants worked hard until they fell ill with fever one after the other; two of them died of typhus. The composition of the patient population reflected the warring parties: Christian refugees, wounded Kurdish irregulars, Turkish and Russian soldiers.[1053] The year 1916 was a difficult one for the hospital. The Assyrian assistant physician and druggist left with their people. Also, all medical students and most servants had fled; in addition, there were no other doctors in town, all had fled. Mrs. Packard and Ms Burgess were morning inspectors of the hospital and Dr. Packard was physician, druggist and general handyman and each had to go to the city to treat patients as well as the Russian force. Dr. Packard saved a village of Christians from slaughter by Kurds by riding with the US flag through the thick of the fight, because the Kurds respected him. Fortunately, at the end of 1916, Dr. Ellis and his wife came, who shared the workload. Dr. Emma Muller came from Tabriz and was put in charge of women's clinic and the female dispensary. Dr. Ellis took over the hospital and the male dispensary.[1054] Together they faced the chaos and horror of Moslems against Christians and the Turkish onslaught. The Mission schools were closed but the hospital remained open. Due to the insecurity prevailing in the province in 1917, roads had become unsafe, so that patients could not travel in large numbers. Especially, patients

---

1051. Presbyterian Church 1914, p. 341
1052. Presbyterian Church 1915, p. 326 (Urmiyeh: Dr. Emma Muller, Mrs. Cochran, Dr. Daniel Werda and Rabi Berkho as druggist).
1053. Presbyterian Church 1916, p. 301.
1054. Presbyterian Church 1917, pp. 306-07; RG 91-20-7, Famous Urumia Hospital to be rebuilt.

from afar didn't come, apart from Sowjbulagh Kurds as in-patients. This meant that the workload that had increased until the beginning of the war, diminished. Emergency cases and gunshots compensated for this, and sometimes there were more patients than the doctors could handle. The Russian Red Cross doctor did much charity work in the city and villages. In return, Dr. Packard did some difficult operations for the Russian doctor. Dr. Dodd went to Sowjbulagh to check whether cholera had broken out there, at the Russian doctor's request.[1055]

Throughout the war years the hospital served thousands of refugees and soldiers, of whatever creed and side. Despite raids, massacres and the Turkish invasion the hospital continued to function. During the early summer of 1918, the hospital was full with 200 in-patients. The flight of the Christians had scattered almost all local hospital helpers and half of the patients. During the night of 30 July 1918, the Turks broke through the Assyrian lines and 80,000 Christians fled; the missionaries learnt about this at 2 a.m. in the morning and they decided to stay. Urmiyeh was pillaged and sacked by the Kurds and death followed them. Most of the Moslem population escaped, but most of those who had stayed behind were killed. One day later the Turks took over the hospital and turned it into a military hospital. Those patients that were not massacred were moved to the school building. The US doctors continued their work in the college buildings, but conditions were unsatisfactory. Also, the Turks brought virulent malaria and other diseases. The nurses continued to care for the sick, and so did Mrs. Cochran and the two American doctors. Sometimes only a cup of cold water could be given, because supplies were lacking. This care continued until 8 October 1918, when the missionaries were deported and had to leave the sick behind. After the missionaries were deported the refugees were all collected in the city yard of the American mission and Dr. Olkhus S. Amrikhus, the best member of the last medical class, assisted by the three nurses in training, took care of the sick and wounded among the refugees and made some house calls in the city among Moslems. They continued to serve the 800 remaining refugees until the massacre of 24 May 1919 in the city yard, when Dr. Olkhus was killed; fortunately, the nurses

---

1055. Presbyterian Church 1918, p. 290; Idem 1920, p. 326.

and refugees were rescued and brought to Tabriz. Dr. Olkhus was the 12th doctor in Urmiyeh to die during the war. After the massacre, the hospital was looted of everything, including all doors and windows. The last medical work in Urmiyeh was done during the captivity of Christians in the governor's yard from May 24 to June 18, 1919. Some 100 patients were cared for, amputations and some minor operations were done, while only one patient died. "The final care of these cases was by a former medical student, a Moslem who failed in his examinations and dropped out of his class before completing half of his work." It was only then that the hospital in Urmiyeh ceased to function. Medical work was continued in Tabriz among the refugees and the Moslems there, because the hospital in Tabriz (see there) was reopened by the Urmiyeh medical staff and operated until the return of the Tabriz missionaries. When the Turks left they took all drugs and equipment and, in February 1919, when Dr. Lamme returned to Tabriz, only the operating room furniture and few locally made tables and chairs were left.

After three years, in the fall of 1922, the Kurds were driven out of Urmiyeh by the Iranian army and the missionaries immediately (in November) returned. Dr. Joseph Cochran Jr. started medical work and the hospital. Thousands came to the dispensary even while hatred against Christians still reigned. Dr. Ellis returned from furlough and relieved Dr. Cochran, who returned to his work in the hospital of Tabriz. Dr. Ellis came with fresh supplies and surgical outfits supplied by friends in the US. The governor closed the missionary school, but the hospital remained open and the missionaries held religious services there. When the hostile governor fell ill, he was treated in the hospital by Dr. Ellis. Thereafter, he totally changed his behavior and became very friendly towards the missionaries.[1056] Although the war was over, its impact on the former war zone had been devastating. "West Persia is still suffering from the effects of the War. In the Sulduz district, south of Urumia, a very small fraction of the land is being cultivated and scores of destroyed villages are not being rehabilitated. The people

---

1056. RG 91-20-7, Famous Urumia Hospital; Presbyterian Church 1920, Presbyterian Church 1920, pp. 326-28.

live in extreme poverty. Scores upon scores of them, men, women, and children, are going through this winter with neither hats, shoes, nor stockings, and with only enough thin cloth to cover their bodies."[1057]

After the missionaries' return to Urmiyeh in November 1922, dispensing work was carried out in the so-called Sardari compound. From November 1922 to December 1925, the totally inadequate hospital was a makeshift operation in the recitation hall of the boys' school. In fact, the dispensary was the most active department of the medical mission until the new hospital was built in 1931. Patients came from very far such as from Khoy, Salmas, Maragheh, Marand, Solduz, Sowjbulagh, and from the mountain regions.[1058] Dispensary attendance was more than the combined ones of Tehran and Hamadan, and its hospital was more used than all other mission hospitals, except Mashhad, which was a class by itself. Half of the out-patients were Moslems, the other half were Kurds, Jews and Christians. A quarter of the patients were Moslem women; there were gynecological exams of 63 Moslem and of 26 Christian women. Dr. Iskander Khan Mirzayoff helped in making work in the dispensary go smoothly.[1059]

By 1925, according to Iranian government figures, there were only 15,000 Assyrian and Armenian Christians remaining in the Urmiyeh and Salmas region, the captive market for the American missionaries. On 12 November 1925, Dr. Cochran Jr., came to Urmiyeh and quietly resumed work. At the end of 1925, the hospital took up quarters in rented quarters in the adjoining compound, which later was purchased. "It was a tumbled down Iranian mansion, memorable because of the 15 different levels to the floors, the wandering nature of its roofs, and the utter lack of modern facilities."[1060] The hospital compound itself remained, but was still occupied by the Iranian army for more than one year after the return of the missionaries. When the Iranian army finally

---

1057. "During 83 years we took care of no less than 300,000 patients, if we included those seen by our graduates in medicine." Presbyterian Church 1920, p. 327.
1058. RG 91-20-7, Report Medical Work Urumia 1924-1925.
1059. RG 91-20-7, Medical Report Urmia 1925-1926.
1060. RG 91-20-7, Cochran Memorial Hospital Report 1932-1933.

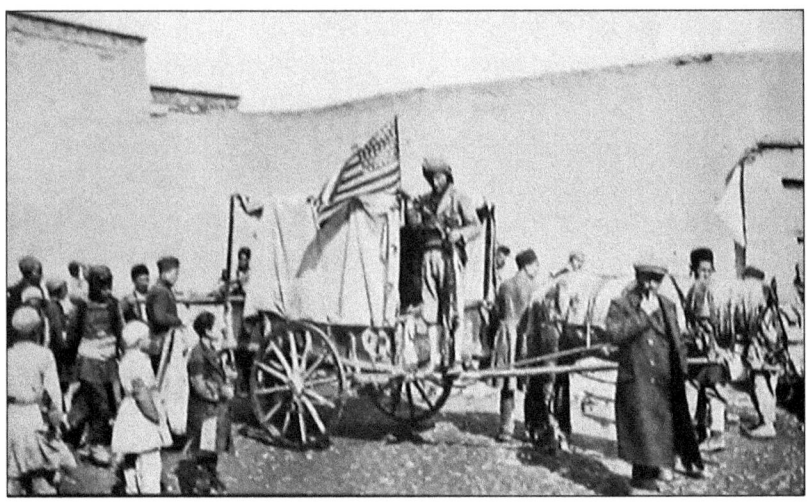

American Red Cross ambulance at Urmiyeh, February 1918

departed it left the hospital in a half ruined state requiring thousands of dollars of repairs. Even so the hospital continued to function. The only available building was the Sardari boys' school and the house built for Kasha Yaku. Until two rooms in the school building could be repaired one room in the house was made into a temporary dispensary. As much work was done as possible in the absence of drugs, equipment and assistants, and Dr. Cochran mainly made house calls, and visited some villages. Hospital admittances were somewhat lower than the average of the other American missionary hospitals.[1061] The average cost per hospital day, including food for servants, was a fraction less than one *shahi* less than two *qrans*. For fuel and light, including that used in the kitchen, a fraction less than a *shahi* less than 15 *shahi*s. For wages not counting that of Dr. Alexander, which was 1.05 *qran*s, was 2.35 *qran*s. Total cost per day, not counting medicines, dressing, foreign salaries, buildings, etc. amounted to 5.05 *qran*s. Although in mid-1925 the hospital was overdrawn, the doctors would try to keep within the limits of their appropriation.[1062]

1061. RG 91-20-7, Report of Medical Work Urumia 1924-1925.
1062. RG 91-20-7, Report of Medical Work Urumia 1924-1925.

After a brief visit to Tabriz, Dr. Cochran Jr. returned in January 1926 to Urmiyeh. A few more school rooms were repaired for hospital purposes, which constituted most cramped and inconvenient quarters. Anna, an Assyrian girl, who had experience in the Relief Hospital in Tabriz helped him, while Dr. Lamme (Tabriz) lent him some instruments and sold him some supplies that he absolutely needed. The Near East Relief donated some bedding, while wooden bedsteads were made locally, and soon Dr. Cochran was able to admit 17 patients. Mrs. Cochran Sr. also came and acted as matron and tried "to make the hospital a place to enjoy rather than to dread. The new [music] records that came with the three phonographs from Westminster Church have had a very important part in her work." From this time onwards the dispensary was open every morning and 40-50 patients were received daily. Many came for surgical work, but due to the lack of instruments they were put off. Dr. Cochran Jr. performed nine major and four minor operations until he returned to Tabriz in April. Most out-patients were Moslem, and of the in-patients half were Moslem. In March 1926, Dr. Alexander Mirzayoff was asked to come from Tabriz to Urmiyeh under a 7-months contract and he was entrusted with medical care of the orphans and some of the work in the dispensary. Since the arrival of Dr. Ellis with a small, but complete supply of instruments and hospital equipment more patients were admitted. The old site with its partially destroyed hospital building nearly three kms from the city was abandoned as a future site. During those four years of experiment in the city the medical staff felt very accessible to the people and was able to reach them as never before, in particular Moslem women. Previously, it was rare to have a Moslem obstetrical case in the hospital, but in 1926 they had them constantly. Women felt afraid to go out of the city to the old hospital, where friends and family only with difficulty were able to visit them and they were fearful to be away from them; now in the city that problem was gone. The Sardari building, which was saved during the war as the various powers used it as a police station, was given to the medical department for one year. Because the school had to return to its original function the hospital had to move into a new building to be erected at a new location, which, therefore, had to be ready by the spring of 1927.

This meant that the Urmiyeh mission needed $40,000 by that time, of a total of $65,000.[1063]

In 1926, the Presbyterian Iran Mission accepted plans for the construction of one residence and the main hospital building to the west of the central compound, on part of the land bought from the Archbishop of Canterbury, i.e. it would be located within the old central compound inside the city. Dr. Ellis wanted to build these two buildings, but he didn't have the funds.[1064] Given the need for a new hospital building, the financier of the original building, the Westminster church, Buffalo, NY, in 1928 pledged $10,000 a year for three years, besides a generous amount for equipment.[1065] However, there was opposition against the proposal, because the Kermanshah mission also wanted funds for its hospital construction plans. Therefore, there was a discussion in Urmiyeh of scaling back and compacting the size of the hospital within the city limits and thus reduce the cost. Dr. Ellis proposed to compress three units into one, and when expansion became necessary the dispensary or the nurses' home could be built as a new unit and the hospital would remain in the original unit. He stressed the need to go ahead with the construction of the approved buildings as soon as possible and asked whether the Westminster church could advance 50% of the investment immediately. However, there was disagreement where to build. Some wanted to rebuild the hospital on the old site, while Dr. Packard wanted it on the German site just outside the city, Dr. Ellis wanted it inside the city and the Mission agreed with that. Dr. Ellis pointed out to Dr. Holmes, the pastor of the Westminster church that he understood that his church had a special link with Dr. Packard, who then was working in the American Mission hospital in Kermanshah.[1066] This last observation

---

1063. RG 91-20-7, Report Medical Work Urumia. Nov. 1922 to June 30, 1923; Idem, Famous Urumia Hospital; Presbyterian Church 1926, p. 221; Presbyterian Church 1931, p. 177.

1064. RG 91-20-7, Ellis to Nesbitt/NY, 08/11/1927.

1065. Presbyterian Church 1929, p. 102.

1066. RG 91-20-7, Dr. W. Ellis/Rezaieh to Dr. Samuel Holmes/Buffalo, 29/11/1926. img1935-36 04/10/1928.

was spot on, because Dr. Packard had written to the Westminster church in January 1929 that, "There has been word twice repeated from Rezaieh [Urmiyeh], to the effect that they very likely will not be able to get their matters in shape in time to avoid the transfer of your interest from there to Kermanshah."[1067]

In November 1927, Dr. Ellis informed the Presbyterian Board in New York that for now only a physician's residence had been built, because the government had laid out poles for a tentative new avenue through the city, which cut right through the intended location of the hospital. Therefore, he had decided not to break ground for its construction.[1068] When the new avenue was constructed, the local authorities demolished the American mission's compound walls. As a result, land prices went up because of the avenue.[1069] Because of this new 'road block' as well as because later an order was issued by the government that no hospital should be built within the city limits, Dr. Ellis suggested to buy the German Orphanage property, as earlier proposed by Dr. Packard. He asked to approve the purchase of the land by telegram.[1070]

What the mission in Urmiyeh had feared came to pass. The Westminster church in Buffalo withdrew its support for the Urmiyeh hospital, transferring it to Kermanshah (see there). Fortunately, other funds were allocated by the Board of Missions of the Presbyterian Church in New York and the approval to buy land was given. For this reason the new hospital building in the city instead of still being called the Westminster Hospital was dedicated as the Cochran Memorial Hospital.[1071] The Urmiyeh mission in September 1929, acquired the

---

1067. RG 91-20-7, Holmes/Buffalo to Speer/NY, 28/02/1929; see also Idem, Ellis/Rezaieh to Speer/NY, 28/08/1929; Idem, Holmes/Buffalo to Speer/NY, 21/11/1929; Idem, Trull to Speer/NY, 04/10/1928.

1068. RG 91-20-7, Ellis/R to Nesbitt/NY08/11/1927; Idem, Ellis/R to Holmes/Buffalo 11/11/1927.

1069. RG 91-20-7, Ellis to Williamson, charge d'affaire Tehran 30/09/1930.

1070. RG 91-20-7, Speer/NY to the Executive Council, 07/06/1929.

1071. RG 91-20-7, Last annual report of the Cochran Memorial Hospital

Salari compound no. 20, the property vacated by the Fiske Seminary. The only problem was that the government had intimated that there was a rule against the building of a hospital within the city limits. Therefore, the Urmiyeh mission planned to build at the site of the German Orphanage, but the government did not want the Americans to buy that land. Therefore, the American mission decided to build the hospital in the city, because the Red Lion and Sun Society, which had intended to build their hospital outside the city, in 1930 had constructed a very nice hospital in the very heart of the city, which had created a precedent. Also, two German doctors had established a small hospital in the busy section of the new avenue right in town. Moreover, the Salari property was next to the Fiske Seminary that was separated from the city wall by just one yard. The Mission was afraid to ask permission to build, because even if the government didn't refuse, permission might be never granted. To assuage possible hurt feelings, the Mission abandoned its plan for building on the German Orphanage property and gave up its rights to claim damages for the loss sustained by the new avenue. The latter also had destroyed the mission's plan to build the hospital there, which obliged it to revert to the first plan and build the hospital at the Salari compound.[1072] Because of the problems raised by Iranian officials against the planned location of the hospital, Dr. Ellis wrote to the American Legation in Tehran. He noted that the government opposed their location to build hospital, because of the noise, given the nearness of the army barracks, which was rather ironic as the inmates of the barracks made a lot of noise! He further observed that although Galla was the old site of the hospital; it was situated some 3 kms outside town. Therefore, before the war, there was little work with women and practically no maternity work, because it was hard for Moslem women to go that far.[1073]

1934.

1072. RG 91-20-7, Ellis/Urmiyeh to Speer/NY, 27/01/1930; Idem, Ellis/Urmiyeh to Speer/NY 25/02/1930; Presbyterian Church 1930, p. 192.

1073. RG 91-20-7, Ellis to Williamson, charge d'affaire Tehran 30/09/1930

In March 1930, the Iran mission formally submitted the building plans to the Board in New York and asked for the approval of the budget ($33,799) and permission to break ground for the construction. The plan was substantially in accordance with the plan earlier proposed by Dr. Ellis in January. However, the Iran Mission proposed to build the hospital in "the German Orphanage property, but with some adjustments to accommodate it for use in the Salari compound," a plan that the government of Iran opposed. The Salari compound adjoined the Sardari, where the Fiske Seminary was situated, in which the dispensary and hospital were then located. The Urmiyeh mission commented that, "It is not fit for a hospital; the dispensary has operated in a yard nearby in rooms temporarily fitted up for that purpose." Therefore, it was intended to purchase another piece of land adjacent to the Salari, which would offer space for all other planned buildings, including the Nurses' Home.[1074] Dr. Ellis, who had been its main designer, had submitted the plans for the hospital to New York. The Urmiyeh staff proposed to build the hospital inside the city, because the old Galla or Kalla [sic; Qal`eh] site, due its location, drew less Moslem patients than desired and possible.[1075] Fortunately for Dr. Ellis and his colleagues, Speer and his collaborators favored to build the hospital inside the city.[1076] During the erection of the new building section by section of the mansion was razed to make room for the new. The women were moved into a small residence in the adjoining yard that the mission was able to buy. There were as yet no trained nurses on the staff and the American nurse had just arrived. Mrs. Cochran Sr. who had been in the hospital business for 25 years bore the brunt of the various upsets in housekeeping and assisted Dr. Ellis and Ms Pease in moving. She did not see the finished product as she died on furlough.[1077] In early 1931, Dr. Cochran reported that: "We have just moved into the new hospital. The second story is not

---

1074. RG 91-20-7, Wilson/Tabriz to Speer/NY. 01/03/1930; Presbyterian Church 1930, p. 192.
1075. RG 91-20-7, Memo Dodd to Speer, 26/03/1930.
1076. RG 91-20-7, Memo Dodd to Speer, 20/05/1930.
1077. RG 91-20-7, Cochran Memorial Hospital Report 1932-1933.

entirely ready, but will be soon."[1078] In early December 1931, Dr. Ellis reported that the hospital was being completed and that they intended to move patients from the current crowded quarters to the first floor before Xmas. The second floor would soon thereafter be available.[1079] The new building presented quite a difference with the premises occupied thus far. In the basement the dispensary was comfortably and accessibly housed in the basement. On the first floor there were two wards and several private rooms; the wards opened to a balcony where patients convalesced. On the second floor were the women's wards, where flowers adorned the bedside tables, and with fresh curtains at the windows. Across the hall was the maternity; the hospital had 86 babies in 1930-31. Also, across the hall was the children's room with white attractive cribs made up with fascinating counterpanes. The walls were tinted and hung with pictures. Next was the babies' room or nursery, where they were tucked in white bassinettes. These had soft coverings made by friends in the US and dainty clothes. When the babies left the hospital instead of in rags the medical staff gave going-away clothes for poor babies.[1080]

So as not lose sight of what else was needed besides a building, Dr. Ellis reminded Speer that "equipment is our prime necessity. Beds are specifically urgent. The patients complain a good deal about the extra inhabitants of the wooden beds we now use."[1081] The Urmiyeh staff returned to this subject one year later when the new hospital had been built. They emphasized the urgent need for new equipment, because the "American hospital must be equipped to modern standards of efficiency to satisfy the demands of progressive Persians themselves." Therefore, they needed adequate lab equipment as neither such government nor private facilities existed in Urmiyeh. An X-ray machine was also a must. Moreover, with all that equipment hospital service could be doubled. Dr. Ellis also argued that they should install the much needed call bell system and electric lighting as well as simpler

---

1078. RG 91-20-7, Memo Tower to Speer/NY 10/04/1931.
1079. RG 91-20-7, Ellis/R to Speer 07/12/1933.
1080. RG 91-20-7, Cochran Memorial Hospital Report 1932-1933.
1081. RG 91-20-7, Ellis to Speer 08/09/1930.

diagnostic and therapeutic apparatus. Since demand for maternity work was on the rise, a proper delivery bed and 12 additional beds for maternity patients were needed. Furthermore, a fracture bed and equipment for the nurses' quarters were a necessity. For the moment, the nurses were temporarily housed in the hospital itself; the beds, carpets and furnishings they needed were to be produced locally.[1082] As of January 1931, when the medical team moved into the new hospital, every month some new equipment was added: 20 iron beds, three children's cribs, four baby baskets from the US, bedside tables and stools, four easy chairs, four benches, instrument cabinets and supply cabinets made locally. Less visible were the improvement made by Ms Pease, the head nurse and her nurses in the use of equipment and supply by bringing order so that each thing had its place, was properly labeled and ready for use. What also helped was the recent arrival of bedding, gauze, dressings, surgical dresses etc. supplied by NY State churches. Meanwhile, Ms Lamme was busy directing the making of curtains, mattresses, pillows, and many other things. In the summer of 1931, the hospital was closed for 10 days and these things then were pushed, the building was cleaned. Later Ms Lamme was relieved as matron and resumed her former duties and Ms Paese became matron.[1083]

The new building was considered a miracle after all the set-backs to get land and having plan after plan rejected. The medical staff was elated. "The American hospitals have been able to maintain a character of work which has kept the confidence of the people in a way which their own hospitals have failed to do in some cases." The American missionaries were also bolstered by the fact that the Urmiyeh Mission had overcome all difficulties (hatred against Christians, difficulty to get land, no nurses). Moreover, the people of the Urmiyeh region kept confidence in the US missionaries, despite the opening of the government Red Lion and Sun hospital, which cared for most of the

---

1082. RG 91-20-7, Hugo Muller, Rezaieh to Cady Allen, Hamadan 22/06/1931.

1083. RG 91-20-7,Cochran Memorial Hospital Rezaieh 1931-1932;Idem, Ruth Elliot to Dr. Ellis 19/03/1932 ("no money for the Nurses' Home we realize you are disappointed.")

poor. The US physicians cooperated closely with them, because they had no surgeon and therefore, the missionary doctors were given a contract to do all their operations. The Cochran Hospital also did the Iranian hospital's sterilizing in its autoclave. Apart from problems (bureaucratic dilatoriness) it made the hospital's statute somewhat more secure, during that time of rising nationalism in Iran. What also helped was that without the missionary physicians there was no surgery, for people were too poor to travel to Tabriz, and emergency cases would die en route.

The second achievement was the work for women and children, and the Urmiyeh staff felt that it was perhaps unsurpassed by any of the US missionary hospitals in Iran. Given the intense fanaticism of the Urmiyeh region, the superstition and ignorance was so dense that it reflected on the confidence in the Christian hospital that it had gained among the Moslem population. In 1932-33, the hospital cared for 67 children under the age of 15 against 22 in the preceding year. Also, the Christian hospital's approach was different from that followed in government hospitals and by other practitioners. In 1932-32, it was for the first time that there were two doctors in the hospital, which made more careful diagnosis and treatment possible. Mrs. Müller taught nurses and assisted in the OR and in the dispensary as recording clerk.[1084]

Drs. Ellis and Cochran Jr. split the work by gender, but not strictly. Cochran had the advantage of speaking Persian and Assyrian, which was especially useful with Assyrian refugees from Russia. They often assisted each other in operations. In November 1933, Dr. Ellis went to Tehran to learn that the hospital in Urmiyeh had to be closed and the Iran Mission thought it best to accede. It was a bitter ending to 100 years of work by US doctors there. The more bitter because apart from the X-ray machine and the nurses' home, funds for which were available, the hospital had finally acquired all its objectives. The hospital building was arranged with well integrated centers for work with out- and in-patients. There were special wards for children, mothers and their babies and plenty of private rooms. The kitchen was

---

1084. RG 91-20-7, Cochran Memorial Hospital Report 1932-1933.

conveniently connected to the serving room on each floor by a food elevator. An adjoining shaft carried the soiled laundry to the basement. The quite complete surgery was in a separate suite, isolated from the wards and yet very accessible. The most modern feature was having running water in Ms Pease's suite, surgery, dispensary, babies bath room, kitchen, two serving rooms and in the two bath rooms on the men's and the women's floors, where there were flush toilets after the native style and other conveniences.

Ms Pease conducted the nurses' school and gave special care to patients; she made the children's room attractive. There was semi-cubical privacy in the wards by curtains strung on wires. Although the hospital served simple food care was given to food brought in by patients' friends. Moreover, there were numerous gadgets for the comfort of patients, sterile supplies for the OR etc. in the hospital. To close the work that the US doctors had tried to perfect for years was beyond belief and painful. If Urmiyeh had an alternative for modern or adequate facilities for surgical care they could leave with grace, but there was not.[1085]

1085. RG 91-20-7, Last annual report Hospital Rezaieh 1934.

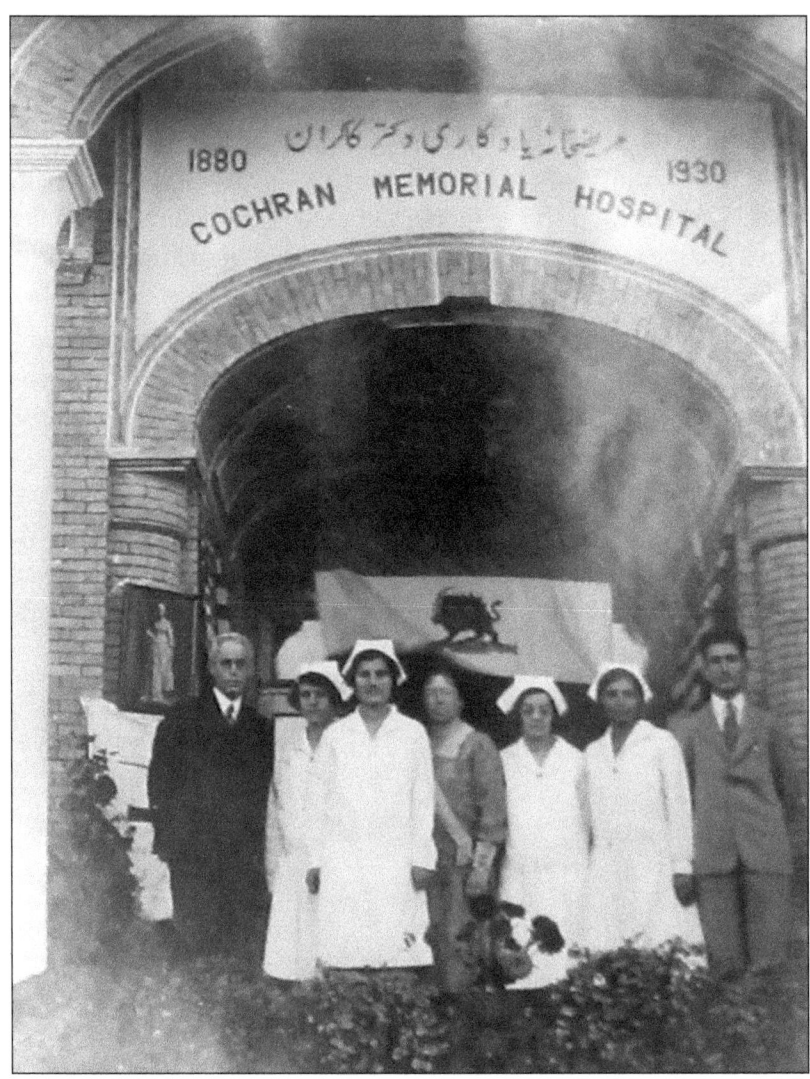

Entrance of the Cochran Memorial hospital, Urmiyeh with Dr. Jos. Cochran Jr. on the left.

Hospitals in Qajar & Pahlavi Iran • 1794–1950

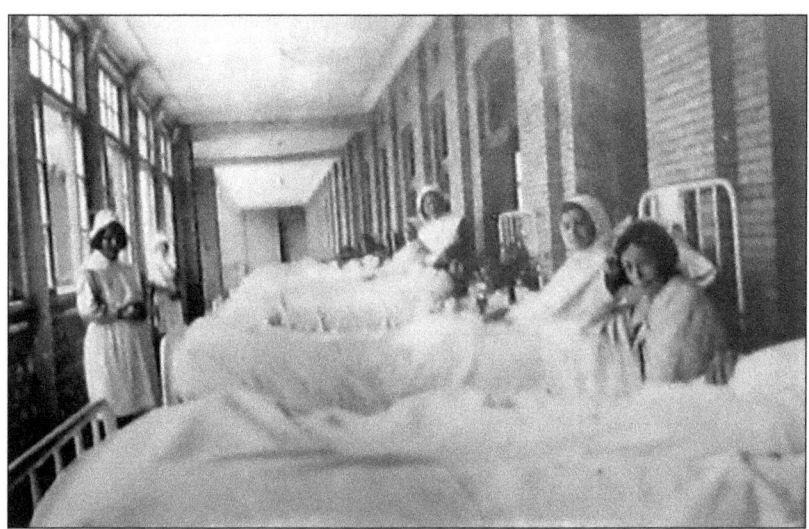

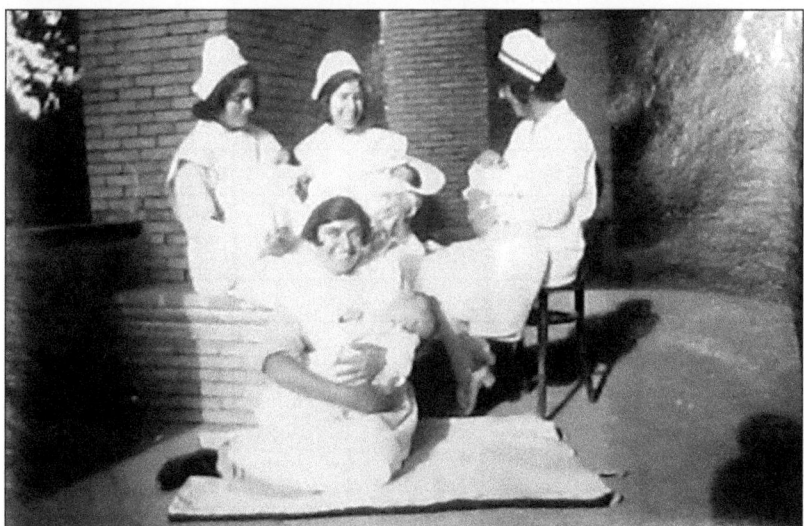

Wards in the Cochran hospital and a group of nurses holding babies.

Table 30: Number of in- and out-patients, house calls and operations at the American Urmiyeh Hospital (1876-1925)

Year	Total patients	Inpatients	Outpatients	House calls	Village visits	Operations
1876	1,500	-	-	-	-	-
1881	7,233					
1882	6,000	100	-	-	-	-
1883	6,341	235	-	-	-	-
1884	Ca. 5.500	>81	-	-	-	-
1885	-	173	-	-	-	40
1886	5,000	-	-	-	-	-
1888	5,000	-	-	-	-	-
1890	-	226	-	-	-	-
1891		337 + 121*				141
1893	7,500	500	-	-	-	-
1894	7,224	361	-	578	-	79
1895	-	202+110*	-	-	-	-
1896	6431	200 +137*	-	-	-	-
1897	-	577	-	-	-	-
1898	9,000	369	-	-	-	-
1899	3,392	16	-	-	-	-
1900	7,341	193+166*	-	-	-	-
1901	3,842	477	-	875	50	-
1902	9,119	238+168*	-	-	-	-
1903	9,662	504	-	-	-	-
1904	12,754	574	10,962	1,128 city +	Village	-
1905	4,527	-	-	-	-	-
1908	7,408	105	4,308	1,812	1,175	-
1910	15,000	360	-	1,123	105 trips	450
1911-24	n.a.	n.a.	n.a.	n.a.	n.a.	n.a.
1925	-		13,250	-	-	-

Source: Presbyterian Church 1882, p. 53; Idem 1886, p. 82; Idem 1911, p. 326; RG 91-20-7, Report Medical Work Urumia 1924-1925.

* = female patients

OTHER HOSPITALS

For a long time the Westminster Hospital in Urmiyeh was the only hospital in Iran, outside Tehran. However, this changed when in 1910, Urmiyeh then had a population of some 20,000, there was a small Russian hospital, of which nothing else is known. It is not mentioned by Aubin, who left an account of foreign activities in Urmiyeh in 1907, which suggest that it was established after that date.[1086] However, it must have been a military establishment, because in August 1914, M. Vedensky, the Russia vice-consul at Urmiyeh,

> hopes before long to establish a Russian school and a public Russian hospital and dispensary in the town, the present military hospital being of little use to the towns people. The matter is under active consideration and the inevitable that will soon be sent round, under the auspices of the Governor. Both these institutions are doubtless designed to counteract the influence of the American mission at Urmia, which has for many years maintained an excellent school and well-equipped hospital in the town.[1087]

Apparently Mr. Vedensky's hospital was never built, because in the following year the Russian consul Nikitine arranged for a sanitary team to visit and help to combat the cholera epidemic of 1915. The leader of that team, Dr. A. Kach, also set up a temporary hospital there. It was the only one sponsored by the Russian Orthodox Church mission. It was discontinued when the Russian troops left in 1918.[1088]

In the fall of 1917, to assist the Russians, a French military field hospital was established in Urmiyeh. This staff abandoned it in April 1918 and with them also left the French nuns, who had been engaged

---

1086. Grothe 1911, p. 131.
1087. Russian Policy on the Turco-Persian Frontier. Capt. A. T. Wilson to Sir W. Townley, Camp Mawana, 15/08/1914, IOR/L/PS/10/451/1, Persia – Policy. British Interests in the South. Russian Policy', no. 13.
1088. Tamaddon 1350, pp. 243-244. Elsewhere in Iran, Russian military physicians and nurses also treated the local population. Andreeva 2007, p. 191.

in medical work. As a result, the American Presbyterian hospital was the only one in remaining Urmiyeh, for the Russian military hospital also had been abandoned with the withdrawal of the Russian troops.[1089] Again, the American missionaries had left and their work had been wiped out by the war, while due to the prevailing insecurity in the area the missionaries did not return until after Reza Khan had re-established central government control.[1090]

In 1930, a government hospital for men was founded by the Red Lion and Sun society. Dr. Wilder P. Ellis acted as consulting physician for the new government hospital. At that time, also a small hospital established by two German physicians is mentioned about which nothing further is known.[1091]

Yazd

In 1892, Dr. and Mrs. Henry White began medical missionary work in Yazd, a town of some 50,000 inhabitants. Unlike in the case of Isfahan, where CMS activities (medical work and evangelization) had run into opposition, in Yazd CMS started with only medical activities. This was the result of a discussion Dr. Carr of Isfahan had with the Persian governor of that city, who told him about the failure of the tobacco regie. He advised him to take things slowly. First, establish a dispensary and hospital and let these get accepted; don't bring your clergy and schools yet; get your hospital first, then bring your clergy and school and begin preaching. This is what the CMS did in Yazd following his advice and it worked.[1092] They first had a dispensary in the open air in a garden and then rented a small house and besides dispensary work they took a few in-patients. Work increased, and in 1899, the Parsi Society at Yazd gave a large ruined caravanserai near

---

1089. Shedd 1922, pp. 212, 246, 258, 273; Mo`tamed al-Vezareh 1379, pp. xxv, 9, 18-27, 74-75, 89-93, 99, 156; Coan 1939, 252, 260, 283; Hellot 1996; Ibid., 2002, pp. 340, 348; for an account of the French medical team in Urmiyeh by a participant, see Zavie 1927.

1090. Speer 1920, p. 69; Presbyterian Church 1920, p. 327; Idem 1921, p. 340; Idem 1922, p. 374.

1091. RG 91-20-7, Ellis Rezaieh to Speer25/02/1930.

1092. Carr 1900, p. 138.

by to the medical mission. In fact, the building was a gift by Mehriban Goodarz, a Zoroastrian merchant,

> and its property including a house that adjoined it. The structure of this erstwhile halting-place for caravans lent itself in a remarkable manner to the uses to which it was now to be put: the central court that was once filled with camels, asses, and pack-mules was turned into a pretty garden; and the old-time lodgings of the camel-drivers and muleteers were transformed into chambers and wards for the Good Samaritan work.[1093]

It was rebuilt costing £400, which Dr. White locally collected. In 1899, Dr. White walled off the stables and an adjoining small house so that he had 12-beds for women, for who medical need was high. In 1900, it had 20 beds and in 1902 this number was increased to 28 beds.[1094] In 1899, the Whites had been joined by Dr. Urania Latham, who later married the Rev. Napier Malcolm (Yazd). They were assisted by Armenian orderlies. In that same year Dr. Latham noted that part of the Women's Hospital was sufficiently ready to be used for 2-3 patients and she hoped that soon more would be admitted who were waiting.[1095]

In 1906, Dr. White felt the need for a bigger, 100-bed hospital in Yazd. His proposal was accepted by the CMS, but it did not have the funds and, therefore, made an appeal to its supporters. Dr. White stressed that in the area of Yazd there was no other access to modern medicine and that traditional Persian physicians had no knowledge of surgery. Also, that of the large patients treated by the CMS hospital some even came from as far as Baluchistan and Afghanistan to seek treatment.[1096]

1093. Jackson 1909, p. 377; Stileman 1902, p. 74; Hume-Griffith 1909, p. 164.
1094. *Mercy and Truth* 1900, vol. 4, p. 188; Idem 1906, vol. 10, pp. 257-58.
1095. *Mercy and Truth* 1902, vol. 6, p. 37.
1096. Stileman 1902, pp. 74-75; Wright 2001, pp. 188, 121; Afshar 1354, vol. 2, p. 803 (text of foundation plaque); Bricteux 1908, p. 235. Dr. Lucy Malony wrote they needed women's skirts, flanellete shirts, T bandages, many-tailed bandages, sheets, draw-sheets, pillowcases, bed-jackets, night socks, and bedroom slippers. *Mercy and Truth* 1906, vol. 10, p. 62.

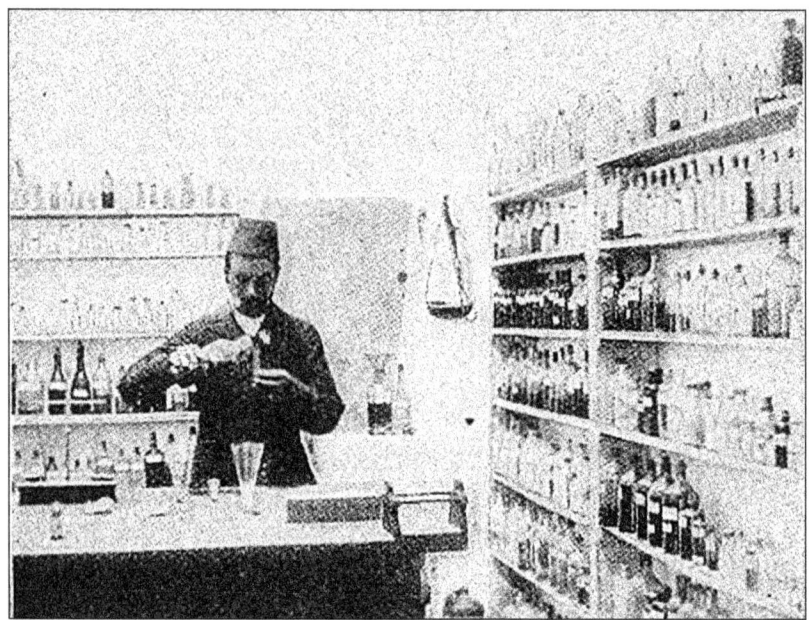

Above: Dispensary in Yazd. *Opposite*: Surgery.

Table 31: In- and Out-Patients Treated in the CMS hospital in Yazd (1898-1905)

Year	In-patients	Visits of out-patients
1898	7	5,401
1899	25	26,018
1900	47	34,171
1901	73	29,462
1902	213	11,280
1903	195	18,293
1904	356	17,541
1905	610	25,122
Total	1,526	167,288

Source: *Mercy and Truth* 1906, vol. 10, p. 258

Moreover, there was an increase in the number of in-patients, which caused the hospital to be too crowded and unsanitary. In particular, the conditions in the small women's hospital had become unsuitable.

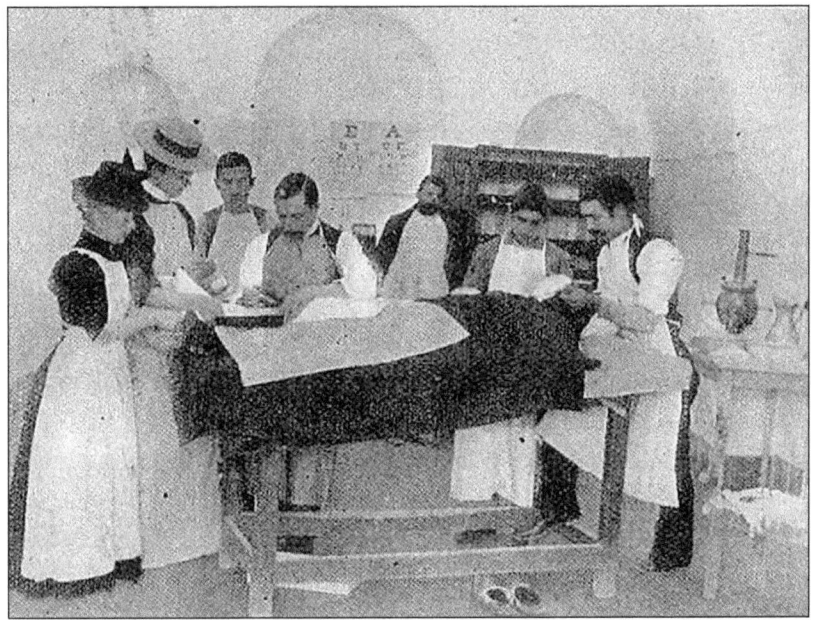

Therefore, the sons of the late Goodarz gave a piece of land, where the CMS staff wanted to build a hospital with 100 beds. If that was realized, the current hospital would become the women's hospital with 35 beds. For the construction of the new hospital £2,000 was needed, of which it was hope to raise £500 locally.[1097] Indeed, "for the erection of this [new] hospital (1907), Parsees in Yezd gave £200, and Muhammadans also made contributions."[1098]

In 1915, the hospital was closed when British subjects had to leave Iran, but it was reopened in 1916, when the political situation became less problematic.[1099] At that time, CMS Yazd had 80 beds in the hospital, which was later called the Gudarz hospital, to which later

---

1097. *Mercy and Truth* 1906, vol. 10, pp. 257-58.

1098. Richter 1910, p. 331. The CMS staff in Yazd in 1906 consisted in the following: Dr. H. White; Dr. Ms L. Malony; Ms A. Macklin, Ms E.A. Thomas, Ms. J. Biggs (evangelist). *Mercy and Truth* 1906, vol. 10, p. 378.

1099. Waterfield 1973, p. 162. On the situation of the hospital of Yazd in 1928, see Cash 1930, p. 57.

the Laal maternity hospital and the nursing school were annexed.[1100] In 1937 and 1938, due to staff shortage the hospital had to be temporarily closed.[1101] In 1941, a flash flood destroyed both the CMS church and hospital.[1102] The hospital was later re-opened and despite political problems and staff shortages continued to operate until 1954, when it closed its doors as did other CMS activities in the city.[1103]

ZABOL

The only modern medical service available in Zabol or Nosratabad, as it was called then, was the British Consular hospital, which probably was established around 1900. In 1906 there was a severe epidemic of plague in Sistan. The British Consulate took anti-plague measures amongst which the establishment of a plague hospital near the Consulate hospital for the isolation and proper treatment of cases. Because the quarantine system that had been put in place did not have any effect on the spread of the disease, the Nosratbadis, incited by local mullahs, rioted and attacked the British Consulate in July 1906. The plague hospital was burnt and the Consulate's hospital was damaged. The British believed that the Russians were behind it and that this attack was not so much an expression of anti-British sentiments, but rather of the conviction that the quarantine and related preventive measures were un-Islamic in nature. Nevertheless, Great Britain asked for and got an apology, punishment of the culprits and permission to buy 10,000 *zar* of land to extend the British dispensary and hospital.[1104] The Zabol hospital was quite popular as indicated by the few data that we have on the

---

1100. Richter 1910, p. 331; RG 231-1-6, Hoffman, Pioneering in Meshed, p. 12.
1101. Waterfield 1973, p. 171.
1102. Waterfield 1973, p. 172.
1103. Waterfield 1973, p. 173.
1104. Mss Eur C600/1, 'A note on the importance of Seistan to India', p. 4; the dispensary of the consulate was practically destroyed. Grant Duff to Mushir-ed-Douleh 31/03/1906, p. 1; IOR/L/PS/10/100, Seistan disturbances and consular guard'. For details see Elgood 1951, pp. 528-29.

number of patients attending it. For example, in November 1909 attendance at the hospital at Zabol was 1,417 patients,[1105] while this number in June 1915 was 1,284 new cases, 1,039 old cases and 18 operations.[1106] British medical presence increased after 1915, when an entire medical column supported the East-Persian Cordon. Of course, this medical unit treated military personnel only, although the British Consular hospitals continued to function as well.[1107]

At an unknown date, probably in 1921, coinciding with the withdrawal of British troops from Iran, the British hospital in Zabol was closed, because in 1925 the British Minister in Tehran urged the government of India "to build a hospital both from a humanitarian and political view in Sistan as proposed by the consul there."[1108] In 1921 when the American missionaries stationed in Mashhad fled the city, because it was feared that a Soviet invasion would take place, they went to Zabol where they did not report the presence of a British Consular hospital. The American missionaries "cleaned up a dirty old building and turned it into a hospital," where every day they treated a large number of people. The missionaries stayed only for about six months, for when the Soviet threat proved to be unfounded they returned to Mashhad.[1109]

Because it was known that the British hospital at Zabol had been very popular,[1110] and it meant political gain at relatively low cost the

---

1105. IOR/L/PS/10/328/1, Reductions in expenditure on Agencies and Consulates', p. 6.

1106. IOR/L/PS/10/210, Sistan and Kain Consulate Diary no. 27, for the week ending 3rd July 1915, p. 2.

1107. IOR/L/MIL/17/15/35, 'Report on the Working of the Line of Communication and on the Withdrawal of the British Military Mission in East Persia, 1919-20. General Staff, India, p. 97, appendix V.

1108. IOR/L/PS/12/3600, No. 78, Percy Lorraine to Secr. GOI/Simla, 18/05/1925.

1109. The old building was that of the former Russian consulate, Miller 1989, pp. 60-64. According to Presbyterian Church 1921, p. 337, these events took place in the second half of 1919.

1110. IOR/L/PS/12/3654, creation of vice consulate; allowances attached to post of Indian Medical Service Officers in East Persia', f. 7; see also Mss Eur C600/1, 'A note on the importance of Seistan to India', f. 6.

British consular hospital was re-opened, probably in 1927. The fact that the Russians were going to open a hospital in Zabol undoubtedly also played a role in that decision. The Russian Consular hospital probably was opened in November 1928, because it is reported that Dr. Morozoff of the Soviet Consulate Hospital "after some delay opened a dispensary, but very soon closed it again as it was discovered by the local authorities that he did not possess the requisite permit from the Ministry of Health."[1111] This is further supported by the fact that in May 1928, the Russian consul in Sistan asked Major Kharegat, IMS to treat the wife of his vice-consul. "Besides paying private fees at full rates, the Soviet Consul has actually donated Tomans 20 to the British hospital, a fact which has created considerable impression."[1112] The two Consular hospitals of the rival powers watched each other's activities and interpreted some of their actions, even the purchase of medicines, as being motivated by ulterior political motives. For example, in April 1929 the British consul reported that "the Soviet hospital Sistan is said to be importing capsules and injections for use of the poor in Sistan." A man was said to have been sent to Bombay to make the purchase.[1113]

Because of Reza Shah's nationalist policy, which restricted the activities of foreigners, in particular of foreign consuls, including those in charge of a dispensary or hospital, this posed real problems for the continuation of medical services. This also held for the British Consulate hospital, which was still open for business, "but it will only do so long as the present sub-Assistant Surgeon, who obtained a license to practice before the days of the boycott, remains. When he goes (and he has been many years there now) the consulate hospital in Zabul, as elsewhere will have to close its doors to the local people." Moreover, in the case of Zabol, the Iranians suspected that the British had ulterior motives in maintaining the vice-consulate there, as they

---

1111. IOR/L/PS/12/3403, Diary of HBM's Consul, Sistan and Kain, for the months of November-December 1928, p. 3.

1112. IOR/L/PS/12/3403, Diary of HBM's Consul, Sistan and Kain, for the months of May 1928, p. 2.

1113. IOR/L/PS/12/3403, Diary of HBM's Consul, Sistan and Kain, for the month of April 1929, p. 2.

believed that there was no economic reason to have a Consulate there. As a result, "the Vice-Consul, almost incarcerated in his house and cut off from all contact with the people, can do nothing to promote Anglo-Iranian friendship."[1114] Fortunately, for the patients, the hospital was not closed down, but the British authorities were considering transferring the Consulate from Zabol to Zahedan. The consul-general in Mashhad, in whose jurisdiction both towns were located, pointed out that, "In S.E. Persia there are no fully qualified Persian or Missionary doctors and the Consular Officers have to rely on their own Consular doctors. The doctor for S.E. Persia has hitherto been an IMS Officer stationed in Sistan [Zabol]. If the Consul is moved to Zahedan his doctor should accompany him. The death of the consul at Birjand and the serious illness of the vice-consul there show the necessity of continuing medical attendance in Sistan."[1115]

When in November 1930, Reza Shah paid a visit to Sistan he had, among other things, an interview with the Russian consul. The Shah asked the Russian consul pointedly whether there were any Russian subjects in Sistan, to which query he replied in the negative. Two days later the Soviet Hospital was closed and a good deal of its furniture auctioned.[1116] Because the Russian Consulate in Zabol also closed somewhat later, in 1932, individuals in Zabol, who supported that the Russian Consulate remain, sent false reports about the British hospital and induced some people to request the government to open an Iranian hospital there. At that time, there was no doctor in Zabol, except for the British Consular medical staff. An Iranian military medical officer sent there was found drunk and knifed in the street and was transferred. Dr. Zahedi, previously municipal medical officer was sent back to Zabul in the same capacity. The British consul commented that: "He is an alcoholic with practically no medical

---

1114. IOR/L/PS/12/3654, 'A note on the importance of Seistan to India', f. 11.

1115. IOR/L/PS/12/3607, HBM's consul-general Meshed, no 325/127/10, 30/03/1932, p. 7.

1116. IOR/L/PS/12/3403, Diary of HBM's Consul, Sistan and Kain, for the month of November 1930, p. 3; Idem, Diary of HBM's Consul, Sistan and Kain, for the months of May 1928, p. 2.

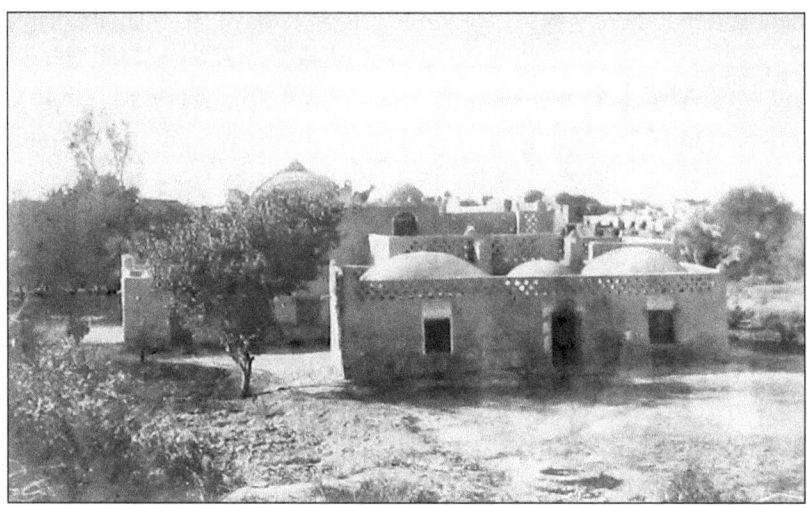
The house in which the missionaries lived in Zabul.

qualifications. The soldiers are forbidden to go to our hospital and therefore can only secretly come or ask the Sub-Surgeon to treat them privately. Therefore, he asked to be dismissed due to lack of medical care. Several soldiers were punished by their CO. Dysentery prevails among the soldiers."[1117] In 1934, the Consulate hospital and dispensary at Zabul was under Capt. G. Fausitt Taylor, IMS with Sub-Assistant Surgeon Jamadar Mian Ghulam Ali as assistant.[1118] In 1935, Dr. Fazal Haq, IMS was in charge of the dispensary. At the end of 1935, the Iranian goverment objected to the post of Vice-Consul being held by the Medical Officer. Therefore, it refused to issue a medical license to Dr. Lt. Col. Pyper, who was to replace Dr. Haq in 1936. This meant that the Consulate hospital probably was closed in 1937, for in that year it was submitted that "it will only do so as long as the present

---

1117. IOR/L/PS/12/3403, HBM's Consul, Sistan and Ka'in, Diary for the month of June 1932, p. 1.

1118. IOR/L/PS/12/3415, Annual Commercial Report for the Province of Khurasan and Zabulistan for the Persian Year 1312 (21st March 1933 to 20th March 1934), p. 6. "The British Consular buildings grounds covered an area of 22 acres. The buildings, including the hospital, were commodious and all mud built, some have a brick face." IOR/L/PS/12/3607, 'General reorganisation of consular posts', p. 1.

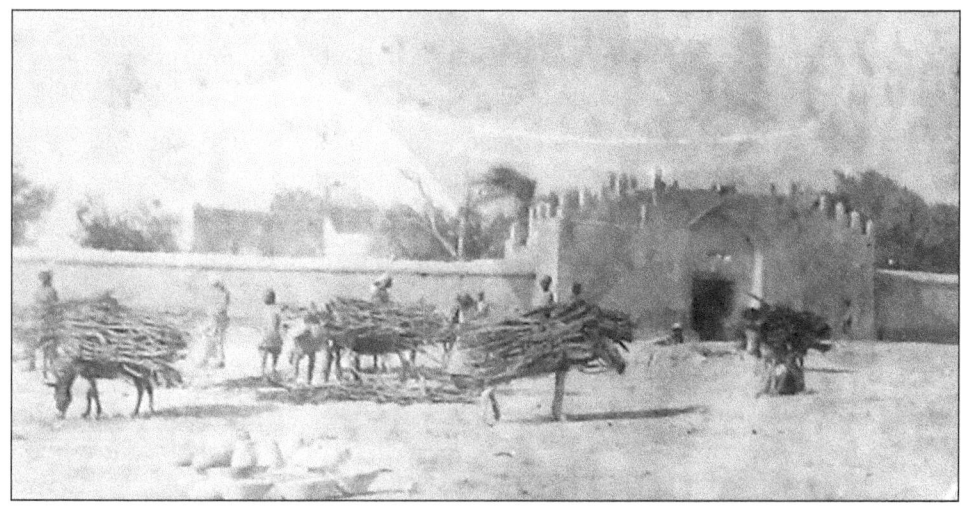

Front entrance of the former Russian Consulate, used as hospital, 1921.

sub-assistant Surgeon, who obtained a licence to practice before the days of the boycott, remains, when he goes (and he has been many years there now) the consulate hospital in Zabul, as elsewhere will have to close its doors to the local people."[1119]

ZAHEDAN

In Zahedan, or Dozdab as it was known until 1930, there was neither a dispensary nor a hospital. With the arrival of the British troops the base hospital of the East-Persia Cordon was established in Zahedan, which only consisted in a number of so-called 'war' huts. After the war, these huts became part of the vice-Consulate that had one of its offices in there.[1120] In 1933, there still was a British Consulate's dispensary. "No less than 44 deaths from Malaria occurred at Zahidan in one month. Malaria still continues in a severe form at Sistan. The

---

1119. A note on the importance of Seistan to India, IOR/L/PS/12/3654, Zabul: creation of vice consulate; allowances attached to post of Indian Medical Service Officers in East Persia', p. 11. The British embassy's annual report for 1937, p. 42 states that it was closed to the public. IOR/L/PS/12/3472A, Annual Report 1937, p. 21 (no. 92).

1120. IOR/L/PS/12/3607, 'General reorganisation of consular posts', f. 238.

appeal of local authorities for Doctors to be sent to deal with this epidemic has remained unanswered, and the only attention sufferers can receive is at the Consulate Dispensary."[1121]

In 1927, the Bible Churchman's Missionary Society came to work in Dozdab and established, among other things, a dispensary. In 1928, Ms Jacobs, a nurse, joined the original group of non-medical missionaries. It was the intention to open a hospital, but due to many delays, Dr. Rice, who had committed to manage it, did not want to wait much longer and instead chose to go to India. In 1929, a Christian Indian physician, Dr. Sitralka came and, with the help of the British Consul, modern medical care really took off. Dr. Sitralka's work area aimed to include Birjand and Bampur as well. In 1934 the missionaries departed due to the great diffulties they encountered in their evangelization work. Dr. Sitralka continued managing the small hospital until 1951, when it was expropriated by the Mossadegh government.[1122]

Zanjan

In 1929, Dr. Cochran Jr. and a graduate nurse visited Zanjan.[1123] A sayyed in Zanjan, just back from pilgrimage in Mashhad warned people against the American physician. He said, when speaking of a man whose foot had been cured by the American doctor, "This doctor has healed the foot of one man and has broken the foot of Islam."[1124] As a result, the people of Zanjan had to limp for quite some time.

In addition to the civil and military hospitals that were established in Iran (some of which are mentioned above) there also was a third category of hospital, viz. that of the so-called non-community organizations. This means that they didn't provide medical care to the community, i.e. general public, but only for specific groups, in this case for personnel employed by the State Railways. Because the Railways

---

1121. IOR/L/PS/12/3406, HMG's Consulate-General, Meshed political diary for the month of August 1933, p. 2.
1122. Waterfield 1973, pp. 175-76. Dr. and Mrs. Sitralka then moved to Tehran where he opened an eye clinic with American support.
1123. Presbyterian Church 1930, p. 194.
1124. Presbyterian Church 1932, p. 175.

had so many hospitals and served a large group of people, I have included this main representative of the non-community hospitals here.

Railway Hospitals

In April 1933, the government of Iran signed a contract with the Danish-Swedish company Kampsax to construct the Transnational Iranian Railway. Because the area in which the railway was to be constructed was large, the government insisted that Kampsax be responsible for the medical care of the people it employed, just as it had required the same from the APOC for its concession area.[1125] Consequently, the contract (art. 4) between Kampsax and the government of Iran states the requirement for the establishment of health centers along the railway for the benefit of the railway workers. As a result, a medical service (*service sanitaire*) was created, headed by Dr. Torfeh, which employed about 500 people, i.e. physicians, nurses and ambulance drivers. Apart from Iranian physicians, many were Italian, probably because Kampsax employed many Italians in its workforce. This medical part of Kampsax operations was financed through a levy of two percent on all enterprise activities.[1126] To implement its medical service Kampsax constructed many hospitals and health posts as shown in Table 32.

Table 32: Location and capacity of the Railway hospitals and dispensaries in 1938

Hospital	Number	Name of location
Hospital with 70 beds	4	Abbasabad, Tnk ?, Gardaneh-ye Nuziyan
Hospital with 50 beds	4	Pol-e Safid, Arak, Borujerd, Bisheh
Hospital with 30 beds	2	Tehran, Shirgah
Hospital with 22 beds	6	Teleh Zanj, Tnk ?, Keshvar, Chamsangar, Sepid-dasht, Karun
Hospital with 20 beds	2	Gaduk, Mazu
Hospital with 15 beds	13	Do Ab, Mahabad, Simin-dasht, Bonkuh, Pishva, Shahryar, Parandak, Anjilavand, Qom, Rahjerd, Nirabad, Azna, Darband

---

1125. Floor 2018 a, pp. 124-25.
1126. Boisen 1946, p. 46, 72; Saxild 1971, p. 93.

Hospital	Number	Name of location
Moveable hospital with 10 beds in tents	4	Tazu, Balarud, Ab-e Sard, Ab-e Garm
Health posts with 2 beds	70	In each area, as required, a building for one to three health posts
Number of physicians and surgeons employed	40	-
Doctors' assistants druggists, nurses, bookkeepers, etc.	400	-
Ambulances	24	-
Passenger cars	n.a.	-

Source: Government of Iran 1317, pp. 139-40.

These various health centers had to see to it that (i) workers remained healthy and did not fall ill and were informed about hygiene and other medical issues; (ii) for their comfort, material help was to be given to the heirs of those who suffered accidents. Therefore, in each area a building with a health post of 15-22 beds and, as needed, a health post with two beds was operated at an interval of 5 km in mountainous terrain and 10 to 15 km in all other terrain.[1127] According to Kampsax information, the railway length was divided into 50 "lots"—i.e. stretches of 12 to 17 kilometers—and each 'lot' had its own field hospital (in Danish: lazaret). In addition, the consortium had built three large hospitals."[1128] In each region where there were 3 to 4 health posts one large central hospital had be erected complete with an OR, a surgeon and instruments and all those employees, who needed surgical work had to be treated there. These central hospitals were also equipped with a laboratory. To ensure that these big and small hospitals could operate independently each one had an ambulance. The health post in each area had a relationship with the hospital of that area. Every day, the hospital director had to visit his area with the ambulance and give instructions to the staff of the health posts

---

1127. Government of Iran 1317, p. 141.
1128. Boisen 1946, p. 46; Saxild 1971, p. 93 (two large hospitals and a number of small hospitals).

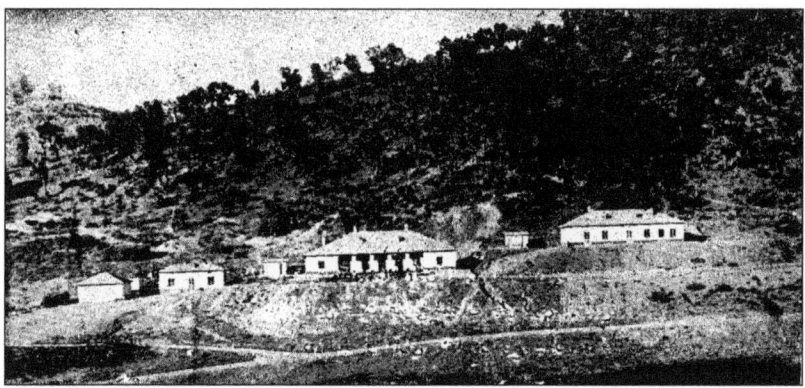

Railway hospital

concerning inspection of houses of the staff, that food and drinking water was given to patients and that sick people were transferred to the hospital. In addition, every day, one physician had to inspect the hospital of his area and correct problems.[1129]

The Kampsax workers, apart from accidents, illness, and hygiene problems, in some part of the country had to cope with malaria epidemics. Ingolf Boisen, who was sent out by Kampsax to Iran in 1937 to make a film about the railway construction, also wrote a book about his experience in Iran, and quotes Karl Olsen, a Danish engineer:

> This [Mazandaran] is by the way one of the worst malaria districts in Iran that we are driving through. When we started building the railway, mortality among the workers was very high. Engineer Wright, who was the head of the construction of the Northern part of the railway, and Doctor Torfeh, the Iranian head of the service sanitaire, organized a tremendous battle against the malaria. The whole workforce received quinine rations. But they didn't want to take it. They preferred to sell it. This was discovered when large quantities of quinine turned up in the market in Teheran. Then something new was tried. Every day the entire workforce was lined up and persons from the service sanitaire stuffed the pills into their mouths. It was, however, discovered that several workers just pretended to swallow the pills and afterwards spat them out. Then workers

---

1129. Government of Iran 1317, pp. 141-42.

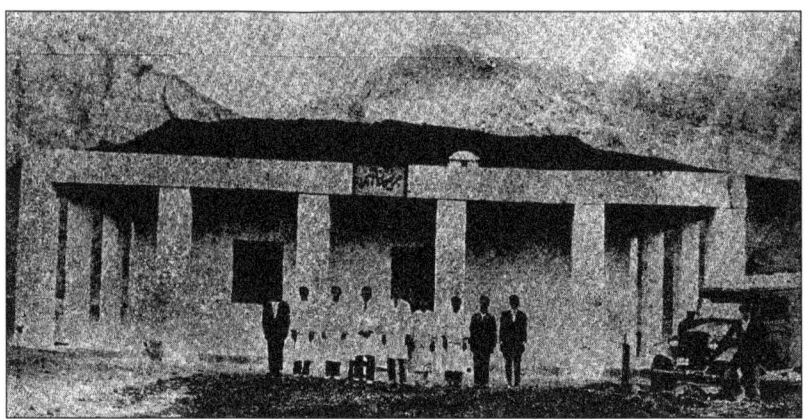

Above and opposite: Railway hospital and health post

had the quinine served in dissolved form with the order to drink it at once. They had to open their mouths so it could be controlled that they had taken the quinine. And in order to make workers themselves control whether other workers had taken the quinine, Dr. Torfeh had put some substance into the dissolved quinine, which caused the urine to become blue. ... The quinine was able counteract the worst consequences of the malaria, but the disease was still widespread. We knew about the origin of the disease - the hundreds of rice fields that were the breeding ground for the malaria mosquitoes. Engineer Wright sent a detailed report to the Ministry with radical proposals to change the situation. The case was decided at the very highest level, and the Shah did not hesitate to make a decision - all cultivation of rice was stopped in those districts through which the railway was being built. The farmers who cultivate the fields in these places had temporarily to move to other places or were offered work at the railway construction. Immediately after the fields were dried out, the incidence of malaria was reduced drastically. This was a harsh but effective measure.[1130]

The orderlies of the health posts had to visit the workers along the line during half a day and dress their wounds, give medicine to the sick

---

1130. Boisen 1946, pp. 72-73. On the incidence of malaria in Northern Iran, see Floor 2018 a, pp. 29-46.

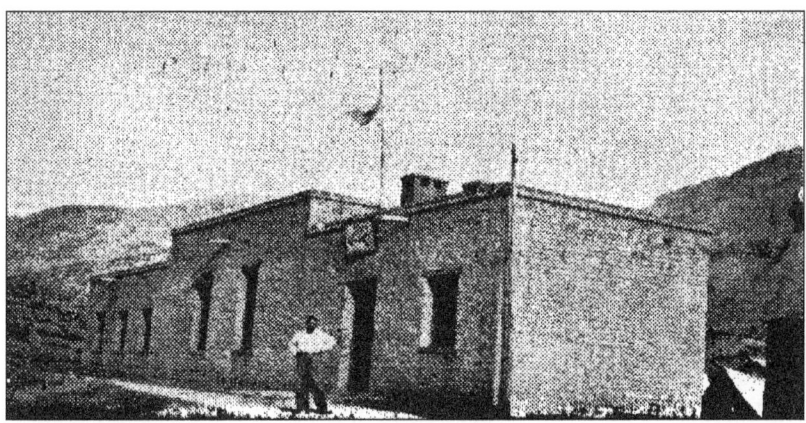

and those wounded or ill had to be transferred to the hospital with the ambulance. The other half of the day they had to be at the health post to treat those who came there. Treatment in the hospitals was without charge; those with a contagious disease were placed in rooms separate from the general wards. Because at Gardaneh-ye Towziyan there are very cold springs and it had a very pleasant climate, in addition to a hospital, a sanatorium was built. The hospitals were equipped with electric fans, refrigerators and cold baths where those suffering from the heat were brought. During the time that workers were in the hospital their wages continued to be paid; if they became invalid they were paid severance pay and in case of death their heirs would receive that. From 1933 to 1938 there were 2,488 accidents, of which 1,137 were healed, 677 men lost a limb, 674 men died. In severance pay more than 2.9 million riyals was paid out. The medical railway headquarters was in Tehran. It had several departments responsible for bookkeeping, inventory, and purchasing all goods and services needed by hospitals, including of all medicines. In some of the larger hospitals there also was a fully equipped dentistry unit. The budget for the health services was ensured by a 2% charge on the operating cost, which resulted in receipts of 25.5 million rials up to 18 Ordibehesht 1317 or 8 May 1938. At that date, 20.3 million rials of that amount had been expended; the remainder was used for the 50-bed hospital near the Tehran railway station.[1131]

Although on paper the healthcare organization of the Railway looked adequate, if not exemplary,[1132] it would seem that at times there was not enough capacity and/or competent medical personnel, or it was felt to be like that, because railway patients and other state employees covered by state health care also were referred to the American missionary hospitals. Kampsax or the R.R. Construction Syndicate in Northern Iran sent quite a few of their more severely injured workers to the American hospitals in Tehran, Hamadan and Rasht and, very important and highly appreciated, paid their bill each month. Most of the injured workers came with more or less infected compound fractures. Dr. Blair (Tehran) not only saved lives but also the limbs of most of them.[1133] A similar situation was found in Hamadan. In 1935, patients of all walks of life and groups, and also Italian and Yugoslav nationals, who worked on the railroad south of the city, although they had a small railroad hospital and few dispensaries in the construction camps.[1134] In 1934, Kampsax offered Dr. Abdollah Khan Vassei, who worked in the American hospital in Tehran, 500 *tumans* per month (over $300) with expenses, but he turned them down.[1135] Unfortunately, I have not been able to find information about the functioning of the railway health system after 1946, but I presume that it continued to function in the same way as it had in the 1930s and

---

1131. Government of Iran 1317, pp. 142-44; Saxild 1971, p. 93; Boisen 1946, p. 46.

1132. "500 people were employed within this part of the organization in their capacity as either doctors, nurses or ambulance drivers." Boisen 1946, p. 46. "Our health service was at their disposal with Iranian and Italian doctors, hospitals, medical orderlies and, in case of an accident, compensation for disability or death." Saxild 1971, pp. 84, 93.

1133. RG 91-19-11-1, Report Medical Work Teheran 1933-1934.

1134. RG 91-19-27, Healing in the Home of Avicenna 1935-1936; Saxild 1971, p. 84.

1135. RG 91-19-11-1, Report Medical Work Teheran 1933-1934.

1940s. This is indicated by data for 1946 and 1947 as to the number of patients treated and examined, and tests made in the laboratory.[1136]

Discussion

From the above, it is clear that there did not exist a system of health care facilities such as hospitals or dispensaries in Iran prior to the 20th century. The few *dar al-shafa*s that were to be found in a small number of cities did not really function as institutions that provided medical services. These traditional institutions mainly served poor and sick pilgrims and travelers. Local inhabitants of the towns where these *dar al-shafa*s were located received medical care at home, where they also preferred to die. However remarkable the potential of the *dar al-shafa*s was, they did not deliver on their promise. For seen within the context of the size of the problem, neither the traditional *dar al-shafa*s nor the nineteenth and twentieth century modern Western hospitals constituted an adequate response to the public health problem in Iran (and elsewhere) in view of their limited impact. For throughout the centuries and until recent times, Iran was an agrarian subsistence economy. We don't have guestimates for the size of the population of Iran before 1500. Even if there would be such figures they cannot be compared with population figures after 1500. This is because: (i) it was only after that year that the country had a territory that in size was only somewhat larger than that of Iran to-day, and (ii) before 1500, Iran was not one country. After the year 1000, the land of Iran was usually divided between two or three states, while the size of the Iranian Empire before 650 was many times bigger, thus making a comparison of population size impossible. During the Safavid period its population was never higher than 9 million during the seventeenth century, a number likely to be much lower in the sixteenth century due to the many wars that were fought. Most of the population (85-90%) was rural in nature, while the pastoral population was never more than about one-third of the total population. There were about 70, mostly small provincial towns in Safavid Iran. In the

---

1136. Overseas Consultants 1949, vol. II, Exhibit A-11.

17th century, Isfahan may have had 500,000 inhabitants, while Tabriz had more than 100,000, may be even more than 200,000, but Qazvin had many less inhabitants, even when it was the capital (until 1590). The urban population, therefore, oscillated around one million during the Safavid period.[1137] No population data are available on the eighteenth century, but, given the wars and oppression that characterized that period, it is likely that the urban population decreased. By 1900, Iran had an estimated population of about 9.8 million. The majority of that population was still rural and engaged in agriculture.[1138] The urban population doubled between 1850 (9%) and 1910 (18%), with three towns having more than 100,000 inhabitants: Tehran with about 280,000, Tabriz with 200,000 and Isfahan with 100,000. Four other towns each had 50,000 inhabitants or more.[1139]

What the above means is that between 550 CE and 1900 CE, some 85% of the population was rural. Therefore, these figures imply that the vast majority of the population had no access to hospitals at all. Because hospitals were only to be found in large cities they were unable to serve most of the rural population (whether sedentary or nomadic), who hardly ever visited the large cities. That still leaves 1 to 1.8 million people in urban areas, where the hospitals were located, but most of these people never saw the inside of a hospital either, because of their small number, their limited staff and means as well as the nature of their function, but, above all, due to their lack of appeal to the public at large. Even as late as the 1950s, the majority of the Iranian population had only access to traditional medicine, which was also their preferred medical treatment. As yet, there was little confidence in Western medicine and/or hospitals and the traditional health care providers (household remedies; herbalists, barbers, bone setters, oculists, *mamas*, and *hakims*) were still the man or woman to see.[1140]

1137. Floor 2000, pp. 2-8.
1138. Floor 2003, p. 45.
1139. Gilbar 1976, pp. 147-149
1140. On these traditional health care providers, see Floor 2004, pp. 80-166.

APPENDIX

List of American Medical Missionaries

Alexander, Edgar W. M.D.	1882–1892 W	
Baber, Eunice R.N.	1948–?	
Bartlett Ms	1898–?	
Bean, Bernice	?	
Benz, Gertrude E.	1920–1952 R	
Bird, Frederick L.	1916–1922 W	
Bird, Mrs. (Myra Sutherland)	1913–1922 W	
Blair, Edward M.D.	1925–1938 W	
Blair, Mrs. (Catherine R. Cooper)	1925–1938 W	
Bradford, Mary Elizabeth M.D.	1888–1909 W	
Brinkman, Harry M.D.	1931–1938 W	
Brinkman, Mrs. (Adriana van Lopik)	1931–1938 W	
Browning, Mrs.	?	
Ms Burgess	?	
Bussdicker, Russell D. M.D.	1922–1955 R	
Bussdicker, Mrs. (Blanche Gillis)	1922–1955 R	
Chambers, Estella M.	1936–1950	
Chase, Ms	?	
Cochran, Dorothy Anne R.N.	1945–1947 W	
Cochran, Ermna G.	1885–1888 W	
Cochran, Katherine	1871–1875 W	
Cochran, Rev. Joseph G.	1847–1871 D	
Cochran, Mrs. (Deborah Plumb)	1847–1871 W	
Cochran, Joseph P. M.D.	1878–1905 D	
Cochran, Mrs. (Katharine Hale)	1879–1895 D	
Cochran, Mrs. (Bertha H. McConaughy)	1900–1907 W	1909–1932 W
Cochran, Joseph P. Jr. M.D.	1920–1958 R	
Cochran, Mrs. (Bernice Gregg)	1920–1958 R	
Cook, Joseph W. M.D.	1912–1920 W 1	929–1932 D
Cook, Mrs. (Alice O. Ensign)	1913–1920	1929–1932 W
Dale, Ms	1898–?	

Degner, Emma A. R.N.	1945–1959 R	
Dodd, Edward M. M.D.	1916–1925 W	
Dodd, Edmund MD	1918–1930?	
Doolittle, Jane Ms	1940?	
Easton, Helen, see Mrs. Hoffman		
Enderson, Anna E.	1931–1956 R	
Fisher, Faye R.N.	1916–1917 W	
Fleming, Mary R. M.D.	1915–1920 W	
Frame, John D. M.D.	1905–1948 D	
Frame, Mrs. (Grace J. Murray 1)	1912–1946 D	
Frame, Mrs. (Adelaide Kibbe 2)	1929–1948 W	
Frame, John D. Jr. M.D.	1947–1952 W	
Frame, Mrs. (Dorothy Anderson)	1947–1952 W	
Fulton, Janet S., B.A., R.N.	1931–1956 W	
Funk, John Arthur M.D.	1903–1939 D	
Funk, Mrs. (Susanna S. Leinbach)	1891–1939 R	
Gudhart, Ms	?	
Harvey, E. Mary R.N.	1937– ?	
Hoffman, Rolla E. M.D.	1915–1957 R	
Hoffman, Mrs. (Helen Easton 1)	1920–1947 D	
Hoffman, Mrs. (Adelaide Kibbe 2)	1950–1957 R	
Holmes, George W. M.D.	1874–1899 W	
Holmes, Mrs. (Eliza A. Wisner 1)	1874–1890 D	
Holmes, Mrs. (Lucy S. Hale M.D. 2)	1892–1899 W	
Jones, Jeanette R.N.	1920–1933 W	
Keller, Ms	1956– ?	
Lamme, Charles W. M.D.	1911–1919 W	1920–1950 R
Lamme, Mrs. (Jessie C. Garman)	1930–1950 R	
Lamme Ms.	1930–?	
Lawrence, T.E. MD	1902–1919 ?	
Lawrence, Mrs. (Jessie C. Wilson)	1892–1919 W	
Lichtwardt, Hartman A. M.D. Rev.	1919–1945 R	
Lichtwardt, Mrs. (Hilda M. Tozier)	1919–1945 R	
McDowell, Philip C. M.D.	1918–1944 W	
McDowell, Mrs. (Sarah E. Wright)	1918–1944 W	1954–1960 R

Miller, Emma T. M.D.	1891–1909 W	
Murray, Thomas A. M.D.	1946– ?	
Murray, Mrs. (Nancy Lounsbury)	1946– ?	
Nicholson, Ellen D.	1924–1955 R	
Norem, Walter M.D.	1939–1947 W	
Norem, Mrs. (Katherine Morrows)	1939–1947 W	
Orcutt, Edna E. M.D.	1911–1914 D	
Packard, Harry P. M.D.	1906–1944 R	
Packard, Mrs. (Julia F. Bayley 1)	1906–1924 D	
Packard, Mrs. (Edna J. Wells 2)	1916–1944 R	
Payne, Mrs. (Grace E. Visher)	1922–1956 R	
Payne Mrs. J.D.	1936?–1947?	
Pease, Wilma E. R.N.	1924–1960 W	
Porter, Dorothy M.D.	1957–?	
Reynolds, Elizabeth M.	?	
Rice, Homer M.D.	1950– 196?	
Rice, Mrs . (Charlotte L. Means)	1950– 196?	
Romig, M.D.	19??–1956?	
Schneider, Arnold J. M.D.	1949–1959 W	
Schneider, Mrs. (Lois Bosworth)	1949–1959 W	
Scott, Ms Fern	1962–?	
Scott, Gordon W. M.D.	1959– ?	
Scott, Mrs. (Lola Madeline Bowman)	1959–?	
Simpson, Ms	?	
Smell, Ms	?	
Smith, Mary J. M.D.	1889–1923 W	
Stead, Rev. Francis M.	1902–1924 W	
Stead, Mrs. (Blanche Wilson M.D.)	1900–1922 D	
Stetner, Mrs.	1956	
Stewart, Ashton, T. M.D.	1947– ?	
Stewart, Mrs. (Natalie Mah1ow)	1947– ?	
Tai11ie, Grace S.	1919–1933 W	
Torrence W. W. M.D.	1881–1891 W	
Torrence, Mrs. W. W.	1881–1891 W	

Appendix •

Van Norden, Rev. Thomas L. M.D.	1866–1873 W	
Van Norden, Mrs. (Mary M. Paterson) 1866–1873 W		
Vanneman, William, S. M.D.	1890–1933 D	
Vanneman, Mrs. (Marguerite A. Fox)	1890–1933 R	
Wallstrom, Ira C. M.D.	1955– ?	
Wallstrom, Mrs. (Doris Elaine Rylander)	1955–?	
Ward, Vera R.N.	1958–?	
Wells, Ms. E. Jean R.N., see Mrs. Packard		
Wheeler, Helen R.N.	1951–1956 W	
Wilder, Ms	?	
Wilson, Ms Mabel F. R.N.	?	
Winkelman, Ms Gertrude R.N.	1941–1945?	
Wishard; John G. M.D.	1889–1899 W	1903–1910 W
Wishard, Mrs. (Annabette Bryan 1)	1893–1899 D	
Wishard, Mrs.	1903–1910 W	
Wright, Robert N. M.D.	1927–1933 W	
Wright, Mrs. (Margaret M. McKay)	1927–1933 W	
Yates, Christina, M.D.	1958–1959 W	
Zarn, Ms Dolores	?	
Zoeckler, Frances Louise M.D.	1949–1970 R	
Zoeckler, Rev. George F.	1909–1948 D	
Zoeckler, Mrs. (Mary D. Allen M.D.)	1912–1948 ?	

Source: Rev. John Elder, *History of the American Presbyterian Mission to Iran 1834–1960*, pp. 98–107 and sources cited in the text. D= died; R= Retired; W= worked

BIBLIOGRAPHY

Archives

Presbyterian Historical Society, Philadelphia (USA).

Birjand

RG 280-1-14, Frances Zoeckler, Report on Medical Itineration, 1963 (Birjand).

Dowlatabad – Malayer

RG 280-1-8, Home Letters (Mary A. Zoeckler, 1917-1950)
Report on 25 Days Itineration, Malayir. July-August 1916
Mary Allen Zoeckler to the Women's Guild, North Church, Buffalo, 16/05/1917.
Mary Allen Zoeckler to the Women's Guild, North Church, Buffalo, 15/02/1921

RG 280-1-10, Medical Reports (Mary Zoeckler) 1914-1949.
    Report of Medical Work for Women, Daulatbad, 1914-1915
    Report of Medical Work Daulatabad, 1915-1916
    Report of Medical Work Daulatbad 1916-1917
    Report of Medical Work Daulatabad, July 1--Nov. 12, 1917
    Medical Report. Daulatabad 1921-22
    Report of Medical Work Daulatabad 1922-23
    American Dispensary Daulatabad [1923-24?]
    Report of Medical Work Daulatabad 1924-1925
    Report of Medical Work, Daulatabad 1925-26
    Report of Medical Work, Daulatabad 1925-26
    Report of Medical Work Daulatabad. July 1-Nov. 1, 1926
    Report of Medical Work Daulatabad May 28-June 20, 1928
    Report of Medical Work Daulatabad 1928-1929

Report of Medical Work Daulatabad 1929-1930
Report of Daulatabad Medical Work 1930-1931
Report of Daulatabad Medical Work 1931-1932
Report of Daulatabad Medical Work 1932-1933
Report of Daulatabad Medical Work 1933-1934
Report of Daulatabad Medical Work 1938-1939
Report of Daulatabad Medical Work 1939-1940
Report of Daulatabad Medical Work 1940-1941
Report of Daulatabad Medical Work 1941-1942

Hamadan

RG 91-19-27, Hamadan Hospital 1927-1956
- Hamadan Medical Report 1932-33
- Hamadan Medical Report 1933-34
- Medical Report Hamadan Station 1934-35
- Healing in the Home of Avicenna 1935-36
- Hamadan Medical Report 1936-37
- Report on Medical Work Hamadan 1937-38
- Christian Healing in Hamadan 1938-39
- Healing in Hamadan 1939-40
- Medical Report Hamadan 1940-41
- Medical Report Hamadan 1941-42
- Medical Report Hamadan 1942-43
- Medical Report Hamadan 1944-44
- Medical Report Hamadan Hospital 1945-46
- Medical Report Hamadan 1946-47
- Medical Report Hamadan 1947-48

RG 280-1-10, Medical Reports (Mary Zoeckler) 1914-1949.
- M. A. Zoeckler, Report of the Women's Medical Work Hamadan 1914
- M. A. Zoeckler, Report of the Medical Department, Hamadan Station, July 1, 1920
- Report of Medical Work Hamadan 1920-21

RG 161-3-44, Institution Chrisitian Hospital Hamadan, 1956-1959
- Ms Francis Gray to Dr. Rice, 26/01/1956;
- Rice to Ms Francis Gray, 12/02/1956.
- [Extract of] Action taken at the Meeting of the Executive Committee of the Iran Mission on 6-8 March, 1956.

Walstrom to Dr. Dodd and Dr. Stevenson, 15/04/1956;
Walstrom to Ms Francis Gray and Dr. Romig, 29/04/1956
Rice to Sundberg, 18/11/1956
Memo Sundberg to Cochran, 30/11/1959
Questionnaire for the medical office 1958. 30/01/1959

Kermanshah

RG 91-19-28, Kermanshah 1919-1926
    Mrs. Stead to [Mission HQ], 30/08/1921
    Trull to Speer, 21/12/1922
    [?] to Mrs. Cyrus McCormick, 11/01/1923
    Letter for the Supporters of the Orphanage at Kermanshah, 1923
    Harry Packard to Dr. Speer, 08/03/1923
    Dr. Packard to [?]. (undated/rec. 15/03/1923)
    Note 14/04/28
    Note 27/07/1927
    Note 29/10/27
    Packard/Kermanshah to Holmes/Buffalo, 15/11/1931
    Packard to Speer, 30/07/1932
    Westminster Hospital Report 07/03/1933
    Packard to Butzer 03/06/1933
    Speer to Butzer, 16/10/1933
    Speer to Butzer, 22/10/1934.
    Note concerning Linens and Laundry [undated].
    Frances Zoeckler to Board of Foreign Missions 08/02/1956
    Bushdicker/Kermanshah to Huntwork/New York, 29/09/1957
    Muradian to Bussdicker, 06/08/1959

RG 91-19-30, Kermanshah Hospital 1927-47
    Westminster Hospital News vol. 1/3 -15/09/1932
    Westminster Hospital Report no. 2, 1932
    Westminster Hospital Report no. 4, 1932
    Report Westminster Hospital 1932-33
    Report of Westminster Hospital 1933-34
    The Westminster Hospital Annual Report 1934-35[mimeo pamphlet]
    Kermanshah Medical Report 1935-36
    Kermanshah Medical Report 1937-38
    Annual Report Westminster Hospital Kermanshah 1938
    The Westminster Hospital Bulletin. vol/. 1/2. May 1938

Bibliography

Annual Report Westminster Hospital Kermanshah 1938-39
The Westminster Hospital Bulletin. vol. 2/1. October 1939
Report Westminster Hospital Kermanshah 1939-40
Report Westminster Hospital Kermanshah 1940-41
Report Westminster Hospital Kermanshah 1942-43
Report Westminster Hospital Kermanshah 1943-44
Annual Report Westminster Hospital Kermanshah 1944-45
Social and Education Project – Kermanshah 1944-45
The out-patient clinic

Mashhad

RG 91-20-2, Mashad Hospital 1925-1948.
Mashad Medical Report 1928-29
Mashad Medical Report 1929-30
Mashad Medical Report 1930-31
Mashad Medical Report 1931-32
Mashad Medical Report 1932-33
Mashad Medical Report 1933-34
Mashad Medical Report 1934-35
Mashad Medical Report 1935-36
Mashad Medical Report 1936-37
Mashad Medical Report 1937-38
Mashad Medical Report 1938-39
Mashad Medical Report 1939-40
Mashad Medical Report 1940-41
Mashad Medical Report 1941-42
Mashad Medical Report 1942-43
Mashad Medical Report 1944-45
Mashad Medical Report 1945-46
Allen to Hoffman 25/06/1946
Hoffman to Allen 03/12/1947

RG 231-1-2, Rolla Hoffman Correspondence 1915-1919
R.E. Hoffman to Friends, Tehran, 26/12/1915
NN [Hoffman] to Friends, Meshed, March 1918
Hoffman to Parents, 16/04/1918
Donaldson? to friends, Mashhad 20/07/1918
NN to friends, Mashhad 30/08/1918
incomplete letter Hoffman to Speer, October 1918

Hoffman to Donaldson, Mashhad 10/10/1918
Murray to Speer, Meshed 12/10/1918
Hoffman to parents, 25/07/1920.
Hoffman to parents, Mashad 02/10/1918
Hoffman to parents. Tehran, 10/10/1919
Hoffman to Friends 10/03/1930
Hoffman to New Castle church 31/07/1934
Hoffman to Mother, 04/10/1936
Hoffman to N.N., no date (probably 1938).

RG 231-1-5, Rolla Hoffman Correspondence 1930-1949
Memo Medical Needs Rasht Hospital undated, probably 1948

RG 231-6, Rolla Hoffman Reports, Memos & Newsletters 1918-1949
Annual Report of the Medical Work at Meshed, Persia. The American Hospital. For the year ending June 30, 1929.
Personal Report 1933
Personal Report Mrs. Hoffman 1929-1930
Report of Famine Relief Work of Meshed Station June 1st 1917 to June 30th 1918

RG 231-1-7.
Rolla Edwards Hoffman, *Pioneering in Meshed, the Holy City of Iran. Saga of a Medical Missionary*. Duarte, California, 1969 (typescript).

Rasht

RG 91-1-12, Report of Resht Station 1910-1911
Report of Resht Station 1910-1911

RG 91-19-9, Resht Medical Reports 1918-1944.
"History of Resht Station."
Resht Medical Report, 10/07/1919
Resht Medical Report 1919-20
Resht Medical Report 1921-22
Resht Medical Report 1923-24
Resht Medical Report 1924-25
Resht Medical Report 1927-28
Resht Medical Report 1928-29
Resht Medical Report 1929-30
Resht Medical Report 1930-31

Resht Medical Report 1931-32
Resht Medical Report 1932-33
Resht Medical Work 1933-34
Report of Resht Medical Work 1934-35
Medical Report Resht 1935-36
Resht Medical Report 1936-37
Resht Hospital Report 1937-38
Resht Hospital Report 1938-39
Resht Hospital Report 1939-40
Resht Hospital Report 1940-1941
Medical Report Resht Hospital 1941- 1942
Resht Hospital Report 1942-43
Resht Hospital Report 1943-44
Resht Hospital Report 1944-45

RG 91-20-8 - Resht Hospital ?-1957
    Frame/Rasht to Speer/NY 17/02/1931
    Resht Hospital Social Service Center 1942-43
    Resht Hospital Social Service Center 1944-45

RG 231-1-5, Rolla Hoffman Correspondence 1930-1949.
    Hoffman/Rasht to Friends, 12/09/1948

RG 231-1-6
    Personal Report 1949 and Hospital Report 1948-1949
    Memo Medical Needs Rasht Hospital undated, probably 1948

TABRIZ

RG 161.3.51, Institutions- Christian Hospital, Tabriz 1956, 1958-1964
    Arnold Schneider M.D. Tabriz. Kirkwood Hospital. Questionnaire for the Medical Office, 1958, Tabriz, 17/01/1959.
    Arnold Schneider (Tabriz) to Stevenson and Sundberg (N.Y.), 04/08/1958,
    Drs. Wallstrom M.D. Questionnaire for the Medical Office 1958, 26/12/1958
    Gloria Simpson, Nurses education
    Christian Hospital Tabriz Report 1962-1963
    N.N. to Stevens (N.Y.), 07/14/1964
    Memo Sundberg to Stevenson and McGilvray, 06/12/1964

Tehran

RG 91-19-11-1: Tehran Medical Work-reports 1922-52
    Notes on medical work of Teheran station Jan. 1922
    S. W. McD. Historical Sketch of Teheran Medical Work
    Teheran Hospital Report 1927-28
    Report of the Medical Work Teheran 1931-1932
    Report of Teheran Hospital 1932-33
    Report of Tehran Medical Work 1934-1935
    Report of Teheran Hospital 1935-36
    Report Teheran American Hospital 1936-37
    Report Medical Work Teheran 1937-1938
    Report American Hospital Teheran 1940-1941
    Teheran Medical Report 1941-1942
    Teheran Medical Report 1942-1943

RG 91-19-17: Medical Committees Reports 1938-41
    Jane Payne, Health Center for Children
    Memo Bussdicker-Blair, 14 May 1938
    Circular letter concerning the Health Center, 11 November 1938.

RG 231-1-2, Rolla Hoffman, no date.
    Hoffman/Tehran to Friends, 26/12/1915
    Report of Medical Work Teheran Station 1934.

RG 231-1-5, Rolla Hoffman, Correspondance 1930-1949
    Gifford [?] to Allen/Wysham, Tehran 17/08/1936, Government Nurses' School Project
    Hoffman/Tehran to Dr. McClanahan/Cairo (31/07/1932).

RG 231-6, Rolla Hoffman Reports, Memos & Newsletters 1918-1949
    Personal Report 1942

Urmiyeh

RG 91-20-7: Rezaieh Hospital 1926-31
    Report of Medical Work in Urumia. Nov. 1922-1923
    Report Medical Work Urumia 1924-1925
    Medical Report Urmia 1925-1926
    Report Jessie Lee Ellis. [1925?]
    Famous Urumia Hospital to be rebuilt - memo

Ellis to Williamson, charge d'affaire Tehran 30/09/1930
Cochran Memorial Hospital Rezaieh 1931-1932
Cochran Memorial Hospital Report 1932-33
Last annual report of the Cochran Memorial Hospital, Rezaieh 1934
Dr. W. Ellis/Rezaieh to Dr. Samuel Holmes/Buffalo, 29/11/1926
Ellis/Rezaieh to Nesbitt/NY, 08/11/1927
Ellis/Rezaieh to Holmes/Buffalo 11/11/1927
? to Speer and Trull, 04/10/1928.
Trull to Speer/NY, 04/10/1928.
Holmes/Buffalo to Speer/NY, 28/02/1929
Speer/NY to the Executive Council, 07/06/1929.
Ellis/Rezaieh to Speer/NY, 28/08/1929;
Holmes/Buffalo to Speer/NY, 21/11/1929
Ellis/Urmiyeh to Speer/NY, 27/01/1930
Ellis/Urmiyeh to Speer/NY 25/02/1930
Wilson/Tabriz to Speer/NY. 01/03/1930
Memo Dodd to Speer, 26/03/1930
Memo Dodd to Speer, 20/05/1930
Ellis to Speer 08/09/1930
Ellis to Williamson, charge d'affaire Tehran 30/09/1930.
Memo Tower to Speer/NY 10/04/1931
Hugo Muller, Rezaieh to Cady Allen, Hamadan 22/06/1931
Ruth Elliot to Dr. Ellis 19/03/1932
Ellis/Rezaieh to Speer 07/12/1933.

RG 231-2 Rolla Hoffman, Photograph album 2,
RG 231-4 Rolla Hoffman, Photograph album 3, 1923-

British Library, India Office (IOR), London (UK).

IOR/L/MIL/17/15/6/1, 'Military Report on Persia. vol. iv, part i,'
IOR/L/MIL/17/15/8, 'Military Report on Southern Persia'.
IOR/L/MIL/17/15/10/1, Military Report on S. W. Persia, 4 vols. Simla, 1909.
IOR/L/MIL/17/15/13, M.T. Routes in Persia
IOR/L/MIL/17/15/24, 'Military Report on Oilfield Area'
IOR/L/MIL/17/15/35, 'Report on the Working of the Line of Communication and on the Withdrawal of the British Military Mission in East Persia, 1919-20. General Staff, India, p. 97, appendix V.
IOR/L/MIL/17/15/40, 'Persia Intelligence Report. May, 1946'
IOR/L/PS/10/100, Seistan disturbances and consular guard'

IOR/L/PS/10/209, Meshed Consular Diary No. 50 for the week ending 11th December 1911

IOR/L/PS/10/209, Diary of the Military Attache, Meshed, no. 30, for the week ending August 3rd, 1912

IOR/L/PS/10/209, Consular Diary HBM's Consul for Sistan and Kain, Diary no. 40 ending 4th October 1913

IOR/L/PS/10/209, Consular Diary HBM's Consul for Sistan and Kain, no. 42, for the week ending 18th October 1913,

IOR/L/PS/10/209, Meshed Consular Diary no. 6, for the week ending 8th February 1913

IOR/L/PS/10/210, Sistan and Kain Consulate Diary no. 27 , for the week ending 3rd July 1915,

IOR/L/PS/10/211, Meshed Diary no. 22 for the week ending the 1st June 1918

IOR/L/PS/10/284, Tehran Sanitary Council

IOR/L/PS/10/328/1, Reductions in expenditure on Agencies and Consulates

IOR/L/PS/10/451/1, Persia – Policy. British Interests in the South. Russian Policy', no. 13. Russian Policy on the Turco-Persian Frontier. Capt. A. T. Wilson to Sir W. Townley, Camp Mawana, 15/08/1914

IOR/L/PS/11/182.

IOR/L/PS/11/182, Finance Department to Secretary of State for India, Simla, 09/09/1921

IOR/L/PS/11/182, R.C. Parr, Britsh Legation to Taqi Esfandiary, Tehran, 12/10/1923.

IOR/L/PS/11/182. Johnston to New Delhi, 02/12/1928.

IOR/L/PS/11/182, Foreign Secretary India, New Delhi to Under-secretary for India, London. 07/01/1930

IOR/L/PS/12/3400, Diary of HBM's Consul for Khuzestan, Ahwaz, no. 1, for the month of January 1931

IOR/L/PS/12/3400, Diary of HBM's Consul for Khuzestan, Ahwaz, no. 6, 1933 for the month of June 1933

IOR/L/PS/12/3400, HBM's Consulate for Khuzistan, Ahwaz, Diary no. 4 for the month of April 1933

IOR/L/PS/12/3400, Diary of HBM's Consul for Khuzestan, Ahwaz, no. 6, 1933 for the month of June 1933

IOR/L/PS/12/3400, Diary of HBM's Consul for Khuzestan, Ahwaz, no. 9 of 1933 for the period of 21st October 1933 to 30th November 1933

IOR/L/PS/12/3400, Diary of HBM's Consul for Khuzestan, Ahwaz, no. 10 of 1933 for the month of December 1933

IOR/L/PS/12/3403, Diary of HBM's Consul, Sistan and Kain, for the months of November-December 1928, p. 3.

IOR/L/PS/12/3403, Diary of HBM's Consul, Sistan and Kain, for the months of May 1928, p. 2.

IOR/L/PS/12/3403, Diary of HBM's Consul, Sistan and Kain, for the month of April 1929,

IOR/L/PS/12/3403, HBM's Consulate, Sistan and Kain, Diary for July 1932

Bibliography

IOR/L/PS/12/3406, Coll 28/10 'Persia. Diaries; Meshed Consular Jany 1931 – May 1940. Secret. Diary for February 1935. HBM ConsGen Khorasan and Sistan, Khorassan Political 1934 – May 1940. Khorassan Fortnightly Reports'

IOR/L/PS/12/3406, Khorasan Political Diary for November 1939, p. 2 [Persia. Diaries; Meshed Consular Jany 1931 – May 1940. Khorassan Political 1934 – May 1940. Khorassan Fortnightly Reports']

IOR/L/PS/12/3413, Diary of HBM's consul, Kerman, no. 10, for the month of December 1931

IOR/L/PS/12/3413, Diary of HBM's Consulate, Kerman, no. 4, for the month of April 1932

IOR/L/PS/12/3413, Diary of HBM's consul, Kerman, no. 11, for the month of November 1933

IOR/L/PS/12/3413, HBM's Consulate Kerman Diary no 11, 1936

IOR/L/PS/12/3415, Annual Commercial Report for the Province of Sistan and the Kainat for the year 1928-29

IOR/L/PS/12/3415, Annual Commercial Report for the Province of Khurasan and Zabulistan for the Persian Year 1312 (21st March 1933 to 20th March 1934)

IOR/L/PS/12/3406, HMG's Consulate-General, Meshed political diary for the month of August 1933

IOR/L/PS/12/3406, Secret. Diary for February 1935

IOR/L/PS/12/3416, Coll. 28/20 'Persia Judicial. Civil, Commercial + Penal Code, and various laws.'

IOR/L/PS/12/3472A, Annual Report 1937

IOR/L/PS/12/3542

IOR/L/PS/12/3561, Personal aspects of life as Vice-Consul, Zabul (December 1941),

IOR/L/PS/12/3592, copy letter no. 540 from vice-consul Mohammarah to Pol. Resident Persian Gulf, 07/06/1935 [Reduction of medical expenditure'].

IOR/L/PS/12/3600, No. 78, Percy Lorraine to Secr. GOI/Simla, 18/05/1925.

IOR/L/PS/12/3607, Meshed Consular Diary no. 24 for the period ending 31at December 1931, General reorganization of consular posts'

IOR/L/PS/12/3607, HBM's consul-general Meshed, no 325/127/10, 30/03/1932

IOR/L/PS/12/3650, Consul Ahvaz to Amb. R.H. Hoare, Tehran, 27/03/1933.

IOR/L/PS/12/3654, creation of vice consulate; allowances attached to post of Indian Medical Service Officers in East Persia'

IOR/L/PS/12/3654, A note on the importance of Seistan to India by Captain Maurice Patrick O'Connor Tandy, HM Vice-Consul, Birjand, 18 September 1939

IOR/L/PS/12/3713, Intelligence Summary no. 22 for the month December 1945

IOR/L/PS/20/7, Report on Fars by Captain A T Wilson, Indian Political Department

IOR/L/PS/20/224, Biographies of the notables of Fars and certain Persian officials who have served at Shiraz. Delhi: Government of India, 1925

Mss Eur C600/1, 'A note on the importance of Seistan to India' Grant Duff to Mushir-ed-Douleh 31/03/1906

National Archives (Kew Gardens)

FO 248/1291, Neligan to M (20/01/1919).

FO 248/1291, Memo on a proposal to secure an English instead of an German administration for the Persian Government Hospital, Tehran, 20 October 1918

FO 248/1291, Sir Percy Cox to Vothuq al-Dowleh, (03/04/1919).

FO 248/1291, Vothugh al-Dowleh to Cox, (11/05/1919).

FO 248/1291, Cox to Vothugh al-Dowleh, (18/09/1919)

FO 248/1291, Memo Neligan 30 November 1922: Comments on McLean's memo

FO 248/1291, Invoice medical instruments

For 248/1291, Lt. Col. Fortescue to Minister, (04/02/1920).

FO 248/1291, Neligan to Overseas Nursing Association (05/08/1919);

FO 248/1291, Memo MacLean (07/08/1920).

FO 248/1291, Curzon to Cox telegram (29/10/1920).

FO 248/1204, Kermanshah report no. 6, 02/08/1918 by Lt. Col. Kennion

FO 248/1204, Kermanshah report no. 9, 01/11/1918 by Lt. Col. Kennion

FO 371/40177, Kermanshah Diary January 1944

FO 371/40177, Kermanshah Diary February 1944

FO 371/40177, Kermanshah Diary March 1944.

FO 371/40177, Kermanshah Diary April 1944

FO 371/9030, Foreign Office: General Correspondance from 1906-1966. Easter, Persia.

FO 371/10131, Foreign Office: General Correspondance from 1906-1966. Easter, Persia.

FO 371/15473, Foreign Office: General Correspondance from 1906-1966. Easter, Persia.

FO 371/21900, Foreign Office: General Correspondance from 1906-1966. Easter, Persia.

Websites:

Iranicaonline.org is the online version of the *Encyclopedia Iranica*.

Books and Articles.

Abbasi-Dezfouli, A.; Daneshvar-Kakhi, A; Arab M.; Javaherzadeh M.; Shadmehr M.B.; Abbasi S. and Nournbala, A.A. 2014. "Development of Thoracic Surgery in Iran," in Azizi ed. 2014, pp. 201-04.

Abbott, Keith Edward, 1855, "Geographical Notes taken during a Journey in Persia in 1840 and 1850." *Journal of the Royal Geographical Society*, XXV, pp. 1-78.

Abbott, Nabia 1968. "Jundishapur: A Preliminary Historical Sketch," *Ars Orientalis* 7, 53-73.

Adamec, Ludwig 1989. *Historical Gazetteer of Iran*. 4 vols. Graz: Akademische Verlag.

Adamiyat, Fereydun 1348/1969. *Amir Kabir*. Tehran: Khvarezmi.

Adhari-Khakestar, GholamReza 1395/2016. *Tarikh-e Pezeshki-ye Novin-e Mashhad*. Tehran: Daneshgah-e Azadi-ye Eslami.

Administration Report = *Administration Report on the Persian Gulf Political Residency for the year (1873 to 1940)* in Government of India. *The Persian Gulf Administration Reports 1873-1947*, 11 vols., Gerrards Cross, Archives Editions, 1986-89.

A Friend of Iran. 1940. *"Dawdson," The Doctor. G.E. Dodson of Iran*. London: Highway Press.

Afshar, Iraj. 1354/1975. *Yadgarha-ye Yazd*. 2 vols. Tehran: Anjoman-e Athar-e Melli.

___, 1371/1992. *Ganjineh-ye `aksha-ye Iran*. Tehran: Farhang.

Afzal al-Molk, Gholam Hoseyn 1361/1982. *Afzal al-Tavarikh* ed. Mansureh Ettehadiyeh and Sirus Sa`vandiyan. Tehran: Tarikh.

Algar, Hamed 1969. *Religion and State in Iran 1785-1906. The role of the Ulama in the Qajar Period*. Berkeley: UCLA Press.

Allen, Terry 1981. *A Catalogue of the Toponyms and Monuments of Timurid Herat*. Cambridge: MIT.

Amanat, Abbas 1998. "E`tezad al-Saltana, `Aliqoli Mirza," iranicaonline.org.

Amir Hoseyni, Karim Nikzad. 1357/1378. *Shenakht-e Sarzamin-e Char Mahall*. Isfahan.

Andreeva, Elena 2007. *Russia and Iran in the Great Game*. London-New York: Routledge.

Andrews, Justin M. 1950. "Planning a malarial control program for Iran." *CDC Bulletin, Malaria Control in Iran*, July, pp. 1-24.

Anonymous 1895. "The Persia and Baghdad Mission. I. Report of the Mission for the Year 1891." *The Church Mission Intelligencer*, vol. 46 (April), pp. 263-66.

Idem 1905. "Royal philanthropy in Persia: a prince and his hospital," *The Graphic* 7 October, p. 458.

Idem 1911. "Traveling in Persia," *Bulletin of Pharmacy*, vol. 25, p. 425.

Idem 1918. "Notes on Current Topics," *The Moslem World*, vol. 8, p. 303.

Idem 1922, "Encouraging contrasts in Persia," *The Missionary Review*, vol. 45 (February), p. 146.

Idem 1924. "Current Topics," *The Moslem World* 14, p. 182.

Idem 1954. *Auguste Rollier, M.D. (1954).The British Medical Journal* 2: (4897): 1169-1170.

Idem 1366/1987. *Tarikh-e Sistan.* ed. Malek al-Sho`ara Bahar. Tehran: Khavar.

Arasteh, A. Reza 1970. *Education and Social Awakening in Iran.* Leiden: Brill.

Ardabili, Ebn Bazzaz 1373/1994. *Safvat al-Safa.* ed. GholamReza Tabataba'i-Majd. Tabriz.

Ardakani, Hoseyn Mahbubi 1368/1989. *Tarikh-e Mo'assesat-e Tamaddoni-ye Jadid dar Iran.* 3 vols. Tehran: Daneshgah-e Tehran.

Arjah, Akram- Hadiyan, Farideh- Soltanifar, Sadiqeh- and Chehrekhand, Zahrah eds. 1371/1992. *Ketabshenasi-e Nosakh-e Khatti-ye Pezeshki-ye Iran* (Tehran: Ketabkhhaneh-ye Melli.

Asaf al-Dowleh, Mirza `Abdol-Vahhab Khan. 1377/1998. *Asnad* 2 vols. ed. `Abdol-Hoseyn Nava'i and Nilufar Kasri. Tehran: Mo'asseseh-ye Motale`at-e Tarikh-e Mo`aser-e Iran.

Asaf, Mohammad Hashem (Rostam al-Hokama). 1348/1969. *Rostam al-Tavarikh* ed. Mohammad Moshiri. Tehran.

`Ataredi, Azizollah 1371/1992. *Tarikh-e Astan-e Qods-e Razavi.* 2 vols. Tehran: Utared.

Aubin, Eugène 1908. *La Perse d'aujourd'hui.* Paris: Armand Colin.

Aubin, Jean. 2000. "Ormuz au jour le jour à travers un register de Luís Figueira 1516-1518, in Françoise Aubin ed. *Le Latin et l'Astrolabe* 2 vols. Lisbon-Paris, vol. 2, pp. 393-415.

Azizi, Mohammad-Hossein; Bahadori, Moslem; Raees-Jalali, Ghanbar-Ali 2014. "In commemoration of Haj Mohammad Nemazee (1895-1972): The Founder of Nemazee Hospital in Shiraz," in Mohammad-Hossein Azizi ed. *A Collection of Essays on the History of Medicine in Iran.* Tehran, 2014, pp. 239-43.

Bafqi, Mohammad Mofid Mostowfi-ye. 1340/1961. *Jame`-ye Mofidi.* 3 vols. ed. Iraj Afshar. Tehran.

Bahadori M. 2014. "A Historical Review of Pathology in Iran," in Azizi M. H. ed. 2014, pp. 143-50.

Baladiyyeh-ye Tehran (Servis-e Ma`aref va Ehsa'iyeh va Nashriyat) 1310/1931. *Dovvomin Salnameh-ye Ehsa'iyeh-ye Shahr-e Tehran.* Tehran.

Balkhi, Hamid al-Din Abu Bakr `Omar b. Mahmudi 1372/1993, *Maqamat-e Hamidi*, ed, Reza Enzabi-nezhad, Tehran: Daneshgahi.

Bamdad, Mehdi 1356. *Tarikh-e Rejal-e Iran qorun-e 12-13-14.* 6 vols. Tehran: Zavvar.

Barbaro, Josef et al., 1873. *Travels to Tana and Persia by Josef Barbaro and Ambrogio Contarini* 2 vols. translated into English by Lord Stanley. London, Hakluyt.

Bast, Olivier "Germany ix: Germans in Persia," iranicaonline.org.

Billings, F. T. 1957. "Dr. Auguste Rollier." *Transactions of the American Clinical and Climatological Association* 68: 52-53.

Boisen, Ingolf 1946. *Jernbanen skal bygges på seks Aar.* København: Nyt Nordisk Forlag Arnold Busck.

Bricteux, Auguste. 1908. *Au pays du lion et du soleil.* Brussels: Falk Fils.

Brown, Simon and Simcock, David C. 2012. "Leprosy in Mesopotamia," *Research on History of Medicine* Nov. 1(4), pp. 147-56.

Brugsch, Heinrich 1863. *Reise der K.Preussischen Gesandtschaft nach Persien 1860 und 1861*. Leipzig: Hinrichs.

___, 1886. *Im Lande der Sonne. Wanderungen in Persien*. Berlin.

Brydges-Jones, Harford 1976. *An Account of the Transactions of His Majesty's Mission to the Court of Persia in the Years 1807-11*. Tehran: Imperial Organization for Social Services.

Burrell, R.M. 1988. "The 1904 epidemic of cholera in Persia: some aspects of Qajar society," *Bulletin of the School of Oriental and African Studies* 51/2, pp. 258-70.

Busse, Heribert 1969. *Chalif und Grosskoenig. Die Buyiden im Iraq (945-1055)*. Wiesbaden: Franz Steiner.

Calmard, Jean 2019. "Le voyage de Louise de la Marnierre en Iran (1836-1837): Introduction, récit, notes," *Studia Iranica* 48/2, pp. 235-97.

CARE 1961. *Resume of Current or Recently Completed Technical Assistance Programs Of Private American Agencies In Iran prepared for Study Group on Technical Assistance Iran of the American Council of Voluntary Agencies for Foreign Service February 1, 1961 prepared by The American Council in cooperation with the Program Research Department of CARE, the Cooperative for American Relief Everywhere*. n.p.

Carr, Dr. D.W. 1900. "What medical missions are doing in Persia," *Mercy and Truth: A Record of C.M.S. Medical Mission Work*, Volume 4, pp. 137-42.

Cash, W. Wilson. *Persia Old and New*. London: CMS.

Chaqueri, C. ed. 1978. *The Condition of the Working Class*. Florence: Mazdak.

Chaqueri, Cosroe 1995. *The Soviet Socialist Republic of Iran, 1920-1921*. Pittsburgh: Univ. Pittsburgh Press

Chardin, Jean. 1811. *Voyages*, ed. L. Langlès, 10 vols. Paris.

Clarke, H.T. 1837. "Sketches on the State of Medical Knowledge in Persia," *London Medical and Surgical Journal* 2, pp. 707-10.

Coan, Frederick G. 1939. *Yesterdays in Persia and Kurdistan*. Claremont.

Cochran, James P. 1899. "Treatment of the Sick and Insane in Persia," *The American Journal of Insanity* 56, pp.105-07.

Collins, Edward Treacher. 1896. *In the Kingdom of the Shah*. London: T. F. Unwin.

Collins, Henry. 1925. W. *From Pigeon Post to Wireless*. London: Hodden and Stoughton.

Coloru, Omar 2017. "Ancient Persia and silent disability," in Chr. Laes ed., *Disability in Antiquity*, London and New York, Routledge, pp. 61-74.

Conrad, Lawrence I.; Neve, Michael; Nutton, Vivian; Porter, Roy; and Wear, Andrew, 1995. *The Western Medical Tradition 800 BC to AD 1800*. Cambridge: CUP.

Cook, Joseph Wright 1932. "In the Heart of Kurdistan," *The Princeton Alumni Weekly* vol. 32/20 (26 February), pp. 458-59.

Cursetjee, C.M. 2001. *A Voyage in the Gulf. The Land of the Date*. San Jose: Author Choice Press.

Curzon, G.N. 1892. *Persia and the Persian Question*. 2 vols. London.

Dailami, Pezhman. "Jangali Movement," iranicaonline.org

Daniel, Rabbi Mooshie G. 1901. *Modern Persia*. Toronto: The Carswell Co.

Daniel, T.M. 2006. "The History of Tuberculosis," *Respiratory Medicine* 2006 Nov;100 (11):1862-70.

DCR (Diplomatic and Consular Reports)

DCR no. 3189, "Trade of Kermanshah and District for the year 1903-04" by Consular Agent H.L. Rabino. London: HMSO, 1904.

DCR 3683, Report for the Year ended March 20, 1906 on the Trade of Kermanshah by Captain H. Cough" (London, 1906), pp. 3-19.

DCR no. 4828, Report from March 21, 1909 to March 20, 1911 on the Trade of the Persian Caspian Provinces by Mr. H.L. Rabino, pp. 1-34.

Dehgan, Ebrahim, 1329/1950, *Tarikh-e Arak*, 2 vols., Arak.

de Gobineau, A. 1923. *Trois Ans en Asie (de 1855 a 1858)* 2 vols. Paris, Bernard Grasset.

De Warzeé, Dorothy. 1913. *Peeps into Persia*. London.

Dickson, W. E. R. 1924, *East Persia. A Backwater of the Great War*. London: Edward Arnold & Co.

Dodge, Bayard 1958. *The American University of Beirut- A Brief History*. Beirut: Khayat.

Dols, M. 1987. "The Origins of the Islamic Hospital: Myth and Reality," *Bulletin of the History of Medicine* 61, 1987, pp. 367-90.

Donaldson, Dwight D. 1920. "On the Persian Border of Afghanistan," *The Missionary Review of the World*. June vol. 43, pp. 533-35.

Donaldson, Bess Allen 1972. *Prairie Girl in Iran and India*. Galesburg, Ill.

Dowlatabadi, Yahya 1336/1957. *Hayat-e Yahya*. 4 vols. Tehran: Mosavvar.

Du Mans, Raphael. 1890. *Estat de la Perse en 1660*. ed. Charles Schefer. Paris: E. Leroux.

Dunsterville, L.C. Maj.General 1920. *The Adventures of the Dunsterforce*. London: Edward Arnold.

Iran Almanac 1963, 1970. Tehran: Echo of Iran.

Eastwick, Edward B. 1976, *Journal of a Diplomat's Three Years' Residence in Persia*, 2 vols. in one, Tehran, Imperial Organization for Social Services.

Ebn Bazaz Ardabili 1373/1994. *Safvat al-Safa*. ed. Gholamreza Tabataba'i-Majd. Ardabil.

Ebrahim, Mohammad b. 1343/1964. *Seljuqiyan va Ghozz dar Kerman*. ed. Bastani Parizi. Tehran: Tahhuri.

Ebrahimnejad, Hormoz. "Introduction de la médecine européenne en Iran au XIXe siècle," *Sciences Sociales et Santé* 16/4 (décembre 1998), pp. 69-96.

Idem 2000, Theory and Practice in Nineteenth-Century Persian Medicine: Intellectual and Institutional Reforms," *History of Science* 38, pp. 171-78.

Idem 2002, "Religion and Medicine in Iran: from Relationship to Dissocation," *History of Science* 40, pp. 91-112.

Idem 2014. *Medicine in Iran. Profession, Practice, and Politics, 1800-1925.* New York: Palgrave-MacMillan.

Ehtesham al-Saltaneh 1366/1987. *Khaterat.* ed. Sayyed Mohammad Mehdi Musavi. Tehran: Zavvar.

Eilers, Wilhelm 1979. *Die Al, ein persisches Kindbettgespenst.* Munich: Bayerischen Akademie der Wissenschaften.

Ekhtiar, Maryam Dorreh 1994. *The Dar al-Funun: Educational Reform and Cultural Development in Qajar Iran.* unpublished thesis, New York University.

Elgood, Cyril 1951. *A Medical History of Persia and the Eastern Caliphate. The Development of Persian and Arabic Medical Sciences from the Earliest Times until the Year A.D. 1932.* Cambridge: CUP.

Encyclopedia Iranica 1989, "Bongah-e hemayat-e madaran o kudakan," iranicaonline.org.

Eshraqi, Firuz. 1383/2004. *Golpeygan dar a'ineh-ye tarikh.* Isfahan: Chahar Bagh.

E`temad al-Saltaneh (Sani` al-Dowleh), Mohammad Hasan Khan. 1345/1967. *Ruznameh-ye Khaterat.* ed. Iraj Afshar. Tehran: Amir Kabir.

___, 1294-97/1877-80. *Mer'at al-Boldan* 4 vols. Tehran: lithograph.

___, 1300/1883. *Montazam-e Naseri.* 3 vols. Tehran: lithograph.

___, 1301-03/1883-86. *Matla` al-Shams.* Tehran: lithograph.

___, 1306/1884. *Ketab al-Athar va'l-Ma'ather.* Tehran: lithograph.

Ettela`at 1329. *Ettela`at dar yek rob`-e qarn.* Tehran: Ettel`at.

Eyn al-Saltaneh, Qahraman Mirza Salur. 1376/1997. *Ruznameh-ye Khaterat.* 10 vols. eds. Mas`ud Salur and Iraj Afshar. Tehran: Asatir.

Ezz al-Mamalek, Amanollah Ardalan 1332/1953. *Avvalin Qiyam-e Moqaddas-e Melli dar jang-e beyn al-millali-ye avval.* Tehran: Ibn Sina.

Fakhra'i, Ebrahim 1353/1974, *Gilan dar jonbesh-e mashrutiyat.* Tehran: Franklin

Farahmandfar, Amir Qoli 1384. "Tolu`-e pezeshki-ye modern va ta'sis-e daneshkadeh dar Shiraz," in Sadeq Homayuni ed. *Yaran-e yekshanbeh.* Shiraz: Novid, pp. 117-28 (with the text of the agreement).

Fardyar, Mehrdad 1395/2016. "Tarikhcheh-ye mariz-khaneh-ye melli-ye Tabriz (1326-1333 Q)," *Faslnameh-ye Pezeshki* 8/26, pp. 192-224.

Farid al-Molk Hamadani, Mirza Mohammad `Ali Khan. 1345/1967. *Khaterat-e Farid* ed. Mas`ud Farid Qaragozlu. Tehran: Zavvar.

Fasa'i, Hajj Mirza Hasan Hoseyni. 1367/1988. *Farsnameh-ye Naseri.* 2 vols. ed. Mansur Rastegar Fasa'i. Tehran: Amir Kabir.

Feuvrier, Dr. 1900. *Trois Ans à la Cour de Perse.* Paris: F. Juven.

Firth, Stanley J. 1927. "Treatment of ringworm by thallium acetate," *The British Medical Journal* 18 July, p. 1097.

Floor, Willem 1999. *The Persian Textile Industry, Its Products and Their Use 1500-1925.* Paris: Harmattan.

Idem 2000, *The Economy of Safavid Persia.* Wiesbaden, Reichert.

Idem 2003. *Agriculture in Qajar Iran.* Washington DC, MAGE.

Idem 2004. *Public Health in Qajar Iran.* Washington DC, MAGE.

Idem 2006. *The Persian Gulf. A Political and Economic History.* Washington DC, MAGE.

Idem 2010. *The Rise and Fall of Bandar-e Lengeh. The Distribution Center for the Arabian Coast, 1750-1930.* Washington DC: MAGE.

Odem 2011. *Bandar Abbas, the natural gateway to southeast Iran.* (Washington DC: Mage

Idem 2012. "Hospitals in Safavid and Qajar Iran: an enquiry into their number, growth and importance," in Fabrizio Speziale ed. *Hospitals in Iran and India 1500-1950s.* Leiden: Brill, pp. 37-116.

Idem 2014. "A Neglected Aspect of the Social History of the Iranian Oil Industry: The Case of Southern Khuzestān's Early Medical Infrastructure." *Studia Iranica* 43/2, pp. 221-47.

Idem 2018 a. *Studies in the History of Medicine of Iran.* Washington DC: MAGE.

Idem 2018 b. *Kermanshah: City, Society and Trade.* Washington D.C.: MAGE.

Idem 2018 c. *Salar al-Dowleh. Delusional Prince and Wannabe Shah.* Washington D.C.: MAGE.

Idem 2020, *The Beginnings of Modern Medicine in Iran.* Washington D.C.: MAGE.

Idem, 'Korsi," iranicaonline. org.

Floor, Willem & Javadi, Hasan 2019. *Persian Pleasures. How Iranians Relaxed Through the Centuries. Food, Drink & Drugs.* Washington DC: MAGE

Forbes-Leith, F.A.C. 1927. *Checkmate: Fighting Tradition in Central Persia.* New York: Robert McBride.

Forsat-e Shirazi, Mohammad Naser. 1312/1894. *Athar-e `Ajam.* Bombay: lithograph.

Fraser, James Baillie 1826. *Travels and Adventures in The Persian Provinces on the Southern Banks of The Caspian Sea.* London: Longman.

Fryer, John. 1909-15. *A New Account of East India and Persia Being Nine Years' Travels, 1672-1681*, 3 vols. London: Hakluyt.

Funk, J. Arthur. 1920. "The Missionary Problem in Persia," *Muslim World* X, pp. 138-43.

Garrison, Fielding H. 1933. "Persian Medicine and Medicine in Persia," *Bulletin of the Institute of the History of Medicine. The Johns Hospkins University*, Vol. 1, No. 4 (May, 1933), pp. 129-153.

Gaube, H. - Wirth, E. 1978. *Der Bazar von Isfahan.* Wiesbaden: Reichert.

Ghani, Qasem. 1367/1988. *Yaddashtha-ye Doktor Qasem Ghani* 9 vols. ed. Sirus Ghani. Tehran: Zavvar.

Ghorban, Zabih 1989. *Medical Education in Shiraz, A Personal Memoir.* n.p.

Gilbar, Gad G. 1976. "Demographic Development in late Qajar Persia, 1870-1906," *Asian and African Studies* 11, pp. 125-56.

Gilmour, John 1924. *Rapport sur la situation sanitaire de la Perse.* Geneva, Société des Nations.

Gleadowe-Newcomen, A.H. 1904. *Report of a commercial mission to Persia.* Calcutta.

Good, Byron J. 1981. "The Transformation of Health Care in Modern Iranian History," in Michael E. Bonine and Nikki Keddie eds. *Modern Iran. The Dialectics of Continuity and Change.* Albany: State University of New York Press, pp. 59-82.

Idem 1945. *Geographical Handbook Series – Persia*. n.p.

Government of France 1914, *Rapports Commerciaux des agents diplomatiques et consulaires de France* – Année 1914 no. 1079 Perse. Paris.

Government of Great Britain 1914. Persia no. 1 (1914). *Further Correspondence respecting the Affairs of Persia*. London: HMSO.

Government of India 1906. *Statistics of British India, Part V. Public Health*. Calcutta.

Idem 1924. *Military Report on Persia* 4 vols. Simla, n.p. (vol. 4, part 2, Fars, Gulf Ports, Yazd and Laristan).

Government of Iran n.d., *Modhakerat-e Majles, Dowreh-ye Dovvom-e Taqniniyeh*. 3 vols. Tehran: Majles.

Idem 1317/1938. *Rahahan-e sarasar-e Iran*. Tehran: Vezarat-e Toruq.

Government of Iran, 1373/1994. *Ruznameh-ye Vaqaye`-ye Ettefaqiyeh*. 4 vols. Tehran.

Griffith, Dr. H. 1902 a."Kirman and the work there I," *Mercy and Truth: A Record of C.M.S. Medical Mission Work*, Volume 6, pp. 10-15.

Idem 1902 b, "Kirman and the work there II," *Mercy and Truth: A Record of C.M.S. Medical Mission Work*, Volume 6, pp. 48-52.

Griscom, Mary W. 1921. "A medical motor trip through Persia," *Asia. The American Magazine on the Orient* March, pp. 233-40.

Grothe, Hugo 1911. *Zur Natur und Wirtschaft von Vorderasien. I. Persien*. Halle: Gebauer-Schwetschke.

Guillaume, Paul 1992. *Vingt ans au service de la mission belge ... en Iran 1886-1967*. Bruxelles: Robert Le Marinel (unpublished typed manuscript).

Gurney, John and Nabavi, Negin 1993. "Dar al-Fonun," iranicaonline.org.

Hajbaghery. Adib M and M. Salsali. A model for empowerment of nursing in Iran. *BMC Health Serv Res*. 2005; 5(1):24. Published 2005 Mar 16. doi:10.1186/1472-6963-5-24.

Hakim al-Mamalek, `Ali Naqi b. Esma`il. 1356/1977. *Ruznameh-ye safar-e Khorasan*. Tehran: Farhang-e Iran-Zamin.

Hale F. 1920. *From Persian Uplands*. New York. E.P. Dutton & Comp

Hamadani, Ayatollah Saberi. 1382/2003. *Tarikh-e Mofassal-e Hamadan*. 3 vols. Qom: Shaker.

Hamadani, Rashid al-Din Fazlollah 2536/1977. *Vaqfnameh-ye Rab`-e Rashidi*. eds. Mojtaba Minovi and Iraj Afshar. Tehran: Anjoman-e Athar-e Melli.

Idem 1358/1979. *Savaneh al-Afkar-e Rashidi*. ed. Mohammad Taqi Daneshpazhuh. Tehran: Daneshgah.

Hamed, Mohammad Sadeq and Habibi, Manuchehr 1376/1997. *Tarikh-e San`at-e Barq dar Iran*. Tehran.

Hamideh Khanim, *Awake*. translated from Azeri by Hasan Javadi and Willem Floor with an Introduction and appendices. Washington D.C.: MAGE, 2016.

Hamilton, Alexander. 1930. *A New Account of the East Indies* 2 vols. London.

Häntzsche, J.C. 1869. "Specialstatistik von Persien," *Zeitschrift der Gesellschaft für Erdkunde zu Berlin*, pp. 429-49.

Hasanbegi, Mohammad Reza 1377/1998. *Tehran-e Qadim*. Tehran: Mansuri.

Hassendorfer, Colonel. 1954. "Les médecins militaries français fondateurs et organisateurs de l'Enseignement Médical et de la Santé Publique en Iran," *Histoire de la médicine* 4/7, pp. 57-63.

Hedayat, Mohammad. 1344/1965. *Khatarat va Khaterat*. Tehran: Zavvar.

Hedayat, Rezaqoli Khan 1338-39/1959-60. *Tarikh-e Rowzat al-Safa*. 10 vols. Tehran: Khayyam.

Hellot, Florence. 1996. "L'ambulance français d'Urmia (1917-1918) ou le ressac de la grande guerre en Perse," *Studia Iranica* 25, pp. 45-82.

___, 2002. "La première guerre mondiale à l'ouest de lac d'Urumiye," in Olivier Bast ed. *La Perse et la Grande Guerre*. Paris: Institut Français de Recherché en Iran.

Hemmati, Abouzardjomehr. n.d. *Die abenländische Medizin in Persien*. Unpublished dissertation University of Bonn.

Hoffmann, Birgitt 2000. *Waqf im Mongolischen Iran*. Stuttgart: Franz Steiner.

Hoffman, Rolla 1916. "A Medical Missionary's Journey to Persia in War Time," *The Cleveland Medical Journal*, vol. 15/1 (January), pp. 576-90.

Holmes, W.R. 1845. *Sketches on the Shores of the Caspian, Descriptive and Pictorial*. London: Richard Bentley.

Horden, Peregrine 2016. *Music as Medicine: The History of Music Therapy Since Antiquity*. London: Routledge.

Hume-Griffith, M.E. 1909. *Behind the Veil in Persia and Turkish Arabia*. Philadelphia, J.B. Lippincott.

Ibn Abu Usaybi`a -2020. *A Literary History of Medicine - The ʿUyūn al-anbāʾ fī ṭabaqāt al-aṭibbāʾ of Ibn Abī Uṣaybiʿah Online*. eds. and transl. E. Savage-Smith, S. Swain, G.J. van Gelder eds., Leiden: Brill, on-line edition.

Ibn Balkhi, 1915. *Description of the Province of Fars in Persia*. tr. Guy Le Strange. London: RAS.

Idem 1374/1995. *Farsnameh*. ed. Mansur Rastgar-Fasa'i. Shiraz: Bonyad-e Darsshenasi.

Ibn Nadim 1970. *The Fihrist of al-Nadim: A Tenth-Century Survey of Islamic Culture*, translated by Bayard Dodge, 2 vols. New York: Columbia University.

Ingram, John T. 1932. "Thallium acetate in the treatment of ringworm of the scalp," *The British Medical Journal* (2 January), pp. 8-10.

Iran Almanac 1963. Tehran: Echo of Iran.

Jaberi-Ansari, Hajj Mirza Hasan Khan. 1373/1994. *Tarikh-e Esfahan*. ed. Jamshid Mozaheri. Isfahan: Bahi.

Jackson, A.V. Williams. 1909. *Persia Past and Present*. New York.

James, Frank 1934, *Faraway Campaign. Experiences of an Indian Army Cavalry Officer in Persia and Russia*. London: Grayson & Grayson.

Janab, Mir Sayyed `Ali 1303/1924. *Kitab al-Isfahan*. Isfahan (litho).

Jarman, R. 1997. *Iran: political diaries, 1881-1965*, 14 vols. n.p. Archive Editions.

Jashemi, Sayyed Mohammad Reza Fazel 1389/2010. "Bimarestan va dar al-shafa' dar haram-e motahhar-e razavi dar a'ineh-ye tarikh," *Nashr-e elektronik-e sazman-e ketabkhnehha va muzehha va markaz-e asnad-e astan-e qods-e razavi*. Nos. 7-8, pp. 1-23.

Johna, Samir 2003. *Twenty-Five Years in Persia: The Memoirs of Mary Allen Whipple*. [Bloomington, IN] : 1st Books Library.

Jorjani, Esma`il 1380/2002. *Dhakhireh-ye Khvarazmshahi*. Moharreri MohammadReza ed. 3 vols. Tehran: Farhangestan-e `olum-e pezeshki.

Jozani, Niloufar 1994. *La Beauté Menacée*. Paris-Tehran: IFRI.

Kaempfer, Engelbert 2018. *Exotic Attractions in Persia: 1684-1688*. Washington DC: MAGE.

Kai Ka'us b. Iskandar 1951. *A Mirror for Princes, The Qabus Nama*. tr. Reuben Levy. New York: E.P. Dutton.

Karamati, Yunos and EIr 1999. "Faculties of the University of Tehran. v. Faculty of Medicine." Iranicaonline.org.

Kazembeyki, Mohammad Ali. 2003. *Society, Politics and Economics in Mazandaran, Iran, 1848-1914*. London: RoutledgeCurzon.

Kedourie, Elie ed.; Haim,Sylvia G.ed. 1980. *Towards a Modern Iran. Studies in Thought, Politics and Society*. London: Frank Cass.

Kermani, Naser a-Din Monshi-ye 1362/1983. *Simt al-`Ula li'l-Hizrat al-`Uliya*. Tehran: Asatir.

Khalifeh, Mojtaba and Najafzadeh, Ali 1390/2011. "Dar ol-Fonun-e Razavi, Ideh'i baraye moqabeleh ba fe`aliyatha-ye hey'at-e tabshiri Presbiterian dar Mashhad," *Motale`at-e Eslami, Tarikh va Farhang*, 43/87, pp. 9-25.

Khvami, Abu'l-Qasem Shehab al-Din Ahmad 1357/1978. *Monsha al-Ensha*. Tehran: Daneshgah-e Melli.

Khvandamir, Ghayath al-Din b.Homam al-Din, 1378/1999. *Makarem al-Akhlaq. Sharh-e Ahval va Zendegani-ye Amir `Ali Shir Nava'i*. ed. Mojammad Akbar `Asheq. Tehran: Ayeneh-ye Mirath.

Linton, J.H. et al. 1921. *Persian Pie. Stories and articles by people who have lived in Persia*. London: CMS.

Linton, J.H. 1923. *Persian Sketches*. London: CMS.

Litten, Wilhelm. 1925. *Persische Flitterwochen*. Berlin: Georg Stilke.

Loghatnameh-ye Dehkhoda.

Lorimer, J. G. 1970. *Gazetteer of the Persian Gulf* (Calcutta, 1915 [Gregg: Westmead, 1970]).

Lycklama à Nijeholt, T.M 1872–75. *Voyage en Russie, au Caucase et en Perse*. 4 vols. Paris-Amsterdam: Aethus Bertrand - C. L. van Langenhuysen.

Mahdavi, Shireen 2009, "Kofri, Mohammad Kermanshahi," iranicaonline.org.

Malcolm, Napier. 1905. *Five Years in a Persian* Town. London: John Murray.

Malcolm, Mrs. Napier. 1911. *Children of Persia*. Edinburgh: Oliphant, Anderson & Ferrier.

Malekzadeh, Elham 1392. *Mo'assesat-e Kheyriyeh-ye Refahi – Behdashti dar Dowreh-ye Reza Shah*. Tehran: Tarikh-e Iran

Idem 1394. *Seyr-e Takvin va Tatavvor-e Herfeh-ye Mama'i dar `Asr-e Qajar va Pahlavi*. Tehran: Pazhuheshgah-e `Olum-e Ensani.

Martin, François. 1990. *Mémoires de -, fondateur de Pondicherry*, 3 vols. ed. A. Martineau (Paris 1931-34), of which vol. 1 and part of vol. 2 have been translated into English by Aniruddha Ray as *François Martin Travels to Africa, Persia & India*. Calcutta.

McClintic, Eleanor Soukup 1917. "With the Russians in Persia," *American Journal of Nursing* vol. 18/1, pp. 34-40; vol. 18/2, pp. 102-06.

Melgunof, Greogorii Valerianiovich. 1868. *Das südliche Ufer des Kaspischen Meeres*. Leipzig: Leopold Voss.

Mercy and Truth: a record of CMS medical mission work. 1897-1921.

Miller, William McElwee. 1989. *My Persian Pilgrimage*. Pasadena: William Carey.

Moghtader, Réza. 1992. "Teheran dans ses murailles (1553-1930)," in Adle, Charyar et Hourcade, Bernard eds. *Téhéran Capitale bicentenaire*, Tehran-Paris: Institut Français de Recherche en Iran (Bibliotheque iranienne, vol. 37), pp. 39-49.

Mohtat, Mohammad Reza 1366/1987. *Sima-ye Arak - Jame`shenasi-ye shahri*. Tehran: Homa.

Momeni, Mostafa. 1976. *Malayer und sein Umland*. Marburg/Lain.

Monshi, Eskander Beg. 1350/1971. *Tarikh-e `Alamara-ye `Abbasi*. Iraj Afshar ed. 2 vols. Tehran, translated into English by R.M. Savory, 1978 as *History of Shah `Abbas the Great* 2 vols. Boulder.

Morton, Rosalie Slaughter. 1940. *A Doctor's Holiday in Iran*. New York: Funk & Wagnalls.

Mostafavi, Mohammad Taqi. 1343/1964. *Eqlim-e Pars*. Tehran: Anjoman-e Athar-e Melli.

Mostowfi, Abdollah 1343. *Sharh-e Zendegani-ye Man ya Tarikh-e Ejtema`i va Edari-ye Dowreh-ye Qajariyeh*. 3 vols. Tehran: Zavvar.

Mo'taman, `Ali 1348/1969. *Rahnama ya Tarikh va Towsif Darbar-e Velayatmadar-e Razavi*. Tehran.

Mo`tamedi, Mohsen. 1381/2002. *Joghrafiya-ye Tarikhi-ye Tehran*. Tehran: Daneshgahi.

Mo`tamed al-Vezareh, Rahmatollah Khan. 1379/2000 *Urumiyeh dar moharabeh-ye `alamsuz*. ed. Kaveh Bayat. Tehran.

Muirhead. A. L. 1913. *Western Medical Review*, XVIII. Omaha: Nebraska.

Mustawfi, Abdullah 1919. *The Geographical Part of the Nuzhat al-Qulub*. tr. Guy Le Strange. Leyde: Brill.

Nafisi, Sa`id. 1325/1946. "Doktor `Ali Akbar Nafisi Nazem al-Atebba," *Yadgar* 3/4, pp. 52-65.

___, 1329-31/1950-52. "Tarikh-e bimarestanha-ye Iran," *Majalleh-ye shir va Khorshid-e sorkh-e Iran* 3/9-10, pp. 12-23.

Najmabadi, Mahmud 1353/1974. *Tarikh-e tebb dar Iran pas az Eslam*. Tehran: Daneshgah.

Idem 1354/1975, "Tebb-e Dar al-fonun va kotub-e darsi-ye an," in Qodratollah Rowshani Za`faranlu ed., *Amir Kabir va Dar al-Fonun*. Tehran, pp. 202-37.

Idem 1364/1985. *A Bibliography of Printed Books in Persian on Medicine and Allied Subjects*. Tehran.

Nakhjevani, Mohammad b. Hendushah. 1964. *Dastur al-katib fi ta'yin al-maratib* 2 vols. in 3 parts. A.A. Ali-zadeh ed. Moscow: Nauka.

Nasiri, Mirza Naqi 2008. *Titles & Emoluments in Safavid Iran.* translated and annotated by Willem Floor. Washington DC: Mage.

Nasiri, Mohammad Ebrahim b. Zeyn al-`Abedin, 1373/1994, *Dastur-e shahriyar*, Mohammad Nader Nasiri Moqaddam, ed., Tehran.

Idem, 2016. *La Révolution constitutionnelle a Tabriz a travers les Archives diplomatiques françaises (1906-1909)*. Strassburg: Connaissances et Savoirs.

Nasrabadi, Mirza Mohammad Taher. 1361/1982. *Takhkereh-ye Nasrabadi*. ed. Vahid Dastgerdi. Tehran.

Neligan, A.R. 1926. "Public Health in Persia. 1914-24," *The Lancet* Part I; Part II-March 27, pp. 690-94; Part III-April 3, pp. 742-44.

Nezam al-Saltaneh 1361. *Khaterat va asnad-e Hoseyn Qoli Khan Nezam al-Saltaneh Mafi*. 2 vols. ed. Mansureh Nezam Mafi, Sirus Sa`dvandiyan and Hamid Rampisheh. Tehran: Nashr-e Now.

al-Nezami al-Aruzi al-Samarqandi, Ahmad b. `Omar b. `Ali 1927., *Ketab-e Chahar Maqalat*. Ed. Mohammad b. Abdol-Vahhab Qazvini. Berlin: Iranschär

Nura'i, Morteza 1385/2006. *Asnad-e Kargodhari-ye Bushehr*. Tehran: Mo'asseseh-ye Motale`at-e Tarikh-e Mo`aser-e Iran.

Overseas Consultants, Inc. 1949. *Report on the Seven Year Development Plan for the Plan Organization of the Imperial Government of Iran.* 5 vols. New York.

Paidar, Parvin 1995. *Women and the Political Process in twenty-century Iran.* Cambridge: CUP.

Persits, M.A.1996. *Zastenchivaia Interventsia.* Moscow: AIRO-XX.

Piemontese, Angelo Michele, "The Statutes of the Qājār Orders of Knighthood," *East and West* 19/3-4, 1969, pp. 431-73.

Idem 1984. "Gli Ufficiali Italiani al servizio della Persia nel XIX secolo," in: G. Borsa and Brocchieri P. Beonio. *Garibaldi, Mazzini et il Risorgimento nel Risveglio dell'Asia e dell'Africa*. Milan: Francio Angeli, 1984, pp. 65-130.

Pigulevskaya N. 1963. *Les Villes de l'Etat Iranien aux epoques Parthe et Sassanide.* La Haye-Paris: Mouton.

Polak, J. E. 1852. "Briefe aus Persien," *Wiener medizinische Wochenschrift* vol. 2, pp. 742-43, 789-90.

Idem 1853. "Briefe aus Persien," *Wiener medizinische Wochenschrift.* vol. 3, pp. 219-21, 509-10.

Idem 1854. "Briefe aus Persien," *Wiener medizinische Wochenschrift.* vol. 4, pp. 59-60, 396-97.

Idem 1855. "Briefe aus Persien," *Wiener medizinische Wochenschrift.* vol. 5, pp. 269-70.

Idem 1859 a. "Briefe aus Persien," *Wiener medizinische Wochenschrift.* vol. 9, p. 765.

Idem 1859 b. "Medicinische Briefe aus Persien (17/11/1858)," *Zeitschrift der k.k. Gesellschaft der Aerzte zu Wien* vol. 15, pp. 138-40.

Idem 1860, "Ueber 158 Stein-Operationen ausgefuehrt in Persien," *Zeitschrift der K.K. Gesellschaft der Aertze zu Wien*, vol. 15, pp. 694-99.

Idem 1862. "Die medizinische Schule und Spitäler in Teheran," *Zeitschrift der k.k. Gesellschaft der Aerzte zu Wien* vol. 12, pp. 235-36, 249-51.

Idem 1863. "Lepra in Persien," *Virchows Archiv für pathologische Anatomie und Physiologie* 27, pp. 175-80.

Idem 1865. *Persien, das Land und seine Bewohner*, 2 vols. Leipzig.

Political Diaries = *Political Diaries of the Persian Gulf* 1904-1947, 17 vols. n.p. Archive Editions, 1990.

Presbyterian Church 1876, The Thirty-Ninth Annual Report of the Board of Foreign Missions. New York.

Presbyterian Church 1877. The Fortieth Annual Report of the Board of Foreign Missions. New York.

Presbyterian Church 1883, The Forty-Sixth Annual Report of the Board of Foreign Missions. New York.

Presbyterian Church 1884, The Forty-Seventh Annual Report of the Board of Foreign Missions. New York.

Presbyterian Church 1886, The Forty-Ninth Annual Report of the Board of Foreign Missions. New York.

Presbyterian Church 1887, Seventeenth Annual Report of Board of Home Missions. New York.

Presbyterian Church 1888. Eighteenth Annual Report of Board of Home Missions. New York.

Presbyterian Church 1889, Nineteenth Annual Report of Board of Home Missions. New York.

Presbyterian Church 1890. Twentieth Annual Report of Board of Home Missions. New York.

Presbyterian Church 1891. Twenty-First Annual Report of Board of Home Missions. New York.

Presbyterian Church 1892. Twenty-Second Annual Report of Board of Home Missions. New York.

Presbyterian Church 1893. Twenty-Third Annual Report of Board of Home Missions. New York.

Presbyterian Church 1894, Twenty-Fourth Annual Report of Board of Home Missions. New York.

Presbyterian Church 1895. Twenty-Fifth Annual Report of Board of Home Missions. New York.

Presbyterian Church 1896. Ninety Fourth Annual Report. Board of Home Missions. New York.

Presbyterian Church 1897. Ninety Fifth Annual Report. Board of Home Missions. New York.

Presbyterian Church 1898. Ninety Sixth Annual Report. Board of Home Missions. New York.

Presbyterian Church 1899. Ninety Seventh Annual Report. Board of Home Missions. New York.

Presbyterian Church 1901. Ninety Ninth Annual Report. Board of Home Missions. New York.

Presbyterian Church 1902. One Hundred and First Annual Report. Board of Home Missions. New York.

Presbyterian Church 1904. *Hundred and Second Annual Report of the Board of Home Missions of the Presbyterian Church in the U.S.A.* New York.

Presbyterian Church 1905. One Hundred and Third Annual Report. Board of Home Missions. New York.

Presbyterian Church 1906. One Hundred and Fourth Annual Report. Board of Home Missions. New York.

Presbyterian Church 1907. One Hundred and Fifth Annual Report. Board of Home Missions. New York.

Presbyterian Church 1908. *Reports of the Missionary and Benevolent Boards and Committees to the General Assembly of the Presbyterian Church in the USA.* New York.

Presbyterian Church 1909. One Hundred and Seventh Annual Report. Board of Home Missions. New York.

Presbyterian Church 1910. One Hundred and Eighth Annual Report. Board of Home Missions. New York.

Presbyterian Church 1911. One Hundred Ninth Annual Report. Board of Home Missions. New York.

Presbyterian Church 1912. One Hundred Tenth Annual Report. Board of Home Missions. New York.

Presbyterian Church 1913. One Hundred Eleventh Annual Report. Board of Home Missions. New York.

Presbyterian Church 1914. One Hundred Twelfth Annual Report. Board of Home Missions. New York.

Presbyterian Church 1915. *One Hundred Thirteenth Annual Report of the Board of Home Mission*s, Reports of the Missionary and Benevolent Boards and Committees to the General Assembly.

Presbyterian Church 1919. *One Hundred Seventeenth Annual Report of the Home Missions of the Presbyterian Church of the U.S.A.*

Presbyterian Church 1919-20. *Annual Report, By Presbyterian Church in the U.S.A. Board of Foreign Missions*, Volumes 82-83, 1919-20, p. 265-266.

Presbyterian Church 1920. One Hundred Eighteenth Annual Report. Board of Home Missions. New York.

Presbyterian Church 1920. *The Eighty-third Annual Report of the Board of Foreign Missions of the Presbyterian Church in the U.S.A.*, 1920.

Presbyterian Church 1921. *The Eighty-fourth Annual Report of the Board of Foreign Missions of the Presbyterian Church in the U.S.A.*

Presbyterian Church 1922 a. *The Eighty-fifth Annual Report of the Board of Foreign Missions of the Presbyterian Church in the U.S.A.*, 1922.

Presbyterian Church 1922 b. *The Presbyterian Hospital Bulletin.* Chicago, Ill. January 1922, no. 48.

Presbyterian Church 1928 a. Annual Meeting Actions of the East Persia Mission of the Presbyterian Church in the USA. Daulatabad, August 1-10, 1928.

Presbyterian Church 1928 b. Minutes to the General Assembly of Presbyterian Church in the USA, Third Series-Volume VIII-1928, Part II. Philadelphia, July.

Presbyterian Church 1930. *Seventh Annual Report of the Board of National Missions of the Presbyterian Church in the USA.* New York.

Presbyterian Church 1932. Minutes to the General Assembly of Presbyterian Church in the USA, Third Series-Volume XI-1932, Part II. Philadelphia, July.

Rahnama-ye Daneshkadeh-ye pezeshki, daru-sazi, dandan-pezeshki. 1333/1954. Tehran: Daneshgah.

Prioreschi, Plinio 2004. *A History of Medicine.* vol. IV. *Byzantine and Islamic Medicine.* Omaha: Horatius Press.

Qazvini, Zeyn al-Din b. Hamdollah Mostowfi-ye 1372/1993. *Dheyl-e Tarikh-e Gozideh.* ed. Iraj Afshar. Tehran: Bonyad-e Mowqufat-e Mahmud Afshar.

Qodsi, Hasan A`zam 1342/1963. *Ketab-e Khaterat-e Man.* 2 vols. Tehran.

Rabino, H.L. 1928. *Mazandaran and Astarabad.* London: Luzac.

Rahnama-ye Daneshkadeh-ye pezeshki, daru-sazi, dandan-pezeshki. 1333/1954. Tehran: Daneshgah.

Rasooli, Jay M. and Allen, Cady H. 1958. *The Life Story of Dr. Sa`eed of Iran* (Grand Rapids: Grand Rapids International Publications.

Rastegar Dr. 1312/1933. "Hefz al-Sehheh-ye `Omumi-ye Atfal," *Salnameh-ye Pars*, part 2, pp. 80-96.

Red Cross 1922. *History of American Red Cross Nursing. American National Red Cross. Nursing Service.*

Report 1920-21 = Government of India, 1987. *The Persian Gulf Trade Reports 1905-1940 – Bushire,* 2 vols. Gerrards Cross: Archive Editions.

Rezai, Omid 2012. "Des particuliers au service du people. Le rôle des *vaqf*s dans la foundation d'hôpitaux en Iran au début di XXe siecle," in Fabrizio Speziale ed. *Hospitals in Iran and India, 1500-1950s.* Leiden: Brill.

Rice, Clara. 1916. *Mary Bird in Persia.* London: CMS.

___, 1923. *Persian Women and Their Ways.* London: Seeley, Service & Co.

Richard, Francis ed. 1995. *Raphael du Mans, missionnaire en Perse au XVIIè s.* 2 vols. Paris.

Richter, Julius. 1910. *A History of Protestant Missions in the Near East.* Edinburgh-London: Oliphant, Anderson & Ferrier.

Rubin, Michael Allen. 1999. *The Formation of Modern Iran, 1858-1909: Communication, Telegraph and Society.* Yale University, unpublished thesis.

Rühling, R. 1934. *Quer durch Persien.* Hamburg: Advent Verlag.

Rusta'i, Mohsen 1382. *Tarikh-e Tebb va Tebabat dar Iran,* 2 vols. Tehran: Asnad-e Melli.

Ruznameh-ye Anjoman-e Tabriz 1374/1995. 2 vols. Tehran: Ketabkhaneh-ye Melli.

Ruznameh-ye Dowlat-e `Aliyeh-ye Iran 1370-72/1991-93. 2 vols. Tehran: Ketabkhaneh-ye Melli (reprint).

Ruznameh-ye Iran 1374-78/1995-99. 5 vols. Tehran: Ketabkhaneh-ye Melli.

Ruznameh-e ye Soltani va Iran 1380/2001. Tehran: Ketabkhaneh-ye Melli.

Sadeq, Isa 1340/1961. *Yadegar-e `Omr*. 3 vols. Tehran: Amir Kabir.

Sadid al-Saltaneh Kebabi, Mohammad `Ali 1342/1963, *Bandar `Abbas va Khalij-e Fars*. Tehran: Amir Kabir.

Idem 1371/1992. *Sarzaminha-ye shomali-ye peyramun-e khalij-e Fars va darya-ye `Oman dar sad sal-e pish 1324-1332 h.q.* ed. Ahmad Eqtedari. Tehran: Jahan-e Mo`aser.

Sa`dvandiyan, Sirus and Ettehadiyeh (Nezam-Mafi), Mansureh. 1368/1989. *Amar-e Dar al-Khelafeh*. Tehran: Nashr-e Tarikh.

Safari, Baba. *Ardabil dar Godhargah-e Tarikh* 3 vols. (Tehran, 1350-62/1971-83).

Sajjadi, Sadegh 1989. "Bimarestan," iranicaonline.org.

Idem 1994. "Dentistry," iranicaonline.org.

Salnameh-ye Pars 1308/1929. Tehran.

Sani` al-Dowleh, Mohammad Hasan Khan 1295-97/1878-81. *Mer'at al-Boldan*. 4 vols. Tehran (lithograph).

Idem 1296/1879. *Ketab al-Ma'ather va'l-Athar*. Tehran (lithograph).

Idem 1300/1883. *Montazam-e Naseri*. 3 vols. Tehran (lithograph).

Savage-Smith, Emilie 2020. "The Practice of Medicine as Seen through the 'Uyūn al-anbā'," in Ibn Abu Usaybi`a -2020, ch. 8 (of the Commentary).

Saxild, Jørgen 1971. *En dansk Ingeniørs Erindringer*. København: Lindhardt og Ringhof.

Sayyah, Hajj. 1347/1968. *Khaterat-e Hajj Sayyah ya Dowreh-ye Khowf va Vahshat* ed. Hamid Sayyah. Tehran: Ebn Sina.

Schlimmer, Joh. L. 1970. *Terminologie Medico-Pharmaceutique*. Tehran: Daneshgah.

Schmidel, Justus. n.d. [1926] *Durch Russland und Persien*. Berlin: Deutscher Wille.

Schwarz, Paul 1993. *Iran im Mittelalter nach den Arabischen Geographen*. 9 vols. in 4. Frankfurt: Inst. f. History of Arabic-Islamic Science.

Sepehr, `Abdol-Hoseyn 1368/1889. *Mer'at al-Vaqaye`-ye Mozaffari va Yaddashtha-ye Malek al-Mo'arrekhin* ed. `Abdol-Hoseyn Nava'i. Tehran: Zarrin.

Sepehr, Mohammad Taqi Lesan al-Molk. 1377/1998. *Nasokh al-Tavarikh* ed. Jamshid Kayanfar 3 vols. Tehran: Asatir.

Serena, C. 1883. *Hommes et Choses en Perse*. Paris: G. Charpentier.

Setudeh, Manuchehr ed. 1366/1987. *Az Astara ta Astarabad* 10 vols. Tehran: Anjoman-e Athar va Mafakher-e Farhang.

Setzler, Lorraine. 1941. "In Iran: The development of a nursing school in Shiraz," *The American Journal of Nursing* 41/5, pp. 520-25.

Shahidi, Hamideh 1388/2009. "Negahi beh Tebb-e Sonnati dar Dar al-Shafa-ye Astaneh-e Qods-e Razavi dar `Asr-e Safavi (Barrasi-ye Haft Ruz az Asnad-e Ruznamehcheh-ye Dar al-Shafa)," *Ganjineh-ye Asnad* 19/3, pp. 63-84.

Shahni, Danesh `Abbasi. 1374/1995. *Tarikh-e Masjed-e Soleyman*. Tehran: Hirmand.

Shahri, Ja`far 1368/1989. *Tarikh-e ejtema`i -Tehran dar qarn-e sizdahom*, 6 vols. Tehran: Farhang-Rasa.

Shedd, Mary Lewis. 1922. *The Measure of a Man*. New York: George H. Doran.

Shepherd, William Ashton, 1857, *From Bombay to Bushire and Bussora: Including an Account of the Present State of Persia and Notes on the Persian War*. London, Bentley.

Shushtari, Mir `Abdol-Latif Khan. 1363/1984. *Tohfat al-`Alam va Dheyl al-Tohfat*. ed. Samad Movvahed. Tehran: Tahhuri.

Skrine, Clarmont 1962. *World War in Iran*. London: Constable & Company.

Slaby, Helmut 1982. *Bindenschild und Sonnenlöwe. Die Geschichte der österreichisch-iranischen Beziehungen bis zur Gegenwart*. Graz: Akademische Druck u. Verlagsanstalt.

Shteglova, O.P. 1975. *Katalog litografirovannykh Knig na persidskom yazyke v sobranii LO IV AN SSSR*. 2 vols. Moscow: Nauka.

Soltani, Mohammad `Ali 1370/1991. *Joghrafiya-ye Tarikhi va Tarikh-e Mofassal-e Kermanshahan*. 3 vols. Tehran.

Speer, Robert E. 1911. *Hakim Sahib, the foreign doctor; a biography of Joseph Plumb Cochran*. New York: Revell.

___, 1920. "Persia," in *Foreign Missions Yearbook of North America 1920*. ed. Roderick Beach. New York: Foreign Missions Conference.

Speer, Robert E. and Carter, Russell. 1922. *Report on India and Persia*. New York: Board of Foreign Missions.

Stead, Blanche Wilson 1907. "Four months in Kermanshah," *Women's Work*, vol. 22, p. 234.

Stead, F.M. 1908. "From Hamadan, Persia," *The Westminster*, vol. 33, 11 January, p. 18.

Stead, Rev. and Mrs. J.M. 1906. "A Medico-Evangelistic Trip in Persia," *Presbyterian Banner*. vol. 93 (18 October), pp. 13-14.

Stileman, Rev. Charles Harvey. 1902. *The Subjects of the Shah*. London: CMS.

St. Joseph, Ange de. 1985. *Souvenir de la Perse safavide et autres lieux de l'Orient (1664-1678)*, translated and annotated by Michel Bastiaensen. Brussels.

Stuart, Emmeline M. n.d. *Doctors in Persia*. London: CMS.

Stuart, Dr. Emmeline 1902. "Preaching and healing among women," (December 1901). *Mercy and Truth: A Record of C.M.S. Medical Mission Work* 6, pp. 115-18.

Idem 1906. "The Women's Hospital in Isfahan," *Mercy and Truth: A Record of C.M.S. Medical Mission Work* 10, pp. 368-70.

Swain, Simon 2020. "The Greek Chapters and Galen," in Ibn Abu Usaybi`a -2020, ch. 7 (of the Commentary).

Tchalenko, John, 2006, *Images from the Endgame. Persia through a Russian Lens 1901-1914*. London.

Sureshjani, Salem Hoseynzadeh 1395/2006. *Tarikh-e Dar al-Shafa-ye Astan-e Qods-e Razavi az dowreh-ye Safavi ta Payan-e dowreh-ye Qajariyeh*. Tehran: Daneshgah-e Azad-e Eslami.

Sykes, Major P. Molesworth, 1905, "Report on the Trade of Khorassan for the Year 1904-05". *Diplomatic and Consular Report no. 3499 Annual Series*. London, HMSO.

Tabataba'i, Modarresi Hoseyn. 2535/1977. *Torbat-e Pakan*. 2 vols. Qom.

Ta`eb, Hasan 1384/2005. *Bimarestanha-ye Rasht az mashruteh ta 1357*. Rasht: Iliya.

Tajbakhsh, Ḥasan, 1379/2000, *Tarikh-e bimarestanha-ye Iran*. Tehran, Pazhuheshgah-e 'olum-e ensani va motale'at-e farhangi.

Tamaddon, Mohammad. 1350/1971. *Owza`-ye Iran dar jang-e avval ya tarikh-e Rezayeh*. Tehran.

al-Tanukhi,al-Muhassin b.`Ali b.Mohammad b.Dawud 1922. *The Table-Talk of a Mesopotamian Judge*. Tr. D.S.Margiolouth. London: Royal Asiatic Society.

Tarbiyat 1377/1998. 3 vols. Tehran, Ketabkhaneh-ye Melli.

Tavassoli, Mahmoud - Naser, Bonyadi, 1371/1992, *Urban Space Design*. Tehran.

Tavernier, Jean-Baptiste, 1930, *Voyages en Perse et description de ce Royaume*. Paris, Éditions du Carrefour.

Tavili, `Aziz. 1371/1992. *Tarikh-e jame`-ye Bandar-e Enzeli* 2 vols. Rasht.

Teixeira Pedro 1991. *The Travels of Pedro Teixeira with his "Kings of Harmuz"*. Nendeln - Liechtenstein: Kraus Reprint.

Teymuri, Ebrahim. 1363/1984. *`Asr-e Bikhabari*. Tehran.

The Michigan Alumnus, 39 (September 1933).

Trade Report = *The Persian Gulf Trade Reports 1905-1940. Bushire*, 2 vols., Gerrards Cross, Archive Editions, 1987.

Ullman, Manfred 1970. *Die Medizin im Islam*. Leiden: Brill.

UNESCO 1963. *Iran-Shahr: a survey of Iran's land, people, culture, government and economy*. 2 vols. Tehran: University.

US Army 1963. *Area Handbook for Iran*, Washington DC.

US Army Medical Service 1976. *Preventive Medicine in World War II*, Washington DC: Office of the Surgeon General, Department of the Army, GPO.

US Government 1956. *United States Operations in Iran, Hearings of the Subcommittee on Government Operations pf the House of Representatives*. Washington DC: GPO.

Ussher, John 1865. *A Journey from London to Persepolis*. London: Hurst and Blackett.

Vaqaye`-ye Ettefaqiyeh 1373-74/1994-95. 4 vols. Tehran: Ketabkhaneh- Melli.

Varjavand, Parviz. 1377/1998. *Sima-ye Tarikh va Farhang-e Qazvin*. 3 vols. Tehran: Ney.

Vaume, Dr. 1866. "La lèpre dans le Kurdistan Persan," *Bulletin de la Société d'Anthropologie de Lyon* 5, pp. 158-62.

Vessal K, Rad. S., Alizadeh A., Jalal-Shokouhi, J. 2014. "Development of Radiology in Iran," in Azizi ed. 2014, pp. 157-64.

Warne, William E. 1956. *Mission For Peace. Point 4 in Iran*. Indianapolis/New York: Bobbs-Merrill.

Wassaf 2010-17. *Geschichte Wassaf's Persisch herausgegeben und Deutsch übersetzt von Hammer-Purgstall*. New ed. Sybille Wentker. 3 vols. Vienna: OAW.

Watelin, Louis-Charles 1921. *La Perse Immobile*. Paris: Chapelot.

Waterfield, Robin E. 1973. *Christians in Persia - Assyrians, Armenians, Roman Catholics and Protestants*. London: George Allen & Unwin.

Wells, R. P. 1878, *A Year in Persia. A discourse in memory of Mrs. Hattie Lyman Stocking*. Holeyoke, Mass.: Transcript Steam Book and Job Printing House.

Werner, Christoph. 2000. *An Iranian Town in Transition*. Wiesbaden: Harrassowitz.

Williams, Molly 1994. *The Rich Persian Tapestry of My Persian Years*. Bendigo: Keith Cole.

Williamson, J.W. 1927. *In A Persian Oil Field. A Study in Scientific and Industrial Development*. London: Ernest Benn.

Wills, C. J. 1893. *In the Land of the Lion and the Sun*. London: Ward, Lock & Bowden, 1893.

Wilson, Arnold T. 1932. *Persia*. London: Ernest Benn.

Idem 1941. S.W.Persia. *Letters and Diary of a Young Political Officer 1907-1914*. Oxford: OUP.

Wilson, S.G. 1895. *Persian Life and Customs*. New York: Fleming. H. Revell.

Idem 1896. *Persia: Western Mission*. Philadelphia: Presbyterian Board of Publication.

Wishard, John G. 1908. *Twenty Years in Persia*. New York: Fleming H. Revell.

Wolff, Joseph 1860-61. *Travels and Adventures of the Rev. Joseph Wolff*. London: Saunders, Otley and Co.

Wood, M. M. 1922. *Glimpses of Persia*. London: CMS.

Wright, Denis. 2001. *The English Amongst the Persians*. London: I.B. Tauris.

Yaghma'i, E. "Madraseh-ye Dar al-Fonun," *Yaghma* 23, 1349/1970-71, pp. 233-38, 361-66, and 423-26.

Yate, C.E. 1900. *Khurasan and Seistan*. London: Blackwood & Sons.

Year Book 1922- Royal Society of Tropical Medicine and Hygiene. London.

Zahereddini, Badri. 1966. *Medizinische Topographie der iranischen Stadt Malayer* Erlangen.

Zavie, Emile 1927. *D'Archangel au Golfe persique*. Paris.

Zabih Ghorban 1989. *Medical Education in Shiraz, A Personal Memoir*. N.p.

Zahir al-Dowleh 1351/1972. *Khaterat va Asnad-e Zahir al-Dowleh*. ed. Iraj Afshar. Tehran: Jibi.

Zarkub Shirazi, Abu'l-`Abbas Mo`in al-Din Ahmad b.Shehab al-Din Abu'l-Kheir 1350/1971. *Shiraz-nameh*. ed. Esma`il Va'ezjavadi. Tehran: Bonyad-e Farhang.

INDEX

A

Abbasak 144
Abdol-Hoseyn Mirza Farmanfarma 225
Abdol-Karim b. Abi Othman Nishapuri 14
Abdollah Khan Monajjami 155
Abu'l-Fazl Mirza Azod al-Soltan 357
Abu'l-Hasan Bajkam 10
Abu Sa`id Nishaburi 19
Ach-tacon 49
acute abdomens 389
adhan 24
Adl Hospital 401
adviyeh-khaneh 20
Afghanistan 460
afiyun 42
Agha Jari 121
Ahmadi 167
Ahmadiyyeh hospital 429
Ahram 162, 163, 167
Ahvaz 121
air-conditioning 170
air cooled 349
Ajari, assistant 341
Akbarbad 120
akhal 24
Alamdasht 290
Alam Hospital 141
alat 24
Alborz College 97
albucid 249
Alem al-Saltaneh 109
Ali Akbar Khan 65
Ali Aqa Nizkad 392
Ali Asghar Hekmat 408

Ali b. `Abbas Majusi Ahvazi 15
Ali b. `Isa 10
Ali b. Rabban al-Tabari 4
Ali Qoli Mirza 63
al-Mu`tadid bi-Allah 9
al-Muqtadir bi-Allah 10
al-Qati` 10
al-Razi 15
American-Iranian Relief Commission 319
American Red Cross 229, 254
American University Beirut 97
Amin al-Dowleh 82, 95
Amir Fakhr al-Din Abu Bakr 21
Amir Kabir 59
Amir Moqarreb al-Din Mas`ud 21
Amir Nezam Garrusi Mosque 253
Amru b. Leyth al-Saffar 11
amuzeshgah-e `ali-ye behdari 410
amuzeshgah-e pezeshkyari 410
anesthesia 101, 304, 306, 343, 347, 384
anjoman-e kheyriyeh 358, 395
Anjoman-e Ravabet-e Farhang-e Iran va Shuravi 302
Anushirvan Mirza 403
APOC xxi, 72, 77, 120, 121, 125, 127, 128, 152, 154, 242, 244, 348, 349, 352, 469
APRC 372, 373, 374, 375, 376, 378, 380
APRRF 161, 168
Aqa Sayyed `Ali Aqa Fumeni 358
Aqdasiyeh hospital 352
arbab-e estehqaq va vazayef 23
Ardabil 38, 381

Aristotle 16
Armenian committee, Rasht 372
Asadollah Alam 140
ash-e parhiz 43
ash-maqam 49
ashribah wa adviyah 13
askenadaukin 5
Assyrian refugees 181
Astarabad 38, 131
Astqiq Hosepian 96
asylum 160, 225
Atabeg Abu Bakr b. Sa`d 21
Atabeg Mozaffar al-Din 20
Atash-ye Sharq 320
atrafil 42
Atta Mohammad, sub-assistant surgeon 125
attar-khaneh 42
Augustinians 45
ayaraj 42
azab 43
Azodi hospital 13

B

badam 43
badgir 27
Baghdad 13, 19
Bagh-e Ettehadiyeh 399
Bagh-e Hakim Khanom 252
Bagherpur, Z. 246
Baha' al-Dowleh-ye Khvarezmi 19
Bahar 172
Bahjat al-Molk 205
Bahmani 160
Bahram Shah 20
Bakandeh 354
Bakhtiari 126
Baku 310, 362, 372, 373, 375, 378, 380
balini 43
Balkan frames 390
Balkh 9, 19
Baluchistan 460
Bam 20
Bampur 468
barber 63
Bardsir 20
Barmaki brothers 8
Baron Hagop 255, 363, 376
Basra 27, 47

Bastam 27
bathhouse 63
bavvab 24
Bawardah 120
bazar-e dar al-shafa 37
Bedouin Arabs 123
behbudestan-e Namazi 406
Behdari 253
Behdari Ostan 224
Behdari Shardari 224
Beirut 244, 273, 321, 407
Ben Esfahan 39
Berjand 468
beyt al-adviyeh 24, 27, 28
Bible Churchman's Missionary Society 468
bimaran-e motafarreqeh 43
bimaran-e sar-pa'i 43
bimardaran 41, 278
bimarestan 4, 27
bimarestan-e Ahmadiyeh 119
bimarestan-e Amir A`lam 113
bimarestan-e Amrika'i 252
bimarestan-e Aqa Sayyed `Ali Aqa 359
bimarestan-e baladiyeh 128
bimarestan-e baladiyeh no. 1 113
bimarestan-e baladiyeh no. 2 113
bimarestan-e doctor Rezanur 115
bimarestan-e dowlati 78, 107
bimarestan-e eslami 205
bimarestan-e Firuzabadi 116
bimarestan-e Hakim 115
bimarestan-e Ibn Sina 78
bimarestan-e Jahanshah Saleh 113
bimarestan-e masihi 252
bimarestan-e melli 358
bimarestan-e Mo`tamed 115
bimarestan-e mobarezeh 224
bimarestan-e Morsalin 405
bimarestan-e Najmiyeh 114
bimarestan-e Pahlavi 118
bimarestan-e Pur Sina-ye Rasht 396
bimarestan-e Rayy 10
bimarestan-e Razi 114
bimarestan-e Ruzbeh 113
bimarestan-e sehamiyeh 357
bimarestan-e Sheikh Hadi 114
bimarestan-e Sina 78
bimarestan-e Tutiya 115
bimarestan-e vagirdarha 295

Index 513

bimarestan-e Vaziri 109
bimarestan-e zahravi 401
bimarestan-e zanan 111
bimarestan-e Zarand 10
bimaresyan-e Farabi 113
bimar-khaneh 41
Bipp 377
blood transfusion xxix
bongah-e hemayat-e maderan va nowzadan 400
Borazjan 162, 166
Borujerd 272
botica 46
bread price 307
British Consulate hospital, Berjand 139
British Consulate hospital, Mashhad 297
British Consulate hospital, Zabol 465
British financial contribution 71
British Residency Dispensary 163
broadcast program 243
Brookline Church 384
Bukhtishu 7
Bun-e Bazar quarter 179
Burburud 274
Bushehr Civil Hospital 144
Bushehr Residency Dispensary and Charitable Hospital 145

C

Captain Bishop, IMS 125
Capt. Crossle, IMS 122
Capt. Taylor, IMS 467
Capt. Warren 374
CARE 409, 410
Carmelites 47
Caspian littoral 131
Caucasus 437
Ceasarian section 141
census 64
central heating 170
Central Midwives Board 220
Chasm-e Ali 353
children 219
China 26
chloroform 306
Choghadak 167
cholera xxi, xxii, xxiii, 82, 83, 84, 107, 109, 125, 134, 136, 170, 182, 208, 226, 232, 307, 308, 350, 351, 352, 358, 361, 373, 374, 413, 425, 432, 442, 458, 495
Church Missionary Society 198
clothes 51
clothes, listed 43
Cochran Memorial 440
Colton-Kirkwood-Whipple hospital 417
Colton Memorial hospital 415
comparative advantage 56, 94, 384
Coulonger, General 159
criminal suits 96
Cuzen, E.M., asst. surgeon 257
Czech physician 106

D

dabbaj 28
Dakin's solution 377
dallak 42
Damghan 39
darabi 52
dar al-`ajazeh 295
Dar al-Fonun 60, 63, 65, 204
dar al- hadith 23
dar al-majanin 119
dar al-marg 49
dar al-marza 6, 23
dar al-masakin 23
dar al-mosaferin 23
dar al-mowt 49
dar al-qoran 23
dar al-shafa 23
dar al-shafa triangle 17
dar al-shafa-ye `Abdollah `Amr 31
dar al-shafa-ye `Ali Shir 31
dar al-shafa-ye jadid-e Naseri-ye tupkhaneh 63
dar al-shafa-ye Malikat Agha 31
dar al-shafa-ye Sahebi 27
dar al-shafa-ye Shahrokh 31
dar al-shafa-ye Soltan Hoseyn 31
dar al-shorb 24
dar al-tabib 26
dar al-ziyafat 10, 23, 25
darban 15
Dar Dasht quarter 199
darmangah 142, 359
darmangah-e shomareh-ye yek 408
daru-khaneh 19, 24, 42
daru-saz 42

Dastak 165
dava-khanehha 64
davasaz 63
dayeh 15
DDT 393, 408
Deghan Yaghut 370
Dehli boils xxvi
Delam 162
dental surgery 121
Deycke Pasha 145
Dezful 123
diabetes 384
diarrhea xxvi
Diathermy 243
diba 28
Dick, K.S., assist. surgeon 125
Dick, K.S., asst. surgeon 352
Dietz lanterns 316
dig al-masakin 23
diphtheria xxvi, 79
diploma 113
disinfector 250
dispensary routine 340, 367
djinn 270
Dorquain 121
Dowlatabad 259
Dozdab 467
Dr. `Abdal`Ali Khan Aresta 253
Dr. `Abdollah Tabib 225
Dr. `Ali Khan Hamidi 138
Dr. `Ali Khan Shafa 395
Dr. `Ali Reza Bahrami 112
Dr. `Ataollah 162
Dr. `Isa `Ali 200
Dr. `Isa Qoli 205
Dr. A`lam al-Molk 428
Dr. Abbas Adham A`lam al-Molk 114
Dr. Abdollah Khan Vassei 474
Dr. Abu'l-Hasan Khan Bahrami 65
Dr. Abu'l-Qasem Bahrami 157
Dr. Abu'l-Qasem Khan Farbod 395
Dr. Abu Torab 119
Dr. Abu Turab 109
Dr. Adelaide Kibbe 317, 390
Dr. Adle 140
Dr. Ahmad Khan 253
Dr. Ahmad Khan Philosopher 222
Dr. Albo 63
Dr. Alexander 170, 176, 445
Dr. Alfred Cohn 190

Dr. Aliasgharzadeh 95, 100
Dr. Ali Khan 157
Dr. Ali Khan Shafa 366
Dr. Allah Khan Mo'ed 253
Dr. Amir A`lam 111
Dr. Amir Khan A`lam al-Mamalek 283
Dr. and Mrs. Schuler 357
Dr. Andreas 179, 190
Dr. Andreos Hovanissian 181
Dr. Aqa Khan Tub 395
Dr. Arezu 130
Dr. Aristu 118
Dr. Aristu Khan 222
Dr. Art Moradian 251
Dr. Art Muradian 194, 393
Dr. Ashraf 138
Dr. Ayob 84
Dr. Badvagan 398
Dr. Baker 79
Dr. Baruch 292
Dr. Basil 81
Dr. Basirian 168
Dr. Bastan 111
Dr. Becker 65
Dr. Bedrosian 84, 353
Dr. Blair 95, 474
Dr. Blanche Wilson 174, 182
Dr. Brinkman 95, 257, 365, 388
Dr. Bruneel 228
Dr. Burton Dyson 251
Dr. Bussdicker 236, 385
Dr. Capt. Bishop 352
Dr. Capt. Campbell 177
Dr. Capt. Sinton 300, 308
Dr. Carr 200, 205, 216, 272, 403, 459
Dr. Casolani 59
Dr. Charis Pigott 218
Dr. Clara H. Field 174
Dr. Cochran 319, 431, 440
Dr. Cochran Jr. 443, 468
Dr. Col. Belt 177
Dr. Collins 198
Dr. Cook 89, 91, 177, 187, 303
Dr. Davies 95
Dr. Dermes 112
Dr. Dias 352
Dr. Dodd 187, 416, 417
Dr. Dodson 207
Dr. D'Souza 129
Dr. Ebrahim Aghajan 253

Dr. Ebrahim Khan Tizabi 253
Dr. Ellis 441
Dr. Emma T. Müller 432
Dr. Emmeline Stuart 200, 404
Dr. Eshoo 423
Dr. E. T. Messe 405
Dr. Fakhr Pezeshkan 253
Dr. Faridun Varjavand 97, 100, 102
Dr. Fazal Haq 467
Dr. Fortescue 73
Dr. Frame 87, 255, 359
Dr. Frame Jr. 192
Dr. Frances Zoeckler 177, 251
Dr. Funk 83, 177, 190
Dr. Gertrude Westlake 210
Dr. Ghani 402
Dr. G. Ovanessian 407
Dr. Grant 430
Dr. Griffith 200, 206
Dr. Griscom 92
Dr. Hagop Kachaturiants 255
Dr. Hammerschlag 291
Dr. Hamzavi 96
Dr. Hargreaves 429
Dr. Hasan Khan Eftekhari 402
Dr. Hasan Zamani 216
Dr. Hoernle 198
Dr. Hoffman 90, 95, 304, 393, 402
Dr. Holmes 173, 411, 430
Dr. Hoseyn Khan Mo`tamed 115
Dr. Hudson 146
Dr. Ibrahim 247
Dr. Ilberg 65
Dr. Ironside 203
Dr. Isaac 432
Dr. Iskander Khan Mirzayoff 445
Dr. Islami 101
Dr. Jahanshah Saleh 112
Dr. J. Coleman 406
Dr. Jenny Crozier Stead 253
Dr. Jenny Stead 244
Dr. Jessie C. Wilson 173, 353
Dr. J. E. Sweeney 136
Dr. Kach 458
Dr. Kaikobad Hormisji Dumree 137
Dr. Karim Hedayat 406
Dr. Khachatur 177, 186
Dr. Kibbe-Frame 390
Dr. Kolnik 65
Dr. Lamme 415, 419, 426

Dr. Laura Müller 416
Dr. Lawrence 353, 357
Dr. Lesan al-Hokama 74
Dr. Lichtwardt 179
Dr. Lindley 87
Dr. Loew 65, 119
Dr. Lt. Col. Pyper 467
Dr. Lustig's serum 432
Dr. MacKay 136
Dr. Mahmud Mo`tamed 225
Dr. Marabelle 204
Dr. Martin 218, 406
Dr. Mary Allen 175
Dr. Mary Bradford 411, 421
Dr. Mary Griscom 91
Dr. Mary Price 216
Dr. Mary R. Fleming 416
Dr. Mary Smith 80, 82, 173
Dr. Mary Zoeckler 180, 186, 259
Dr. McDowell 88
Dr. McPherson 148
Dr. Mehdi Malekzadeh 110
Dr. Meyer 174
Dr. Milani Hospital 401
Dr. Mir 110
Dr. Mirza Ali Khan Irani 222
Dr. Mohammad A`zam Zanganeh 250
Dr. Mohammad Ali Khan Moayed Hikmat 136
Dr. Mohammad Ali Khan Tutiya 115
Dr. Mohammad Daftari 249
Dr. Mohammad Hesabi 110
Dr. Mohammad Kar 391
Dr. Mohammad Khan Ala'i 74
Dr. Mohammad Khan Faqihi 258
Dr. Mohammad Khan Kofri 65
Dr. Moir 125
Dr. Moloney 216
Dr. Moosa Khan 306
Dr. Morel 107
Dr. Morozoff 464
Dr. Mozayyan al-Soltan 205
Dr. Mrs Malcolm 206
Dr. Mrs. Stead 227
Dr. Ms Baillie 217
Dr. Ms Charis Pigott 217
Dr. Ms D. M. Howgate 218
Dr. Ms G. A. (Stella) Henriques 218, 406
Dr. Ms Hodgkinson 216
Dr. Ms K. Blackwood 218

Dr. Muller 66
Dr. Muniri 158
Dr. Murray 322
Dr. Musa Khan 74, 222
Dr. Musa Khan (Hakim A`lam) 115
Dr. Neligan 67, 72, 87
Dr. Niku 401
Dr. Niri 401
Dr. No-ee 317
Dr. Norem 102, 319
Dr. Nur al-Din Pezeshki 168
Dr. Nurollah Hakim-A`lam 321
Dr. Nurolllah Hakim-A`lam 393
Dr. Odling 81
Dr. Olkhus 442
Dr. Orcutt 413
Dr. Ost 226
drought 307
Dr. Packard 181, 190, 234, 440
Dr. Petros 90
Dr. Piggott 217
Dr. Polak 60, 62
Dr. Post 89, 92, 372
Dr. Rastan 275
Dr. Rezanur 116
Dr. R.H. Carpenter 218
Dr. Rice 193, 468
Dr. Roland 110
Dr. Rustam Sarfeh 244
Dr. Sa`id Malek Loqman al-Mamalek 112
Dr. Saeed Khan 91
Dr. Sayyed Mohammad Khan 395
Dr. Schlimmer 61
Dr. Schneider 419
Dr. Scott 68, 72, 87, 91
Dr. Sharp 405
Dr. Siadat 161
Dr. Sirus 401
Dr. Sitralka 468
Dr. Sohrab Barkhordar 223
Dr. Sterlini 360
Dr. Stewart 419
Dr. T. `Oyun 407
Dr. Tashchiyan 373, 395
Dr. Tashjiantz 361
Dr. Tholozan 83
Dr. Torfeh 469
Dr. Torrence 79
Dr. Urania Latham 460

Dr. Vahan 428
Dr. Vakili 224
Dr. Vanneman 411, 421
Dr. van Orden 430
Dr. Vartan 398
Dr. Vartan Oganessian 367
Dr. Vassei 95
Dr. Vaughn 405
Dr. Walstrom 193
Dr. Westlake 208
Dr. White 206, 458
Dr. Wild 218
Dr. Wilhelm 110
Dr. Wishard 82
Dr. Wolf 109
Dr. Woollatt 73
Dr. Wright 430
Dr. Yadollah Khan 395
Dr. Yahya Mirza Lesan ol-Hokama 111
Dr. Yohanan Sayaed 402
Dr. Young 348
Dr. Zabih Ghorban 406
Dr. Zahedi 466
Dr. Zeyn al-`Abedin Khan Loqman al-Mamalek 66
Dunsterforce 371
duran 11
dysentery xxvi, xxvii, 61, 62, 74, 124, 166, 225, 301, 374, 390, 392

E

E`tezad al-Saltaneh 63
Edessa 1
Egypt 26
Ehtesham al-Atteba 205
ejazeh 26
electricity 217, 238, 386
endowment, misuse of 49
English hospital. 77
Eno's fruit salts 158
Enzeli 373
Eqbal al-Saltaneh 64
erysipelas 95, 249, 272
Esfahanak 39
Eskandar Mirza 204
European trained doctors in Tabriz 425
evangelization 94, 459, 468
eye diseases 124, 135, 350

Index

F

fairy 270
falasafeh 42
faluniya 24
family wards 316
famine 92, 372
Farid al-Din `Attar 19
Farmanfarma 98
farrash 15, 24
Fath `Ali Shah 59
Favus 273
Fazl Elahi, hospital-assistant 123
Fazl Elahi, sub-assistant surgeon 125
fee-for service system 260
felchers 229
female physicians 100
Ferry hospital 83
Feylosuf al-Saltaneh Mirza `Abd al-Karim 107
field hospital 458
filles de charité 108
Firuzabad 14
Fiske Seminary 449
foluniya 42
food 43
food elevator 455
fracture cases 389
free hospital 263
Friends of Arabia Mission 188

G

Gach Qaragoli 121
Gach Saran 121
Ganaveh 121, 162
Garland, J. R. 170
gas gangrene 377
Gaz 131
German hospital, Urmiyeh 449
German nurses 291
German 'professors' 291
German roentgenologist 291
Ghazan Khan 23
Ghinaw 46
ghoraba 38
girls 219
gonorrhea 407
Gorgan 13
grant from government of India 151, 156, 163
Greek physician 360
Greenway, IMD 135
Griffiths, British chemist 82
Gudarz hospital 461

H

Haft Kel 353
Haji Sheikh Ahmed Galledary 135
Hajj `Ezz al-Molk 404
Hajj Dhu'l Faqr Khan Bayat Samsam al-Molk 197
Hajj Mahmud Khan Kermani 205
Hajj Mohammad Hasan Mirza Montaser al-Molk 294
Hajj Mohammad Hoseyn Namazi 405
Hajj Sayyah 107
Hajj Sheikh `Abdol-Karim 118
Hajj Sheykh Hadi Najmabadi 109
hakim 47
Hakim al-Dowleh 70
hakim-bashi 41
hakim-e kheyri 39
Hakim Oshanna Badal 432
Hakim Yar `Ali Tehrani 39
Halileh 167
hallaj 43
Hamadan 27, 170
Hargreaves, Henry E. 130
Harran 9
Harun al-Rashid 9
Hasan Zahir al-Dowleh 403
Health Department 161, 163, 168
Herat 31, 310
hernia operation 90
Heshmatiyeh hospital 402
Hikowe Boghasian 96
Hill, E.R., asst. surgeon 258
hojreh 26
Hormoz 45
Hoseyn Sohbati 246
hospice 2, 7, 10, 17, 21, 25, 26, 28, 31, 33, 37, 38, 39, 40, 41, 43, 45, 48, 51, 52, 276, 278, 279, 282, 284, 285, 294
Hospital, Borazjan 161
hospital, new 163
hot springs 46, 163
house for invalids 253
Howard Annex 435
howzkhaneh 27

hubbha 42

I

Ibn Abu Usaybi`ah 5
Ibn Mandavayh al-Isfahani 14
Ibn Sina 16
IETD xv, 157, 165, 209, 221, 405
Imperial Iranian Pharmaceutical Institute 250
India 26
Indian army hospital unit 102
Indian medicine 8
Indian Military Hospital 153
Indo-European Telegraph Department xv
infirmary, municipal 160
influenza xxv, 81, 125, 165, 170, 223, 232, 270, 308, 352, 377, 387
insulin 384
Iowa Synodical Society 314
Isa b. Maseh 11
Isfahan 14, 19, 20, 45, 198
Israel Karam 426
itinerating xxiv, 94, 175, 182, 255, 354, 360, 361, 370, 377, 413, 424

J

Jalayarids 28
Jamadar Mian Ghulam Ali, sub-asst. surgeon 467
Jangalis 362, 372, 374
jarrad 24
jarrah 42, 278
jarrahiyyun 13
javarshat 42
Jemadar Abdur Rahim IMD 137
Jewish xviii
Jiroft 20
Jolfa 200, 201
Jundishapur 1, 4, 7

K

Kababian quarter 176
kafil 43
kahhalan 13, 24
Kahn test 218
Kamal al-Din Abu'l-Ma`ali 28
Kamareh 274

Kampsax 469
Kandeh 272
Kangan 162
Kerman 20
khadameh-ye `owrat-e bimar 41
khadem 24
khadem-e bimaran 41
Khalili hospital 408
Khanom Sharifeh 311
Kharegat, Major IMS 464
Khark 167
khashkhash 42
khatam al-atibba 16
Khatoun, medical assistant 173
khazanehdar 15, 43
khazin 24
khazzan 13
Khisht 167
khoddam al-marza 26
Khormuj 162, 163
Khoshab 167
Khosrow Anushirvan I 1, 3
Khvajeh Ruhollah Mowlana Faraj 28
Kirschner Traction Pin outfit 390
Konartakhteh 167
Kuhgilu 126
Kurds 441
Kut Abdollah 121

L

la`uqat 42
Laal maternity hospital 462
lepers 160
leprosarium 7
Lilahan 272
Loqman al-Mamalek 68
Luristan 126
Lyman Memorial 436

M

ma`ajin 24, 42
Mackay, IMD 135
madraseh-ye dar al-shafa 37, 59, 198, 356
Mahareh Nuri, matron 141
mahbas-e majanin va marza 27
Mahdavi 290
Mahmud Muradi 246

makhzan al-adviyeh 25
malaria xxvi, 78, 112, 124, 135, 165, 308, 350, 390, 393, 468
malaria survey 275
Malek al-Atteba 307
Malek Taj Firuz Najm al-Saltaneh 114
malpana 4
Mankah 9
marahim 24
maraz-khaneh 41
Mardin 33
marestan 33, 38
mariz-khaneh 41
mariz-khaneh-ye Amini 356
mariz-khaneh-ye baladiyeh or melli 427
mariz-khaneh-ye dowlati 59, 63, 109
mariz-khaneh-ye Mahdavi 403
mariz-khaneh-ye melli 137, 365, 386, 395
Marv 11
maser 43
Mashhad changing 287
Mashhad-e Sar 360
Masih al-Saltaneh 307
Masih Khan 204
masjed-e dar al-shafa 37, 39, 198
mastoiditis 249
matbakh 24
maternity hospital 158
maternity hospital, Rasht 401
maternity service 106
matron 83, 187, 217, 327, 349, 376, 433, 446
matron, British 72, 74
Mazandaran 381
measles 79, 166, 274
Medical School for Women 112
medicines 42
medicines, listed 24
medico-legal issues 272
Mehriban Goodarz 459
mental asylum 119, 253, 295
Meydan-e Naftun 353
midwifery 159
midwives 113, 162
military field hospital 261
military hospital 60, 62, 70, 119, 128, 141, 160, 205, 376, 399, 405, 406
military hospitals, Turkish 231
Minab 136

Miryam Khanom 367
Mirza `Isa Tafarroshi Vazir 109
Mirza Abdol-Baqi 204
Mirza Abdol-Karim 204
Mirza Ali 426
Mirza Ali Akbar Khan Nazem al-Atteba 205
Mirza Ayub Hakim 170
Mirza Habib 204
Mirza Habib Tabib-e Fowj 205
Mirza Hajji Agha 306
Mirza Hasan Khan Moshir al-Dowleh 62
Mirza Hoseyn Khan 205
Mirza Mahmud Hakkak-bashi 428
Mirza Masih Khan 205
Mirza Meyer 174
Mirza Mohammad Baqer Hakim-bashi Sadr al-Atteba 204
Mirza Mohammad Nazem al-Atebba 64
Mirza Mohammad Vali Hakim-bashi 59
Mirza Molla Hoseyn Hakim-Bashi 294
Mirza Morteza 306
Mirza Musa 88
Mirza Musa Khan Hafez al-Sehheh 204
Mirza Qavam 88
Mirza Sa`id 171
Mirza Sheikh Mohammad Khan 205
Mirza Shimoil 411
Mirza Tatevos 174
Mirza Ya`qub 172
Mirza Yusof Hakim 170
missionaries opposed 171, 199, 303, 412
miveh-ye akhar-e ruz 43
Mme Fraskina 112
mo`id 39
Mo`in al-Tojjar 149
mobasher 63
mobile dispensary 167, 168
modarres 39
modir 43
Mohammad `Ali Amini 356
Mohammad `Ali Najmi, I.M.D. 159
Mohammad b. Arsalanshah 20
Mohammad b. Mozaffar 28
Mohammad Hasan Mirza 205
Mohammad Sadeq Khan 277
Mohammad Vali Khan Asadi 287
Mohammarah 120
moharrer 43
mohtaseb 107

mojabberan 26
Mokhtar al-Saltaneh 107
Montasariyeh Hospital 294
moqava-ye qardun 169
Moqavvar, Mirza Hoseyn Khan 128
moqtada 28
morestan 20
morgue 389
Moshir al-Dowleh 107
moshref 15, 43
mota'allem 26
motaraddedin 38
motassarefan 28
motavalli 13, 15, 109, 276, 283, 286
Mozaffar al-Din Mirza 421
mozavareh 43
mozavvarat 24
Mr. and Mrs. Whipple 412
Mr. A. Robertson 217
Mr. B. W. Stead 227
Mr. G.N. Oddy 217
Mr. Jessup 425, 426
Mr. Naus 107
Mr. Oldfather 421
Mrs. Arthur Muller R.N. 191
Mrs. Bussdicker R.N. 236
Mrs. Bussey 176
Mrs. D.P. Cochran 433
Mrs. George Howard 435
Mrs. Henry White 458
Mrs. Lillie Reid-Holt 412
Mrs. McCormick 86
Mrs. Müller 455
Mrs. Norem, lab technician 319
Mrs. Packard 441
Mrs. Stetner 193
Mr. Steinhoff, asst. surgeon 221
Mrs. Vanneman 425
Mrs. W.H. Ferry 80, 411
Mrs. Whipple, donation 176
Ms Amerman 364
Ms Baber 393
Ms Bartlett 353
Ms Benz 392
Ms Burgess 441
Ms Carrick 210
Ms Cochran 430
Ms Dale 83, 353
Ms Easton 415
Ms E. C.H. Stratton 219

Ms E.J. Petley 217
Ms E.M. Robinson 220
Ms E.M. Seton-Adamson 207
Ms Enderson 191
Ms Estelle Chambers RN 244
Ms Evert Harutunian 192
Ms Fulton 103
Ms Gertrude Winkelman R.N. 191
Ms Grace Murray 362
Ms Haikows Minassian 96
Ms Helen McKin 201
Ms Hioanoosh Muradian 338
Ms Jeanette Jones R.N. 187
Ms Keller 193
Ms Kelley 188
Ms Keyhan Ghorban 407
Ms Magdaleta Essa 246
Ms Maimanat Dana 407
Ms Margaret Yohanna 246
Ms Mary Bird 199
Ms Mary Edna Burgess 236
Ms M. James 217
Ms Murray 181
Ms Nicholson 382, 392
Ms Oxley 74
Ms Parry 210
Ms Pease 193, 450
Ms Phillips 201
Ms Proctor 203
Ms Setzlar 409
Ms Shamsi Borumand 319
Ms Soghra Namazi 410
Ms Sutherland 90
Ms Taillie 95, 186, 376
Ms Taku'i 395
Ms Verinder 404
Ms W.A. Westlake 207
Ms Wells 187
Ms. Wells 416
Ms Wheeler 193
Ms Williams 410
Ms Willmott 206
Ms Woodruff 221
mu'id 24
mujabbirun 13
Mumtaz Ali Khan, surgeon 301
municipal hospital 139, 295
municipal hospital Hamadan 196
Musawaih 7
music therapy 20

Index

Mutawwakil `ala Allah 9

N

nafkheh-khaneh 41
Namazi hospital 408
Namse, pharmacy 101
Naser al-Din Shah 60, 62
Naseri 123
Nasr b. Harun 13
Nastine treatment 145
navan-khaneh 295
Navvab al-Towliyeh Yazdi 231
nazer 15
nazeran 43, 63
Near East Foundation 393
Nehavand 265
neosalvaran 251, 363
Nestorian refugees 177
Nezam al-Molk 19
Nezami Aruzi 16
Nezamiyeh 19
Nineveh 437
Nishapur 14, 19
Nisibis 1, 3, 4, 9, 26
Nobel barracks 399
Northumberland Presbytery 384
nosokomeion 2
Nosratabad 462
notables 150
nuns 108, 458
Nuriyeh Hospital 222
Nurollah Khan Zahir al-Mamalek 222
nurse, British 72
nurses 82, 97, 184, 375, 397
nurses, Russian 169

O

Oljaytu 23
omen xix
operations 135, 145, 247, 262, 273, 306, 346, 375, 377, 387
opposition to showers 224
orderlies xiv, 15, 24, 41, 51, 63, 69, 78, 120, 195, 231, 278, 287, 400, 434, 460, 472
orphanage 187, 296, 396
Ostad Ramazan 238
ovariotomies 200

Overseas Nursing Assocation 72
owqaf 11, 38, 43

P

Pahlavi hospital, Hamadan 197
Pahlavi hospital, Rasht 394
Pahlavi hospital, Sari 403
parestar 41, 63
Park hospital 266
Parsi Society, Yazd 459
parvareshgah-e atfal 296
parvareshgah-e aytam-e dar al-tarbiyeh 296
pathology lab 349
pathology laboratory 121
pathology work 217
Pay-e Mosalla 177
pharmacies, unreliable 310
pharmacists 254
pharmacy 59, 101
piano 362
piped water 195, 328
plague 352, 462
pneumonia 165, 249
Polish refugees 102
Portuguese 45
Poulos Sagda 338
Presbyterian Church, New Castle, Penn. 305
prontosil 249
provedor do esprital e defuntos 46
puerperal fever 249, 272
Pur Sina hospital 398

Q

Qabusnameh 15
qa'em 15
Qa'en 310
qanat 28
qayyim 24
Qazvin 38, 355
qorz-e benefsheh 42
qorzha la`uq 42
Qotlogh Torkan Khatun 20
quarantine xv
quinine 61, 169, 257, 407, 471

R

Rab'-e Rashidi 23
rabbaita 3
Rabbi Yona Alie 246
radiology 349
railway hospital 128
Ra'is al-Tojjar 352
ra'is-e behdasht 224
ra'is-e bimarestan 5
ra'is-e edareh-ye hefz al-sehheh 204
ra'is-e maliyeh 155
ra'is-e sehhiyeh 223
Rajab Ali Khan Nozar 237
Rashid al-Din 23
record system 101, 338, 368
Red Lion and Rising Sun Society 158
Red Lion and Sun hospital 141, 248, 454
Red Lion and Sun Society 118, 129, 295, 449
refinery 120
refref 52
refugees 373, 374, 441
Reid-Holt Hospital for Men 183
Reid Memorial Hospital 182
relapsing fever 308, 344, 373
relief fund 307
respiratory diseases xxvi, 350
Rev. Carless 207
Rev. Esselstyn 303
Rev. Geo. Zoeckler 177
Rev. Napier Malcolm 460
rheumatic affections 350
Rishar 165
rivaq al-adviyeh 26
rivaq al-morattabin 26
rivaq dar al-shafa 26
rivaq-e beyt al-adviyeh 26
Rokn al-Haqq va'l-Din Mohammad b. Nezam al-Hoseyni 28
rowghan-e zamat 169
R.R. Construction Syndicate 473
running water 238
Russian dispensary 363
Russian hospital 108, 131
Russian hospital, Mashhad 301
Russian hospital, Rasht 399
Russian hospitals 230
Russian hospital, Urmiyeh 457
Russian Orthodox Sisters 355
Russian physicians 169
Russian Red Cross 67, 108, 185, 442
Russian Road Company 355

S

Sa'di Hospital 408
sa'i 39
sa'ur 13, 28, 45
sabat 26
Sabzabad 162, 166
sabzi 43
Sadr-ol-Atteba 306
Safavid 45
saffat 27
sahib-e tahvil 28
Salt, asst. surgeon 209
salvarsan 408
Salvatori xiii
Samsamiyeh hospital 197
sanatorium 473
sanitars 229
Sanitary Council 284
saqqa 24
Sarakhs 64
Sara-ye Naseri 277
Sayyed Mirza Ja'far Khan Moshir al-Dowleh 276
scarlet fever 79
Schick test xxvi
sefufat 42
sehhat-khaneh 38
Sehhiyeh Baladiyeh 137
septic tank 194, 195, 242, 326
Seventh Day Adventists 130
Seyf al-Dowleh 263
Shaghab hospital 10
Shahdokht Maternity Hospital 159
Shahpur I 1
Shahpur II 1
Shahr-e Rashidi 25
Shah Reza hospital 289
Shah Shoja' Mozaffari 29
Shamakhi 33
sharabdar 24
sharab-khaneh 24
sharbatdar 40, 41
sharbat-khaneh-ye kheyriyeh 39
Sheikh Abdol-Karim Ha'eri 357
Sheikh Khaz'al 150, 352
Sheikh Nur al-Din Bimarestani 29

Shekeri 161
Sheverin 172
Shiraz 13, 14, 20, 29, 39
shirkhvargah 396
Shir va Khorshid organization 231
shiyaf 42
shiyafat 24
shower 238
shurba 43
Shushtar 123
Sifat al-bimarestan 15
Sistan 64
skin diseases xxvi, 135, 350
small 124
small-pox 166, 209
soldiers 441
Soltanabad 130, 219
Soltaniyeh 23
Soviet Consulate Hospital, Zabol 464
spinal anesthesia 90
staff 13, 15, 48, 51, 63, 78, 121, 208, 246, 278, 287, 291
Stead Memorial Chapel 240
sterility 273, 274
sterilizer 243
strikes 159
sulfanilimide 249
sulfapyridine 249
sun-treatment 224
surgeon 63, 64, 78, 109, 121, 349
surgery 77, 97
Susruta-samhita 9
Swedish mission, Turkistan 357
Swiss physician 106
syphilis xxvi, 363, 407
Syria 26

T

taba'i'iyyin 13
tabbakh 43, 63
tabib 24, 42
Tabriz 23, 33, 38
Tahir b. al-Hoseyn 11
tahvildar 285
tanabi 27
taraqiyat 42
taryaq-e arba'eh 42
taryaq-e faruq 24, 42
tas neshastan 270

Tavus, medical assistant 173
TB ward 95
tebb-e ruhi 20
Tehran 60, 64, 107, 108
Tehran hospital 103
Tehran hospital closed 103
Tehran University 78
Tembi 353
Terrill, Mr. 171
tetanus 377
thavab xv
Theodore Child 412
Theodore Roosevelt, Col. 242
throat clinic 95
ticket system 269, 337
timarchi-bashi 45
timardar 19, 45
timarestan 295
Timothy, Syrian Patriarch 4
toilets 194, 238, 397, 455
Tonakebun 381
Tooba Rezail 319
toshak 44
tuberculosis xxvi, 350
Tun and Tabas 310
Turanshah I `Emad al-Dowleh 20
Turghabeh 295
Turks 183, 228, 231, 372, 373, 416, 426, 442
typhoid xxvi, 209, 274, 308, 373
typhoid fever xix
typhus 61, 92, 224, 249, 274, 308, 373, 401, 408
typhus vaccine 102

U

urban population 476
Urumiyeh 430
US Army 103
US White Cross 98
Utica Presbyterian Society 176, 184
Uzun Hasan 33

V

vaccinations 135, 161, 166, 362
vaccine, anti-cholera 136
Vajihollah Mirza Sepahsalar 109
vakil 15

Vartanush Minasian 96
venereal diseases 350
Vothuq al-Dowleh 66, 68, 69, 71, 492

W

wages 43, 51
Walid I 7
washers of the dead 107
Wasserman test 115
Westminster church Buffalo, N.Y. 237, 433, 447
Westminster Hospital 248, 433
Whipple Hospital 413
Whipple-Kirkwood hospital for women 414
Whipple Memorial Hospital 176
Whipple Memorial Hospital for Women 183
White Cross 314
whooping cough 125, 209, 270, 274
windmill 316
women 83, 85, 94, 104, 184, 199, 211, 219, 253, 257, 272, 423
Women's Hospital, Rasht 386
Woodsell, J.W., asst. surgeon 258
workmen's compensation 389

X

xenodeikh 3
xenodokheion 2, 3, 6, 17

Y

Yazd 27, 28, 38
Yengi Donya 309
Yezneek 377
Yusofabad 119

Z

zabet 43
Zabol 313
Zanjan 381
Zemsky Zayust 230
Zemsky Zayust hospital 355
zereshk 43
zovvar 38

www.ingramcontent.com/pod-product-compliance
Ingram Content Group UK Ltd.
Pitfield, Milton Keynes, MK11 3LW, UK
UKHW040612030426
469645UK00004B/51